HANDBOOK OF MINDFULNESS

HANDBOOK OF
MINDFULNESS

Theory, Research, and Practice

Edited by

Kirk Warren Brown
J. David Creswell
Richard M. Ryan

THE GUILFORD PRESS
New York   London

© 2015 The Guilford Press
A Division of Guilford Publications, Inc.
370 Seventh Avenue, Suite 1200, New York, NY 10001
www.guilford.com

Printed in the United States of America

This book is printed on acid-free paper.

Last digit is print number: 9 8 7 6 5 4 3 2 1

The authors have checked with sources believed to be reliable in their efforts to provide information that is complete and generally in accord with the standards of practice that are accepted at the time of publication. However, in view of the possibility of human error or changes in behavioral, mental health, or medical sciences, neither the authors, nor the editors and publisher, nor any other party who has been involved in the preparation or publication of this work warrants that the information contained herein is in every respect accurate or complete, and they are not responsible for any errors or omissions or the results obtained from the use of such information. Readers are encouraged to confirm the information contained in this book with other sources.

Library of Congress Cataloging-in-Publication Data
Handbook of mindfulness : theory, research, and practice / edited by Kirk Warren Brown, J. David Creswell, Richard M. Ryan.
     pages cm
  Includes bibliographical references and index.
  ISBN 978-1-4625-1890-6 (hardback)
  1. Attention. 2. Awareness. 3. Meditation—Therapeutic use. I. Brown, Kirk Warren, editor. II. Creswell, J. David, editor. III. Ryan, Richard M., editor.
  BF327.H366 2015
  158—dc23
                                2014020504

About the Editors

Kirk Warren Brown, PhD, is Associate Professor of Psychology at Virginia Commonwealth University, where he studies the role of attention to and awareness of internal states and behavior, with a particular interest in the nature of mindfulness, and the role of mindfulness and mindfulness-based interventions in emotion regulation, behavior regulation, and mental health in healthy and clinical populations. He has received fellowships from several foundations and from the Social Sciences and Humanities Research Council of Canada. Dr. Brown regularly lectures on mindfulness at universities across the United States and Europe and has been a Visiting Professor at the University of Paris.

J. David Creswell, PhD, is Associate Professor of Psychology at Carnegie Mellon University, where he conducts research on stress and coping, with a focus on pathways linking mindfulness meditation training with stress reduction and stress-related disease outcomes. He serves as an academic editor for the journal *PLoS ONE*. Dr. Creswell is a recipient of the American Psychological Association Distinguished Scientific Award for an Early Career Contribution to Psychology.

Richard M. Ryan, PhD, is a clinical psychologist and Senior Research Professor at the Institute for Positive Psychology and Education at Australian Catholic University, with a secondary appointment at the University of Rochester. He is a codeveloper of self-determination theory, an internationally researched theory of human motivation and personality development that has been applied in schools, clinics, sports teams, virtual environments, and work organizations around the world. Dr. Ryan is a fellow of several professional organizations, an honorary member of the German Psychological Society, and the recipient of distinguished career awards from several societies and fellowships from the Cattell and Leverhulme foundations. He has also been a Visiting Professor at the Max Planck Institute, the University of Bath, and Nanyang Technical University.

Contributors

Joanna J. Arch, PhD, Department of Psychology and Neuroscience, University of Colorado, Boulder, Boulder, Colorado

David S. Black, PhD, MPH, Department of Preventive Medicine, Keck School of Medicine, University of Southern California, Los Angeles, California

Sarah Bowen, PhD, Department of Psychiatry and Behavioral Sciences, University of Washington, Seattle, Washington

Kirk Warren Brown, PhD, Department of Psychology, Virginia Commonwealth University, Richmond, Virginia

Linda E. Carlson, PhD, RPsych, Department of Psychosocial Resources, Tom Baker Cancer Centre, Calgary, Alberta, Canada

James Carmody, PhD, Division of Preventive and Behavioral Medicine, University of Massachusetts Medical School, Worcester, Massachusetts

Haley Carroll, BS, Department of Psychology, University of Washington, Seattle, Washington

Jennifer S. Cheavens, PhD, Department of Psychology, Ohio State University, Columbus, Ohio

J. David Creswell, PhD, Department of Psychology, Carnegie Mellon University, Pittsburgh, Pennsylvania

Jake H. Davis, MA, Philosophy Program, The Graduate Center, City University of New York, New York, New York

Edward L. Deci, PhD, Department of Clinical and Social Sciences in Psychology, University of Rochester, Rochester, New York

Elissa S. Epel, PhD, Department of Psychiatry, University of California, San Francisco, San Francisco, California

Norman A. S. Farb, PhD, Department of Psychology, University of Toronto, Toronto, Ontario, Canada

Rupert Gethin, PhD, Department of Religion and Theology, University of Bristol, Bristol, United Kingdom

Robert J. Goodman, MA, Department of Psychological Sciences, Northern Arizona University, Flagstaff, Arizona

Steven C. Hayes, PhD, Department of Psychology, University of Nevada, Reno, Reno, Nevada

Sarah A. Hayes-Skelton, PhD, Department of Psychology, University of Massachusetts Boston, Boston, Massachusetts

Julie Anne Irving, PhD, Mood and Anxiety Disorders Program, Centre for Addiction and Mental Health, Toronto, Ontario, Canada

Hooria Jazaieri, MFT, Department of Psychology, Institute of Personality and Social Research, University of California, Berkeley, Berkeley, California

Lauren N. Landy, MA, Department of Psychology and Neuroscience, University of Colorado, Boulder, Boulder, Colorado

Sophie A. Lazarus, MS, Department of Psychology, Ohio State University, Columbus, Ohio

Emily K. Lindsay, MS, Department of Psychology, Carnegie Mellon University, Pittsburgh, Pennsylvania

Douglas M. Long, MA, Department of Psychology, University of Nevada, Reno, Reno, Nevada

Thomas R. Lynch, PhD, Personality and Emotion Biobehavioural Laboratory, School of Psychology, University of Southampton, Southampton, United Kingdom

Benjamin W. Nelson, BA, Department of Psychology, University of Oregon, Eugene, Oregon

Christopher P. Niemiec, PhD, Department of Clinical and Social Sciences in Psychology, University of Rochester, Rochester, New York

Suzanne C. Parker, PhD, Department of Psychology, American University, Washington, DC

Michael I. Posner, PhD, Department of Psychology, University of Oregon, Eugene, Oregon

Jordan T. Quaglia, MS, Department of Psychology, Virginia Commonwealth University, Richmond, Virginia

C. Scott Rigby, PhD, Immersyve, Inc., Celebration, Florida

Richard M. Ryan, PhD, Institute for Positive Psychology and Education, Australian Catholic University, Sydney, Australia, and Department of Clinical and Social Sciences in Psychology, University of Rochester, Rochester, New York

Patricia P. Schultz, MA, Department of Clinical and Social Sciences in Psychology, University of Rochester, Rochester, New York

Zindel V. Segal, PhD, Department of Psychology, University of Toronto, Toronto, Ontario, Canada

Shauna L. Shapiro, PhD, School of Education and Counseling Psychology, Santa Clara University, Santa Clara, California

Daniel J. Siegel, MD, Mindful Awareness Research Center, University of California, Los Angeles, and Mindsight Institute, Los Angeles, California

Thomas G. Szabo, PhD, BCBA-D, School of Behavior Analysis, Florida Institute of Technology, Melbourne, Florida

Yi-Yuan Tang, PhD, Department of Psychological Sciences, Texas Tech University, Lubbock, Texas

Evan Thompson, PhD, Department of Philosophy, University of British Columbia, Vancouver, British Columbia, Canada

Marieke K. van Vugt, PhD, Institute of Artificial Intelligence and Cognitive Engineering, University of Groningen, Groningen, The Netherlands

Cassandra Vieten, PhD, Institute of Noetic Sciences, Petaluma, California

Matthieu Villatte, PhD, Evidence-Based Practice Institute, University of Washington, Seattle, Washington

Lauren P. Wadsworth, MA, Department of Psychology, University of Massachusetts Boston, Boston, Massachusetts

Edward R. Watkins, PhD, Mood Disorders Centre, Department of Psychology, College of Life and Environmental Sciences, University of Exeter, Exeter, United Kingdom

Katie Witkiewitz, PhD, Department of Psychology, University of New Mexico, Albuquerque, New Mexico

Fadel Zeidan, PhD, Department of Neurobiology and Anatomy, Wake Forest School of Medicine, Winston-Salem, North Carolina

Contents

PART III

THE BASIC SCIENCE OF MINDFULNESS

PART IV

MINDFULNESS INTERVENTIONS
FOR HEALTHY POPULATIONS

PART V

MINDFULNESS INTERVENTIONS
FOR CLINICAL POPULATIONS

CHAPTER 1

Introduction

The Evolution of Mindfulness Science

Kirk Warren Brown, J. David Creswell, and Richard M. Ryan

A decade ago, when each of us began to give academic talks on mindfulness, a few members of our audiences—mainly clinical psychologists and the occasional cognitive scientist—would nod their heads knowingly when mindfulness was described, even if they had not heard the term before. Most others found the whole idea of mindfulness unfamiliar in the context of their scientific training. A lot has changed in a decade. Today, mindfulness is among the hottest topics in both clinical and basic psychological science. Research on the topic regularly appears in journals across the spectrum of the behavioral sciences, federal grant agencies devote considerable sums to its study, a number of behavioral interventions include mindfulness training in treating a variety of mental and physical health conditions, and many in the general public know something about mindfulness from the considerable number of books, online media, courses, and workshops on the subject.

The current widespread theoretical and scientific interest in mindfulness is particularly remarkable when seen in historical context of psychology, psychiatry, and related disciplines. Whereas psychological science has conventionally focused in one way or another on the contents of consciousness (e.g., cognitions, emotions, and their somatic and behavioral consequences), mindfulness fundamentally concerns consciousness itself. While there is no single definition of mindfulness (Anālayo, 2014), fundamental to classical and other definitions is clear-eyed attention to the workings of the mind, body, and behavior (e.g., Bodhi, 2011). This attentiveness to what is present appears to yield corrective and curative benefits in its own right. These benefits have placed this quality of consciousness squarely in a scientific spotlight.

1

Theoretical and Empirical Advances in the Field

One testament to the burgeoning interest in mindfulness is the exponential growth in research papers and books on the topic; as Figure 1.1 shows, publications (articles and books) containing the term *mindfulness* were few through to the 1980s and 1990s but have increased exponentially over time since the early 2000s. Over a 30-year span, the science of mindfulness has seen significant developments along four major fronts, each represented in this volume: conceptualization, psychological theory, basic science, and applied science. We briefly discuss each of these areas in turn.

Conceptualization

Within Western psychology, interest in conscious awareness of, or attention to, what occurs—as both a way of being and a tool for inquiry—is long-standing, dating at least to the writings of William James (1890/1950). Over the course of the 20th century, consciousness came to figure prominently in one form or another in a number of schools of psychology, ranging from Gestalt, humanistic, and existential

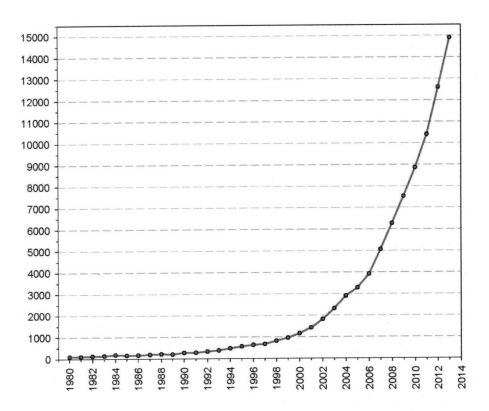

FIGURE 1.1. Number of publications containing the word *mindfulness* in Google Scholar, 1980–2013. Each point represents the citation count for a single year.

phenomenology to, more recently and perhaps most surprisingly, cognitive behaviorism. However, these historical interests pale by comparison to the intensity of interest in consciousness today. The receptive attentiveness featured in mindfulness has conceptual affinity with other modes of attending that are actively investigated in contemporary psychology, including *concrete* and *experiential processing* (Teasdale, 1999; Edward R.Watkins, 2008 and Chapter 6, this volume), *first-order phenomenal experience* (Lambie & Marcel, 2002; Marcel, 2003), *interest taking* (Edward L.Deci, Richard M. Ryan, Patricia P. Schultz, & Christopher P. Niemiec, Chapter 7, this volume), and *psychological distancing* (Ayduk & Kross, 2010).

Although research on mindfulness has connections with these contemporary interests, it has nonetheless been most deeply informed by the rich "inner science" (Cabezon, 2003) developed over many centuries in the Buddhist traditions. Wallace (2003, 2007) and others (e.g., Hut, 2003) suggest that there is a deep complementarity between Western scientific and Buddhist contemplative approaches to the study of the mind and behavior. The methods employed by each approach differ, of course— one experimental, the other experiential—but the refinement of attention cultivated in Buddhist contemplative practices has made it a powerful tool for the direct observation of mind and behavior. In this sense, Buddhism represents a mode of inquiry bridging "rigorous logical analysis (as in philosophy) and empirical investigation (as in science)" (Wallace, 2003, p. 27).

Yet for much of the brief history of mindfulness science, the Buddhist intellectual influence on research has been, with notable exceptions, rather distant—simply referenced rather than actively engaged. In recent years, active dialogue between Buddhist scholarship and Western science has grown, and with it efforts to clarify our understanding of what mindfulness is, its cognitive expressions, and its psychological effects. Part I of this book, with chapters from Buddhist scholar Rupert Gethin (Chapter 2), philosophers Jake H. Davis and Evan Thompson (Chapter 3), and psychologist James Carmody (Chapter 4), offers insights that have accrued from this rich cross-disciplinary dialogue.

Psychological Theory

Another marker of the evolution of mindfulness science is its increased embeddedness in psychological theory. For much of its brief scientific history, researchers in the area have drawn from Buddhist theory (or clinical theories drawing from Buddhism) regarding the salutary effects of mindfulness. Buddhist psychological theory was not developed to make predictions about specific outcomes of interest to Western science, so much research has explored the neurophysiological, subjective, and behavioral correlates and consequences of mindfulness without comprehensive, scientifically grounded theoretical frameworks. Part II of this volume addresses this agenda with chapters that seek to understand mindfulness and its operation from within four major contemporary theoretical perspectives focused on largely different but interrelated levels of analysis. These bear on networks of attention (Yi-Yuan Tang and Michael I. Posner, Chapter 5), on modes of perceptual processing (Edward R. Watkins, Chapter 6), on motivation (Deci et al., Chapter 7), and on learning-supportive environments (Thomas G. Szabo, Douglas M. Long, Matthieu Villatte, & Steven C. Hayes, Chapter 8).

Basic Science

Mindfulness research had its origins in the clinic, on the front lines of suffering, wherein questions were framed in terms of mindfulness-based treatment effectiveness. For much of the history of the field, basic scientific questions about mindfulness were not addressed: What is mindfulness anyway, and how can we measure it? To which psychological phenomena is it similar and to which does it differ? What effects does mindfulness itself have, stripped of the components that accompany its training in treatment programs (e.g., group and instructor support)? Through what neural and psychological processes or mechanisms do these effects occur? In recent years, questions such as these have received considerable study, and the chapters in Part III of this handbook present state-of-the-science research on the measurement of mindfulness (Jordan T. Quaglia, Kirk Warren Brown, Emily K. Lindsay, J. David Creswell, & Robert J. Goodman, Chapter 9), and on the expressions and consequences of mindfulness for neural structure and functioning (Fadel Ziedan, Chapter 10), cognition (Marieke K. van Vugt, Chapter 11), emotion (Joanna J. Arch & Lauren N. Landy, Chapter 12), interpersonal behavior (Suzanne C. Parker, Benjamin W. Nelson, Elissa S. Epel, & Daniel J. Siegel, Chapter 13), and the nature of the self (Richard M. Ryan & C. Scott Rigby, Chapter 14). Using a suite of methods to study mindfulness—trait and state subjective measures, brief experimental inductions, mindfulness training programs, and comparison of advanced mindfulness practitioners to matched controls—this science is probing deeply into the character and action of mindful states and traits, with a yield of findings that enhance our understanding of the nature of mindfulness while also providing insights that help clinical researchers to target symptoms and populations likely to benefit from mindfulness training.

Applied Science

From its beginnings in the early 1980s the research base of mindfulness-based and mindfulness-integrated psychoeducational and clinical treatment programs has expanded into a wide variety of populations, while at the same time uncovering mechanisms of their effectiveness. Applied mindfulness science can be grouped into that which targets healthy populations, discussed in Part IV of this volume, and that which addresses symptomatology in clinical populations, discussed in Part V.

In healthy populations, mindfulness training programs for adults dealing with stress have spread around the world, and with them, a growing body of research demonstrating benefits for a range of psychological outcomes, as Shauna L. Shapiro and Hooria Jazaieri discuss (Chapter 15). Recently, training programs have been developed to address the particular developmental stresses of healthy children and adolescents, as well as psychiatric symptomatology in clinical youth populations, and David S. Black (Chapter 16) discusses this incipient growth area of research. Such training has not been limited to correcting deficits or normalizing psychological functioning, however. Training in mindfulness and other contemplative practices has long been thought to push the capacities for well-being into the range of what might be considered optimal functioning, and Brown (Chapter 17) discusses the evidence for this claim.

There is now a family of mindfulness-based and mindfulness-integrated treatments being applied to a wide range of psychiatric and biomedical populations. This body of literature has become large enough to warrant a volume of its own (Didonna, 2009). In this book we highlight research on mindfulness treatment that, first, addresses clinical conditions impacting a large number of adults in the West and second, has a strong and growing evidence base. Chapters in Part V concern the application of mindfulness training to the treatment of emotion dysregulated and overregulated problems (Thomas R. Lynch, Sophie A. Lazarus, & Jennifer S. Cheavens, Chapter 18), chronic depression (Julie Anne Irving, Norman A. S. Farb, & Zindel V. Segal, Chapter 19), anxiety disorders (Sarah A. Hayes-Skelton & Lauren P. Wadsworth, Chapter 20), addictive disorders (Sarah Bowen, Cassandra Vieten, Katie Witkiewitz, & Haley Carroll, Chapter 21), and a number of biomedical conditions (Linda E. Carlson, Chapter 22). A final chapter in this section describes how mindfulness might get under the skin to influence this broad range of mental and physical health outcomes, via stress buffering pathways (J. David Creswell, Chapter 23).

Conclusions

As we observed earlier in this Introduction, it is remarkable that broad research interest in mindfulness exists at all. Equally remarkable is the breadth of investigation that has taken place in the comparatively brief span of 30 years that the topic has received study. The research discussed in this volume highlights many of the most recent developments in the field, of course, but it is telling that the vast majority of all research on mindfulness has been carried out in the last decade. The science continues to grow rapidly but also, and more importantly, is collectively taking a multilevel approach that allows us to ask sophisticated questions about the predisposing factors, correlates, mechanisms, and consequences of mindfulness, and training in it, at neurophysiological, subjective, and overt behavioral levels, and in a range of functional domains—including neural, cognitive, conative, affective, physical, and social—that are of interest to scholars, researchers, and health care providers in a variety of disciplines.

While we have learned a great deal about mindfulness in the past 30 years, unquestionably the field of mindfulness science is still maturing, and in the chapters herein the authors have taken pains to point out how the current research is limited in its methods and conclusions, and to point to specific ways in which future research studies can overcome these limitations. That said, the work represented in this handbook is among the best conducted to date, measured in terms of scientific creativity, sophistication, and insight. Our hope is that this volume offers readers both a panoramic view of the current science of mindfulness and a compass to help guide its ongoing evolution.

REFERENCES

Anālayo, B. (2014). *Perspectives on Satipatthāna.* Birmingham, UK: Windhorse Publications.

Ayduk, Ö. & Kross, E. (2010). From a distance: Implications of spontaneous self-distancing for adaptive self-reflection. *Journal of Personality and Social Psychology, 98*(5), 809–829.

Bodhi, B. (2011). What does mindfulness really mean?: A canonical perspective. *Contemporary Buddhism, 12*(1), 19–39.

Cabezon, J. I. (2003). Buddhism and science: On the nature of the dialogue. In B. A. Wallace (Ed.), *Buddhism and science: Breaking new ground* (pp. 35–70). New York: Columbia University Press.

Didonna, F. (2009). *Clinical handbook of mindfulness.* New York: Springer.

Hut, P. (2003). Life as a laboratory. In B. A. Wallace (Ed.), *Buddhism and science: Breaking new ground* (pp. 399–422). New York: Columbia University Press.

James, W. (1950). *The principles of psychology.* New York: Dover. (Original work published 1890)

Lambie, J. A., & Marcel, A. J. (2002). Consciousness and the varieties of emotion experience: A theoretical framework. *Psychological Review, 109*(2), 219–259.

Marcel, A. J. (2003). Introspective report: Trust, self-knowledge and science. *Journal of Consciousness Studies, 10,* 167–186.

Teasdale, J. D. (1999). Emotional processing, three modes of mind and the prevention of relapse in depression. *Behaviour Research and Therapy, 37,* 53–77.

Wallace, B. A. (2003). Introduction: Buddhism and science—breaking down the barriers. In B. A. Wallace (Ed.), *Buddhism and science: Breaking new ground* (pp. 1–30). New York: Columbia University Press.

Wallace, B. A. (2007). *Contemplative science: Where Buddhism and science converge.* New York: Columbia University Press.

Watkins, E. R. (2008). Constructive and unconstructive repetitive thought. *Psychological Bulletin, 134,* 163–206.

PART I

HISTORICAL AND CONCEPTUAL OVERVIEW OF MINDFULNESS

CHAPTER 2

Buddhist Conceptualizations
of Mindfulness

Rupert Gethin

While we, of course, know otherwise, it is all too easy in the context of the contemporary discussion of mindfulness to find ourselves talking as if "mindfulness" were some particular thing out there in the world that Buddhism first discovered over 2,000 years ago and 21st-century science is now investigating, such that soon we will finally be able to say exactly what it is. But *mindfulness* is a word, and like other words, *mindfulness* is used in a variety of ways. That is, different people, whether ancient Buddhists or contemporary neuroscientists, may use and define *mindfulness*—or Pali *sati*, Sanskrit *smṛti*, Chinese *nian*, and Tibetan *dran pa*—in different ways and it is not clear what standard we might use to judge any given account of mindfulness as either wanting or fitting.

Insofar as those who developed such therapeutic approaches as mindfulness-based stress reduction (MBSR; Kabat-Zinn, 1990) and mindfulness-based cognitive therapy (MBCT; Segal, Williams, & Teasdale, 2002) point to Buddhist traditions of mindfulness as a significant source and inspiration, the modern therapeutic and scientific discussions of mindfulness claim a connection with traditional Buddhist discourse. The nature of this connection has yet to be fully investigated and analyzed, although some useful observations on mindfulness and modernity have been made by McMahan (2008).

Certainly there has been an explosion in academic studies and discussions of mindfulness in the last 20 years, spanning fields as diverse as Buddhist studies, cognitive psychology, neuroscience, and clinical psychology (Williams & Kabat-Zinn, 2011a). In Buddhist studies, although there have been both important monographs (Anālayo, 2003; Kuan, 2008) and collections of essays (Gyatso, 1992; Williams & Kabat-Zinn, 2011b) outlining specific Buddhist perspectives on mindfulness, attempts either to assess the full range of these Buddhist perspectives or to consider their relationship to the perspectives on mindfulness that have emerged in modern neuroscientific studies and the therapeutic contexts of MBSR and MBCT are to date more limited (Gethin, 2011a; Gilpin, 2008). Thus, in this discussion I attempt to take in the earliest Buddhist conceptions of mindfulness (fourth to second centuries B.C.E.), the technical accounts of mindfulness in Indian Buddhist systematic thought (second century B.C.E. to fifth century C.E.), and some characteristic examples of different approaches to mindfulness in Buddhist meditation practice in China (seventh century), Tibet (10th to 15th centuries), and Burma (20th century), before concluding with some assessment of the tensions found in Buddhist notions of mindfulness and how these relate to modern scientific and therapeutic accounts of mindfulness.

It seems to have been T. W. Rhys Davids (1881), one of the pioneers of the Western study of Pali texts, who first translated the Buddhist technical term *sati* by the English word *mindfulness* (pp. 144, 147, 150, 306). Although the translation *mindfulness* has since become more or less standard in English, it is not clear that it is suited to every context; the semantic range of Pali *sati* does not correspond precisely with that of English *mindfulness*. The situation is complicated by the manner in which the words *mindful* and *mindfulness* have in English themselves assimilated a particular modern reception of ancient Buddhist notions. Thus, the *Oxford English Dictionary Online* (2011) concludes its entries for *mindful* and *mindfulness* by citing their usage "with reference to Yoga philosophy and Buddhism" in the sense of respectively "fully aware of the moment, whilst self-conscious and attentive to this awareness" and "the meditative state of being fully aware of the moment." Clearly when Rhys Davids first chose the word as a translation of *sati*, he must have had in mind the broader range of usage already established in English at that time: "possessing a good memory," "full of care," "heedful," "thoughtful," and "being conscious or aware" (*Oxford English Dictionary Online*, 2011). Thus, whereas in this chapter I shall generally use *mindfulness* as the accepted English translation of a Buddhist technical term, the reader should bear in mind that this is a matter of expedience in the absence of an exact English equivalent of Pali *sati* or Sanskrit *smṛti*.

Mindfulness and Remembering

Broadly, the earliest surviving stratum of Buddhist literature takes the form of the collections (*nikāaya* or *āgama*) of discourses (Sanskrit *sūtra*, Pali *sutta*) of the Buddha extant today principally in the Pali canon of the Theravāda school, in Sanskrit fragments mostly from the canon of the Sarvāstivāda school, and in ancient Chinese translations of Indian texts probably from the canons of both the Sarvāstivāda and Dharmaguptaka schools. This literature was composed in India probably between the fourth and second centuries B.C.E.

In one of the earliest English language discussions of the notion of "mindfulness" in early Buddhist literature, Rhys Davids and Rhys Davids (1910) pointed out that etymologically Pali *sati* means *memory* and then suggested that the way the term comes to be used in Buddhist texts to characterize a way of paying attention represents something of an reinterpretation (p. 322). Some (e.g., Bodhi, 2011, pp. 22–23) have taken this double meaning of *smṛti* as the starting point, while others (Cox, 1992; Griffiths, 1992) have questioned such a bifurcation of *smṛti*. The problem has to do, of course, with how we understand English "memory." If we think of *memory* primarily as the ability to remember the past or of *a memory* as what is remembered, then the Buddhist use of *sati* in the context of various meditation exercises can seem puzzling insofar as these are not *prima facie* envisioned as exercises in memory in the sense of recalling the past. On the other hand, if we think of *memory* as more generally holding or keeping something in mind, the specific Buddhist use of *smṛti* and its development seem less puzzling.

Alongside *remembrance, reminiscence,* and *memory,* the widely used Sanskrit dictionary of Monier-Williams (1899) gives as possible meanings for *smṛti* "thinking of or upon" and "calling to mind." In keeping with this kind of usage, the term *sati* is in the first place used in early Buddhist texts simply to mean "keeping or holding in mind"—that is, not forgetting—any subject of contemplation or meditation. In many places in early Buddhist texts we find a standard list of six subjects designated by the closely related term *anu-smṛti*: the Buddha, the Dharma, the Sangha, virtue, generosity, the gods. Sometimes appended to this we find "mindfulness of breathing in and out" (*ānapāna-(anu)smṛti*), "mindfulness of death" (*maraṇa-(anu)smṛti*), and "mindfulness connected with the body" (*kāyagatā-(anu)smṛti*). The prefix *anu* indicates that these subjects are for "repeatedly thinking on" or "recollecting." While we can, then, translate *ānāpānasmṛti* as "mindfulness of breathing in and out," we might equally translate it is as "keeping in mind breathing in and out." Consonant with this usage, the Pali *Metta-sutta* refers to the cultivation of kindness (*maitrī/ mettā*) as a *sati,* that is, an exercise in keeping kindness in mind (Sn 151; see Appendix 2.1). The preeminent subjects for "keeping in mind" are those designated the four "places"—that is, objects—of mindfulness (*sati-paṭṭhāna/ smṛt-upasthāna*): the body, feelings, states of mind, and mental qualities. In summary, as Paul Griffiths (1992) concluded, the semantic range of *smṛti* "spans that of memory-words and attention-words in English" (p. 115). Similarly Cox (1992) points out that she chooses *mindfulness* as a translation of *smṛti* not

> to avoid confusion with the psychological function of *smṛti* as memory, but precisely for the opposite reason: that is, to indicate at the outset . . . that the contexts for the operation of *smṛti* suggested by the term *mindfulness* actually encompass the psychological functions of memory as they were understood within Indian Buddhism. (pp. 67–68)

This means that Buddhist texts may slip between talk of "mindfulness" as "memory" of the past and as "paying attention" to an object of meditation without a sense of disjunction. In fact, some of the tensions between *smṛti* as memory and attention may be resolved if we think of the Buddhist understanding of *smṛti* as having more affinity with modern discussions around the notion of "working memory" (Baddeley & Hitch, 1974) than, say, "long-term memory."

The Practice of Mindfulness in Early Buddhist Texts

Mindfulness is one of a number of virtues or qualities whose cultivation is presented as fundamental to the Buddhist path to "enlightenment" or "awakening." It is therefore

included in various lists of such qualities and in accounts of the practice of meditation. Mindfulness is counted one of five basic faculties: faith (śraddhā), vigor (vīrya),
mindfulness (smṛti), concentration (samādhi), and wisdom (prajñā). It is one of seven
constituents of awakening: investigation of dharma (dharmapravicaya), mindfulness,
vigor, joy (prīti), tranquillity (praśrabdhi), concentration, and equanimity (upekṣā).
It is one of the eight constituents of the eightfold path: right view (samyagdṛṣṭi), right
intent (samyaksaṃkalpa), right action (samyakkarmānta), right speech (samyagvāk),
right livelihood (samyagājīva), right effort (samyagvyāyāma), right mindfulness, and
right concentration. The list of the four applications of mindfulness is also the first of
an important list of seven sets of items—four applications of mindfulness, four right
efforts, four bases of success in meditation, five faculties, five powers, seven constituents of awakening, the eightfold path—that are collectively taken as constituting the
essential practices that make up the Buddhist path and later come to be designated
"the thirty-seven qualities that contribute to enlightenment" (Gethin, 1992). While
there is no doubt that mindfulness has a prominent place among the virtues and
qualities to be developed by the Buddhist monk, there is no suggestion in the earliest
literature that mindfulness is somehow the key or central virtue.

Little is said in these texts by way of explicit definition of mindfulness. What
is understood as mindfulness must be gleaned from descriptions of its application
in practice. As a faculty and a constituent of awakening, the quality of mindfulness
is said to be exemplified by someone who is "mindful, possesses perfect mindfulness and understanding, one who remembers, one who recollects things done and
things said long before" (D 3.268, 3.286; M 1.356; S 5.198, 5.200, 5.225, 5.226; A,
2.35, 3.11, 4.4, 4.111, 4.234, 5.25, 5.28, 5.91[1]: satimā hoti paramena satinepakkena
samannāgato cirakatam pi cirabhāsitam pi saritā anussaritā; see Appendix 2.1).
While this might be taken as simply referring to anyone with a good memory, Buddhist tradition understands it in terms of remembering things said and done by oneself or others that are specifically connected with religious practice; recalling them is
therefore part of one's practice (Ps 3.30; Spk, 3.234; Śrāv-bh 132).

As a constituent of the eightfold path and as a faculty, mindfulness is also characteristically expanded on by reference to a set of four meditations already mentioned: the four "applications of mindfulness" (satipaṭṭhāna/smṛtyupasthāna). This
important expression seems early on to have been understood in two alternative
ways: both "the act of applying mindfulness" and "the place where—that is, object
to which—mindfulness is applied."[2] The practice of the applications of mindfulness
is very frequently elaborated using the following stock formula:

> A monk lives observing (1) the body as body; ardent, knowing fully, mindful, he
> overcomes his longing for and discontent with the world. He lives observing (2) feel-
> ings as feelings . . . (3) mind as mind . . . (4) mental qualities as mental qualities;
> ardent, knowing fully, mindful, he overcomes his longing for and discontent with
> the world. (D 2.290, M 1.55, MPS 200)

This summary description is expanded and explained in Buddhist literature,
especially in a discourse of the Buddha known in Pali as the Satipaṭṭhāna-sutta (Sanskrit Smṛtyupasthāna-sūtra). This sūtra survives in three principal versions, one in

Pali and two in Chinese translation.[3] The *sūtra* proceeds by explaining in some detail how a monk should watch the body, feelings, one's general mental state, and specific mental qualities and emotions. There is some variation in the way each exercise is elaborated in the Pali version (preserved by the Theravāda school) and the principal version surviving in Chinese translation (probably belonging to the ancient Sarvāstivāda school), but also significant common ground. Among the exercises suggested for observing the body in both versions are the following:

- Observing the breath.
- Being aware of one's posture (walking, standing, sitting, or lying).
- Being aware when one is involved in everyday activities (in moving forward and turning back; in looking ahead and looking around; in bending and straightening the limbs; in wearing the monk's robes; in carrying an alms bowl; in eating, drinking, chewing and swallowing; in defecating and urinating; in walking, standing, sitting, falling asleep, waking up, speaking, and keeping silent).
- Reviewing the various organs and parts of the physical body (31 are listed).
- Considering the body as consisting of the four elements (earth, water, fire, air).
- Considering the body as being like a corpse at various stages of decay.

To observe feelings the *sūtra* suggests paying attention to feelings as pleasant, unpleasant, and neutral. To observe one's state of mind, the *sūtra* suggests paying attention to the mind as, for example, affected by desire or by aversion, or by delusion. To observe mental qualities, the *sūtra* suggests paying attention to, for example:

- The presence or otherwise of five qualities that obstruct meditation (desire for the objects of the senses, ill-will, sleepiness, excitement and depression, doubt).
- The way in which the mind becomes ensnared by the senses and their respective objects.
- The presence or otherwise of the seven particular qualities that together bring about and constitute enlightenment (mindfulness, investigation of dharma, vigor, joy, tranquillity, concentration, and equanimity).

The exercise of mindfulness here is thus presented in the first place not so much as a specific *way* of paying attention as a matter of *what* we pay attention to. Thus, in the practice of mindfulness of the body, the Buddhist monk is instructed to pay attention to precisely things he might not normally pay attention to, that is, things that we do unconsciously or with little attention: breathing, walking, standing, sitting, lying, eating, drinking, and so on. This attention should ultimately encompass everything: what is "within" (our own bodies and those mental states that are directed inward) and what is "without" (the bodies of others and those mental states that are directed outward through the five senses). Thus, the body is deconstructed and reduced to breathing in and out, various postures and activities, its constituent parts and organs. Likewise feelings are seen as various kinds of pleasant, unpleasant, and neutral feeling. Mental states, capacities, and emotions are simply qualities that are bound up with the operation of the senses and therefore come and go. The assumption appears to be that in directing attention to these things, we begin to see them in a different way, that is, for what they truly are: just physical and mental qualities or phenomena (*dharma*) that come and go according to certain conditions. When we see them as such, they lose their hold over us:

> In this way he lives watching the body . . . feelings . . . mind . . . qualities within . . . without . . . within and without as body . . . feelings . . . mind . . . qualities. He lives watching the way things arise . . . the way things pass . . . the way things arise and pass in the case of the body . . . feelings . . . mind . . . qualities. Furthermore his mindfulness that there are body . . . feelings . . . mind . . . qualities is established so that there is knowledge and recollection in full measure; he lives independently, not holding on to anything in the world. (D 2.292, 2.298, 2.299–300, 2.301; M 1.56, 1.59–60; Gethin, 2008, pp. 143, 146–148)

The *sūtra* ends by suggesting that anyone who practices in the way described for even just 7 days will surely attain either awakening or, if not awakening, the state of "non-return." That is, either one will attain freedom from the round of rebirth in this very life, or one will be reborn in one of the heavens known as the Pure Abodes and there attain such freedom.

Little is said explicitly about mindfulness as a way of paying attention, although certain things might be gleaned from the account of its practice in the *Smṛtyupasthāna-sūtra* and other passages. Generally the application of mindfulness implies a deliberate directing and placing of attention on certain objects of consciousness; this is perhaps brought out especially by the term here translated as "ardent" (*ātāpin*), which is taken by the later tradition to indicate application and effort. As already suggested, the exercises in the application of mindfulness are closely associated with the Buddhist goal of seeing things as they are as opposed to being taken in by how they may superficially appear. As such, mindfulness is closely associated with developing understanding or wisdom (*prajñā*), as is indicated in the *Smṛtyupasthāna-sūtra* by the cognate term *samprajāna*, "knowing clearly or fully"; *samprajanya*, "full or clear knowledge," is a term frequently coupled with *smṛti* in the Nikāyas and Āgamas and taken by later Buddhist tradition to connote understanding or wisdom.

We should note also that not all the exercises in mindfulness described in this text appear to involve the simple observation of objects directly present to the senses:

> A monk reviews this body from the soles of his feet upwards and from the ends of the hair on his head downwards, as enveloped in skin and full of various kinds of impurity: "Here in this body there are head hairs, body hairs, nails, teeth, skin, flesh, sinews, bones, bone marrow, kidneys, heart, liver, diaphragm, spleen, lungs, large intestine, small intestine, gorge, faeces, bile, phlegm, pus, blood, sweat, fat, tears, grease, saliva, snot, oil of the joints, and urine." As if there were a sack with an opening at either end full of various sorts of grain, which a man with good eyes should review thus: "Here are rice grains, here mung beans, here kidney beans, here sesame seeds." (M 1.57; cf. T 1.583b 5–583b17; Kuan, 2008, pp. 149–150)

Such a practice would seem to involve both the exercise of the imagination and basic memory, certainly, of the list of body parts but also, perhaps, of prior observation of the various parts of the body. Moreover the meditator is directed not just to observe the body parts, but to hold them in mind as "impurities" (*asucin*). This is a good illustration of the way memory and sustained attention are taken as two facets of the same mental capacity: The monk who has memorized the parts of the body, recalls and pays attention to each of the parts in turn (Vism VIII 42–144; Ñāṇamoli, 1964, pp. 259–285), in a similar manner perhaps to the way a musician, say, might play a piece of music from memory with full attention. In similar fashion, "a monk should consider his body as though he were looking at a body left in a charnel ground, as white bones looking like shells, as piled up bones more than a year old, as rotten crumbling bones," and he should reflect that his own body is "of the same nature, of the same constitution, it has not got beyond this" (M 1.58–59; cf. T 1.583c17– 583c21; Kuan, 2008, pp. 150–151). Later Buddhist tradition sometimes describes such a practice being undertaken as a visualization (Abhidh-k-bh VI 10; Pruden, 1988, pp. 918–919) or using an actual corpse or bones as a visual prompt (Vism VI 78; Ñāṇamoli, 1964, p. 198). In any case, exercising the imagination in relation to what is observed in one's own body once again goes beyond simple observation.

The Role of Mindfulness in the Buddhist Path

Early Buddhist texts conceive of the Buddhist path to enlightenment by way of a threefold scheme comprising the progressive development of, first, moral conduct (*śīla*); second, deep states of meditative concentration (*samādhi*); and third, understanding (*prajñā*) of the nature of reality. The underlying psychology here is transparent enough: The transforming knowledge (*prajñā*) that constitutes awakening can only be achieved by a mind that is first settled in a state of clarity and stillness (*samādhi*); such a state can in turn only be established and maintained on the basis of strict moral restraint (*śīla*). The monastic rule (Prātimokṣa) as set out in the Vinaya provides the framework for achieving moral restraint, while the two separate achievements of concentration and understanding come to be articulated in terms of two different emphases in the practice of meditation: calm (*śamatha*) and insight (*vipaśyanā*). Calm meditation refers to the practice of meditation orientated toward the cultivation of deep states of concentration styled "absorptions" (*dhyāna*), where the mind, having become unified and absorbed in the contemplation of some simple object of meditation, such as the breath, temporarily remains completely still and calm. Insight meditation, on the other hand, refers to the practice of meditation orientated toward seeing the complex of mental and physical phenomena (comprising in Buddhist thought the five *skandhas* or collections of physical form, feeling, perception, volitional forces, and consciousness) that constitute both our selves (experiencing subjects) and the world (experienced objects) as impermanent (*anitya*), unsatisfying (*duḥkha*) and not self (*anātman*). The development of and relationship between these two styles of meditation in the history of Buddhist practice is complex and remains disputed in the scholarly literature.

The close association of "mindfulness" with "understanding" in some of the formulations found in early Buddhist texts has led to the suggestion in both modern scholarly literature and modern Buddhist literature that the practice of mindfulness is to be seen as particularly characteristic of "insight" meditation as opposed to "calm" meditation. Indeed, insight meditation and the practice of the four applications of mindfulness are sometimes straightforwardly identified with each other (e.g., Griffiths, 1981, pp. 814–815; Soma, 1967, p. xv). Such an identification is problematic. The terminology of calm and insight is in fact absent from the *Satipaṭṭhāna-sutta* itself (in all versions), and it seems clear that for those who composed and compiled the early collections of Buddhist literature (fourth to second century B.C.E.), "mindfulness" was considered as much a feature of calm meditation as it was of insight meditation. Moreover, the specific practice of the applications of mindfulness was itself understood to be as much about the cultivation of calm as insight. This follows from a number of passages in the corpus of early literature. In the first place, when the section of mindfulness of body is expanded in the Pali *Kāyagatāsati-sutta* (*Discourse on Mindfulness of Body*), the four progressive stages of absorption are straightforwardly included as part of the practice of mindfulness of body (M 3.92–94). The corresponding Sarvāstivāda versions of both the *Satipaṭṭhāna-sutta* and *Kāyagatāsati-sutta* preserved in Chinese similarly both present pervading the body with the feelings of joy, happiness, and purity characteristic of the attainment of the four *dhyānas* as examples of exercises in developing mindfulness of body (T 1.582c–583a; T 1.555b–555c; Kuan, 2008, pp. 148–149, 158–159). The practice of the four applications of mindfulness is said to result in the mind becoming properly concentrated and settled (D 2.216); underlining this point, their practice is even said to be the basis for the development of the various "yogic" powers (*iddhi*), such as passing through walls, flying through the air, walking on water, which ancient Buddhist texts regard as being developed from the mastery of concentration exercises (S 5.303; Gethin, 2011b). More generally, we can note that when the eight constituents of the Buddha's Eightfold Path are considered by way of the three main divisions of the Buddhist path—morality, concentration, and wisdom—right mindfulness is grouped with right concentration under the general heading of concentration (M 1.301; Anālayo, 2011, Vol. 1, pp. 279–280). Significantly the four applications of mindfulness are said to be the "signs" (*nimitta*), that is, meditation objects, for concentration, and their repeated practice constitutes the way to cultivate concentration (M 1.301; Anālayo, 2011, Vol. 1, p. 281). All this seems to reflect an outlook in which cultivating both concentration (*samādhi*) and even the absorptions (*dhyāna*) requires mindfulness and itself develops and strengthens mindfulness. In line with this, the ancient and often repeated description of the fourth of the four *dhyānas* or "absorptions" characterizes it as a state in which mindfulness has been completely purified.[4]

This way of understanding the applications of mindfulness as embracing both calm and insight is taken up in, for example, the Theravāda exegetical tradition. Here the various exercises set out under the heading of the first of the four ways of applying mindfulness—paying attention to the body—are approached initially as a means of developing deep states of concentration by way of the attainment of the four *dhyānas*. Thus, Buddhaghosa's commentary (fourth to fifth century C.E.) to the *Satipaṭṭhāna-sutta* explains that as the meditator trains by paying attention to the breath in the manner set out in the *sūtra*, the four successive absorptions are attained, with the inbreaths and outbreaths as the object of concentration (Sv 3.764; Ps 1.248–249; Sp 2.415; Paṭis-a, 2.494; cf. Vism VIII 186; Ñāṇamoli, 1964, p. 299). The practice of the three remaining ways of applying mindfulness—namely, paying attention to feelings, state of mind, and mental qualities—is then understood in terms of developing insight by bringing the mindfulness and concentration established by the practice of the absorptions to bear on these objects.

The beginning and end of the *Satipaṭṭhāna-sutta* characterizes the practice of the applications of mindfulness as a path that is *ekāyana* (D 2.290, M 1.55). Early English translations took this to mean that the applications of mindfulness are presented here as the *only* path leading to the purification of beings (e.g., Horner, 1954, p. 71; Rhys Davids & Rhys Davids, 1910, p. 327; Soma, 1967, p. 1). This has perhaps contributed to the modern reception of mindfulness. The term *ekāyana* is occasionally applied in the ancient literature to other forms of practice, including the eightfold path (NiddI 455–456), and while its precise interpretation in this context remains uncertain, it seems unlikely that it should be taken in the sense of "only." Probably its meaning is "going to just one place," and it can therefore be rendered "direct": "this path leading to the purification of beings, namely the four applications of mindfulness, is direct and clear" (Gethin, 1992, pp. 59–66). Of course, the overall significance of the expression also depends on whether we understand the applications of mindfulness as inclusive of forms of Buddhist practice that involve the attainment of meditative absorption (as I have suggested the earliest Buddhist texts and the Theravāda commentarial tradition did) or as exclusive of those forms of practices (as some modern interpreters do).

In the context of the practice of the applications of mindfulness, mindfulness is presented as a basic tool of Buddhist meditation. The role of mindfulness in keeping an object of meditation in mind in order to observe it clearly, and also the manner in which the practice of the applications of mindfulness involves directing the mind to attend to particular objects, mean that mindfulness and the applications of mindfulness come to be understood as playing a special role in guarding and protecting the mind from wandering into unhelpful and even dangerous pastures. In a number of places in early Buddhist literature, the practice of the applications of mindfulness is given by way of explanation of how to realize the instruction to live "taking no other refuge but yourselves, as an island of safety and a place of refuge; taking no other refuge but the Dharma, as an island of safety and place of refuge" (D 2.100; MPS 200).

Two similes vividly illustrate the theme of the four applications of mindfulness as the protection and refuge of the monk. These similes oppose the applications of mindfulness as a "resort" (*gocara*) that is the monk's own home ground (*sako pettiko visayo*) to the objects of five senses as somewhere outside the monk's resort (*agocara*), and so the ground of others (*para-visaya*). Thus, the fowl that wanders away from the protection of the clods of earth in a ploughed field is prey to the hawk, just as the monk who wanders from the protection of the applications of mindfulness into the domain of the objects of the senses is prey to Māra; or the monkey held in a monkey trap by his four limbs and head is at the mercy of the hunter, just as the monk captivated by the objects of the five senses is at the mercy of Māra (S 5.146–149; T 2.172c24–173a28, 2.173b20–173c11). Furthermore, practicing the applications of mindfulness is seen not only as a way of protecting oneself but as a way of protecting others; this is compared to two acrobats working together, one standing on the shoulders of the other (S 5.168–169; T 2.173b5–173b19).

In these passages the expression "application of mindfulness" is taken as primarily referring to the recommended objects of mindfulness; that is, as far as is possible, one should protect and guard the mind by keeping one's mind occupied with observing the body, feelings, states of mind and mental qualities, and stopping the mind straying away. Elsewhere, mindfulness itself seems to take on the role of standing guard and noticing when unhelpful thoughts threaten to upset the mind. Thus, a monk's prevention of bad, unwholesome qualities, such as longing and discontent, from overwhelming him is compared to living in a forest where one is surrounded by thorns and has to come and go mindfully in case one is scratched (S 4.189; cf. A 5.110–11; Kuan, 2008, pp. 42–44). This appears to echo a frequently occurring passage describing the guarding of the "gates" of the senses:

> How does a monk guard the gates of the senses? In this, when he looks at a visible object with his eyes, he does not hold on to the general experience nor particular aspects. Since someone who lives with the sense of sight unchecked might be affected by longing and discontent, by bad, unwholesome qualities, he tries to practice checking the sense of sight; he guards it, and achieves restraint. When he hears a sound with his ears . . . smells a smell with his nose . . . tastes a taste with his tongue . . . touches an object with his body . . . is conscious of a thought in his mind, he does not grasp at the general experience nor at particular aspects. Since someone who lives with the mind unchecked might be affected by longing and discontent, by bad, unwholesome qualities, he tries to practice checking the mind; he guards it, and achieves restraint. (e.g., D 1.70; cf. SBV 240; T 1.84c13–84c20)

This passage is often repeated in the early texts as a prelude to the exercise of establishing mindfulness and clear understanding with reference to everyday ordinary activities, such as eating, drinking, urinating, defecating, and so forth. A simile found elsewhere (S 4.194) explicitly likens mindfulness to a gatekeeper guarding a city (the body) with six gates (the senses). The characterization of mindfulness as guarding and as like a gatekeeper can be seen as closely related to mindfulness's general capacity of remembering and keeping in mind. The suggestion seems to be that if the monk has mindfulness then he will not forget his practice, and thus when feelings, perceptions, emotions, and states of mind that might interfere with this arise, he will have the presence of mind not to let them enter and overwhelm his mind. As a gatekeeper mindfulness remembers qualities for what they are and so does not let in those that are unwelcome. In sum, in guarding his mind with mindfulness a monk is said to have a unique guard (*ekārakkha*) (D 3.269; A 5.30).

The Elaboration of Mindfulness
in Indian Buddhist Systematic Thought

Between the second century B.C.E. and the fifth century C.E., Buddhist thinkers produced a body of exegetical and commentarial literature that attempted to explain and systematize the material contained in the discourses of the Buddha. This body of literature comprises especially the Abhidharma ("on the Dharma") works and various collections of commentaries and manuals. A feature of these works is the attempt to take further the limited explanations of psychological terms found in the Nikāyas in order to provide exact definitions of terms that identify them as specific mental qualities with specific characteristics.

Among the earliest exegetical texts of the Buddhist tradition is the *Milindapañha* (*Milinda's Questions*), which survives in both Pali and Chinese versions (Demiéville, 1924). The *Milindapañha* takes the form of a no doubt fictionalized dialogue between a Buddhist monk, Nāgasena, and King Milinda, that is, Menander, ruler of the kingdom of Bactria during the second century B.C.E. At one point relatively early in their conversation, Milinda asks Nāgasena for a definition of, among other qualities, mindfulness. Nāgasena explains that mindfulness has two distinctive characteristics: "recalling" (*apilāpana*) and "keeping hold" (*upagaṇhana*). The precise meaning of these terms, especially the former, is elusive and must in part be surmised from the two extended similes given by way of illustration (Mil 37; cf. Demiéville, 1924, pp. 112–113). The first is as follows:

> It is like the Wheel-Turning King's steward who reminds (*sārapeti*) the king evening and morning of his glory. He recalls (*apilāpeti*) the king's property saying, "So many, lord, are your elephants, so many your horses, chariots, foot soldiers, so much your gold, wealth, and property. Let my lord remember! (*saratu*)." In the same way, when mindfulness arises, it recalls various qualities and their opposites— skilful and unskilful, with faults and faultless, inferior and refined, dark and pure— [reminding the practitioner], "These are the four applications of mindfulness, these the four right endeavours, these the four bases of success, these the five faculties, these the five powers, these the seven constituents of awakening, this the noble eightfold path, this calm, this insight, this knowledge, this freedom." As a result the practitioner resorts to qualities that should be resorted to and not to those that should not be resorted to; he embraces qualities that should be embraced and not those that should not be embraced.

What this account suggests is that in "recalling," mindfulness can remember the full range of qualities; mindfulness therefore becomes a reminder of how any quality, good or bad, that may arise exists in relation to a whole variety of qualities. In this way, mindfulness helps the practitioner to remember the relative value of mental qualities and which to cultivate and which not to cultivate.

Initially the second characteristic of mindfulness highlighted in the *Milindapañha*, namely, "keeping hold," might seem to be merely a reiteration of mindfulness as keeping an object before the mind, but the connotations of the word *upagaṇhana* and the simile suggest something rather more is intended:

> It is like a Wheel-Turning King's precious adviser. Knowing what is beneficial and unbeneficial to the king, [he thinks] "These things are beneficial, these unbeneficial, these helpful, these unhelpful." As a result he gets rid of the unbeneficial things and keeps hold of the beneficial. In the same way, when mindfulness arises, it follows the course (*gati*) of beneficial and unbeneficial qualities, [and sees] "These qualities are beneficial, these unbeneficial; these helpful, these unhelpful." As a result the

practitioner gets rid of unbeneficial qualities and keeps hold of beneficial qualities; he gets rid of unhelpful qualities and keeps hold of helpful qualities.

This simile suggests that in holding things before the mind, mindfulness is understood to follow the course or outcome of mental qualities, and so keep track of which are beneficial and which unbeneficial. As a direct consequence the practitioner "takes possession" of what is beneficial. Mindfulness, from this perspective, cannot but involve the acquiring of what is beneficial. Both of these *Milindapañha* similes therefore draw out significant implications of keeping things in mind, making of mindfulness something more than simply sustaining attention.

One of the earliest exegetical works of the Theravāda tradition is the *Niddesa* (*Exposition*), a text that attempts to elucidate certain portions of another canonical text, the *Suttanipāta* (*A Collection of Sūtras*). In keeping with the early understanding of "mindfulness" as keeping and holding in mind objects of meditation, the *Niddesa* begins by defining *sati* by referring to the practice of the four applications of mindfulness and then to the set of six recollections (*anussati*)—of the Buddha, the Dharma, the Sangha, virtue, generosity, and the gods—supplemented by mindfulness of death, of breathing in and out, of the body, and recollection of peace. Finally a list of expository terms is given: recollection (*anussati*), remembrance (*paṭissati*), remembering (*saraṇatā*), keeping in mind (*dhāraṇatā*), lack of forgetfulness (*asammussanatā*), the faculty of mindfulness, the power of mindfulness, right mindfulness, the constituent of awakening that is mindfulness, the direct path (NiddI 9–10; cf. NiddII 347, 506). These terms reinforce the basic understanding of mindfulness as holding or keeping in mind, especially directed toward the objects specified in the exercises of the applications of mindfulness. But the list also includes the first of the two terms used in the *Milindapañha*: *apilāpana*, which is given in several early Pali texts as the special characteristic of mindfulness (Nett 15, 28, 54; NiddI 10, 347, 506; NiddII (Be) 30; Peṭ 187).

In the *Milindapañha*, context requires that *apilāpana* means something like "recalling." Exploiting the possibility of an alternative etymology, however, the Theravāda canonical Abhidharma texts interpret *apilāpanatā* rather differently.[5] They create a pair of opposites, *apilāpanatā* and *pilāpanatā*, which are used to explain mindfulness and "absentmindedness" (*muṭṭha-sati*), respectively, and seem to mean "not floating about" and "floating about" (Dhs 11, 232; Pugg 21; Vibh 360, 373). As the ancient Pali commentaries explain, mindfulness is therefore characterized as the mind's "not floating about," that is, its "immersion in" (*ogāhana*) or "going right into" (*anupavisana*) the object of awareness. This is to be contrasted with the "floating about" characteristic of "absentmindedness," when the mind floats on objects of awareness, like a gourd bobbing about on the surface of water (As 147, 405).

The Theravāda commentaries (fourth to fifth century C.E.) sum up the definition of mindfulness in the following manner:

Sati is that by means of which [the qualities that constitute the mind] remember, or it itself remembers, or it is simply remembering. Its characteristic is not floating about, its property absence of forgetting, its manifestation guarding or being face to face with an object of awareness; its basis is steady perception (*thirasaññā*) or the application of mindfulness of the body, and so on. Because of its being firmly set in the object of awareness, it should be seen as like a post and, because it guards the gates of the eye and other senses, as like a gatekeeper. (As 121–122; Vism XIV 141)

Such a definition keys into the various themes found in the earlier texts I have been reviewing. The summary definitions found in the exegetical traditions of other Buddhist schools are generally more succinct, highlighting mindfulness as simply not losing (*asaṃpramoṣa, avipramoṣa*) an object of awareness and recalling or calling to mind (*abhilapana*). The fifth-century Vaibhāṣika-Sarvāstivāda *Abhidharmadīpa* (*Light on Abhidharma*) defines mindfulness as "a type of function of the mind; it is recalling (*abhilapana*) the mind's purpose; it has the characteristic of not losing an action, whether it is something done, to be done or being done."[6] Asaṅga (fourth century), one of the founders of the Yogācāra school of Buddhist thought, defines mindfulness in his *Abhidharmasammucaya* as "not mentally losing a familiar object" and "in effect non-distraction."[7]

The contrast between the more restricted Vaibhāṣika and Yogācāra definitions, and the broader Theravāda definitions of mindfulness highlights a tension in the history of the Buddhist conceptualization of "mindfulness." In drawing up definitive lists of mental qualities (*caitasika, caitta*) that arise in association with consciousness (*citta*), the Abhidharma systematizers classified certain qualities as always and in every instance "wholesome" or "skillful" (*kuśala*), others as always and in every instance "unwholesome" or "unskillful" (*akuśala*), yet others as potentially either, depending on circumstances. Some mental qualities presented no problems: All agreed that "greed" (*lobha*) and "hatred" (*dveṣa*) are always and in every instance unwholesome; all agreed that "concentration" (*samādhi*) might be either. In the case of "mindfulness," however, there was a basic disagreement. For the Theravādins, "mindfulness" is an intrinsically skillful quality. That is, it is not found to be associated with consciousness rooted in greed, hatred, and delusion, only with consciousness rooted in nonattachment and friendliness. In fact, they suggested, it is a feature of all wholesome consciousness. For the Sarvāstivādins, however, mindfulness is one of 10 qualities considered characteristic of any kind of consciousness (*cittamahābhūmika*); that is, it is always present in the mind, and so may on occasion be either skillful or unskillful.

The considerations that led the Theravādins and Sarvāstivādins to classify mindfulness in these two different ways are not clear. Both schools seem to have started from a basic conceptualization of mindfulness as the capacity of consciousness to hold or keep in mind an object of awareness. Common sense may have suggested to Sarvāstivādin thinkers that a minimal "keeping in mind" should be a prerequisite of all consciousness. Moreover, if this "keeping in mind" is what allows us to remember things, then it must be conceded that we seem to be able to remember, at least sometimes, states of mind that are associated with unwholesome qualities, such as greed, hatred, and delusion, and also what we did when in those states. Furthermore, the authority of the earliest Buddhist texts, which not infrequently contrast "right mindfulness" with "wrong mindfulness" (*mithyāsmṛti*), may have persuaded them that *smṛti* should certainly not be regarded as a quality of mind only found to be associated with a wholesome mind. The thinkers of another school of Abhidharma, the Yogācāra, adopted yet another position. They disagreed with the Sarvāstivādin view that mindfulness is present in all consciousness, yet they did not take up the position of the Theravādins that it is always and only associated with wholesome states of mind. For the Yogācārins, mindfulness was one of several qualities of mind limited (*viniyata*) to specific circumstances. That is, it might occur in both unwholesome and wholesome states of mind, depending on conditions.

The extent to which and the manner in which mindfulness should be identified as playing the crucial role in acts of memory was the subject of some discussion. Asked whether those in unwholesome states of mind remember their past actions, the Theravādin author of the *Atthasālinī* (*Exposition of Meaning*) responded that they do, "but this is not called mindfulness," it is simply the occurrence of unwholesome consciousness in the aspect of memory (As 250); he goes on to explain that the expression "wrong mindfulness" in the Sūtras merely indicates how unwholesome states of mind are deprived of and opposed to mindfulness; "wrong mindfulness" is spoken of merely by way of completing an eightfold wrong path that parallels the noble eightfold path.

In his subcommentary (sixth century?), Ānanda explains further that when we bear some grudge, say, and we "remember" some perceived wrong done to us by reflecting on things done long ago, this memory should be understood not as being facilitated by its association with mindfulness but rather its association with clear and sharp *saṃjñā*, that is, "conceptual identification" (Dhs-mṭ 120; Nyanaponika, 1992). Of relevance here is that from the perspective of mindfulness, it is apparent that many of one's "memories," far from being accurate reflections of the way things truly were, are rather simply conceptions and ideas that are the products of a mind affected by greed, hatred, and delusion (Gethin, 1992, pp. 41–42).

In all systems of Indian Buddhist psychology, *saṃjñā* is understood as a further distinct quality of consciousness that is associated with all states of mind. How precisely it was understood in the earliest Buddhist texts is perhaps problematic, but in Buddhist systematic thought it is said to perform the function of learning (*udgrahṇa*) the "signs" or "marks" (*nimitta*) of objects of awareness.[8] The Yogācārin Asaṅga (fourth century) describes *saṃjñā* as thereby providing the means of giving conventional expression to things that have been experienced through the senses or conceived by the mind.[9] The Theravādin Buddhaghosa (fourth to fifth century) describes it as labeling or marking objects of experience so that they can be recognized again as the same (Vism XIV 130; cf. As 110; Abhidh-av 18). An exact English translation is difficult, and it is often rendered simply as "perception," although this must be considered insufficiently precise; some scholars have suggested "apperception" (Hamilton, 1996), though the specific technical usage of this in modern psychological literature makes this problematic; it seems to embrace something of the semantic range of English *conception, identification,* and *recognition* (Wayman, 1976). But as understood in Buddhist Abhidharma thought, *saṃjñā* clearly has some relevance to the operation of memory. Thus, in explanation of how one might remember or recognize something previously experienced, Vasubandhu sums up an act of memory as a specific instance of consciousness consequent upon—to borrow Jaini's (1992, p. 49) rendering of *saṃjñā* in this context—"a conceptual identification" of an object of memory (that is, something already experienced) (Abhidh-k-bh 472.17–18; Pruden, 1988, Vol. 4, p. 1339).

In this context it is worth noting a disagreement between the Sarvāstivādins and others, including Yogācārins, on the question of whether the object of "mindfulness" may be present or past. For the Sarvāstivādins, mindfulness "recalls" (*abhilapati*) objects of awareness in the present moment, thereby creating one of the conditions for objects to be subsequently remembered (Cox, 1992, p. 84). For the Yogācārins, on the other hand, mindfulness should be seen as only "recalling" an object of consciousness that has been previously apprehended. This understanding of the operation of mindfulness is set out in some technical detail in Sthiramati's (sixth century) commentary to Vasubandhu's succinct *Triṃśikā* (*Thirty Verses*):

> Mindfulness is not losing a familiar object; it is the mind's recalling [of that object]. A familiar object is one that has been previously experienced. There is no losing of this object because [in mindfulness] there exists a cause that prevents its apprehension from fading away. Recalling is repeatedly remembering the previously apprehended object's appearance as a mental support. . . . Moreover, mindfulness has the effect of non-distraction. That is, when an object is being recalled, this has the effect of non-distraction because there is no distraction either by a different object of consciousness or by a different aspect.[10]

What this explanation makes clear is that the Yogācāra insistence that the object of mindfulness is always one that has been previously apprehended should not be misconstrued as a claim that mindfulness has only to do with recollecting things done and said long before. On the contrary, the explanation seems intended to show how mindfulness facilitates continued and unbroken awareness of an object in the present: Once an object has become known to the mind, mindfulness repeatedly "recalls" it to mind and prevents the mind from being distracted by other objects of consciousness (Griffiths, 1992, pp. 111–112). We therefore have once more to do with the fundamental idea of mindfulness as keeping or holding an object of awareness in mind in the context of meditation practice.

This begins to bring out how, for Buddhist thinkers, the psychology of "mindfulness" should be articulated in the context of an account of the interaction of various ways of paying attention. In fact, in addition to mindfulness and "conceptual identification," I should mention at least a further five mental qualities that are distinguished as playing specific functions in the act of being aware of an object of consciousness: attention (*manaskāra*), concentration (*samādhi*), understanding (*prajñā*), application of thought (*vitarka*), and examining (*vicāra*).

While the different Abhidharma schools may not understand each of these mental qualities in precisely the same way, there is broad agreement. Thus, *attention* refers to the mind's turning toward the object of awareness in each moment of consciousness; *concentration*, to the mind's various mental capacities, qualities, and emotions becoming unified and resting, either momentarily or for a longer period, on a single object of awareness; *application of thought*, to the mind's deliberately and actively thinking about the object; *examining*, to the mind's careful examination of the different aspects of an object; and *understanding*, to the mind's forming some understanding of the value or significance of the object. Whereas according to the different Abhidharma schools not all of these mental qualities are necessarily active at all times and in every moment of consciousness, according to all schools they may be.

This raises the question of what determines the shape of these technical Abhidharma accounts of the mind and attention. Here we have to do with a complex interaction of tradition, reason and introspection. All the terms just given are received from the earliest Buddhist tradition and so are established as part of Buddhist thinking on such matters and must be included. The manner in which they are then presented as mental qualities that are both distinct and related is then determined by a continuing tradition of both logic and introspection.

We can illustrate this in part by the way Vasubandhu explains "application of mindfulness." For Vasubandhu, the application of mindfulness is essentially (*svabhāva*) understanding (*prajñā*). This is because the *Sūtras* describe its practice as a form of "observation" (*anupaśyanā*), and according to Vasubandhu's (or rather the tradition he follows) reading of the *Sūtras*, this involves some form of seeing or insight into how things are, in other words, understanding. Borrowing from the Abhidharma commentaries available to him (Cox, 1992, pp. 75–77), he then offers two alternative explanations of the role mindfulness plays in this kind of observation. According to the first explanation, mindfulness plays the leading role in holding whatever is being observed before the mind; understanding is then able to operate:

> Why does the Buddha speak of understanding as "presence of mindfulness"? Those who follow the Abhidharma Commentary say that it is because of the dominance of mindfulness [in the practice of the application of mindfulness]. What they mean is that it is because of the circumstance of the application of the power of mindfulness. It is like holding together splitting wood with a peg.[11]

According to his second, preferred, explanation, understanding observes how the object actually is, and mindfulness then has the role of "recalling" this (*abhilapana*): "But the following explanation is the appropriate one. Mindfulness applies itself through understanding, so the application of mindfulness is understanding because [mindfulness] recalls things as seen [by understanding]."[12]

In part, Vasubandhu's two accounts of the functioning of mindfulness illustrate the tension inherent in the basic meaning of *smṛti* that I noted at the start of this discussion. According to the first explanation, mindfulness simply holds the present object of consciousness firmly in attention. According to the second, mindfulness, literally, "speaks about" (*abhilapati*), that is, recalls, records, notes, or even remembers what has just been observed.

For Buddhist thinkers such as Vasubandhu, mindfulness can function both as the means by which we hold on to what is seen by understanding and more generally as the means by which we keep in mind what has been perceived. But in terms of modern cognitive psychology, it appears to be envisioned more in terms of working memory and short-term memory than long-term memory. As the *Abhidharmadīpa* (*Light on Abhidharma*), another fifth century Sarvāstivādin manual, puts it, "With reference to the body, and so on, as discerned by understanding, the faculty of mindfulness is not losing [what is perceived], both as undistorted recalling—that is, recognition—and as the means by which there is no loss of a mental object once ascertained."[13]

Some Later Conceptualizations in China, Tibet, and Burma

A common theme of Buddhist theory and practice at different times and in different places has been the suggestion that the way we ordinarily see and understand the world is at the root of our problems. Enlightenment, the goal of the Buddhist path, has therefore been conceived as involving a fundamental transformation in how an individual understands and relates to the world. The theoretical statement of precisely what is wrong with our ordinary unenlightened way of looking at the world and the method we need to employ in order to put it right have varied to greater or lesser extents. A significant idea that had some bearing on how these matters were understood and expressed is the notion that the mind is naturally pure, and that our delusion is in some sense secondary. The idea is occasionally expressed in the earliest stratum of Buddhist literature, but it is in certain Indian Mahāyāna Buddhist texts that it is developed and exploited. Here the idea is expressed in the suggestion that all beings have within them the Tathāgata (*tathāgatagarbha*) and that the essence of our minds is the Buddha Nature (*buddhadhātu*). As Buddhist thought took root in China, certain ideas and practices resonated with certain Daoist ideas and practices, inspiring in particular a tradition of discourse and practice centered on the Buddha Nature (*foxing*), that is, our True Nature (*zhenxing*) or True Mind (*zhenxin*) (McRae, 1986, pp. 138–140). Connected with this was an outlook that viewed our ordinary way of thinking as simply distracting us and keeping us from realizing our True Nature. These ordinary activities manifest in the mind's tendency to discriminate and make distinctions. If we attempt to interfere in these activities by discriminating between "good" and "bad" thoughts, we are drawn into these activities, thereby reinforcing the illusions of the everyday mind rather than seeing through them. Our strategy should instead be one of simply watching mental activities until they settle and cease to obscure our True Mind.

The usual Chinese translation of *smṛti* or "mindfulness" is *nian* (念), "to think of" or "recall," but some early Chinese translations of Buddhist texts use the expression *shouyi* (守 意), "maintaining or guarding consciousness."[14] This latter expression resonates with several expressions that come to play a significant role in the articulation of early Chan (Zen) Buddhist practice, including *shouxin* (守心), "guarding the mind" and *shouyi* (守一), "guarding the one" (Buswell, 1989, pp. 137–157; McRae, 1986, 136–144; Sharf, 2002, pp. 182–184, 2014). Such expressions are associated with an approach to meditation in which the emphasis is placed on watching the mind itself in order to experience directly its intrinsically pure nature. While such an approach to meditation was not universally accepted among Chinese Buddhist practitioners, it is worth considering briefly here because it highlights an approach to meditation and mindfulness that is not fully expressed in the Indian materials and that may have had some influence on the modern Western reception of mindfulness.

The teachings of the fifth Chan patriarch, Hongren (601–674) were compiled in the *Xiuxin yao lun (Treatise on the Essentials of Cultivating the Mind).*[15] According to this treatise, "Sentient beings . . . are all deluded as to the True Nature and do not discern the fundamental mind. Because they cognize the various [*dharmas*] falsely, they do not cultivate correct mindfulness [*zhengnian* 正念]. Since they do not cultivate correct mindfulness, thoughts of revulsion and attraction are activated [in them]" (McRae, 1986, p. 123).

For Hongren, "correct mindfulness" is crucial: "To never fail in correct mindfulness—even when one's body is being torn apart or at the time of death—is to be a buddha" (McRae, 1986, p. 131). And correct mindfulness is conceived in terms of *shouxin*, "to maintain the mind" or, as McRae has explained the expression, "to maintain constant, undiscriminating awareness of the absolute mind or Buddha Nature within oneself" (p. 136). It is to be practiced as follows:

> Make your body and mind pure and peaceful, without any discriminative thinking at all. Sit properly with the body erect. Regulate the breath and concentrate the mind so it is not within you, not outside of you, and not in any intermediate location. Do this carefully and naturally. View your own consciousness tranquilly and attentively, so that you can see how it is always moving, like flowing water or a glittering mirage. After you have perceived this consciousness, simply continue to view it gently and naturally . . . until its fluctuations dissolve into peaceful stability. This flowing consciousness will disappear like a gust of wind. (McRae, 1986, p. 130)

Interestingly there are in Hongren's treatise apparent echoes of the *Smṛtyupasthāna-sūtra* itself. The *Smṛtyupasthāna-sūtra* envisions the practice of mindfulness of the body in terms of a monk who, "when walking, knows he is walking; when standing, knows he is standing; when sitting, knows he is sitting; when lying down, knows he is lying down" (Kuan, 2008, pp. 146–147; M 1.56–57; T 1.582b). Hongren urges his followers similarly: "During all your activities—walking, standing still, sitting, and lying down—you should simply maintain awareness of your fundamental Pure Mind."[16] And just as the *Smṛtyupasthāna-sūtra* ends with the observation that the practice of the applications of mindfulness can lead to awakening in a matter of 7 days (M I 62–63), and, according to the version preserved in Chinese translation, to at least significant progress even in a brief moment (Kuan, 2008, p. 154; T 1.584b16–584b27),[17] we are told at the conclusion of Hongren's treatise that "anyone who practices according to this text will achieve buddhahood immediately" (McRae, 1986, p. 132; T 48.397b7–397b8).

Discussions around the kind of approach to meditation advocated in early Chan developed, in China in the seventh and eighth centuries, into debates around the nature of Buddhist enlightenment as sudden or gradual. Such debates hinged not primarily on how fast one might reach enlightenment, but rather on whether enlightenment is something innate and intrinsic to the mind or something to be constructed and acquired by the mind (Gómez, 1987).

During the eighth century, when Buddhism was establishing itself in Tibet, there is evidence of influence from both India and China, and the so-called Lhasa debates at the end of the eighth century hinged once more on the notions of sudden or gradual enlightenment. How far we should see a direct relationship between the approaches to Buddhist meditation characteristic of Chinese Chan and certain approaches that came to flourish in Tibet is perhaps unclear, but there is a certainly an affinity. Thus, for the practitioner of "Great Perfection" or Dzogchen (*rdzogs chen*), a system of practice particularly associated with the Nyingma (*rnying ma*) school of Tibetan Buddhism, getting caught up in meditation in identifying certain thoughts as good and others as bad and trying to promote the former and block the latter hinders the very process of meditation (van Schaik, 2004).

In turn, Dzogchen practice has some affinity with the "Great Seal" (Sanskrit *mahāmudrā*, Tibetan *phyag chen*) tradition particularly associated with the Kagyu (*bka' brgyud*) school, such that the two traditions of practice can sometimes be brought together as Chag-Dzog (*phyag rdzogs*), as in the work of the 17th century Karma Chagme (Chags med), *An introduction to the practice of great compassion according to the fusion of Dzogchen and Mahāmudrā (Thugs rje chen po'i dmar khrid phyag rdzogs zung 'jug)*. Like Hongren's practice of "guarding the mind," both Dzogchen and Mahāmudrā practice start from the assumption that the mind is naturally pure. They also both target as our problem the manner in which our minds habitually and routinely discriminate and conceptualize. The following comments on Dzogchen and Mahāmudrā draw from Lutz, Dunne, and Davidson (2007, pp. 510–517) and especially Dunne (2011).

Dzogchen and Mahāmudrā practices aim at a radical deconstruction of the mental apparatus of conceptualization and discrimination, such that the mind is returned to a natural pristine awareness (sometimes called *rig pa* in Tibetan). This pristine awareness can be characterized as "non-dual" insofar as the normal way the mind operates based on polarities and opposites—in particular the conceptual apparatus of a perceiving subject and a perceived object—is, as it were, switched off. This approach to meditation draws on the traditions of the Indian "Great Adepts" (*mahāsiddha*) such as Saraha (10th century?) and Tilopa (988–1069). Their practices involved a certain subversion of the traditional Buddhist terms used to describe the functions of consciousness, among them "mindfulness" and "attention" (*manaskāra*). Thus, Saraha can write:

Though true understanding varies with knowledge interests,
In non-mindfulness (*dran med*), there has never been anything false.
Though the goal varies according to efforts on the path,
In mindfulness (*dran pa*), there has never been anything true.[18]

Here mindfulness is apparently construed as part of the apparatus of discrimination and conceptualization, so it is part of the problem rather than the solution: What we need to do is somehow get behind "mindfulness" to a nondual, nonconceptual awareness. But such a way of talking needs to be understood as in dialogue with the Buddhist tradition. The language of the earlier Buddhist tradition, which may previously have conveyed a message of liberation from our conceptual prison, has from the perspective of Mahāmudrā become part of it. Nevertheless, in practice at least some Mahāmudrā teachers, such as Wangchug Dorje (dBang phyug rdo rje) (1556–1601) in his *The Ocean of Certainty (Nges don rgya mtsho)*, continue to exhort us to "set up the spy of mindfulness and carefully examine our mental continuum, thinking, 'Is my mind stable, or not? Is it agitated or dull?'" (Dunne, 2011, p. 88). Yet this mindfulness is seen as provisional. True mindfulness is "the mindfulness of mere non-distraction" (*ma yengs tsam gyi dran pa*), which is something deeper, more natural, and effortless, but which we are inevitably caught up in striving to attain. As Wangchung Dorje again puts it in his *Eliminating the Darkness of Ignorance (Ma rig mun sel)*:

> Do not self-consciously try to accomplish anything, rather fix your mind like an eagle soaring. Be completely free from all expectations and worries. When you have no mental wandering thoughts will not come. But when mental wandering occurs, then because your thoughts will come one after the other, try to recognise them for what they are as soon as they arise. In other words, stare right at them and then fix your mind as before. No matter what thoughts arise in this way, just recognise them for what they are. Place your attention right on them without thinking anything like, "I must block them," or feeling happy or unhappy. (Berzin, 1978, p. 52)

But as Dunne (2011) has observed, the "spy" of conventional mindfulness is not entirely unrelated to the ultimate "mindfulness of mere non-distraction"; it is "a gross, conceptual manifestation of this fundamental capacity of consciousness" (p. 84).

From the perspective of earlier systematic Buddhist thought, certainly as articulated in the Theravāda and Sarvāstivāda Abhidharma, escaping into some pure, nonconceptual, nondual awareness is not possible. All consciousness, even at the moment of enlightenment itself, is understood as occurring by way of certain fundamental mental capacities—including feeling (*vedanā*) and recognition (*samjñā*)—directed toward the object. That this is so may suggest the existence of a clear fault line between Buddhist systems and theories that seek to analyse consciousness in terms of such mental capacities and those that speak of some form of pristine awareness beyond, or deeper, than all such capacities. Alternatively, we may think in terms of there being a continuum rather than a stark fault line. As I have already noted, Buddhist systems of meditation characteristically aim in some way at deconstructing our perceptual and mental process as a means to escaping from a distorted and self-centred view of the world. Buddhist meditation tends to be articulated within a theoretical framework that is fundamentally suspicious of the mind's capacity to proliferate concepts that we mistake for reality and see as reflecting the way the world is. The dynamics of the theories may vary, as may the approach to neutralizing the capacity of our mental and perceptual processes to fool us.

At the other end of the spectrum, perhaps, from Chan, Dzogchen, and Mahāmudrā are the methods of 'insight' (*vipassanā*) meditation as taught by U Ba Khin (1899–1971) and Mahasi Sayadaw (1904–1982), two Burmese teachers in the tradition of modern Burmese insight mediation, whose techniques have had considerable influence on contemporary Theravāda meditation internationally (Braun, 2008, 2013; Hout-man, 1985, 1997; Kornfield, 1977). For Mahasi (1971/1979), mindful awareness appears to be understood as, or is at least approached through, a mental "noting." The meditator is instructed initially to be fully aware of the rising and falling of the abdomen in connection with breathing. As practice progresses, awareness is extended from the movement of the body to the movements of the mind.

> If you are thirsty while contemplating, notice the feeling, *thirsty*. When you intend to stand, *intending*. Keep the mind intently on the act of standing up, and mentally note, *standing*. When you look forward after standing up straight, note *looking, seeing*. Should you intend to walk forward, *intending*. When you begin to step forward, mentally note each step as *walking, walking*, or *left, right*. It is important for you to be aware of every moment in each step from the beginning to the end when you walk. Adhere to the same procedure when strolling or when taking walking exercise. Try to make a mental note of each step in two sections as follows: *lifting, putting, lifting, putting*. When you have obtained sufficient practice in this manner of walking, then try to make a mental note of each step in three sections: *lifting, pushing, putting*; or *up, forward, down*. (pp. 17–18)

Mahasi's method is often talked of loosely as a method of "labeling," yet there appears to be in the instructions a wariness of words and conceptualization: "Continue with this exercise in full awareness of the abdomen's rising and falling movements. Never verbally repeat the words *rising, falling*, and do not think of *rising* and *falling* as words. *Be aware only of the actual process of the rising and falling movements of the abdomen* (Mahasi, 1971/1979, pp. 12–13, original emphasis).[19]

The European monk Nyanaponika (1901–1994), a follower of Mahasi's method (Bodhi, 1995), seems to present Mahasi's "noting" in terms of what he calls "bare attention," which he understands as an "elementary manifestation" of mindfulness, to be distinguished from fully developed "right mindfulness," a constituent of the eightfold path (1962, pp. 24, 30–31).

Nyanaponika contrasts "bare attention" with our habitual manner of perceiving things "in the light of added subjective judgements" that are bound up with our preconceived sense of ourselves, our personality and ego (1962, pp. 30, 45). Bare attention is seen as a way of beginning to counteract the process whereby with every act of awareness we reinforce habits of mind and preconceived ideas that prevent us from seeing things as they truly are. As countering preconceptions and habitual patterns of thought, Nyanaponika's "bare attention" might be understood as appealing to some form of pure, nonconceptual, and even pristine awareness of the kind assumed in Chan, Dzogchen, and Mahāmudrā (Sharf, 2014). Nyanaponika himself, however, refers his understanding to the technical account of the process of perception (*citta-vīthi*) found in Theravāda systematic thought: he equates bare attention with the initial "turning [of the mind] toward" (*āvajjana*) an object of awareness, a stage in the process of perception that is characterized by a simple attention (*manasikāra*) to an object (1962, pp. 24, 112). In Theravāda systematic thought, this attention is not technically "nonconceptual" (it is associated with at least rudimentary conceptualization in the form of *saññā*), but is prior to the complete mental processing of the object by way of "receiving" (*sampaṭicchana*), "investigating" (*santīraṇa*), determining (*votthapana*), and the consequent mental "impulsion" (*javana*) that underlies "actions" (*karma*). Strictly the stage of turning toward the object is not associated with mindfulness at all, nor is it possible to halt the perceptual process at this stage (Wijeratne & Gethin, 2002, pp. 124–138). Nonetheless Nyanaponika presents "bare attention" as a preliminary practical approach to mindfulness practice (Wallace & Bodhi, 2006).

U Ba Khin's method, which has become widely practiced in the West especially in a form taught by S. N. Goenka (1924–2013), is characterized not so much by a particular understanding of mindfulness as by what mindfulness is directed toward. Thus, the practice of mindfulness of breathing is developed with the specific focus of perceiving directly the fundamental impermanence (*aniccatā*) of things. This is achieved by a particular technique of mindfulness of the body that involves scanning the body while focusing on the sense of touch. Using a specific formula of instruction, the meditator is told to begin "the practice of sweeping the attention through the body, part by part, feeling the impermanence of all touch and sensation": "As the awareness of impermanence continues, the meditator will see how the power of his concentration and mindfulness can unblock the flow of energy in the body. Then the sweeping becomes more rapid and more clear" (Kornfield, 1977, p. 251).

The experience of the flow of energy is interpreted according to a framework adapted from the Theravāda Abhidharma theory of matter (*rūpa*) as constituted by "clusters" (*kalāpa*) or "atoms" (the smallest indivisible instances of matter) consisting of earth ("extension"), water ("cohesion"), fire ("heat and cold") and air ("motion"), along with other secondary qualities (Kornfield, 1977, p. 251):

> A *kalāpa* is the minutest particle in the physical plane—still beyond the range of science today. . . . The life span of a *kalāpa* is termed a "moment," and a trillion such moments are said to elapse during the wink of a man's eye. These *kalāpas* are all in a state of perpetual change or flux. To a developed student in Vipassanā meditation they can be felt as a stream of energy.

Both Mahasi's and U Ba Khin's methods of meditation look back to the *Smṛtyupasthāna-sūtra* and appeal in part to the authority of the Buddha. And yet straightforwardly relating either method directly to the instructions in the *Smṛtyupasthāna-sūtra* is clearly problematic. Certainly the *Smṛtyupasthāna-sūtra* talks of a monk "acting with full awareness" (*sampajānakārin*):

> In moving forward and turning back . . . in looking ahead and looking around . . . in bending and straightening his limbs . . . in wearing his inner and outer robes and carrying his alms bowl . . . in eating, drinking, chewing and swallowing . . . in defecating and urinating . . . in walking, standing, sitting, falling asleep, waking up, speaking and keeping silent.

Yet it is not at all clear that such acting with full awareness assumes the kind of "noting" advocated in Mahasi's practice, or that mindfulness of breathing as described in the *Satipaṭṭhāna-sutta* involves the focus on the impermanence of bodily sensations in the manner envisaged by U Ba Khin's method.[20]

Conclusions

The following are two frequently cited definitions of *mindfulness* in the modern mindfulness literature:

1. "Mindfulness means paying attention in a particular way: on purpose, in the present moment, and nonjudgmentally" (Kabat-Zinn, 1994, p. 4).
2. "A kind of nonelaborative, nonjudgmental, present-centered awareness in which each thought, feeling, or sensation that arises in the attentional field is acknowledged and accepted as it is" (Bishop et al., 2004, p. 232)

Such definitions are in part the product of over a century of the Western reception of Buddhist ideas. To what extent do they coincide with how Buddhists have conceptualized mindfulness?

Certainly mindfulness is understood in Buddhist texts as a way of paying attention and as a kind of awareness, but its domain in traditional Buddhist discussions is not restricted to present thoughts, feelings, or sensations as they occur. Indeed such formulations, especially that of Bishop and colleagues (2004), seem to exclude certain of the mindfulness practices traditionally described under the heading "mindfulness of the body" (e.g., mindfulness of the ugliness of a rotting corpse, or of the 30+ parts of the body). Such practices seem not to be adequately described as "present-centered awareness in which each thought, feeling, or sensation that arises in the attentional field is acknowledged and accepted as it is." While they clearly assume not getting lost in thoughts about the past or the future, they at the same time assume the recollection of a list of body parts, as well as in some measure the exercise of the imagination.

The suggestion that mindfulness involves accepting each thought, feeling, or sensation as it is may have a particular resonance with some of the Buddhist approaches to the practice of mindfulness outlined earlier (especially Chan, Dzogchen, and Mahāmudrā), but from the perspective of Buddhist texts more generally, this is to restrict the scope of mindfulness. That is, Buddhist texts quite clearly see mindfulness as having a role in deliberately and purposefully holding the attention on a chosen object of meditation. To this extent, Jon Kabat-Zinn's "on purpose" is apposite, but from the perspective of traditional Indian Buddhist thought, the modern operational definitions of mindfulness used in the context of MBSR and MBCT, for example, tend to conflate the manner of paying attention with particular objects recommended for attention. This is in part a result of the tendency, noted earlier, to equate the practice of mindfulness with the practice of insight (*vipassanā*).

Here, we are concerned not so much with different Buddhist conceptualizations of mindfulness as with how mindfulness is to be employed in different practices and at different stages of the Buddhist path. That is, mindfulness seems always to be understood as a holding of attention on something; in some practices this involves holding the attention on the breath or the emotion of friendliness; in others, the emphasis is on holding attention on the way the mind works, that is, on the process of attention itself. In the practice of the fourth application of mindfulness as described in the ancient *Smṛtyupasthāna-sūtra*, this involves observing the mental and physical qualities (*dharma*) that constitute the process of our experience of the world in its entirety as just qualities—insubstantial phenomena that come and go. In Chan, Dzogchen, and Mahāmudrā, holding attention becomes the ability to sustain a nonconceptual, nondual awareness of reality.

Modern discussions of Buddhist meditation have distinguished between practices that cultivate a kind of "meta-awareness" or "open monitoring" on the one hand, and those that rely on "focused attention" on the other. *Focused attention* has been defined as "voluntary focusing attention on a chosen object in a sustained fashion" (Lutz, Slagter, Dunne, & Davidson, 2008, p. 163) and open monitoring as "nonreactively monitoring the content of experience from moment to moment, primarily as a means to recognize the nature of emotional and cognitive patterns" (p. 163). The general tendency has been to assimilate "mindfulness" to the latter and the practice of calm (*śamatha*) and concentration (*samādhi*) to the former, although some have drawn attention to the fact that this does not neatly fit the usage of terminology in traditional Buddhist discourse (Lutz, Dunne, & Davidson, 2007). This certainly seems to be the case. My reading of the Indian Buddhist systematic thought suggests that its authors would not regard this distinction between "open monitoring" and "focused attention" as hinging on "mindfulness" at all. That is, from their perspective, both practices would require the exercise of mindfulness in equal measure: Both practices would require mindfulness in order to sustain the attention and keep the mind focused on the exercise. According to this interpretation of the Buddhist materials, mindfulness is primarily conceived of as a kind of lucid sustaining of attention on the object of awareness, in which the mind is both aware of the object and, in some sense, aware that it is aware, with all that implies (that the object is the object the mind should be aware of, and that the manner of awareness is appropriate). If this encompasses the monitoring of attention, it is not restricted to an "open monitoring" of the way the mind attends to objects. Rather, sustaining the attention in this manner is as relevant to cultivating focused absorption (*dhyāna, samādhi*) when contemplating a single and simple object as it is to monitoring the coming and going of objects of perception and the mind's reaction to them.

Accepting each thought, feeling, or sensation as it is also is related to the characterization of mindfulness as "nonelaborative" and "nonjudgmental." A problem here is the imprecision of such English expressions. As we have seen, Buddhist systems of meditation tend to view our mental habits as unhealthy and in need of attention. A common Buddhist strategy might be identified as trying to *see* what is going on, rather than to *think* we know what is going on. The latter means reinforcing our delusional take on the world, the former patiently watching. Furthermore, something of a practical common ground of Buddhist psychology might be expressed by saying that although—or precisely because—the aim is to rid ourselves of greed, hatred, and delusion, getting angry when we observe our own greed, hatred and delusion, or conversely, being pleased when we observe our own nonattachment, friendliness and wisdom, is clearly something of a trap.

According to ordinary English usage, telling someone that he or she is *judgmental* is not a compliment. Hence, to the extent that mindfulness is considered a virtue it cannot, according to the same English usage, be defined as *judgmental*. But from at least some Buddhist perspectives, an unqualified emphasis on mindfulness as "non-judgmental" might be seen as implying that there are no values in being mindful, that greed is somehow as good as nonattachment, and friendliness as bad as anger. The question of the ultimate "value" of our fleeting mental states takes us into complex areas of Buddhist thought and ethics, in which different Buddhist traditions will express themselves differently. But Buddhist meditation has generally been taught and practiced within an ethical and conceptual framework where certain mental states and actions are valued as good (wholesome) and others as bad (unwholesome). Even when this framework has been challenged by Buddhist traditions advocating antinomian practices, the challenge takes place within the context of a discussion that appeals to broader Buddhist principles about the relationship of ignorance to greed and attachment. This discussion explores in turn questions about the relationship of our theoretically constructed ideas about "good" and "bad" thoughts to actual good and bad thoughts.

The distinction that Dunne (2011) makes between "constructivist" and "innatist" tendencies in Buddhist understandings of enlightenment is helpful here. From the constructivist perspective, the manner in which our unenlightened minds misunderstand the way things are is cured by cultivating a new, different understanding to take the place of the old. From the innatist perspective, the way our unenlightened minds misunderstand the way things are cured is not by cultivating some new understanding, but by allowing the misunderstanding simply to fade away and cease.

In summary, we have identified three areas in which there is a certain tension in Buddhist conceptualizations of mindfulness. The first is its relationship to memory. Here, Buddhist conceptualizations imply a bringing together of attentiveness and remembering of the sort that might occur when one performs certain tasks with full awareness, such as reciting a *sūtra* or poem learned by heart. Second is mindfulness's relationship to conceptual and discursive types of thinking. Here, Buddhist conceptualizations imply a distinction between self-consciously thinking about what one is doing and being fully aware and attentive to what one is doing. The reciter of *sūtras*, like the concert pianist, the tightrope walker, and the racing driver, must all be fully aware and fully present to perform well, but self-consciously thinking about what they are doing is likely to interfere with this awareness and presence and, even worse, interfere with the successful completion of their respective tasks.

Finally there is mindfulness's relationship to ethical action. At least *prima facie*, the starkest contrast in the Buddhist conceptualization of mindfulness is between the Theravāda understanding of it as an exclusively wholesome (*kuśala*) quality (i.e., a quality that is exclusively characteristic of states of consciousness associated with nonattachment, friendliness and understanding), and the Sarvāstivāda and Yogācāra understanding of it as potentially a quality of both the wholesome and unwholesome mind (i.e., it may be associated with *either* nonattachment, kindness, and understanding *or* greed, hatred, and delusion). In saying that mindfulness is exclusive to and always present in wholesome states of mind, the Theravādins seem to want to suggest that there is something about the very activity of maintaining attention that affects the quality of awareness; unwholesome states are somehow intrinsically lacking in awareness. But what is the nature of the unwholesome mindfulness of the

Sarvāstivādins and Yogācārins? The answer might be, perhaps, the kind of mindfulness that is present when one carefully, deliberately, and with full attention carries out some action motivated by greed, hatred, and delusion: murder or theft. The defender of the Theravāda position might respond that to the extent that one is mindful (i.e., remains attentive to body, feeling, mental states, and emotions), one is protected from doing anything unwholesome.

According to Theravādin systematic thought, it is strictly not possible to be mindful of greed, hatred, and delusion as things *present* in the mind. From the perspective of the Theravādin model of the mind, being aware of greed, say, as something present in the mind must be understood in terms of the intermittent occurrence of relatively clouded and relatively lucid moments of consciousness, where greed is present in one moment, and mindfulness of greed's *former* presence is present in the next moment. Thus, to become aware, mindful, of the presence in the mind of emotions such as greed and hatred is already to step back from them. Conversely, in the moment of fulfilling some unwholesome purpose, mindfulness must inevitably desert us, and the mind be taken over by greed, hatred, and delusion. Such an outlook begins to take on the character of an innatist perspective: We do not have to *make* our actions wholesome, so much as always be fully aware of and present in them, for it is impossible to be fully aware of and present in actions motivated by greed, hatred, and delusion without beginning to see them for what they are—the cause of our own and others' suffering. In speaking like this, one begins to evoke the imagery and metaphors of Buddhist discourse: The awareness of the unwholesome, unskillful mind is the impaired awareness of a mind that is obscure, dark, clouded, blind; the awareness of the wholesome, skillful mind, on the other hand, is the awareness of a mind that is bright, clear, lucid. And so in practice, whatever the underlying scholastic position, Buddhist conceptualizations of mindfulness tend to focus on "right mindfulness": a way of paying attention to and sustaining attention that, when combined and developed with other wholesome qualities of mind, both facilitates and is characteristic of what Buddhism calls "enlightenment" or, better, "awakening" (*bodhi*).

ACKNOWLEDGMENTS

The research for this chapter was in part funded by the Leverhulme Trust as part of a project entitled "Abhidharma: The Buddhist Model of the Mind." I am grateful to Anālayo Bhikkhu, Erik Braun, Kirk Warren Brown, John Dunne, Giuliano Giustarini, Rita Langer, Robert Sharf, and Paul Williams for their criticisms and suggestions. Any mistakes and misunderstandings that remain are my own.

NOTES

1. See Appendix 2.1 for abbreviations of Pali, Sanskrit, and Chinese Buddhist texts used throughout this chapter.

2. It seems likely that the element *paṭṭhāna* in Pali *sati-paṭṭhāna* should be taken as a contraction of *upaṭṭhāna* (= Sanskrit *upasthāna*), which can refer either to "the act of standing

near" or "the place something stands near" (cf. Monier-Williams, 1899, p. 211, s.v. [sub verbo, or "under the word"] *upasthāna*). The ancient Theravāda commentators sometimes also take *paṭṭhāna* in this context as equivalent to Sanskrit *prasthāna*, which is then understood similarly as either "the act of standing forth" or "the place where something stands forth" (cf. Monier-Williams, 1899, p. 699, s.v. *prasthāna*). See Sv 752–753; Ps 1.238; Spk, 3.179; Paṭis-a 695–696; Vibh-a 214–215; Kv-a 52–53; Abhidh-k-bh 342.5–17 (VI 15 a–b).

3. The Pali version is found in both the Digha Nikāya (D 2.290–315) and, in a slightly abbreviated form, the Majjhima Nikāya (M 1.55–62); for the two versions in Chinese translation, see T 1.582b–584b and T 2.568a–569b. The Pali versions have been frequently translated into English (e.g., Gethin, 2008, pp. 141–151; Ñāṇamoli & Bodhi, 1995, pp. 145–155; Nyanaponika, 1962, pp. 117–135; Rhys Davids & Rhys Davids, 1910, pp. 327–346); for a translation of the first Chinese version see Kuan (2008, pp. 145–154).

4. Pali *upekkhāsatipārisuddhi*; in Buddhist Sanskrit texts we find *upekṣāsmṛtipāriśuddhi*, *-pariśuddhi*, *-pariśuddha*. On the analysis of the expression, see Trenckner et al. (1924–2011), s.v. *upekkhāsatipārisuddhi*, and Sastri (1978, pp. 394–395).

5. The *Milindapañha* seems to assume a derivation from *api-lapati* (= Sanskrit *abhi-lapati*), "to talk or speak about"; the Theravāda Abhidharma texts assume a derivation from *pilavati* (= Sanskrit *plavate*), "to float or swim." See Cone (2001); Cox (1992, pp. 79–82); Gethin (1992, pp. 38–39); Norman (1988, pp. 49–51).

6. Abhidh-dī 69: *cittavyāpārarūpā smṛtiḥ | cittasyārthābhilapanā kṛtakartavyakriyamāṇak armāntāvipramoṣalakṣaṇā ||.*

7. Abhidh-sam 16.3–4: *smṛtiḥ katamā | saṃstute vastuni cetaso 'saṃpramoṣaḥ | avikṣepakarmikā ||.*

8. Trimś-bh 57: *saṃjñā viṣayanimittodgrahaṇam | viṣaya ālambanam | nimittaṃ tadviśeṣo nīlapītādyālambanavyavasthākāraṇam | tasyodgrahaṇaṃ nirūpaṇaṃ nīlam etan na pītam iti.*

9. This portion of Abhidh-sam survives only in Chinese and Tibetan; see Rahula (2001, p. 3), T (1605) 31.663b5–663b7.

10. Trimś-bh 72: *smṛtiḥ saṃstute vastuny asaṃpramoṣaś cetaso 'bhilapanatā | saṃstutaṃ vastu pūrvānubhūtam | ālambanagrahaṇāvipraṇāśakāraṇatvād asaṃpramoṣaḥ | pūrvagṛhītasya vastunaḥ punaḥ punar ālambanākārasmaraṇam abhilapanatā | . . . sā punar avikṣepakarmikā | ālambanābhilapane sati cittasyālambanāntara ākārāntare vā vikṣepābhāvād avikṣepakarmikā |.*

11. Abhidh-k-bh 342.9–10 (VI 15 a–b): *kasmāt prajñā smṛtyupasthānam ity uktā bhagavatā | smṛtyudrekatvād iti Vaibhāṣikāḥ | smṛtibalādhānavṛttitvād iti yo 'rthaḥ | dārupāṭakilasaṃdhāraṇavat |* (Reading with Abhidh-k-vy 530).

12. Abhidh-k-bh 342.11 (VI 15 a–b): *evaṃ tu yujyate | smṛtir anayopatiṣṭhata iti smṛtyupasthānaṃ prajñā yathādṛṣṭasyābhilapanāt |.*

13. Abhidh-dī 360: *smṛtindriyaṃ nāma kāyādiṣu prajñayopalakṣiteṣu yā khalv aviparītābhilapanā pratyabhijñānam yenāvadhārite viṣayasammoṣaś cetasi na bhavati sa khalv asammoṣaḥ smṛtindriyam.*

14. For example, see An Shigao's second century CE translations of the *Shibaofa jing* (*Daśottara-sūtra*) (T 1.236b24) and the *Da anban shouyi jing* (*Great Discourse on Maintaining Awareness of Breathing In and Out*) (T 15.163a3–173a24 passim); McRae (1986, p. 136).

15. Translated by McRae (1986, pp. 121–132) on the basis of a text found at Dunhuang; it is found in the Taisho edition (No. 2011) under the title *Zuishangsheng lun (Treatise on the Supreme Vehicle)*, T 48.377a14–379b14.

16. Adapted from McRae (1986, pp. 124, 316 [n. 66]); the Taishō edition (at 48.377c11) lacks the explicit reference to the standard Buddhist list of four modes of deportment (*īryāpatha*); but these are given in the unpaginated edition appended to McRae.

17. In the Pali version the formula ends with seven days, but the commentary (Ps 1.302) adds that this is said with reference to a practitioner of average ability; someone of keen understanding might receive instruction in the morning and be successful in the evening, or receive instruction in the evening, and be successful the next morning. A similar formula is used in the *Bodhirājakumāra-sutta* (M 1.96), which ends with one day and seems closer to the formula found in the Chinese *Smṛtyupasthāna-sūtra*.

18. Adapted from the *Kāyakośāmṛtavajragīti* as quoted and translated by Higgins (2008, p. 278); Higgins translates *dran med* and *dran pa* as "nonreflection" and "reflection," respectively; for a brief discussion, see his note 51.

19. Mahasi's *Practical Insight Meditation* (1971/1979) represents an English translation of instructions originally given and published in Burmese in 1944. The Burmese word translated as "noting" is *hmat'*, which can mean "mark," "note," "keep in mind," "remember." (I am grateful to Erik Braun for this information.)

20. Anālayo (2006) has argued for a direct historical connection between the way of focusing on bodily sensations in mindfulness of breathing in the U Ba Khin tradition and the account of mindfulness of breathing found in the *Zuochan sanmei jing (Dhyānasamādhi-sūtra)*; see T 15.275b25. Nonetheless, the *theoretical* framework of U Ba Khin's method does not appear to be found in the *sūtra*.

REFERENCES

Anālayo. (2003). *Satipaṭṭhāna: The direct path to realization.* Birmingham, UK: Windhorse.

Anālayo. (2006). The ancient roots of the U Ba Khin Vipassanā meditation. *Journal of the Centre for Buddhist Studies, Sri Lanka, 4,* 259–269.

Anālayo. (2011). *A comparative study of the Majjhima-nikāya* (Vols. 1–2). Taipei, Taiwan: Dharma Drum.

Baddeley, A. D., & Hitch, G. (1974). Working memory. *Psychology of Learning and Motivation, 8,* 47–89.

Berzin, A. (1978). *The Mahāmudrā: Eliminating the darkness of ignorance.* Dharamsala, India: Library of Tibetan Works and Archives.

Bishop, S. R., Lau, M., Shapiro, S., Carlson, L., Anderson, N. D., Carmody, J., et al. (2004). Mindfulness: A proposed operational definition. *Clinical Psychology: Science and Practice, 11*(3), 230–241.

Bodhi. (1995). Life sketch of Venerable Nyanaponika. In Bodhi (Ed.), *Nyanaponika: A farewell tribute* (pp. 8–14). Kandy, Sri Lanka: Buddhist Publication Society.

Bodhi. (2011). What does mindfulness really mean?: A canonical perspective. *Contemporary Buddhism, 12*(1), 19–39.

Braun, E. (2008). *Ledi Sayadaw, Abhidhamma, and the development of the Modern Insight Meditation Movement in Burma.* Doctoral dissertation, Harvard University, Cambridge, MA.

Braun, E. (2013). *The birth of insight: Meditation, modern Buddhism, and the Burmese monk Ledi Sayadaw.* Chicago: University of Chicago Press.

Buswell, R. E. (1989). *The formation of Ch'an ideology in China and Korea: The Vajrasamādhi-Sūtra, a Buddhist Apocryphon.* Princeton, NJ: Princeton University Press.

Cone, M. (2001). *A Dictionary of Pāli: Part I a–kh.* Oxford, UK: Pali Text Society.

Cox, C. (1992). Mindfulness and memory: The scope of *smṛti* from early Buddhism to the Savāastivādin Abhidharma. In J. Gyatso (Ed.), *In the mirror of memory: Reflections on mindfulness and remembrance in Indian and Tibetan Buddhism* (pp. 67–108). Albany: State University of New York.

Demiéville, P. (1924). Les versions chinoises du Milindapañha [The Chinese versions of the Milindapañha]. *Bulletin de l'Ecole Française d'Extrême-Orient, 24*(1), 1–258.

Dunne, J. (2011). Toward an understanding of non-dual mindfulness. *Contemporary Buddhism, 12*(1), 71–88.

Gethin, R. (1992). *The Buddhist path to awakening: A study of the Bodhi-Pakkhiyā Dhammā.* Leiden, The Netherlands: E. J. Brill.

Gethin, R. (2008). *Sayings of the Buddha: A selection of suttas from the Pali Nikayas.* Oxford, UK: Oxford University Press.

Gethin, R. (2011a). On some definitions of mindfulness. *Contemporary Buddhism, 12*(1), 263–279.

Gethin, R. (2011b). Tales of miraculous teachings: miracles in early Indian Buddhism. In G. H. Twelftree (Ed.), *The Cambridge companion to miracles* (pp. 216–234). Cambridge, UK: Cambridge University Press.

Gilpin, R. (2008). The use of Theravāda Buddhist practices and perspectives in mindfulness-based cognitive therapy. *Contemporary Buddhism, 9,* 227–251.

Gómez, L. O. (1987). Purifying gold: The metaphor of effort and intuition in Buddhist thought and practice. In P. N. Gregory (Ed.), *Sudden and gradual: Approaches to enlightenment in Chinese thought* (pp. 67–165). Honolulu: University of Hawaii Press.

Griffiths, P. (1981). Concentration or insight: The problematic of Theravāda Buddhist meditation-theory. *Journal of the American Academy of Religion, 49,* 605–624.

Griffiths, P. J. (1992). Memory in classical Indian Yogācarā. In J. Gyatso (Ed.), *In the mirror of memory: Reflections on mindfulness and remembrance in Indian and Tibetan Buddhism* (pp. 109–131). Albany: State University of New York.

Gyatso, J. (Ed.). (1992). *In the mirror of memory: Reflections on mindfulness and remembrance in Indian and Tibetan Buddhism.* Albany: State University of New York.

Hamilton, S. (1996). *Identity and experience: The constitution of the human being according to Early Buddhism.* London: Luzac Oriental.

Higgins, D. (2008). On the development of the non-mentation (*amanasikāra*) doctrine in Indo-Tibetan Buddhism. *Journal of the International Association of Buddhist Studies, 29*(2), 255–303.

Horner, I. B. (1954). *Middle length sayings* (Vol. 1). London: PTS.

Houtman, G. (1985). The Burmese wipathana meditation tradition self-conscious: A history of sleeping texts and silent Buddhas. *Groniek, 92,* 87–105.

Houtman, G. (1997). Beyond the cradle and past the grave: The biography of Burmese meditation master U Ba Khin. In J. Schober (Ed.), *Sacred biography in the Buddhist traditions of South and Southeast Asia* (pp. 310–344). Honolulu: University of Hawaii Press.

Jaini, P. S. (1992). *Smṛti* in the Abhidharma literature and the development of Buddhist acconts of memory of the past. In J. Gyatso (Ed.), *In the mirror of memory: Reflections on mindfulness and remembrance in Indian and Tibetan Buddhism* (pp. 47–59). Albany: State University of New York.

Kabat-Zinn, J. (1990). *Full catastrophe living: Using the wisdom of your body and mind to face stress, pain, and illness.* New York: Bantam Dell.

Kabat-Zinn, J. (1994). *Wherever you go, there you are: Mindfulness meditation for everyday life.* London: Piatkus.

Kornfield, J. (1977). *Living Buddhist masters.* Santa Cruz, CA: University Press.

Kuan, T. (2008). *Mindfulness in early Buddhism: New approaches through psychology and textual analysis of Pali, Chinese, and Sanskrit sources.* London: Routledge.

Lutz, A., Dunne, J. D., & Davidson, R. J. (2007). Meditation and the neuroscience of consciousness: An introduction. In P. D. Zelazo, M. Moscovitch, & E. Thompson (Eds.), *The Cambridge handbook of consciousness* (pp. 499–551). New York: Cambridge University Press.

Lutz, A., Slagter, H. A., Dunne, J. D., & Davidson, R. J. (2008). Attention regulation and monitoring in meditation. *Trends in Cognitive Sciences, 12*(4), 163–169.

Mahasi. (1979). *Practical insight meditation: Basic and progressive stages.* Rangoon, Burma: Department of Religious Affairs. (Original work published 1971)

Mahasi. (1979). *The Satipatthana Vipassanā meditation: A basic Buddhist mindfulness excercise [sic].* Rangoon, Burma: Department of Religious Affairs.

McMahan, D. L. (2008). *The making of Buddhist modernism.* Oxford, UK: Oxford University Press.

McRae, J. R. (1986). *The Northern School and the formation of early Ch'an Buddhism.* Honolulu: University of Hawaii Press.

Monier-Williams, M. (1899). *A Sanskrit-English dictionary.* Oxford, UK: Oxford University Press.

Ñāṇamoli. (1964). *The path of purification (Visuddhimagga) by Bhadantācariya Buddhaghosa.* Colombo, Sri Lanka: Semage.

Ñāṇamoli & Bodhi. (1995). *The middle length discourses of the Buddha: A new translation of the Majjhima Nikāya.* Boston: Wisdom.

Norman, K. R. (1988). Pāli lexicographical studies V. *Journal of the Pali Text Society, 12,* 49–61.

Nyanaponika. (1962). *The heart of Buddhist meditation: A handbook of mental training based on the Buddha's way of mindfulness.* London: Rider & Company.

Nyanaponika. (1992). The omission of memory in the Theravādin list of dhammas: On the nature of *saññā.* In J. Gyatso (Ed.), *In the mirror of memory: Reflections on mindfulness and remembrance in Indian and Tibetan Buddhism* (pp. 61–65). Albany: State University of New York.

Oxford English Dictionary Online. (2011) Retrieved January 6, 2012, from *www.oed.com.*

Pruden, L. M. (1988). *Abhidharmakośabhāyam by Louis de La Vallée Poussin: English translation by Leo M. Pruden* (Vols. 1–4). Berkeley, CA: Asian Humanities Press.

Rāhula, W. (2001). *Abhidharmasamuccaya: The compendium of the higher teaching (philosophy) of Asaṅga* (S. Boin-Webb, Trans.). Fremont, CA: Asian Humanities Press.

Rhys Davids, T. W. (1881). *Buddhist Suttas translated from Pāli.* Oxford, UK: Clarendon Press.

Rhys Davids, T. W., & Rhys Davids, C. A. F. (1910). *Dialogues of the Buddha: Part II.* London: Henry Frowde.

Sastri, N. A. (1978). *Satyasiddhiśāstra of Harivarman: Vol. II. English translation.* Baroda, MI: Oriental Institute.

Segal, Z. V., Williams, J. M. G., & Teasdale, J. D. (2002). *Mindfulness-based cognitive therapy for depression: A new approach to preventing relapse.* New York: Guilford Press.

Sharf, R. H. (2002). *Coming to terms with Chinese Buddhism: A reading of the treasure store treatise.* Honolulu: University of Hawaii Press.

Sharf, R. H. (2014). Mindfulness and mindlessness in early Chan. *Philosophy East and West, 64*(4), 933–964.

Soma. (1967). *The way of mindfulness: Being a translation of the Satipaṭṭhāna sutta of the Majjhima nikāya; its commentary, the Satipaṭṭhāna sutta vaṇṇanā of the Papañcasūdanī of Buddhaghosa Thera, and excerpts from the Līnatthapākasanā ṭīkā, marginal notes, of Dhammapāla Thera on the commentary* (3rd ed.). Kandy, Sri Lanka: Buddhist Publication Society.

Trenckner, V., Andersen, D., Smith, H., Hendriksen, H., Alsdorf, L., & Norman, K. R. (1924–2011). *A critical Pāli dictionary.* Copenhagen: Royal Danish Academy of Sciences and Letters.

van Schaik, S. (2004). *Approaching the great perfection: Simultaneous and gradual approaches to Dzogchen practice in Jigme Lingpa's Longchen Nyingtig.* Boston: Wisdom.

Wallace, B. A., & Bodhi (2006). The nature of mindfulness and its role in Buddhist meditation: A correspondence between B. Alan Wallace and the Venerable Bhikkhu Bodhi. Retrieved from the International Shamatha Project website at *http://shamatha.org/sites/default/files/bhikkhu_bodhi_correspondence.pdf.*

Wayman, A. (1976). Regarding the translation of the Buddhist terms saññā/samjñā viññāṇa/vijñāna. In O. H. D. A. Wijesekera (Ed.), *Malalasekera commemoration volume* (pp. 325–335). Colombo, Sri Lanka: Malalasekera Commemoration Volume Editorial Committee.

Wijeratne, R. P., & Gethin, R. (2002). *Summary of the topics of Abhidhamma (Abhidhammatthasaṅgaha) by Anuruddha and exposition of the topics of Abhidhamma (Abhidhammatthavibhāvinī) by Sumangala.* Oxford, UK: Pali Text Society.

Williams, J. M. G., & Kabat-Zinn, J. (2011a). Mindfulness: Diverse perspectives on its meaning, origins, and multiple applications at the intersection of science and dharma. *Contemporary Buddhism, 12*(1), 1–18.

Williams, J. M. G., & Kabat-Zinn, J. (Eds.). (2011b). Special issue: Mindfulness: Diverse perspectives on its meaning, origins, and multiple applications at the intersection of science and dharma. *Contemporary Buddhism, 12.*

APPENDIX 2.1.
Abbreviations of Pali, Sanskrit, and Chinese Buddhist Texts

A = R. Morris & E. Hardy (Eds.). (1885–1900). *Anguttara Nikāya* (Vols. 1–5). London: PTS.

Abhidh-av = A. P. Buddhadatta (Ed.). (1915). *Abhidhammāvatāra*. London: PTS.

Abhidh-dī = P. S. Jaini (Ed.). (1959). *Abhidharmadīpa*. Patna, India: Kashi Prasad Jayaswal Research Institute.

Abhidh-k-bh = P. Pradhan (Ed.). (1967). *Abhidharmakośa-bhāṣya*. Patna, India: Kashi Prasad Jayaswal Research Institute.

Abhidh-k-vy = Wogihara, U. (Ed.). (1936). *Sphuṭārthā Abhidharmakośavyākhyā*. Tokyo: Publishing Association of Abhidharmakosavyākhyā.

Abhidh-sam = V. V. Gokhale (1947). Fragments from the Abhidharmasamuccaya of Asaṃga. *Journal of the Bombay Branch of the Royal Asiatic Society, New Series, 23*, 13–38.

As = E. Müller (Ed.). (1897). *Atthasālinī*. London: PTS.

D = T. W. Rhys Davids & J. E. Carpenter (Eds.). (1890–1911). *Dīgha Nikāya* (Vols. 1–3). London: PTS.

Dhs = E. Müller (Ed.). (1885). *Dhammsaṅgaṇi*. London: PTS.

Dhs-mṭ = *Dhammsaṅgaṇi-mūlaṭīkā*. (1960). Rangoon: Buddhasāsana-samiti.

Kv-a = N. A. Jayawickrama (Ed.). (1979). *Kathāvatthuppakaraṇa-aṭṭhakathā*. London: PTS.

M = V. Trenckner & R. Chalmers (Eds.). (1887–1902). *Majjhima Nikāya* (Vols. 1–3). London: PTS.

Mil = V. Trenckner (Ed.). (1880). *Milindapañha*. London: PTS.

Mp = M. Walleser & H. Kopp (Eds.). (1936–1957). *Manorathapūraṇī* (Vols. 1–5). London: PTS.

MPS = E. Waldschmidt. *Das Mahāparinirvāṇasūtra*. (1951). Berlin: Deutschen Akademie der Wissenschaften.

Nett = E. Hardy (Ed.). (1902). *Nettippakaraṇa*. London: PTS.

NiddI = L. de La Vallée Poussin & E. J. Thomas (Eds.). (1916–1917/1978). *Mahāniddesa*. London: PTS.

NiddII = W. Stede (Ed.). (1918). *Cullaniddesa*. London: PTS.

Paṭis = A. C. Taylor (Ed.). (1905–1907/1979). *Paṭisambhidāmagga*. London: PTS.

Paṭis-a = C. V. Joshi (Ed.). (1933–1947). *Saddhammappakāsinī: Commentary on the Paṭisambhidāmagga* (Vols. 1–3). London: PTS.

Peṭ = A. Barua (Ed.). (1949). *Peṭakopadesa*. London: PTS.

Ps = J. H. Woods, D. Kosambi, & I. B. Horner (Eds.). (1933–1938). *Papañcapasūdanī* (Vols. 1–5). London: PTS.

Pugg = R. Morris (Ed.). (1883). *Puggala-paññatti*. London: PTS

S = L. Feer (Ed.). (1884–1898). *Saṃyutta Nikāya* (Vols. 1–5). London: PTS.

SBV = R. Gnoli & T. Venkatacharya (Eds.). (1977–1978). *Saṅghabhedavastu*. Roma: Istituto Italiano per il Medio ed Estremo Oriente.

Sn = D. Andersen & H. Smith (Eds.). (1913). *Sutta-Nipāta*. London: PTS.

Sp = J. Takakusu & M. Nagai (Eds.). (1924–1947). *Samantapāsādikā* (Vols. 1–7). London: PTS.

Spk = F. L. Woodward (Ed.). (1929–1937). *Sāratthappakāsinī* (Vols. 1–3). London: PTS.

Srāv-bh = K. Shukla (Ed.). (1973). *Śrāvakabhūmi*. Patna, India: K. P. Jayaswal Research Institute.

Sv = T. W. Rhys Davids, J. E. Carpenter, & W. Stede (Eds.). (1886–1932). *The Sumaṅgala-vilāsinī: Buddhaghosa's commentary on the Dīgha nikāya* (Vols. 1–3). London: PTS.

T = J. Takakusu & K. Watanabe (Eds.). (1924–1932). *Taishō Shinshū Daizōkyō* (Vols. 1–85). Tokyo: Taishō issaikyō kanko kwai.

Trimś-bh = H. Buescher (Ed.). (2007). *Triṃśikāvijñaptibhāṣya*. Vienna: Verlag der Österreichischen Akademie der Wissenachaften.

Vibh = C. A. F. Rhys Davids (Ed.). (1904). *Vibhaṅgā*. London: PTS.

Vibh-a = A. P. Buddhadatta (Ed.). (1923). *Sammohavinodanī Vibhaṅga-aṭṭhakathā*. London: PTS.

Vism = H.C. Warren & D. Kosambi (Eds.). (1950). *Visuddhimagga*. Cambridge, MA: Harvard University Press.

CHAPTER 3

Developing Attention and Decreasing Affective Bias

Toward a Cross-Cultural Cognitive Science of Mindfulness

Jake H. Davis and Evan Thompson

Wisdom and consciousness, friend—these states are conjoined, not disjoined. . . .
For what one wisely understands, one is conscious of, and what one is conscious
of, that one wisely understands.

—MAJJHIMA NIKĀYA 43[1]

The study of consciousness was banished from respectable science with the rise of behaviorism in the early 20th century. Beginning in the 1980s, however, researchers in cognitive science began to return to the topic (e.g., Baars, 1988; Chalmers, 1996; Crick & Koch, 1990; Dennett, 1991), In recent decades, there has been an explosion of research on the neurophysiological processes underlying conscious experience (Tononi & Koch, 2008), as well as the ways in which attention (Mole, Smithies, & Wu, 2011) and emotion (Barrett, Mesquita, Ochsner, & Gross, 2007) shape conscious experience. We think that this research climate is beneficial for understanding the nature and benefits of mindfulness meditation because advances in the cognitive science of consciousness provide an important but as yet underused resource for deepening our understanding of how contemplative attention-training practices function in traditional Buddhist and modern clinical contexts.

Mindfulness meditation is traditionally said to be part of a process of "awakening" (*bodhi*). In keeping with this idea, many teachers characterize mindfulness as involving one's becoming more conscious of subtle bodily stimuli and emotional reactions. For example, Bhante Gunaratana (2002, p. 108) stresses the importance of developing mindfulness such that mental habits of fear and grasping run their course "in the arena of conscious attention." As he puts it, "we can make the unconscious conscious, slowly, one piece at a time" (p. 9). Similarly, Jon Kabat-Zinn (2005) notes that simple experiences of seeing or tasting or walking become vivid and transformative when one becomes mindful of them: "Sentience is closer than close. . . . Cultivated and strengthened, sentience lights up our lives and it lights up the world, and grants us degrees of freedom we could scarcely imagine even though our imagination itself stems from it" (pp. 319–320). The reason that resting on the level of bare sentience is said to be transformative is that often we are caught up in distortive interpretation and analysis: "Thinking and memory come in a bit later, but very quickly, on the heels of an initial moment of pure sense contact. Thinking and memory can easily color our original experience in ways that distort or detract from the bare experience itself" (p. 199).

Meditation teachers, and practitioners of meditation more generally, draw from their first-person experience in explaining how the forms of attention training they practice may result in health and other benefits. Yet our earlier comments on the relationship between attention training and consciousness are more poetic than precise. Specifically, they do not aim at the kind of theoretical sophistication and controlled, third-person perspective needed for a scientific understanding of how attention training may result in psychological and behavioral changes. Similarly, the statement quoted at the outset of this chapter that "consciousness and wisdom are conjoined" might seem—like many descriptions of the relationship between attention, consciousness, wisdom, and ethical action found in traditional texts—to aim more at practical inspiration than at theoretical precision. Although other textual descriptions from traditional Buddhist psychological theory do offer systematic and fine-grained accounts of the interrelations among attention, consciousness, and emotional reactivity (see Anālayo, 2003), these accounts have only recently begun to be tapped by the scientific community (e.g., Grabovac, Lau, & Willett, 2011). One reason for this state of affairs may be that it is unclear how such traditional accounts could be empirically operationalized using constructs from cognitive science. This uncertainty about how to proceed scientifically may be especially true in the case of traditional claims about the development of wisdom, such as the suggestion that developing mindfulness results in "seeing and knowing things as they are." Hence, our aim in this chapter is to show how cognitive science may be able to illuminate mindfulness by detailing some of the ways that attention, affect, and consciousness interrelate. In this way, we hope to contribute to a more rigorous scientific and philosophical understanding of precisely how consciousness and wisdom relate to each other in the cultivation of mindfulness.

To study the effects of therapeutic interventions, such as mindfulness training, on the brain and the rest of the body, scientists need to employ conceptual constructs of the phenomena under investigation that guide where and how they will look. Thus, in studying the health benefits and physiological mechanisms of mindfulness meditation, scientists have had to ask what precisely mindfulness is (Davidson, 2010). In describing "what mindfulness is, what it isn't, and its role in healthcare and medicine" Kabat-Zinn (1996) suggests that two Buddhist canonical texts in which the practice "is elaborated most thoroughly" (pp. 161–162) are the *Anapanasati-sutta* and the *Mahāsatipaṭṭhāna-sutta*. Each text consists of a discourse attributed to the Buddha and recorded among the canonical texts of the Theravāda Buddhist tradition. Scholars call the body of dialogues and discourses to which these texts belong to the Pāli *Nikāyas*. In order to focus our discussion in this chapter on one example of an approach integrating textual and scientific perspectives, among the many different conceptions of mindfulness, we draw inspiration mainly from the accounts found in the Pāli Nikāyas, without thereby meaning to privilege the particular notion of mindfulness found there over different notions of mindfulness found in other Buddhist traditions, or in later texts of the Theravāda Buddhist tradition. Likewise, for the sake of simplicity, we make reference especially to Pāli textual sources and terminology.

It has been noted sometimes in the scientific literature that "mindfulness" is a translation of the Pāli term *sati*. The broad usage of the term *sati* in the Pāli Nikāyas is perhaps best captured by the colloquial English notion of "minding." The Pāli texts employ *sati* in reference to everything from "minding" one's livestock (MN.I.117) to "minding" one's meditation object in practices such as loving-kindness (Sn 26), in addition to using *sati* specifically in the context of mindfulness meditation, or, more literally, in the establishment of *sati* (*sati-upaṭṭhāna*).[2] It is important to note at the outset, however, that even focusing just on accounts of the specific form of meditation termed *satipaṭṭhāna*, the prescriptions for practice and descriptions of its effects found in the Pāli Nikāyas are subject to multiple possible readings. The account of relations between consciousness and wisdom that we develop here is one of a number of possible readings, and the value we see in this account lies not in its claim to historical authenticity, but instead in its suggestion of new and fruitful avenues for scientific research by drawing on suggestions consistent with both the broad thrust of the Buddha's teachings in the Pāli Nikāyas and with recent empirical results.

Toward a Cross-Cultural Cognitive Science of Mindfulness

Scientific investigations of practices derived from Buddhist traditions have focused to date primarily on how various forms of attention training alter cognitive and affective processes (see Lutz, Slagter, Dunne, & Davidson, 2008, for a review). Yet Buddhist teachings include many other methods for training practitioners' habits of mind. The strong emphasis on moral conduct, for example, can be seen as a means for protecting oneself from unwholesome states, such as greed, hatred, and delusion. Modern clinical presentations, out of practical necessity, have often separated practices of ethical restraint from practices of meditation. Traditionally, however, behavioral restraint is taken to be both foundational for and an essential outcome of meditative development.

The term *meditation* generally refers to a category of practices involving attention-training techniques aimed directly at cultivating particular positive mental states. Many Buddhist techniques of reflection, such as reflection on the inevitability of death (*maraṇasati*), act as a complement to ethical training. Other practices range from cultivating states such as loving-kindness, or literally friendliness (*mettā*), to practices aimed simply at cultivating a settled and unified state of mind (*samādhi*) through concentration on a sensory or mental object. In these forms of meditation, practitioners counteract mind-wandering by repeatedly bringing the mind back to the object of meditation.

The use of such methods of attention training for developing strong concentration appears to have been widespread at the time of the Buddha. Buddhist texts relate that the Buddha, before his enlightenment, studied techniques for concentrating the mind under teachers such as Āḷāra Kālāma and Uddaka Rāmaputta (M.36). These early Buddhist texts also emphasize that the method of mind training that the Buddha went on to discover for himself was novel, with results that differed importantly from those that were being taught by his contemporaries.

Over the course of Buddhist history, there have been substantive debates within and between various Buddhist traditions about what precisely the unique and revolutionary aspect of the Buddha's teaching was or is. Within the Theravāda Buddhist tradition of South and Southeast Asia, it is commonly held that the establishment of mindfulness (*satipaṭṭhāna*) is essential for realizing the liberating insights described in the canonical texts of this tradition. Nevertheless, it should not be assumed that there is a single, unequivocal concept of mindfulness to be found in this or any Buddhist tradition. For example, in the recent literature, there has been an emerging debate over what role, if any, cognitive factors such as memory, evaluation, and intellectual analysis play in mindfulness meditation (see the collection of articles in the June 2011 issue of *Contemporary Buddhism*). In some cases, this debate may reflect differences in emphasis and understanding between the early Buddhist texts and later commentarial developments within the Theravāda (Anālayo, 2013). In other cases, these debates may reflect differences in emphasis and understanding between modern presentations of mindfulness in clinical contexts and the various Buddhist traditions from which these modern presentations are partly derived.

Perhaps the most influential clinical presentation of mindfulness is the 8-week mindfulness-based stress reduction (MBSR) program pioneered by Jon Kabat-Zinn at the University of Massachusetts Medical School in the 1980s. This program has been replicated and adapted widely, and is now offered in the secular context of hospitals and clinics around the world. It has also been the subject of a growing body of empirical research. Studies comparing participants in the MBSR program to control groups have shown that mindfulness practice correlates with significant reductions in suffering associated with various illnesses, and with structural and functional changes in the brain (for a relatively recent review, see, e.g., Hölzel et al., 2011).

In addition to being influenced by the Theravāda Buddhist sources noted earlier, Kabat-Zinn's presentation was also influenced by Korean Zen Buddhist teachings, as well as by other Asian spiritual traditions, such as Yoga (Kabat-Zinn, 2011). As Kabat-Zinn noted in a recent article, he used the term *mindfulness* "as a placeholder for the entire dharma," that is, as an umbrella term meant to point in a secular, accessible way toward the many varied techniques employed in a diverse array of Buddhist traditions (2011, p. 290). Perhaps in part for this reason, attempts in the scientific literature to formulate what mindfulness is often have proceeded without serious engagement from theoretical formulations of mindfulness practice contained in Buddhist textual traditions. In the absence of references to such traditional canonical sources, many researchers have focused on one particular phrase Kabat-Zinn used in his introductory guide for practitioners to describe mindfulness, namely, the phrase "paying attention in a particular way: on purpose, in the present moment, and nonjudgmentally" (1994, p. 4). Thus, Bishop and colleagues (2004), in proposing an operational definition of mindfulness for clinical psychology, summarize the literature by noting that "mindfulness has been described as a kind of nonelaborative, nonjudgmental, present-centered awareness in which each thought, feeling, or sensation that arises in the attentional field is acknowledged and accepted as it is" (p. 232).

In this modern conception of mindfulness as present-centered, mindfulness does not itself involve memory or evaluation. In contrast to this modern notion, Dreyfus (2011) argues that *sati* comprises "retentive focus," the ability of the mind to hold its object and not float away from it. This conception seems close to the cognitive science construct of working memory. Like Dreyfus, we believe that the technical vocabularies used in cognitive science can provide a greater degree of precision for characterizing mindfulness than can the operational definition of mindfulness in clinical psychology (notwithstanding the usefulness that definition may have for therapeutic purposes). Indeed, the vocabulary of cognitive science can help to capture for modern practitioners of mindfulness the care and precision with which the Buddhist terms are used in their native philosophical context. For this reason, careful understanding of the traditional Buddhist textual sources in the context of recent scientific research can benefit both scientific understanding of psychological changes involved in mindfulness practice and the Buddhist project of understanding what these texts can mean for us today. Making this point in an earlier article, we suggested that integrating third-person empirical observation of the brain and behavior with ancient and modern accounts based on first-person meditative exploration may prove mutually beneficial to both the scientific project of understanding the mind and the Buddhist project of transforming it (Davis & Thompson, 2013). In particular, we proposed that building bridges between traditional Buddhist models of the mind and contemporary cognitive science may lead toward a more precise understanding of the respective roles of attention, consciousness, and memory in mindfulness meditation. In this chapter, we take that project one step forward, drawing on scientific and philosophical work on consciousness and attention in order to move toward a rigorous, precise, and empirically testable account of the relationship between consciousness and wisdom as suggested by traditional accounts of mindfulness.

Phenomenal Consciousness and Cognitive Awareness

An important step toward a cross-cultural cognitive science of mindfulness is to clarify some of the different senses of the term *consciousness* in contemporary cognitive science so that they can be related to various Buddhist concepts (for further discussion see Davis & Thompson, 2013; Thompson, 2014). One general or comprehensive way to indicate what is meant by *consciousness* is to say that consciousness "consists of inner, qualitative, subjective states and processes of sentience and awareness" (Searle, 2000, p. 559). When we try to refine our understanding of terms such as *inner, qualitative, subjective, sentience,* and *awareness,* however, we need to make at least two important conceptual distinctions.

First, we can distinguish between what philosophers of mind call creature consciousness and state consciousness (Bayne, 2007). Whereas *creature consciousness* pertains to the whole subject of experience, the person or animal, *state consciousness* pertains to a particular mental state. A creature is conscious if, and only if, there is something it is like to be that creature (for that creature) (Nagel, 1974). Notice that creature consciousness, so defined, does not mean being awake because consciousness—that is, inner, qualitative, subjective states and processes of sentience and awareness—occurs during other states besides wakefulness, such as dreaming. Moreover, patients in a vegetative state apparently lack or have highly diminished qualitative awareness of themselves and their environment while nonetheless being awake (they undergo a sleep–wake cycle). Thus, when we say that someone is awake but unresponsive or awake and alert, or asleep and dreaming, it is consciousness in the sense of creature consciousness with which we are concerned. In contrast, when we talk about a person being conscious of a given stimulus versus not being conscious of the stimulus, it is state consciousness with which we are concerned. Thus, in the case of state consciousness, we are concerned with the content and qualitative character of the particular mental states of the subject.

If we now ask what exactly it means to say that the person is conscious of the stimulus or that the content of a given mental state is conscious, we find ourselves needing to make another conceptual distinction (see Block, 1995, 2007). On the one hand, we can say that the person is conscious of the stimulus if the person subjectively experiences the stimulus as being a certain way, that is, as having a certain qualitative appearance. In this sense of *conscious,* a given mental state or bodily state is conscious if, and only if, there is something it is like for the subject to be in that state. Philosophers call this concept of consciousness "phenomenal consciousness" (*phenomenal* here means how things seem or appear in experience). On the other hand, we can also say that the person is conscious of the stimulus if the person can report or describe it, or reason about it, or use it to guide how he or she acts or behaves. Philosophers call this concept "access consciousness" (*access* here means available for use in thought and action). In summary, *consciousness* can mean awareness in the sense of subjective experience (*phenomenal consciousness*) or awareness in the sense of cognitive access (*access consciousness* or *cognitive awareness*).

One reason philosophers draw this distinction is to make the point that to explain consciousness in the sense of cognitive awareness is not necessarily to explain consciousness in the sense of subjective experience. As David Chalmers (1995, p. 206) writes:

Even when we have explained the performance of all the cognitive and behavioral functions in the vicinity of experience—perceptual discrimination, categorization, internal access, verbal report—there may still remain a further unanswered question: *Why is the performance of these functions accompanied by experience?* A simple explanation of the functions leaves this question open.

Another reason for making the distinction between phenomenal consciousness and cognitive awareness is to allow for the possibility that one could subliminally or implicitly experience something without being able to report or describe the experience, at least not fully or explicitly. In other words, one could have an experience with a subjectively felt character—for example, a bodily feeling elicited by a memory or a perceived situation—without being able to report and describe that experience or feeling, at least not fully or easily. Moreover, some cognitive scientists and philosophers argue that in certain experimental situations one can experience an image or a stimulus array but without being able to form the kind of memory needed for a verbal report of exactly what it was (see Block, 2008). Although the interpretation of such results is controversial (Block, 2011; Cohen & Dennett, 2011; Kouider, de Gardelle, Sackur, & Depoux, 2010), it seems reasonable to suppose that it is possible for one's subjective experience (phenomenal consciousness) at a given time and in certain conditions to outstrip the cognitive capacities or resources one has for accessing the experience at that time and in those conditions.

In our earlier article (Davis & Thompson, 2013), we drew a tentative parallel between this cognitive science distinction between phenomenal consciousness and cognitive access and another distinction found in the Buddhist texts in which mindfulness practice is described. One central model of the mind found in the Pāli Nikāyas distinguishes between *viññaṇa*, which is often glossed as "consciousness," and *saññā*, which is defined as involving identification and reportability of what one has experienced. These Pali texts thus define *saññā* in terms remarkably similar to the cognitive science notion of cognitive awareness. The *Nibbedhika Sutta* (AN.III.413), for example, defines *saññā* as that which results in spoken communication (*vohara*): "As one identifies (*sañjānāti*) it, so one says 'I saw thus.'" In the *Khajjaniya Sutta* (SN. III.87), *saññā* is defined as cognizing (*sañjānāti*) that there is blue, that there is red, yellow, or white. Although *saññā* is often glossed as "perception," this interpretation is inadequate. As Pali scholar Peter Harvey (1995, p. 141) explains, "the word '*saññā*' and its verbal form '*sañ-jānāti*' clearly refer to some kind of knowledge or knowing which is done in an associative, connective, linking (*sa-*) way."

Modern meditation teachers often employ this traditional distinction between *viññaṇa* and *saññā* implicitly in their presentations of mindfulness. We noted above Kabat-Zinn's suggestion that "thinking and memory come in a bit later, but very quickly, on the heels of an initial moment of pure sense contact" (2005, p. 199). The practitioner–scholar Bhante Gunaratana (2002) offers a similar but more detailed interpretation of Buddhist theory on this point:

> Mindfulness registers experiences, but it does not compare them. It does not label them or categorize them. It just observes everything as if it was occurring for the first time. It is not analysis which is based on reflection and memory. It is, rather, the direct and immediate experiencing of whatever is happening, without the medium of thought. It comes before thought in the perceptual process. (p. 168)

Although it is difficult to draw out a precise definition of consciousness from the Pāli Nikāyas, given these modern presentations, it is tempting to relate *viññaṇa* to the concept of phenomenal consciousness. According to this interpretation, *viññaṇa*, defined as a moment of visual, auditory, tactile, olfactory, gustatory, or mental experience, would be analogous to phenomenal consciousness, whereas *saññā*, defined as a recognitional ability, would be analogous to cognitive awareness.

Whether phenomenal consciousness and cognitive awareness are separable or whether one depends constitutively on the other is an issue of considerable debate in current cognitive science (see Block, 2011; Cohen & Dennett, 2011). We cannot enter these debates here (for further discussion, see Davis & Thompson, 2013). It is important to note, however, that whereas some philosophers have argued that phenomenal consciousness cannot be characterized in functional terms (Block, 2007, 2008; Chalmers, 1996), our account of the difference between *viññaṇa* and *saññā* does not depend on this claim. On the contrary, given the relation we are suggesting between consciousness and wisdom, our account requires that consciousness have predictable downstream effects on psychological functioning. At a minimum, the way we propose to interpret the textual distinction between *viññaṇa* and *saññā* requires that the function and effects of phenomenal consciousness, or *viññaṇa*, be importantly different from the function of cognitive awareness, or *saññā*, and the effects it has on recall, report, and deliberation.

In spelling out this requirement, we think it is helpful to draw on neuroscientists Parvizi and Damasio's (2001) proposal that there is a basal or core level of consciousness, dependent on the thalamus and brainstem, that occurs independently of selective attentional processes in higher cortical areas. This core or ground-floor level of consciousness depends on a basic kind of alerting function distinct from the higher-level mechanisms of selective attention that come into play in determining what one is conscious of. In our reading of this view, the fact that there is felt experience—the fact that there is something it is like for the subject—depends on the basic alerting function. In contrast, the particular contents of consciousness—what it is like for the subject—depends also on how this consciousness is directed to particular objects and properties through selective attention. Put another way, the particular contents of phenomenal state consciousness can be seen as modifications or modulations of a basal level of creature consciousness dependent on the alerting function (see also Searle, 2000).

Given this viewpoint, we propose that *viññaṇa* corresponds more closely to the basal level of consciousness, whereas *saññā* corresponds more closely to the cognitive awareness of particular phenomenal contents via working memory and selective attention (Davis & Thompson, 2013). This interpretation suggests ways that the two kinds of mental phenomena could be functionally interrelated. On the one hand, one role of phenomenal consciousness may be to make experiential content accessible for encoding in working memory, and hence for the purposes of identification, recall, deliberation, and report (Prinz, 2005, 2012; see also Block 2011, p. 567). On the other hand, one central commentarial text in the Theravāda Buddhist tradition, the *Atthasālinī*, suggests that mindfulness (*sati*) has as its immediate cause (*padaṭṭhāna*) firm identification (*thirasaññā*). *Saññā* here seems to play the role of directing attention toward an object and maintaining it there.[3] Our account suggests one way to understand this proposed function of *saññā*, namely, that by holding in working memory a conceptual representation—say, of the abdomen or of the breath—attentional processes thereby allow more interoceptive and somatosensory stimuli from the body, as it moves with the breath, to be consciously experienced. To explore this idea more fully we need to consider the relation between attention and consciousness, seen especially in the light of mindfulness practice.

Attention and Consciousness

Cognitive neuroscientists distinguish between two types of attention that not only rely on distinct neural systems but also share a common neural network (Corbetta & Shulman, 2002). If we ask you to switch your attention from the words on this page to the sensations in your right hand, and you comply, you are employing so-called top-down, endogenous orienting. Scientists distinguish this voluntary form of attention from so-called bottom-up, stimulus-driven attention, which is activated when a strong or salient stimulus, such as a loud siren or a flash of light, grabs your attention. Top-down attention depends on generating and maintaining a "control set" that specifies in advance what you are to select; thus, when you switched your attention to the sensations in your right hand, you did so by forming an attentional control set on the basis of our instructions. The maintenance of an attentional control set depends crucially on *working memory*, the ability to retain task-relevant information on a short-term basis.

Working memory has been shown to play an important role in visual selective attention (de Fockert, Rees, Frith, & Lavie, 2001) and seems to play a similar role in directing bodily awareness. In a paradigm developed by Ruth Schubert and colleagues, subjects are instructed to attend either to the left or right hand, while tactile stimulation is applied to left and right index fingers with the mechanical pins of a Braille stimulator (Schubert, Blankenburg, Lemm, Villringer, & Curio, 2006; Schubert, Haufe, Blankenburg, Villringer, & Curio, 2009; Schubert, Ritter, Wüstenberg, Preuschhof, Curio, Sommer, et al., 2008). In a series of studies integrating behavioral tasks with multiple neuroimaging methods, Schubert and colleagues found evidence that selective, top-down spatial attention, for instance, to the left hand, functions to increase subjects' ability to detect and report on weak stimuli by directly amplifying early sensory responses to stimuli in this area of the body and inhibiting responses to other areas. More recent studies have shown what are called "mind-only" effects of bodily attention. Jones and colleagues (2010) reported evidence that directing subjects with a visual word cue to attend either to the hand or to the foot exerts effects on the primary somatosensory cortex (S1) even in the absence of tactile stimulation to these areas. Moreover, the degree of attentional modulation of S1 was predictive of detection of tactile stimuli, when they were applied. In further studies, Kerr and colleagues (2011) found that these effects of bodily attention were enhanced in groups undergoing MBSR training compared to a control group. Even in the absence of any tactile stimulus, meditators showed faster response to visually presented directions either to attend to the hand or foot and a greater differentiation between neural responses to these attentional cues. This finding is consistent with results showing that, following a course in the MBSR program, participants show increased performance on tasks measuring such top-down orienting (Jha, Krompinger, & Baine, 2007), as well as enhanced activity in brain areas specific to interoceptive attention (Farb, Segal, & Anderson, 2013a, 2013b).

Desimone and Duncan's (1995) well-known "biased-competition" model of attention makes sense of such results by suggesting that representations in early sensory areas compete with one another for access to downstream resources, such as those involved in the ability to have conscious access to the sensory response and to report on it, while top-down modulation by attentional control sets serves to bias these competitions in favor of certain sensory responses. In a more recent proposal, Rolls (2008, p. 442) drew on the biased-competition model to suggest that attention is an emergent process, in which feedback and feedforward effects between working memory areas and sensory processing areas settle into an optimal configuration for energy minimization. In this light we may hypothesize that when meditators apply instructions to attend to the sensations of the breath in mindfulness practice, working memory plays a role in specifying how attention is to be directed. Indeed, many forms of mindfulness meditation begin in this way, by employing working memory in directing selective attention – for instance, to the sensations of breathing.

In the most central and detailed account in the Pāli Nikāyas of how mindfulness is to be established (D.22, M.10), meditators are instructed to pay attention to every aspect of daily life. In going, the ardent meditator knows clearly, "I am going"; in breathing in or out long or short, he or she knows "I am breathing in short," and so on. Likewise, one knows clearly when there is a pleasant feeling or a painful one; when there is anger in the mind, one knows clearly "there is anger in the mind," and reciprocally when the mind is without anger. Likewise, one knows when concentration or equanimity is not present, and one knows when these are strong. One influential form of mindfulness practice descended from the Mahasi Sayadaw of Burma, and popularized by American teachers such as Joseph Goldstein and Sharon Salzberg, employs a closely related practice of mental noting. At introductory stages of practice, meditators are instructed to use mental labels to note everything from the movement of the breath to perceptual processes such as seeing and hearing, and even mental states such as boredom, interest, restlessness, or joy. Such minimal conceptual labels might seem insufficient for developing the penetrative understanding, *paññā*, that mindfulness is said to bring. In light of the cognitive science of attention reviewed earlier, however, we can understand meditators' use of labels, such as "I am going," not as a phenomenological analysis of experience, or as a metaphysical analysis of the nature of reality, but rather as holding in working memory a mental representation that functions to direct top-down attention in ways that can have transformative effects.

A number of recent studies have shown increased awareness associated with mindfulness practice. Most prominently, following a 3-month mindfulness meditation retreat, participants showed a decrease in what is referred to as the "attentional blink." In this experimental paradigm, subjects have to identify two visual targets presented within 200 to 500 milliseconds of each other in a rapid sequence of other distracting visual stimuli. Subjects often notice the first target but fail to notice the second one, as if their attention had blinked. The standard explanation is that detecting the first target uses up the available attentional resources, so the second target is missed and not reported. A recent study indicated that the ability to detect the second target was greatly improved after a 3-month intensive Theravāda mindfulness meditation retreat, and that this improvement correlated with electrocortical measures showing more efficient neural responses to the first target (Slagter et al., 2007). Importantly, in this study, the participants were instructed not to meditate during the task, so the improved performance indicates that mindfulness meditation had lasting effects on attention outside the context of meditation practice. The authors of this study suggest that mindfulness meditation may lead to less elaborative cognitive processing of the first visual target—less "mental stickiness" to it—and that this reduction facilitates the ability to identify and report the second rapidly occurring target.

The philosopher Jesse Prinz (2005, 2011, 2012), marshaling recent empirical research, has proposed that attention, in particular the occipitoparietal activity associated with endogenous orienting to a particular stimulus, is required for phenomenal consciousness of that stimulus. Yet evidence from recent investigations of meditation, in conjunction with other empirical and theoretical considerations, may require a refinement of such views. For example, in the attentional blink study, long-term mindfulness meditators seem better able to detect the second target precisely because they do not fixate on the first one. Moreover, in recent pilot testing in a group of Zen meditators, subjects did better on the attentional blink task at times when they reported having stopped caring about the task (C. Kerr, personal communication, August, 11, 2014). This finding is consistent with the "biased competition" model of attention noted earlier, in which the function of endogenous orienting is precisely to inhibit stimulus representations outside the focus of attention, in addition to amplifying those representations in the selected set. Our suggestion is that by reducing top-down orienting, and instead cultivating a general and receptive awareness, individuals can become conscious of more subtle and fleeting stimuli than they would be able to otherwise. In other words, mindfulness practice may involve enhancing the processes involved in sustaining the basal alert consciousness instead of acting simply on selective attention (as more concentrative type meditation practices are likely to do).

We can relate this idea to another influential cognitive psychology model of attention—the attention network theory of Posner and colleagues (Fan, McCandliss, Sommer, Raz, & Posner, 2002; Fan, McCandliss, Fossella, Flombaum, & Posner, 2005; Petersen & Posner, 2012; Posner & Petersen, 1990).[3] This model delineates three intereacting attentional networks—alerting, orienting, and executive control. Using the terms of Corbetta and Shulman's (2002) model of top-down versus bottom-up attention (mentioned earlier), we can understand the executive control network as top-down influence on selective attention, the orienting function as the hub of top-down and bottom-up convergence, and the alerting network as a potential bottom-up influence. The alerting function can be further subdivided. On the one hand is *phasic alertness*, a task-specific sensitivity to a particular class of stimuli, such as when a radar operator watches vigilantly for indications of incoming aircraft. There is emerging evidence that cultivating this phasic type of alertness can also raise what is called *intrinsic* or *tonic alertness*, the general level of arousal and sensitivity to stimuli across a range of sense modalities that is characteristic of being minimally conscious (Robertson, Mattingley, Rorden, & Driver, 1998). This finding suggests that developing focused attention, for instance, on the breath or mental states, may help to cultivate a more general alertness to a range of stimuli across perceptual modalities, thereby increasing the scope of the basal phenomenal consciousness.

Two Factors in Mindfulness Meditation

Considering the different types of attention that cognitive science distinguishes can help us to better understand Buddhist textual accounts of the nature of mindfulness practice and how to go about practicing mindfulness ourselves. *Satipaṭṭhāna* has an intimate relation with attention in the early Buddhist dialogues, yet the notion of attention (Pāli: *manasikāra*) found in these texts is not clearly specified. One suggestion that is consistent with later Buddhist Abhidharma theory is to understand *manasikāra* as a kind of endogenous orienting to a particular stimulus, such that one is conscious of only one object at a time. Yet, to the degree that Abhidharma theory also posits that *manasikāra* is necessary for each moment of conscious experience, understanding *manasikāra* as a form of endogenous orienting becomes incompatible with the results of mindfulness practice. First, to the degree that mindfulness involves an open and receptive awareness of unanticipated and rapidly changing stimuli at all the senses, endogenous orienting processes as understood in cognitive science seem too slow and too narrowly focused to perform this function. Second, as noted earlier, endogenous orienting may actually get in the way of being conscious of stimuli that are outside the narrow area of selected focus. Hence, we have proposed that from the perspective of a cross-cultural cognitive science of mindfulness, the relation between *manasikāra* and *satipaṭṭhāna* be taken to indicate that by cultivating a heightened alertness, one consciously experiences more of the internal and external stimuli reaching one's sense organs (Davis & Thompson, 2013). This proposal is consistent with results finding increased alertness in mindfulness interventions (Britton, Lindahl, Cahn, Davis, & Goldman, 2014; Jha et al., 2007). It is also consistent with Parvizi and Damasio's view (2001), noted earlier, that there is a basic, core level of consciousness, dependent on the thalamus and brainstem, that occurs independently of selective attentional processes in higher cortical areas.

Moreover, the development of alertness may counteract biases of attention by broadening the awareness of incoming stimuli to include aspects that attention would otherwise have been biased away from and, in particular, by making our habitual reactions themselves more conscious (cf. Anālayo, 2003, p. 229). One early Buddhist dialogue suggested that the stages of affective appraisal (Pāli: *vedanā*) and cognitive appraisal (*saññā*) serve as the basis of thought (*vitakka*) and conceptual proliferation (*papañca*) (MN 18 and its parallels, in Anālayo, 2011, p. 136). According to this model, initial distortions of attention and memory affect later conceptualizations of the experience. Likewise, in the recent psychological literature, biases of attention and memory have been suggested as affecting the trajectory of psychological reactions to emotionally salient stimuli (Todd, Cunningham, Anderson, & Thompson, 2012). Drawing on such suggestions, Brewer, Elwafi, and Davis (2013) suggest that mindfulness, besides leading to increased awareness of one's own emotional reactions, may lead to more accurate awareness, in particular by attenuating affective biases that underlie distortions of attention and memory (Elliott, Zahn, Deakin, & Anderson, 2010).

A variety of experimental results support this idea. Recent findings showing that mindfulness training is associated with decreases in negative biases in word-recall tasks (Roberts-Wolfe, Sacchet, Hastings, Roth, & Britton, 2012) support the hypothesis that mindfulness attenuates memory biases. Another finding that a group receiving mindfulness training exhibited a decrease in the attentional blink for emotional face stimuli (Van Dam, 2012) supports the suggestion that mindfulness decreases attentional biases (for discussion of the paradigm, see Van Dam, Earleywine, & Altarriba, 2012). In addition, whereas a control group showed small decreases or modest increases in subjective distress as a result of the Trier Social Stress Test (TSST; Kirschbaum, Pirke, & Hellhammer, 1993), the mindfulness group showed large decreases in subjective distress. Further analysis suggested that mindfulness decreased psychological symptoms, in part by improving awareness of emotional imagery, as well as by generating emotional stability in response to psychosocial stress. Using this same psychosocial stress test, Britton, Shahar, Szepsenwol, and Jacobs (2011) found that the perseveration of emotional response was reduced in a group receiving mindfulness training, but not the intensity of the response. Wait-list control subjects showed an increase in anticipatory anxiety, indicating a stress sensitization effect, while the prestressor levels of the subjects receiving Mindfulness-based cognitive therapy (MBCT; Segal, Williams, & Teasdale, 2002) did not change. Moreover, the MBCT group showed decreased emotional reactivity during the poststressor phase. Specifically, the time course (duration) of the affective response, but not the amplitude, was decreased following MBCT. One explanation for these results is that affective biases increase the tendency of attention to return again and again to mental images that spark negative affect, and that mindfulness decreases proliferation by attenuating affective biases of attention and memory.

In summary, we propose that the establishment of mindfulness, *satipaṭṭhāna*, be understood as involving two critical and mutually supportive factors—increased alertness on the one hand, and the attenuation of affective biases of attention and memory on the other. Increased alertness results in increased consciousness of internal and external stimuli that would otherwise not be consciously experienced. Yet without a concomitant reduction in emotional fixation due to affective biases of attention and memory, generalized increases in alertness can lead to pathological symptoms, as in an panic attack when one fixates on an unpleasant stimulus. Conversely, by attenuating affective biases, mindfulness practitioners may become conscious of a broader range of stimuli and also reduce emotional proliferation following pleasant or unpleasant experience. Reciprocally, the extension of one's conscious experience to include a broader range of current stimuli may counteract affective biases by reducing fixation on one stimulus or one recurrent memory.

Full and Accurate Awareness

Both by increasing altertness and by attenuating affective biases, establishing mindfulness may lead to increases in emotional awareness in a variety of forms. Decreased attentional blink, especially in conjunction with more general emotional awareness, might predict increased awareness in interpersonal interactions. For example, increased awareness of visual, nonverbal responses such as "microfacial expressions" can facilitate detection of suppressed or repressed responses (Todd et al., 2012). Such expressions are normally detectable only with slow-motion video or by observers trained to detect such microfacial expressions (Ekman & Friesen, 1969). Yet even without explicit training, decreases in attentional blink predict increased awareness of others' emotional expressions. In this way, the two mutually supportive factors of increased alertness and decreased affective bias may result in better awareness of others' emotions.

Equally important, recent evidence suggests that mindfulness training may result in increased awareness of one's own emotional state by virtue of increased conscious experience of interoceptive changes involved in one's physiological reactions. In a recent study, mindfulness meditators showed significantly more coherence between physiological changes and their subjective awareness of emotional responses than did either professional dancers (ballet and modern dance) or control subjects with no meditation or dance experience (Sze, Gyurak, Yuan, & Levenson, 2010). Mindfulness meditators were more aware of their visceral responses and thereby more aware of their emotions. In another study, Silverstein, Brown, Roth, and Britton (2011) reported evidence of increased interoceptive awareness in female undergraduates engaged in mindfulness training. They suggested that women who were distracted by emotionally driven self-evaluative thoughts were much slower in registering their bodily reactions, as measured by reaction time in rating physiological response to sexual stimuli, whereas mindfulness meditation training increased awareness of bodily reactions by decreasing self-evaluative thoughts.

Such instances in which awareness increases access to information about one's own and others' emotional situation provide examples of how mindfulness might lead to fuller, more accurate cognitive understanding by virtue of cultivating a broad and receptive field of conscious experience. On the one hand, if expressions of one's own or others' emotional reactions are not consciously experienced, then they cannot be encoded in working memory so as to be available for recall, consideration, or report. Thus, by increasing phenomenal consciousness of subtle internal and external stimuli, one makes one's cognitive awareness more complete. On the other hand, to the degree that attention and memory are affectively biased, one is less likely to consciously experience subtle emotional stimuli that do not fit one's biases. Thus, by decreasing affective biases and increasing alertness, cognitive understanding is enhanced.

This perspective suggests an intimate relation between perceptual and cognitive changes involved in mindfulness. In the Pāli Nikāyas, latent craving and aversion are said to result in perceptual distortions (*saññā-vipallāsa*), which when elaborated lead to distortions of both thought (*citta-vipallāsa*) and view (*diṭṭhi-vipallāsa*) when such thought patterns become habitual (see the translator's introduction to Olendzki, 2010). Given the contemporary focus on the present-centered, nonevaluative aspects of mindfulness, it is worth emphasizing that evaluative conceptual understandings informed by mindfulness practice may often be crucial in making decisions that are skillful, in the sense of not setting one up for suffering. Cognitive aspects of mindfulness training may therefore play an important role in generating the beneficial outcomes of mindfulness. As Kabat-Zinn (2011, p. 291) notes, "non-judgmental does not mean . . . that there is some ideal state in which judgments no longer arise." Indeed, early Buddhist definitions of mindfulness (Anālayo, 2013) suggest that mindfulness transforms evaluative and ethical judgments but does not eradicate them.

For example, according to one early Buddhist dialogue, the attraction of sensual pleasures is based on a distorted cognition, and such cognitive distortions can only be corrected through wise attention. The simile given here is that of a leper who takes delight in cauterizing his wounds over fire, but when healed, accurately takes this burning to be painful (MN 75 and its parallels, in Anālayo, 2011, p. 410). To the degree that sensual pleasures do not in fact provide lasting satisfaction, as the Pāli Nikāyas suggest, having expectations of gaining satisfaction in this way and making decisions based on these expectations will inevitably set one up for frustration and sorrow. Thus, a future-focused understanding that no object of experience will bring lasting satisfaction may have important effects on decision making about how to live and act.

On this account, the cognitive effects of establishing mindfulness rest on a lack of affective biases and an increased ability to face hard truths. Some have suggested that the salutary effects of mindfulness may be due to increases in positive reappraisal of life situations (Garland, Gaylord, & Fredrickson, 2011; Garland, Gaylord, & Park, 2009). Garland and colleagues (2011, p. 60) give the example of mindfulness allowing clients' reappraisal of a serious heart condition as "an opportunity to change their lifestyle and health behaviors rather than as a catastrophe portending imminent doom." But the Pāli Nikāyas do not support a conception of mindfulness as biasing subjects' conscious experience or cognitive considerations specifically toward positive aspects of a situation. Rather, we have suggested that satipaṭṭhāna functions to decrease affective biases of attention and memory toward pleasant as well as unpleasant stimuli. In accord with this suggestion, Ortner, Kilner, and Zelazo (2007) found that both mindfulness training and relaxation training groups decreased arousal to negative images, but that only mindfulness training decreased arousal to positive images.

Conclusion: "Seeing and Knowing Things as They Are"

Together, increases in alertness and attenuation of affective biases suggest how mindfulness may achieve the traditional goal of "seeing and knowing things as they are" (yathābhūtañāṇadassana). One function of mindfulness is to counteract not knowing. Under normal attentional circumstances, we miss much of what is going on. By increasing phenomenal consciousness of subtle changes in our bodies, minds, and in our environments, we may make this information available to be encoded in working memory and thus to be identified, deliberated on, and expressed to others. A second function of mindfulness is to counteract knowing wrongly. Through attenuating affective biases, we can gradually replace emotionally distorted perceptions, thoughts, and views with undistorted cognitions. These two functions of mindfulness are mutually reinforcing.

Psychological states induced by nonconscious primes or by expectations, fears, and hopes can cause individuals to misidentify perceptual stimuli in two ways. First, biases of attention may cause certain objects or features to be preferentially selected or deselected for conscious experience. Second, biases of memory may cause certain experiences to be preferentially selected or deselected for uptake into belief-forming processes. Siegel (2012) proposes that such selection effects can make the resulting beliefs less worthy of being called knowledge because these selection effects cause individuals to improperly ignore information that should not be ignored given their purposes, or to improperly bypass experience that bears rationally on the beliefs they form. In Siegel's terms, selection effects "epistemically downgrade" resulting beliefs. We have surveyed recent research suggesting that Buddhist-derived practices of cultivating mindfulness can counteract biases of both attention and memory. If so, cultivating mindfulness can epistemically upgrade certain beliefs, making them more worthy of being called knowledge.

In this chapter, we have sketched an account of two mutually reinforcing factors involved in mindfulness meditation: first, an increased phenomenal consciousness of subtle, fleeting stimuli; and second, decreases in affective biases of attention and memory. By acting on perceptual and cognitive levels, the sharpening of attention and the decrease in affective biases can function to dispel incomplete and biased interpretations. On this account, affective biases function to fixate attention such that we are not conscious in a broad and open manner; reciprocally, being receptive in an alert and open way results in a broad field of conscious experience that includes stimuli that would normally escape awareness. These include fleeting and subtle sensory clues about external conditions, as well as stimuli from interoceptive changes involved in one's emotional reactions that often influence behavior without being consciously experienced. Accordingly, we can understand the cultivation of mindfulness as resulting in fuller and more accurate awareness of external and internal conditions, and of our own and others' psychological states. To the degree that such effects of attention training result in a more accurate and more precise understanding of what leads to suffering in ourselves and in others, this chapter offers an account of how mindfulness training-based increases in the breadth and subtlety of conscious experience could result in better practical understanding of how one ought best to live. Thus, this approach offers one precise and empirically grounded way in which we can understand the claim made in the *Majjhima* text quoted at the outset, that consciousness and wisdom are conjoined.

NOTES

1. Sutta references are to collection (e.g., *Majjhima Nikāya* [MN], *Suttanipāta* [Sn]), and then either to sutta number (in the case of DN, MN, and Iti), saṃyutta and sutta number

(SN), nipāta and sutta number (AN), verse number (Dhp), vagga and sutta number (Ud, Sn).

2. The term *satipaṭṭhāna* has commonly been rendered as a (plural) noun, the (four) "foundations of mindfulness." But the primary sense of the term is verbal and refers to the active practice of establishing mindfulness, as noted recently by prominent translators such as Bhikkhu Bodhi (2011, p. 25) and Thanissaro Bhikkhu (2011). For a critique of the more standard gloss of *satipaṭṭhāna* as "foundations of mindfulness" and the commentarial derivation of the term from *paṭṭhāna* on which this gloss is based, see Anālayo (2003, pp. 29–30).

3. We would like to thank Nicholas Van Dam for helpful discussion on this point.

REFERENCES

Anālayo. (2003). *Satipaṭṭhāna: The direct path to realization.* Birmingham, UK: Windhorse.

Anālayo. (2011). *A comparative study of the Majjhima-nikāya.* Taipei: Dharma Drum.

Anālayo. (2013). *Satipatthāna in comparative perspective.* Birmingham, UK: Windhorse.

Baars, B. (1988). *A cognitive theory of consciousness.* Cambridge, UK: Cambridge University Press.

Barrett, L. F., Mesquita, B., Ochsner, K. N., & Gross, J. J. (2007). The experience of emotion. *Annual Review of Psychology, 58,* 373–403.

Bayne, T. (2007). Conscious states and conscious creatures: Explanation in the scientific study of consciousness. *Philosophical Perspectives, 21*(1), 1–22.

Bhikkhu Bodhi. (2011). What does mindfulness really mean?: A canonical perspective. *Contemporary Buddhism, 12*(01), 19–39.

Bishop, S. R., Lau, M., Shapiro, S., Carlson, L., Anderson, N. D., Carmody, J., et al. (2004). Mindfulness: A proposed operational definition. *Clinical Psychology: Science and Practice, 11*(3), 230–241.

Block, N. (1995). On a confusion about a function of consciousness. *Behavioral and Brain Sciences, 18,* 227–247.

Block, N. (2007). Consciousness, accessibility, and the mesh between psychology and neuroscience. *Behavioral and Brain Sciences, 30*(5–6), 481–548.

Block, N. (2008). Consciousness and cognitive access. *Proceedings of the Aristotelian Society, 108,* 289–317.

Block, N. (2011). Perceptual consciousness overflows cognitive access. *Trends in Cognitive Sciences, 15*(12), 567–575.

Brewer, J. A., Elwafi, H. M., & Davis, J. H. (2013). Craving to quit: Psychological models and neurobiological mechanisms of mindfulness training as treatment for addictions. *Psychology of Addictive Behaviors, 27*(2), 366–379.

Britton, W. B., Lindahl, J. R., Cahn, B. R., Davis, J. H., & Goldman, R. E. (2014). Awakening is not a metaphor: The effects of Buddhist meditation practices on basic wakefulness. *Annals of the New York Academy of Sciences, 1307,* 64–81.

Britton, W. B., Shahar, B., Szepsenwol, Q., & Jacobs, W. J. (2011). Mindfulness-based cognitive therapy improves emotional reactivity to social stress: Results from a randomized controlled trial. *Behavior Therapy, 43,* 365–380.

Chalmers, D. J. (1995). Facing up to the problem of consciousness. *Journal of Consciousness Studies, 2*(3), 200–219.

Chalmers, D. J. (1996). *The conscious mind: In search of a fundamental theory.* New York: Oxford University Press.

Cohen, M. A., & Dennett, D. C. (2011). Consciousness cannot be separated from function. *Trends in Cognitive Sciences, 15*(8), 358–364.

Corbetta, M., & Shulman, G. L. (2002). Control of goal-directed and stimulus-driven attention in the brain. *Nature Reviews Neuroscience, 3*(3), 201–215.

Crick, F., & Koch, C. (1990). Towards a neurobiological theory of consciousness. *Seminars in the Neurosciences, 2*, 263–275.

Davidson, R. J. (2010). Empirical explorations of mindfulness: conceptual and methodological conundrums. *Emotion, 10*(1), 8–11.

Davis, J. H., & Thompson, E. (2013). From the five aggregates to phenomenal consciousness. In S. M. Emmanuel (Ed.), *A companion to Buddhist philosophy* (pp. 585–597). Hoboken, NJ: Wiley.

de Fockert, J. W., Rees, G., Frith, C. D., & Lavie, N. (2001). The role of working memory in visual selective attention. *Science, 291*, 1803–1806.

Dennett, D. (1991). *Consciousness explained*. Boston: Little, Brown.

Desimone, R., & Duncan, J. (1995). Neural mechanisms of selective visual attention. *Annual Review of Neuroscience, 18*(1), 193–222.

Dreyfus, G. (2011). Is mindfulness present-centred and non-judgmental?: A discussion of the cognitive dimensions of mindfulness. *Contemporary Buddhism, 12*(01), 41–54.

Ekman, P., & Friesen, W. V. (1969). Nonverbal leakage and clues to deception. *Psychiatry, 32*(1), 88–106.

Elliott, R., Zahn, R., Deakin, J. F. W., & Anderson, I. M. (2010). Affective cognition and its disruption in mood disorders. *Neuropsychopharmacology, 36*(1), 153–182.

Fan, J., McCandliss, B. D., Fossella, J., Flombaum, J. I., & Posner, M. I. (2005). The activation of attentional networks. *NeuroImage, 26*(2), 471–479.

Fan, J., McCandliss, B. D., Sommer, T., Raz, A., & Posner, M. I. (2002). Testing the efficiency and independence of attentional networks. *Journal of Cognitive Neuroscience, 14*(3), 340–347.

Farb, N. A., Segal, Z. V., & Anderson, A. K. (2013a). Attentional modulation of primary interoceptive and exteroceptive cortices. *Cerebral Cortex, 23*(1), 114–126.

Farb, N. A., Segal, Z. V., & Anderson, A. K. (2013b). Mindfulness meditation training alters cortical representations of interoceptive attention. *Social Cognitive and Affective Neuroscience, 8*(1), 15–26.

Garland, E., Gaylord, S., & Fredrickson, B. L. (2011). Positive reappraisal mediates the stress-reductive effects of mindfulness: An upward spiral process. *Mindfulness, 2*(1), 59–67.

Garland, E. L., Gaylord, S., & Park, J. (2009). The role of mindfulness in positive reappraisal. *EXPLORE: The Journal of Science and Healing, 5*(1), 37–44.

Grabovac, A. D., Lau, M. A., & Willett, B. R. (2011). Mechanisms of mindfulness: A Buddhist psychological model. *Mindfulness, 2*(3), 154–166.

Gunaratana, H. (2002). *Mindfulness in plain English*. Boston: Wisdom Publications.

Harvey, B. P. (1995). *The selfless mind: Personality, consciousness and Nirvana in early Buddhism*. New York: Routledge.

Hölzel, B. K., Lazar, S. W., Gard, T., Schuman-Olivier, Z., Vago, D. R., & Ott, U. (2011). How does mindfulness meditation work?: Proposing mechanisms of action from a conceptual and neural perspective. *Perspectives on Psychological Science, 6*(6), 537–559.

Jha, A. P., Krompinger, J., & Baime, M. J. (2007). Mindfulness training modifies subsystems of attention. *Cognitive, Affective, and Behavioral Neuroscience, 7*(2), 109–119.

Jones, S. R., Kerr, C. E., Wann, Q., Pritchett, D. L., Hämäläinen, M., & Moore, C. L. (2010). Cued spatial attention drives functionally relevant modulation of the mu rhythm in primary somatosensory cortex. *Journal of Neuroscience, 30*, 13760–13765.

Kabat-Zinn, J. (1994). *Wherever you go, there you are: Mindfulness meditation in everyday life*. New York: Hyperion.

Kabat-Zinn, J. (1996). Mindfulness meditation: What it is, what it isn't, and its role in health care and medicine. In Y. Ishii, M. Suzuki, & Y. Haruki (Eds.), *Comparative and psychological study on meditation* (pp. 161–170). Delft, The Netherlands: Eburon.

Kabat-Zinn, J. (2005). *Coming to our senses: Healing ourselves and the world through mindfulness*. New York: Hyperion.

Kabat-Zinn, J. (2011). Some reflections on the origins of MBSR, skillful means, and the trouble with maps. *Contemporary Buddhism, 12*(1), 281–306.

Kerr, C. E., Jones, S. R., Wan, Q., Pritchett, D. L., Wasserman, R. H., Wexler, A., et al. (2011). Effects of mindfulness meditation training on anticipatory alpha modulation in primary somatosensory cortex. *Brain Research Bulletin, 85*(3), 96–103.

Kirschbaum, C., Pirke, K.-M., & Hellhammer, D. H. (1993). The "Trier Social Stress Test"—a tool for investigating psychobiological stress responses in a laboratory setting. *Neuropsychobiology, 28*(1–2), 76–81.

Kouider, S., de Gardelle, V., Sackur, J., & Depoux, E. (2010). How rich is consciousness?: The partial awareness hypothesis. *Trends in Cognitive Sciences, 14*(7), 301–307.

Lutz, A., Slagter, H. A., Dunne, J. D., & Davidson, R. J. (2008). Attention regulation and monitoring in meditation. *Trends in Cognitive Sciences, 12*(4), 163–169.

Mole, C., Smithies, D., & Wu, W. (2011). *Attention: Philosophical and psychological essays*. Oxford, UK: Oxford University Press.

Nagel, T. (1974). What is it like to be a bat? *Philosophical Review, 83*(4), 435–450.

Olendzki, A. (Trans.). (2010). Vipallasa Sutta: Distortions of the mind. Retrieved from *www.accesstoinsight.org/tipitaka/an/an04/an04.049.olen.html*.

Ortner, C., Kilner, S. & Zelazo, P. D. (2007). Mindfulness meditation and reduced emotional interference on a cognitive task. *Motivation and Emotion, 31*(4), 271–283.

Parvizi, J., & Damasio, A. (2001). Consciousness and the brainstem. *Cognition, 79*(1), 135–160.

Petersen, S. E., & Posner, M. I. (2012). The attention system of the human brain: 20 years after. *Annual Review of Neuroscience, 35*(1), 73–89.

Posner, M. I., & Petersen, S. E. (1990). The attention system of the human brain. *Annual Review of Neuroscience, 13*(1), 25–42.

Prinz, J. (2011). Is attention necessary and sufficient for consciousness? In C. Mole, D. Smithies, & W. Wu (Eds.), *Attention: Philosophical and psychological essays* (pp. 174–204). Oxford, UK: Oxford University Press.

Prinz, J. J. (2005). A neurofunctional theory of consciousness. In A. Brook & K. Atkins (Eds.), *Cognition and the brain: The philosophy and neuroscience movement* (pp. 381–396). Cambridge, UK: Cambridge University Press.

Prinz, J. J. (2012). *The conscious brain*. Oxford, UK: Oxford University Press.

Roberts-Wolfe, D., Sacchet, M., Hastings, E., Roth, H., & Britton, W. (2012). Mindfulness training alters emotional memory recall compared to active controls: Support for an emotional information processing model of mindfulness. *Frontiers in Human Neuroscience, 6*, 15.

Robertson, I. H., Mattingley, J. B., Rorden, C., & Driver, J. (1998). Phasic alerting of neglect patients overcomes their spatial deficit in visual awareness. *Nature, 395*, 169–172.

Rolls, E. T. (2008). *Memory, attention and decision-making*. Oxford, UK: Oxford University Press.

Schubert, R., Blankenburg, F., Lemm, S., Villringer, A., & Curio, G. (2006). Now you feel it—now you don't: ERP correlates of somatosensory awareness. *Psychophysiology, 43*(1), 31–40.

Schubert, R., Haufe, S., Blankenburg, F., Villringer, A., & Curio, G. (2009). Now you'll feel it, now you won't: EEG rhythms predict the effectiveness of perceptual masking. *Journal of Cognitive Neuroscience, 21*(12), 2407–2419.

Schubert, R., Ritter, P., Wüstenberg, T., Preuschhof, C., Curio, G., Sommer, W., et al. (2008). Spatial attention related SEP amplitude modulations covary with BOLD signal in S1—a simultaneous EEG—fMRI study. *Cerebral Cortex, 18*(11), 2686–2700.

Searle, J. R. (2000). Consciousness. *Annual Review of Neuroscience, 23,* 557–578.

Segal, Z., Williams, J., & Teasdale, J. (2002). *Mindfulness-based cognitive therapy for depression: A new approach to relapse prevention.* New York: Guilford Press.

Siegel, S. (2012). Can selection effects on experience influence its rational role. In T. Gendler (Ed.), *Oxford studies in epistemology* (4th ed.). Oxford, UK: Oxford University Press.

Silverstein, R. G., Brown, A.-C. H., Roth, H. D., & Britton, W. B. (2011). Effects of mindfulness training on body awareness to sexual stimuli: Implications for female sexual dysfunction. *Psychosomatic Medicine, 73*(9), 817–825.

Slagter, H. A., Lutz, A., Greischar, L. L., Francis, A. D., Niewenhuis, S., Davis, J. M., et al. (2007). Mental training affects distribution of limited brain resources. *PLoS Biology, 5*(6), e138.

Sze, J. A., Gyurak, A., Yuan, J. W., & Levenson, R. W. (2010). Coherence between emotional experience and physiology: Does body awareness training have an impact? *Emotion, 10*(6), 803–814.

Thanissaro, B. (Trans.). (2011). Maha-satipatthana Sutta: The great frames of reference. Retrieved from *www.accesstoinsight.org/tipitaka/dn/dn.22.0.than.html.*

Thompson, E. (2014). *Waking, dreaming, being.* New York: Columbia University Press.

Todd, R. M., Cunningham, W. A., Anderson, A. K., & Thompson, E. (2012). Affect-biased attention as emotion regulation. *Trends in Cognitive Sciences, 16*(7), 365–372.

Tononi, G., & Koch, C. (2008). The neural correlates of consciousness. *Annals of the New York Academy of Sciences, 1124*(1), 239–261.

Van Dam, N. T. (2012). *The impact of meditation on stress and psychopathology: Attentional allocation as a mechanism of active change.* Garrison, NY: Mind and Life Summer Research Institute.

Van Dam, N. T., Earleywine, M., & Altarriba, J. (2012). Anxiety attenuates awareness of emotional faces during rapid serial visual presentation. *Emotion, 12*(4), 796–806.

CHAPTER 4

Reconceptualizing Mindfulness

The Psychological Principles of Attending in Mindfulness Practice and Their Role in Well-Being

James Carmody

Mindfulness training (MT) has long played a key role in a Buddhist system designed to reduce mental suffering. It has now become integrated into Western medicine and psychology, based on research demonstrating the efficacy of several MT programs to reduce stress and distress in healthy people, in a number of diagnosed patient groups and in clinicians (Chiesa & Serretti, 2009, 2010; Hofmann, Sawyer, Witt, & Oh, 2010; Irving, Dobkin, & Park, 2009). Yet there are problems inherent in applying a construct and training approach from a non-Western, fully formed religious system to serve secular Western scientific, psychoeducational, and clinical purposes. In particular, this meeting of cultures and traditions has resulted in seemingly intractable disagreements about the nature and definition of mindfulness, the best means by which to conduct MT, and the conceptual nature of the pathways through which MT has its effects.

In this chapter I attempt to address these issues, drawing on 45 years of practice in the three main Buddhist traditions, along with years of experience researching the clinical effects and mechanisms of MT, and finally teaching mindfulness practice to patients and clinicians. I first briefly describe the role that mindfulness and MT plays in the Buddhist religious and philosophical system, then comment on the disagreements and confusions that result from carrying over Buddhist conceptualizations of human suffering into Western science and clinical settings. I then describe the effect of this on both the development of MT research and the training of people in need. In an effort to offer solutions to these dilemmas, I address the basis of mental suffering using a Western scientific framework rather than a Buddhist one as a basis for explaining the value of mind training programs such as MT. I do this in two ways:

First, I attempt to circumvent disagreements about both the meaning of mindfulness and the role of MT within a larger system of training by presenting an operational and needs-based conceptualization, based on evolutionary psychology, and of how practices typically taught in MT can reduce distress and increase well-being, including the genetically driven imperatives that make MT challenging and the value of mindfulness practice in diminishing their role in ongoing distress.

Second, I discuss the commonalities that MT has (and does not have) with other evidence-based psychological and mind–body trainings. I argue for the clinical and scientific advantages of this approach, highlighting (1) the clinical utility of using concepts already familiar to many Western patients and clinicians; (2) the provision of a stronger empirical foundation for how mindfulness can best be explained and taught, instead of relying on traditional assumptions and/or presumed expert testimony; and (3) the contribution of this approach to the development of a unified theory of the mechanisms underlying psychological and mind–body programs designed to reduce distress and increase well-being. I close this chapter with a discussion of several challenges that this approach faces.

The Buddhist Roots of Mindfulness

The Buddhist narrative is rooted in the primarily introspective approaches to knowledge in India at the time of Gautama the Buddha approximately 2,500 years ago. It places the root of the problem of human suffering in ignorance of the moment-by-moment construction of a sense of ownership of experience in the mind, and the dissatisfaction (suffering) that arises from the resultant craving and aversion. The cultivation of *mindfulness*, a term derived in the late 19th century as the translation for the Pali language word *sati* (see Gethin, Chapter 2, this volume), is one of the elements of a systematic eightfold path claimed to have been put forward by the historical Buddha as a way out of this ignorance and suffering. Recognition of the common goal that Buddhism, medicine, and psychology each have in reducing suffering has helped to pave the way for the entry of mindfulness and Buddhist MT exercises into Western medicine and psychotherapeutic programs.

Mindfulness Makes the Leap from Religious System to Science and Clinical Practice

The introduction of mindfulness practice into the secular world has involved passage from a religious setting wherein it serves as a heuristic/phenomenological tool for insight into the workings of one's own mind, into the world of empirical research and clinical practice. In making this transition, mindfulness itself has, inevitably, become an object of investigation. And since measurement is fundamental to scientific enquiry, operational definitions have been developed to serve as foundations for reliable and valid measures, and to test that outcomes attributed to mindfulness and MT are verifiable and reproducible.

This definition and measurement endeavor has not been without controversy. It has exposed significant disagreements in approaches to the construct, and specifically where and how a "true" understanding of mindfulness is to be found (Brown, Ryan, Loverich, Biegel, & West, 2011; Grossman, 2008, 2011). Disagreement is to be expected for two reasons. First, the Pali language is no longer understood outside the Indian scholarship community, and the term mindfulness has other, non-Buddhist meanings in English. Second, drawing a term from a religious system inevitably results in arguments about its "true" nature, and about where investigators should turn to establish its criterion and discriminant validity. For some investigators and instructors, mindfulness and Buddhism are inextricably coupled ideas; they identify as dharma practitioners on a path of "transformation," and members of a community of mindfulness practitioners. Others come to it principally through Western psychology and may have no more personal connection to Buddhism than as a helpful lens through which to understand the origins of mindfulness and MT. For the former, correct understanding of mindfulness can come only from extended and correctly guided practice of it, and "true" exemplars of the concept are principally to be found within Buddhist texts and traditions. It can also extend to the assumption that mindfulness is sufficiently subtle and unique that it cannot be conceptualized or measured outside of an understanding of its broader Buddhist system—that is, without compromising or diminishing its "true" experiential meaning (Grossman, 2008, 2011; Rapgay & Bystrisky, 2009).

While such convictions are understandable from a religious standpoint, they do not form a fruitful basis for exploring mindfulness in the clinical and scientific arena. Progress in scientific enquiry entails some measure of skepticism; thus, research into mindfulness must allow that because mindfulness is part of an age-old system, or an unquestioned part of a lineage, does not necessarily mean it has been correctly understood or is immune to further investigation, understanding, or development. An overly reverential attitude toward mindfulness and mindfulness practice can result in seeing them as something unique and "other," and lead to orthodoxy, as is alluded to in the well-known Zen story about focusing on the finger rather than the moon toward which the finger points. But, as in any debate that bears upon matters of meaning, there will be the orthodox, those who insist upon the wisdom of taking refuge in traditional forms, transmissions, and narratives to safeguard what is seen as the true understanding, and those more willing to innovate. Such is the history and progress of human understanding. But if an attitude of orthodoxy is carried into the scientific arena, it raises legitimate concerns as to whether the research conducted from such a narrative is being undertaken as a genuine and open enquiry, or as an exercise to provide scientific credence for a pursuit already assumed to be unique, complete, and beneficial to all. Yet in the midst of these debates, progress has been made in defining and operationalizing mindfulness (Baum et al., 2010; Brown, West, Loverich, & Biegel, 2011), and in supporting the clinical effects of training in it. For example, MT has predicted higher levels of self-reported mindfulness, which in turn has been related to minutes of formal mindfulness practice (Carmody & Baer, 2008) and reductions in stress and distress (Baer, Carmody, & Hunsinger, 2012; Kuyken et al., 2010). Furthermore, there is evidence that the increased mindfulness and associated reductions in stress and distress are enduring (Pbert et al., 2012). Yet this endeavor has also resulted in challenges to prevailing orthodoxies about mindfulness and MT.

Specifically, a number of the assumptions derived from contemplative traditions about what is required to obtain meaningful benefits from MT are not supported in clinical studies; these findings include the comparatively minimal length of training programs and amount of practice required to demonstrate significant change (Carmody & Baer, 2009; Jain et al., 2007; Pbert et al., 2012); the evidence that mindfulness can be taught without personal instruction (Gluck & Maercker, 2011); and evidence that increases in mindfulness resulting from therapeutic modalities not explicitly mindfulness-based can occur (Shelov, Suchday, & Friedberg, 2009; Tanner et al., 2009). Additionally, patient distress reduction has been demonstrated with therapeutic systems incorporating mindfulness that vary in their understandings of the construct such as dialectical behavior therapy and acceptance and commitment therapy, and guided by therapists with what some would consider limited experience of formal mindfulness practice. These findings contribute to the dialogue about "true" mindfulness by indicating that it appears to be an evolving concept, and that MT can be creatively explored and adapted without losing its value to enhance well-being. They counsel us also to empirically test traditional assumptions required for teaching and learning mindfulness.

The language used in definitions of mindfulness has also presented a challenge for scientific research and clinical work, as they use both traditional and contemporary terms that reflect the authors' theoretical orientation and experience with MT. These include a present-centered attention to and awareness of all accessible events and experiences (Brown & Ryan, 2004); paying attention in a particular way: on purpose, in the present moment, and nonjudgmentally (Kabat-Zinn, 1994); and a nonelaborative, nonjudgmental, present-centered awareness in which each thought, feeling, or sensation that arises in the attentional field is acknowledged and accepted as it is (Bishop et al., 2004). Such elusive language, as well as cryptic descriptive terms such as *beginner's mind, being in the moment, embodiment, a being mode rather than a doing mode,* and so on, have made more difficult the job of introducing the construct and its possible benefits in a straightforward way to patients and clinicians, and present problems for the operational definitions required for research.

So it is useful to ask whether mindfulness can be placed in a frame that (1) honors its roots while describing it through more readily familiar principles; (2) provides a clear and parsimonious conceptualization of the construct that accommodates trainees' reports of its practical use in their everyday lives; and (3) can serve as a foundation for empirical hypotheses about causal relationships in advancing the psychology and biology of well-being.

To begin addressing these challenges, it is useful to place them in a larger context by revisiting the more fundamental question of why we should need something like mindfulness in the first place. For while it may be apparent that we have craving and aversion, and that they keep us ill-at-ease, as the Buddhist narrative describes, this does not explain the origins of the ignorance at the root of this suffering. Why is this ignorance present in a healthy human? Why is some level of dis-ease so prevalent, even among people with material needs well met? Why are we not naturally at ease?

Why Is Ease Not a Default Condition of the Mind?

The Role of Mindfulness in This Predicament

Attention plays a central role in interacting with the environment in ways that lead to the satisfaction of needs and their resultant desires, and attention training is the initial and central cognitive exercise in the cultivation of well-being through MT. This central role of attention was recognized by William James (1890) and confirmed by later experimental studies demonstrating the key role that effortful focusing of attention plays in well-being-supportive emotion regulation and self-regulated behavior (Baumeister & Heatherton, 1996; Kirschenbaum, 1987; Thayer, Friedman, & Borkovec, 1996). Given its importance, it is curious that we treat the regulation of attention as a naturally formed capacity; an assumption evident in the exhortations to our children to "just pay attention" when learning material in school. But patients report having difficulty in keeping attention focused during MT exercises (Segal, Williams, & Teasdale, 2002), and it is useful to ask why this should be a challenge. Why should attention require any training at all in the cultivation of day-to-day well-being?

The Buddhist explanation for suffering often evokes concepts of craving, aversion, and attachment, and is the lens sometimes used by MT instructors and clinicians. But an explanation using evolutionary principles may provide a culturally more familiar explanation for why attention should keep highlighting what we crave and seek to avoid, even to the detriment of well-being. From a standpoint of evolutionary adaptation, a key role of attention is to highlight in awareness features of the internal and external environment related to physical and reproductive survival needs. As such, it serves to highlight real and imagined opportunities for, and threats to the fulfillment of those needs. In the evolutionary past in which our central nervous system developed, physical danger was ever-present in the external environment, and the capacity of attention to highlight threats and opportunities would have had obvious survival value. And in the service of swift responding, evolutionary pressures appear to have resulted in automatic neural processes to direct attention—that is, in ways not requiring comparatively slow conscious, deliberate decisions. Such default, automatic movements of attention would have clear safety and survival value, and since most threats were likely to be physical in nature, attention was probably predominantly oriented to sensory processes that monitor the physical environment.

As threats to physical safety have been minimized in many modern societies, attention appears now to default to highlighting both real and imagined threats and opportunities for the satisfaction of higher order needs, such as those for relationship, status, and power. And while the satisfaction of these needs requires some level of sensory monitoring, it also requires a great deal of cognitive planning and reflection (Andrews-Hanna, 2012). This is evident from even limited observation of the way attention keeps leaving the sensory realm to favor cognitions that take the form of the ongoing commentary experienced as an internal narrative about oneself, others, and the larger world. This movement of attention in response to the planning and vigilance required to meet social demands in modern societies may well be continuing to evolve through epigenetic (Keverne & Curley, 2008) and cultural processes.

Based in memory and imagination, the internal narrative insistently plans, compares, judges, and regrets. Its role in the meeting of relationship, status, power, and other needs is experienced as the everyday concerns, worries, joys, and other emotionally tinged thoughts and images about such matters as the welfare of family and friends, work, money, and one's own social standing, well-being, and health. Attention preoccupied with this cognitive monitoring is experienced as rumination. As I describe in the following section, when these thoughts and images in attention are threat-based, their associated sensations will be constriction- or tension-related and the associated feeling tone will be an unpleasant one. The degree of constriction and unpleasantness will depend on the level of perceived threat and the perceived capacity to meet it. The ironic result of attention placed in the service of meeting needs by repeatedly dwelling on threat-based cognitive themes is the less-than-pleasant felt sense characterizing so much of life, and at times the real mental suffering that can result from this tendency.

In contrast to the sense of personal separation that characterizes cognitively oriented attention, the perceptible sensory world is held in common with others and is predominant in the pleasantness of delight. MT exercises recognize this principle in cultivating the capacity to make attention available to the senses and the perceptible world, and supporting this orientation in everyday life. For when attention is focused on current activities, experience once again becomes predominantly sense-based, with cognition secondary and immediate task-related (also called *concrete processing*; see Watkins, Chapter 6, this volume). At these times, the internal narrative recedes and the felt sense is less affected by its threat- and opportunity-oriented memories and imaginings. This is nicely demonstrated in an ambulatory study by Killingsworth and Gilbert (2010), who found that people reported being more happy when their attention was focused on what they were currently doing than when their minds were "wandering." Contrast this orientation with the preoccupation that results from attention being focused on the idiosyncratic memories and imaginings of the internal narrative. At those times, awareness of the sensory world is minimized, a situation that results in not only unpleasant everyday experience but also reduced opportunities for joy and connection with others.

With this evolution-based account of attention as background, I suggest three psychological principles that describe how MT and similar programs encourage trainees to attend to sense-based experience, whether bodily sensations or sensory experiences of the perceptible world, and I show how this orientation, together with the recognition of mental processes that accompany it, can reliably lead to the enhancement of well-being.

Using Psychological Principles to Describe MT and Its Benefits

My experience researching, practicing, and teaching mindfulness leads me to suggest that there are just a few psychological principles underpinning the benefits that accrue from MT, and that these can be explained thorough fairly simple and perhaps familiar terms, some of which are also embedded in other therapeutic modalities.

First Principle: Recognition of the Components of Experience

The construction of the experience of ourselves and the world begins in childhood in the realm of sensation and affect, while development of the cognitive component is gradual, implicit, and incremental (Blair, 2002). As development proceeds, these components become so fully integrated that the distinction between them is not apparent to our usual awareness (Pessoa, 2008). This blindness to the components, and the conditioned cycles of association they form, represents one face of the ignorance at the root of suffering referred to in the Buddhist narrative. This is not willful neglect but lack of recognition of how our experience is being created from moment to moment through the conditioned patterns we have acquired and the behaviors we are acting out—a condition that can result in feelings of helplessness in the face of ongoing mental distress.

It can metaphorically be compared to the kind of ignorance fish have about water. If it were possible to ask a talking fish about the water in which it lives, it would very likely respond, "What's water?" The fish can see objects in the water, but the water itself is less visible because the fish has never known any other perceptual medium. In relation to the apparently seamless components comprising experience, and their background of awareness, we are in a position similar to that of the fish. For while the effects of one or another overt behavior or cognition on our life may be more or less apparent, the more subtle conditioned associations forming the core of everyday experience that began before we had the capacity to reflect often remain unperceived. This undifferentiated experience that can lead to distress is illustrated in Figure 4.1. It is often the place at which people come to MT, or into psychotherapy—recognizing that life is not working in a way they find satisfactory, but not fully aware of the role their mental processes are playing in creating or maintaining the situation.

The challenge in the psychoeducational and therapeutic encounter then becomes: How does a person learn about the mental environment in which he or she lives? One way draws upon classical Greek philosophy, a method of investigation that was

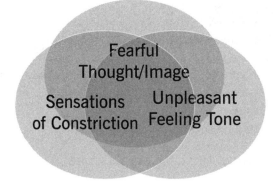

Patient reports:
"I feel tense/anxious/stressed/uptight all the time . . ."

FIGURE 4.1. When the components of experience are undifferentiated, it appears seamless and the cycle of distress is maintained.

developing around the same time that mindfulness-based inquiry was developing in another part of the world. The classical Greek approach is concerned with the use of reason to investigate underlying principles in observed phenomena. In the present context, it is the dynamics of the person's cognitions and beliefs, and whether they are moving the person toward a satisfying life. Therapy may involve helping to uncover and recognize the implicit narrative that the cognitions form, and working to resolve conflicts embedded in the narrative, as in Freudian and other psychodynamic psychotherapies; or it may concern itself with the identification of dysfunctional elements, such as self-defeating or irrational thoughts and behaviors, and the replacement of them with more functional ones. This approach is well developed in cognitive-behavioral therapy (CBT).

In contrast, MT is less concerned with the content of dysfunctional cognitions than with the experiential recognition of how all felt experience is constructed through the normally perceptually undifferentiated components (thoughts, sensations, and pleasant/unpleasant/neutral feeling tone), and the mental dynamics by which those components coalesce from moment to moment to create both functional and dysfunctional responses. This recognition results first from curiosity about these processes and then practice of the mindfulness exercises that bring close attention to, and discriminate between, the components of experience.

Support for the experiential recognition of these processes can be seen in what is usually the initial MT exercise taught in mindfulness-based stress reduction (MBSR; Kabat-Zinn, 1990), known as the *body scan*. In this exercise, the trainee is asked to direct attention systematically to each part of the body and to notice any sensations that may be present there, including the more subtle and neglected sensations escaping awareness in everyday life, while refraining from the attempt to change them in any way. This bare noticing represents an implicit acceptance of the experience. The instructions also ask the trainee to notice the difference between the sensations, and any thoughts and pleasant or unpleasant feeling tone associated with them. In endeavoring to keep attention on the bodily sensations, the trainee typically notices that it does not stay there, and through an awareness of which components attention goes to, such as thoughts about the sensation or its feeling tone, the trainee learns to distinguish between the three major components of experience, and their conditioned cycles of associations become apparent. This is illustrated in Figure 4.2. This

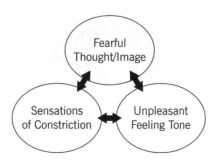

FIGURE 4.2. Components of experience recognized as differentiated and connected. Opportunity arises for self-regulation.

recognition is sometimes supported by encouraging a basic naming of the component in focal attention as a thought, sensation, or feeling.

Second Principle: Emotional Arousal Can Be Self-Regulated through Attention Regulation

Arousal tends to follow the valence of the object of attention—whether the object has positive, negative, or neutral emotional associations. This, too, becomes experientially apparent through the body scan exercise, when the first area of sensations to which the instructions direct attention are those associated with breathing—sensations that, for the most part, are an arousal-neutral object of attention and so associated with a benign affective state. This facility, often referred to as "awareness of the breath," is established at the outset because it provides readily available access to a more calming experience to which one can return in moments of stress.

As practice proceeds, the trainee becomes more aware of those experiential objects to which attention is characteristically drawn, and also becomes aware that attention itself can be better regulated through training. By learning to notice which component(s) of experience attention is focused on at any given moment, the trainee can choose to keep it there or to redirect it to a more arousal-neutral perceptual object. Now, instead of passively allowing the usually automatic cycle of associations maintaining distress to occupy attention, the trainee has the option of interrupting cycles when they are not productive, by deliberately redirecting attention to an arousal-neutral object, such as the sensations of breathing, thereby creating greater calm. Self-reports of a large majority of MBSR trainees indicate that they attach high importance to this simple attention redirection skill in moments of stress/distress (Kabat-Zinn, 1987). Figure 4.3 illustrates how the regulation of attention creates an opportunity for some internal control in the face of stress and distress. This redirection of attention can be distinguished from experiential avoidance, which involves a compulsive mental (or physical) turning away from difficult experiences (Hayes, Wilson, Gifford, Follette, & Strosahl, 1996).

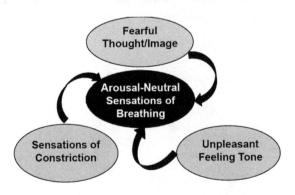

FIGURE 4.3. Cycle maintaining distress is interrupted by self-regulation of attention from differentiated components to arousal-neutral sensations of breathing.

Third Principle: The Development of a Decentered Perspective

The recognition that the thought/image, sensation, and feeling components of experience are simply events occurring in awareness is also implicitly developed through this process. It has been referred to as *decentering* (Segal et al., 2002) and *metacognition* (Bishop et al., 2004), and suggests the development of an "observing self" (Deikman, 1982) that notices experiential processes occurring but is apparently separable from them. This principle is illustrated in Figure 4.4, using as an example a thought commonly reported during panic attacks.

These three principles all center on the process of attending to experience, and their role in MT is supported by three lines of evidence. Consistent with the first principle, while MT participants initially report finding mindfulness exercises challenging (Segal et al., 2002), studies of MT effects on attention processes show an increase in volitional orienting of attention (Chan & Woollacott, 2007; Jha, Krompinger, & Baime, 2007) and improved performance on sustained attention tasks (Lutz et al., 2009); performance on such tasks has also been related to length of mindfulness practice experience (Valentine & Sweet, 1999). Brain imaging studies also show that the default processes of attending are amenable to change with MT (Brewer et al., 2011; Chiesa & Serretti, 2010; Hölzel et al., 2010). Consistent with the second principle, MT has been shown to reduce self-reported rumination (e.g., Campbell, Labelle, Bacon, Faris, & Carlson, 2012), an indicator of attention uncomfortably wandering from immediate tasks to become captivated by the internal narrative. MT program graduates also show less activation of brain regions involved in narrative processing of self-relevant stimuli and greater activation of regions implicated in "experiential" processing, relative to novices (Farb et al., 2007). Finally, and consistent with the third principle, decentering appears to increase with participation in MT programs (Carmody Baer, Lykins, & Olendzki, 2009; Feldman, Greeson, & Senville, 2010; Teasdale et al., 2002), although such change has not yet been shown to predict stress and distress-related outcomes.

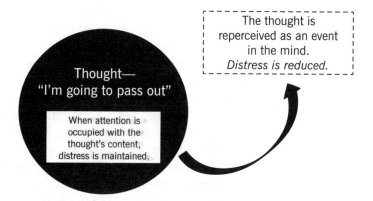

FIGURE 4.4. Reperceiving reduces distress through a perceptual/attentional shift from what the thought is about—"I'm going to pass out"—to "This is a thought." The thought is recognized as an event in the mind/awareness.

While these conceptually straightforward principles of attending can form a use-ful foundation for a clinical explanation of MT and its benefits to well-being, simply describing them does not appear sufficient to evoke changes in habits of attending; the biological and learning-based imperatives driving attention are of such strength as to require experiential practice to derive benefits (Carmody & Baer, 2008). How much MT and mindfulness practice is required for significant benefit remains an open question. The typical 30- to 45-minute daily practice periods in MBSR and related programs have been assumed to be the necessary amount, but studies (e.g., Tang et al., 2007, 2009; see also Tang & Posner, Chapter 5, this volume) indicate that much shorter instruction and practice time is enough to produce positive neurobio-logical changes and subjectively perceived benefits, at least over the very short-term periods in which outcomes have been measured.

Commonality and Uniqueness of Mindfulness with Other Clinical Trainings

Identifying the psychological principles of attending embedded in MT reveals those features that are unique to mindfulness, and also the degree to which the principles and practices are shared with other therapeutic programs. The first principle, in which MT allows participants to recognize and discriminate between the compo-nents that aggregate to form mental constructions and their conditioned associations, is not unique to MT. CBT, for example, focuses on the recognition of self-defeating thoughts/beliefs and their downstream effects in the patient's life, and progressive muscle relaxation is largely an exercise in noticing sensations, similar to the body scan exercise. Mindfulness training is unique, however, in the completeness of the deconstruction of the components, its focus on rediscovering the broader realm of sensation rather than just those associated with the musculature, and in the accep-tance of experience that is implicit in refraining from the attempt to change the thoughts, sensations, and feelings that are noticed in the training exercises.

The second principle, in which patients recognize that arousal levels follow the valence of the object of attention, together with the possibility of redirecting atten-tion to more arousal-neutral objects, is common to a number of other therapeutic and mind–body systems. So while attention to the sensations of breathing, or the broader sensory realm serves this function in MT, other therapeutic programs and religious practices promote the use of other arousal-neutral (or affectively positive) atten-tional objects, such as mantras, prayers, affirmations, visualizations, statements of self-compassion, and so forth. Deliberately bringing attention to one of these affect-neutral/positive mental objects achieves a similar purpose to that of MT by interrupt-ing the internal monologue and the cycle of conditioned components maintaining distress, with purportedly positive effects on felt experience. The third principle, the development of decentering, is implicit also in CBT but the generalizable attention training exercises of MT facilitate decentering in a way that CBT's focus on dysfunc-tional cognitive content likely truncates.

Probably the most unique contributions that MT has introduced to clinical and community-based programs are in the training exercises themselves. For despite the centrality of attention regulation to well-being (Posner & Rothbart, 2007), Western therapeutic systems have not developed intensive attention training exercises. MT has most fruitfully filled this gap through the support that the exercises provide in actualizing important qualities of attending, with the consequent positive psychological changes that support mental health in everyday life.

Clinical and Scientific Advantages in Reconceptualizing Mindfulness and MT

Conceptualizing mindfulness and its training in the way I have presented here has a number of scientific and clinical advantages. First, basing it on the phenomenology of the activities involved in typical MT exercises honors the roots of mindfulness and its training without being caught in deliberations on what is "true" mindfulness or arguments about the wisdom embedded in orthodoxy. Second, placing the habits of attention in an evolutionary frame and employing familiar psychological principles and constructs about attention training takes advantage of Western scientific advances, and embeds the problem of suffering within the ecology of a mind that has developed over millenia to serve ancestral human needs. As such, it can provide a modern frame for people in both therapeutic and psychoeducational settings to better understand the everyday working of the mind and its propensity toward suffering, why changing its functioning is such a challenge, and how MT may help in meeting this challenge. Understanding that these mental tendencies are working for the person's benefit means they can be regarded as processes to be reguided rather than an enemy to be grappled with, and so can foster patience in working with them when they are encountered in MT.

A third advantage of portraying MT as an integrated collection of attending-related trainings is that the problem of psychological suffering and healing is approached through the more general question: What qualities of attending to experience are associated with well-being and the reduction of distress? Focusing on common therapeutic processes in this way rather than the uniqueness of MT improves our understanding of the more general psychological processes by which distress is created and maintained. As such, it encourages development of a unified theory of the mechanisms by which mind–body and other therapeutic programs have their beneficial effects that, in turn, provides a conceptual foundation for informed innovation and adaptation of treatments for specific conditions. Also important is framing MT and other attending-based trainings in simple, familiar, and empirically supported terms that provide a basis for a coherent explanation of the training to patients that can be adapted to their individual circumstances, temperament, and education level.

Challenges to Reconceptualizing Mindfulness and MT

A number of pressures work against a Western psychological science-based conceptualization such as this. When mindfulness fulfills a quasi-religious function, there is the understandable impulse to emphasize and demonstrate the uniqueness of the phenomenon and the training exercises. In this respect, the term *mindfulness* may have become problematic to the degree that it is seen as a way of being that requires a singular training that is fundamentally different from other therapeutic constructs and modalities. Furthermore, competition for research funding dollars, and the maintenance of enterprises and organizations in the self-help and therapeutic marketplace, may depend on their offerings being seen as unique. These pressures can lead to conceptual silos, and the parallels and overlap that MT, the relaxation response, transcendental meditation, tai chi, yoga, CBT, and other interventions have with one another tend not to be made apparent. The effect on research of this pressure to highlight the uniqueness of each modality is evident in the small number of trials that directly compare these therapeutic programs and their mechanisms. Approaching intervention research in this way impedes progress in understanding and does a disservice to prospective participants and therapists by presenting them with a potentially confusing array of treatment options and no clear conceptual basis to choose among them.

A focus on psychological processes also faces pressure from the contention that its dependence on evidence from self-report instruments makes it scientifically "soft" compared to the deceptively "hard" science of biochemical (e.g., Daubenmier et al., 2012) and neural (e.g., Hölzel et al., 2011) approaches to understanding the effects of this or that program. While neurobiological studies are a rich source of knowledge about the biological correlates of MT, and provide value in addressing questions about therapeutic mechanisms, the view that they are fundamentally more objective—and by implication more scientifically and clinically useful—than psychological studies is not necessarily accurate. For even the most sophisticated brain imaging studies of mindfulness-related trainings rely ultimately upon subjects' self-reports of their adherence and fidelity to the training, or that they are generating a particular mental state while in the scanner. Subjects' understanding of their training will also be idiosyncratic, and training modalities will have unique neurobiological effects associated with their regimens not necessarily related to cognitive and emotional benefits.

Identifying neurobiological treatment mechanisms is likely to be a long and challenging endeavor, and giving such outcomes primacy may result in a view that biological explanations are the only empirically useful ones. But it is the intimacy of the psychological that brings people to enroll in psychoeducational and therapeutic programs, not their complaints about, for example, a poverty of amygdala–prefrontal cortical connections. A focus on psychological mechanisms that address phenomenological processes using constructs familiar in everyday experience can provide a more meaningful and accessible explanation about how MT and other interventions work to reduce distress than does a biological or neural narrative. As such, the psychological approach is more likely to be immediately profitable in harnessing participants' motivation to change and their understanding about how it can be done.

Conclusions

Conceptualizing mindfulness, and training in it, through the lens of evolutionary theory, the processes of attending, and familiar psychological principles can illustrate how the lack of ease in everyday life results from a biological imperative, separable from patients' particular personal circumstances. An evolutionary approach recognizes human attentional tendencies as part of a mental ecology that steadfastly, if sometimes unhelpfully, works to meet our needs. This understanding may foster patience in working with these tendencies by regarding them as processes to be reguided rather than an enemy with which to grapple. Though attention regulation is central to well-being and other valued outcomes (Posner & Rothbart, 2007), mainstream Western therapeutic modalities rarely used exercises to cultivate attention skills—a gap that MT can fill to great effect in supporting adaptive functioning (see Parts IV and V of this volume). Focusing on the underlying principles of MT that are associated with well-being provides both an opportunity to simplify treatment descriptions and explanations, and common ground for better understanding the conceptual overlaps relative to the role of attending, for example, that may exist across a variety of therapeutic approaches. In the end, this can only benefit those in need.

REFERENCES

Andrews-Hanna, J. R. (2012). The brain's default network and its adaptive role in internal mentation. *Neuroscientist, 18*(3), 251–270.

Baer, R., Carmody, J., & Hunsinger, M. (2012). Weekly change in mindfulness and perceived stress in a mindfulness-based stress reduction program. *Journal of Clinical Psychology, 68*(7), 755–765.

Baum, C., Kuyken, W., Bohus, M., Heidenreich, T., Michalak, J., & Steil, R. (2010). The psychometric properties of the Kentucky Inventory of Mindfulness Skills in clinical populations. *Assessment, 17*(2), 220–229.

Baumeister, R. F., & Heatherton, T. F. (1996). Self-regulation failure: An overview. *Psychological Inquiry, 7*(1), 1–15.

Bishop, S., Lau, M., Shapiro, S., Carlson, L., Anderson, N. D., Carmody, J., et al. (2004). Mindfulness: A proposed operational definition. *Clinical Psychology: Science and Practice, 11*(3), 230–241.

Blair, C. (2002). School readiness: Integrating cognition and emotion in a neurobiological conceptualization of children's functioning at school entry. *American Psychologist, 57*(2), 111–127.

Brewer, J. A., Worhunsky, P. D., Gray, J. R., Tang, Y. Y., Weber, J., & Kober, H. (2011). Meditation experience is associated with differences in default mode network activity and connectivity. *Proceedings of the National Academy of Sciences, 108*(50), 20254–20259.

Brown, K. W., & Ryan, R. M. (2004). Perils and promise in defining and measuring mindfulness: Observations from experience. *Clinical Psychology: Science and Practice, 11*(3), 242–248.

Brown, K. W., Ryan, R. M., Loverich, T. M., Biegel, G. M., & West, A. M. (2011). Out of the armchair and into the streets: Measuring mindfulness advances knowledge and improves interventions: Reply to Grossman (2011). *Psychological Assessment, 23*(4), 1041–1046.

Brown, K. W., West, A. M., Loverich, T. M., & Biegel, G. M. (2011). Assessing adolescent mindfulness: Validation of an adapted Mindful Attention Awareness Scale in adolescent normative and psychiatric populations. *Psychological Assessment, 23*(4), 1023–1033.

Campbell, T. S., Labelle, L. E., Bacon, S. L., Faris, P., & Carlson, L. E. (2012). Impact of mindfulness-based stress reduction (MBSR) on attention, rumination and resting blood pressure in women with cancer: A waitlist-controlled study. *Journal of Behavioral Medicine, 35*(3), 262–271.

Carmody, J., & Baer, R. A. (2008). Relationships between mindfulness practice and levels of mindfulness, medical and psychological symptoms and well-being in a mindfulness-based stress reduction program. *Journal of Behavioral Medicine, 31*(1), 23–33.

Carmody, J., & Baer, R. A. (2009). How long does a mindfulness-based stress reduction program need to be?: A review of class contact hours and effect sizes for psychological distress. *Journal of Clinical Psychology, 65*(6), 627–638.

Carmody, J., Baer, R. A., Lykins, E. L. B., & Olendzki, N. (2009). An empirical study of the mechanisms of mindfulness in a mindfulness-based stress reduction program. *Journal of Clinical Psychology, 65*(6), 613–626.

Chan, D., & Woollacott, M. (2007). Effects of level of meditation experience on attentional focus: Is the efficiency of executive or orientation networks improved? *Journal of Alternative and Complementary Medicine, 13*(6), 651–658.

Chiesa, A., & Serretti, A. (2009). Mindfulness-based stress reduction for stress management in healthy people: A review and meta-analysis. *Journal of Alternative and Complementary Medicine, 15*, 593–600.

Chiesa, A., & Serretti, A. (2010). A systematic review of neurobiological and clinical features of mindfulness meditations. *Psychological Medicine, 40*(8), 1239–1252.

Daubenmier, J., Lin, J., Blackburn, E., Hecht, F. M., Kristeller, J., Maninger, N., et al. (2012). Changes in stress, eating, and metabolic factors are related to changes in telomerase activity in a randomized mindfulness intervention pilot study. *Psychoneuroendocrinology, 37*(7), 917–928.

Deikman, A. J. (1982). *The observing self.* Boston: Beacon Press.

Farb, N. A. S., Segal, Z. V., Mayberg, H., Bean, J., McKeon, D., Fatima, Z., et al. (2007). Attending to the present: Mindfulness meditation reveals distinct neural modes of self-reference. *Social Cognitive and Affective Neuroscience, 2*(4), 313–322.

Feldman, G., Greeson, J., & Senville, J. (2010). Differential effects of mindful breathing, progressive muscle relaxation, and loving-kindness meditation on decentering and negative reactions to repetitive thoughts. *Behaviour Research and Therapy, 48*(10), 1002–1011.

Gluck, T. M., & Maercker, A. (2011). A randomized controlled pilot study of a brief web-based mindfulness training. *BMC Psychiatry, 11*(1), 175.

Grossman, P. (2008). On measuring mindfulness in psychosomatic and psychological research. *Journal of Psychosomatic Research, 64*(4), 405–408.

Grossman, P. (2011). Defining mindfulness by how poorly I think I pay attention during everyday awareness and other intractable problems for psychology's (re)invention of mindfulness: Comment on Brown et al. (2011). *Psychological Assessment, 23*(4), 1034–1040.

Hayes, S. C., Wilson, K. G., Gifford, E. V., Follette, V. M., & Strosahl, K. (1996). Experiential avoidance and behavioral disorders: A functional dimensional approach to diagnosis and treatment. *Journal of Consulting and Clinical Psychology, 64*(6), 1152–1168.

Hofmann, S. G., Sawyer, A. T., Witt, A. A., & Oh, D. (2010). The effect of mindfulness-based therapy on anxiety and depression: A meta-analytic review. *Journal of Consulting and Clinical Psychology, 78*(2), 169–183.

Hölzel, B. K., Carmody, J., Evans, K. C., Hoge, E. A., Dusek, J. A., Morgan, L., et al. (2010). Stress reduction correlates with structural changes in the amygdala. *Social Cognitive and Affective Neuroscience, 5*(1), 11–17.

Hölzel, B. K., Lazar, S. W., Gard, T., Schuman-Olivier, Z., Vago, D. R., & Ott, U. (2011). How does mindfulness meditation work?: Proposing mechanisms of action from a conceptual and neural perspective. *Perspectives on Psychological Science, 6*(6), 537–559.

Irving, J. A., Dobkin, P. L., & Park, J. (2009). Cultivating mindfulness in health care professionals: A review of empirical studies of mindfulness-based stress reduction (MBSR). *Complementary Therapies in Clinical Practice, 15*(2), 61–66.

Jain, S., Shapiro, S. L., Swanick, S., Roesch, S. C., Mills, P. J., Bell, I., et al. (2007). A randomized controlled trial of mindfulness meditation versus relaxation training: Effects on distress, positive states of mind, rumination, and distraction. *Annals of Behavioral Medicine, 33*(1), 11–21.

James, W. (1890). *The principles of psychology.* New York: Holt.

Jha, A., Krompinger, J., & Baime, M. J. (2007). Mindfulness training modifies subsystems of attention. *Cognitive Affective and Behavioral Neuroscience, 7*(2), 109–119.

Kabat-Zinn, J. (1990). *Full catastrophe living.* New York: Bantam Doubleday Dell.

Kabat-Zinn, J. (1994). *Wherever you go, there you are.* New York: Hyperion.

Keverne, E. B., & Curley, J. P. (2008). Epigenetics, brain evolution and behaviour. *Frontiers in Neuroendocrinology, 29*(3), 398–412.

Killingsworth, M. A., & Gilbert, D. T. (2010). A wandering mind is an unhappy mind. *Science, 330*, 932.

Kirschenbaum, D. S. (1987). Self-regulatory failure: A review with clinical implications. *Clinical Psychology Review, 7*(1), 77–104.

Kuyken, W., Watkins, E., Holden, E., White, K., Taylor, R. S., Evans, A., et al. (2010). How does mindfulness-based cognitive therapy work? *Behaviour Research and Therapy, 48*(11), 1105–1112.

Lutz, A., Slagter, H. A., Rawlings, N. B., Francis, A. D., Greischar, L. L., & Davidson, R. J. (2009). Mental training enhances attentional stability: Neural and behavioral evidence. *Journal of Neuroscience, 29*, 13418–13427.

Pbert, L., Madison, J. M., Druker, S., Olendzki, N., Magner, R., Reed, G., et al. (2012). Effect of mindfulness training on asthma quality of life and lung function: A randomised controlled trial. *Thorax, 67*(9), 769–776.

Pessoa, L. (2008). On the relationship between emotion and cognition. *Nature Reviews Neuroscience, 9*(2), 148–158.

Posner, M. I., & Rothbart, M. K. (2007). Research on attention networks as a model for the integration of psychological science. *Annual Review of Psychology, 58*, 1–23.

Rapgay, L., & Bystrisky, A. (2009). Classical mindfulness. *Annals of the New York Academy of Sciences, 1172*(1), 148–162.

Segal, Z. V., Williams, J. M. G., & Teasdale, J. D. (2002). *Mindfulness-based cognitive therapy for depression: A new approach to preventing relapse.* New York: Guilford Press.

Shelov, D. V., Suchday, S., & Friedberg, J. P. (2009). A pilot study measuring the impact of yoga on the trait of mindfulness. *Behavioural and Cognitive Psychotherapy, 37*(5), 595–598.

Tang, Y., Ma, Y., Fan, Y., Feng, H., Wang, J., Feng, S., et al. (2009). Central and autonomic nervous system interaction is altered by short-term meditation. *Proceedings of the National Academy of Sciences USA, 106*, 8865–8870.

Tang, Y., Ma, Y., Wang, J., Fan, Y., Feng, S., Lu, Q., et al. (2007). Short-term meditation training improves attention and self-regulation. *Proceedings of the National Academy of Sciences USA, 104*, 17152–17156.

Tanner, M. A., Travis, F., Gaylord-King, C., Haaga, D. A. F., Grosswald, S., & Schneider, R. H. (2009). The effects of the transcendental meditation program on mindfulness. *Journal of Clinical Psychology, 65*(6), 574–589.

Teasdale, J. D., Moore, R. G., Hayhurst, H., Pope, M., Williams, S., & Segal, Z. V. (2002). Metacognitive awareness and prevention of relapse in depression: Empirical evidence. *Journal of Consulting and Clinical Psychology, 70*(2), 275–287.

Thayer, J. A., Friedman, B. H., & Borkovec, T. D. (1996). Autonomic characteristics of generalized anxiety disorder and worry. *Society of Behavioral Psychiatry, 39*, 255–266.

Valentine, E. R., & Sweet, P. L. G. (1999). Meditation and attention: A comparison of the effects of concentrative and mindfulness meditation on sustained attention. *Mental Health, Religion and Culture, 2*(1), 59–70.

PART II

MINDFULNESS IN THE CONTEXT OF CONTEMPORARY PSYCHOLOGICAL THEORY

CHAPTER 5

Mindfulness in the Context of the Attention System

Yi-Yuan Tang and Michael I. Posner

In research and clinical contexts, *mindfulness* is often defined as nonjudgmental attention to experiences in the present moment (Kabat-Zinn, 1990). Despite the centrality of attention in mindfulness, very little research has examined how mindfulness is expressed in terms of the well-studied networks of attention. This is an important issue because it bears on the meaning of mindfulness and its relation to the components of the attention system, the framing of scientific hypotheses about mindfulness, and the interpretations of research findings about it. In this chapter, we discuss the place of mindfulness in the context of the attention system, particularly drawing upon recent evidence of changes in attention networks after mindfulness training.

The Networks of the Attention System

We begin with a brief overview of the neurally mediated components of the attention system. Three attentional networks have been defined in both functional and anatomical terms. The functions involve alerting, orienting, and executive attention (Petersen & Posner, 2012). *Alerting* concerns an alert state of vigilance to impending stimuli. It involves a network of brain regions that are modulated by noradrenaline. The source of the brain's noradrenaline is the locus coeruleus, a clump of cells in the midbrain. The *orienting* network involves the selection of information from sensory inputs and involves several cortical brain areas, including the frontal eye fields, the superior parietal lobe and the temporal parietal junction, as well as the superior colliculus and pulvinar, which are subcortical areas. Finally, executive control of attention, or simply, *executive attention*, involves more complex mental operations that

81

monitor and resolve conflict between mental activities (Bush, Luu, & Posner, 2000). This network involves the anterior cingulate cortex (ACC), areas of the prefrontal cortex, the anterior insula, and part of the basal ganglia (Petersen & Posner, 2012).

The efficiency of each of these three networks can be measured by the Attention Network Test (ANT; Fan, McCandliss, Sommer, Raz, & Posner, 2002). By *efficiency*, we refer to not only the speed and accuracy of carrying out the network functions, as measured by the ANT, but also the underlying activation of the brain areas involved and their connectivity; this has been studied through brain imaging while carrying out the ANT (Fan, McCandliss, Fossella, Flombaum, & Posner, 2005). The ANT uses a flanker task to introduce conflict between the target and surrounds to measure executive attention, and uses precues to measure alerting and orienting. Reaction times in different conditions are subtracted from each other to measure the efficiency of the three networks (Fan & Posner, 2004). Executive attention operations are also measured by other conflict tasks that require a person to withhold a dominant response in order to perform a subdominant response (Posner & Rothbart, 2007), such as various versions of the Stroop task (Bush et al., 2000). Neuroimaging research has shown that the ANT activates the anatomical areas for alerting, orienting, and executive networks described earlier. These results also suggest anatomically separate networks related to the three functions of attention (Fan et al., 2005).

Executive Attention and Self-Regulation

Executive attention, and executive attention neural networks, may be a central attention-based mechanism of mindfulness. In a recent review, Hölzel and colleagues (2011) proposed that mindfulness meditation includes at least four mechanisms through which it has its effects: (1) attention regulation; (2) body awareness; (3) emotion regulation; and (4) change in perspective on the self. Executive attention may shape how each of these mechanistic pathways unfolds: Executive attention may foster one's ability to control one's attention (attention regulation), to maintain attention on the body (body awareness) and on the self (change in self-perspective), and to facilitate emotion regulation. We return to the evidence on mindfulness and the effect of mindfulness training on executive attention in the next section, but here we aim to draw a broader link to executive attention and self-regulation. Specifically, executive attention may describe the general capacity to self-regulate one's behavior (e.g., Carver & Scheier, 2011).

Self-regulation concerns the ability to control one's own cognition, emotion, and behavior so as to direct behavior toward internal or external goals. We propose that executive attention is particularly important to self-regulation. The correlation between the efficiency of the executive attention network and parental ratings on their child's self-regulatory ability provides support for this idea (Rothbart, 2011). The ACC appears to play a key role in self-regulation. Functional imaging studies show that the ACC is active in many studies of functional imaging, especially during executive attention and self-regulation tasks (e.g., Posner, Rothbart, Sheese, & Tang, 2007). The sensitivity of the ACC to both reward and pain, and evidence for ACC coupling (functional connectivity) to cognitive and emotional areas during task performance support this identification.

Self-regulation is a very broad concept and provides a framework for examining the role of the executive attention network in development (Posner & Rothbart, 2007). In our work we have examined how genes and experience influence the development of brain networks of attention (Posner & Rothbart, 2007). The orienting network is present in infancy and appears to serve as the main control network through interaction with caregivers (Posner, Rothbart, Sheese, & Voelker, 2012). The executive network is present at least by age 7 months (Berger, Tzur, & Posner, 2006) but undergoes a long developmental process during which long connections to remote brain areas develop (Fair et al., 2007). From late childhood, the executive network provides the major means of control, but the orienting network remains involved in the control of looking behavior (Posner et al., 2012).

Both parenting and specific kinds of attention training are useful in improving the efficiency of the executive attention network (Posner & Rothbart, 2007). Adapting computerized training programs used to train monkeys for NASA experiments (Rueda, Rothbart, McCandliss, Saccamanno, & Posner, 2005), Rueda and colleagues (2005; Rueda, Checa, & Cómbita, 2012) have found that the programs improved the efficiency of the executive attention network and also generalized to changes in IQ and ability to delay reward. In summary, executive attention network plays a key role in executive control and self-regulation, which also supports the mental process of mindfulness (Tang & Posner, 2009).

Attention Networks and Mindfulness Training

All accounts of mindfulness implicate attention as a central feature; after all, mindfulness is about turning attention from thoughts about the past or the future toward the direct experience of the present moment (Tang & Posner, 2009). The centrality of attention is also present in all forms of meditation practice. For example, focused attention (FA) forms of meditation require one to focus attention voluntarily on a chosen object in a sustained way (Lutz, Slagter, Dunne, & Davidson, 2008). But it is also true in the other major category of meditation, namely, open-monitoring (OM) practices, which more explicitly aim to foster mindfulness and involve nonreactively monitoring the content of experience from moment to moment (Lutz et al., 2008). This monitoring process involves vigilance for distractions that can pull attention away from present moment experience (e.g., becoming lost in thought), and disengaging attention from those stimuli to return attention to one's object(s) of meditation. Examining these two types of meditation in the context of the three attention networks, it appears that both FA and OM particularly involve the executive, and to a degree, the alerting networks of attention (Tang, Rothbart, & Posner, 2012).

To test this proposition, several studies have been conducted. For example, comparing graduates of an 8-week mindfulness-based stress reduction (MBSR) program to wait-listed control participants, Farb, Segal, and Anderson (2013) found that mindfulness training improved interoceptive awareness, which appears to be related to alerting attention (Matthias, Schandry, Duschek, & Pollatos, 2009). In another study (Jha, Krompinger, & Baime, 2007), MBSR course graduates were compared to individuals experienced in concentrative (FA) meditation who participated in a 1-month intensive mindfulness retreat, and to meditation-naive control participants. The experienced meditators before retreat training demonstrated better conflict-monitoring performance relative to the MBSR and control groups. However, the MBSR graduates showed significantly higher orienting performance in comparison with the control and experienced, postretreat groups. In contrast, the experienced, postretreat group demonstrated better performance on the alerting component, with improvements in exogenous stimulus detection in comparison with the two groups.

In our work, we have applied one form of mindfulness-based meditation, integrative body–mind training (IBMT; Tang et al., 2007) that originates from an ancient Eastern contemplative tradition and involves body relaxation, mental imagery, and mindfulness training. Jha and colleagues' (2007) findings are consistent with one of our studies indicating that 1 month of IBMT (10 hours in total) improved the efficiency of executive attention and also alertness, as measured by the ANT (Tang, Rothbart, et al., 2012). In comparison with a book listening control group, the group receiving 4 days of meditation training was shown to exhibit enhanced ability to sustain attention—benefits that had previously been reported with long-term meditators (Zeidan, Johnson, Diamond, David, & Goolkasian, 2010).

In another study (Tang et al., 2007), Chinese undergraduates were randomly assigned to an experimental group (IBMT) or a control group (relaxation training) for 5 days of short-term training (20 minutes per day). The IBMT group showed significantly greater improvement of performance in executive attention, as measured by the ANT. They also reported lower anxiety, depression, anger and fatigue, and higher vigor on the Profile of Mood States (POMS; Shacham, 1983). In addition we found that after a stressful task, IBMT participants showed significantly reduced stress responses, as measured by salivary cortisol secretion, and increased immunoreactivity, as measured by salivary immunoglobulin A (IgA) (Tang et al., 2007).

Research has also examined how developing expertise in mindfulness meditation alters the involvement of the attention networks. We believe not only in the early stages of practice but also in the middle stages of expertise development, trainees must exert an appropriate degree of effort to deal with distractions and the wandering mind. Effort involves the subjective experience of striving for a goal and is one of a cluster of motivational concepts involved in task performance (Posner, Rothbart, Rueda, & Tang, 2010). Effortful regulation of attention may be expected to involve the executive attention network. It may be also possible that this capacity to keep bringing attention back (when it wanders) to a meditative object trains the orienting attention network, as shown in one mindfulness training study (Jha et al., 2007).

As Figure 5.1 illustrates, neuroimaging research has shown that high effort on a task (voluntary control) recruits the executive attention network, including the lateral prefrontal cortex (LPFC) and parietal cortex (PC) (Petersen & Posner, 2012). One potentially interesting observation that comes from the emerging mindful attention literature is that attentional effort may moderate neural activity in attention networks. Studies of trainees in the early stages of mindfulness training (both FA and

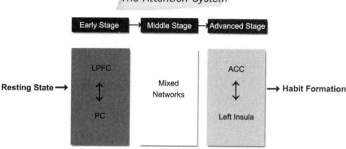

FIGURE 5.1. Early, intermediate, and advanced stages of meditation involving different neural networks. From Tang, Rothbart, and Posner (2012). Reprinted with permission from Elsevier.

OM) indicate that these same regions are engaged, namely, higher activations in the LPFC and PC areas (Farb et al., 2007; Tang, Rothbart, et al., 2012). In the middle stage of practice, the participant exerts the appropriate effort to deal with distractions and the wandering mind, which would be expected to continue to involve executive control networks. Varying the degree of effort during state transitions may involve different attentional networks (Jensen, Vangkilde, Frokjaer, & Hasselbalch, 2012; Petersen, van Mier, Fiez, & Raichle, 1998). If practitioners exert strong attentional control to achieve the meditative state, these same attentional networks are active (Brefczynski-Lewis, Lutz, Schaefer, Levinson, & Davidson, 2007; Farb et al., 2007; Tang et al., 2009). When less effort is required to maintain present-focused attention, such as in the advanced stage of meditation, there is less activity in the portions of the executive network related to mental effort (Hölzel et al., 2011; Tang, Rothbart, et al., 2012); instead the meditative state (FA or OM) is maintained by activity in the ACC and striatum (see Figure 5.1), mainly related to autonomic or/and emotional control (Tang, Rothbart, et al., 2012). Connections among the ACC, striatum, and the autonomic nervous system are also enhanced by mindfulness training and are potentially important in achieving a state of parasympathetic dominance (i.e., a relaxation response). Thus, this interaction between brain and body may help to maintain the meditative state and promote relaxation (Tang et al., 2009).

It bears noting that IBMT stresses minimal or no effort to control thoughts, and the achievement of a state of restful alertness that allows a high degree of awareness and balance of the body, mind, and environment. The meditation state is facilitated through training and trainer–group dynamics, harmony, and resonance. Whether different training strategies, meditation styles (FA or OM), or levels of effort engage the attention networks differently warrant further investigation (Hölzel et al., 2011; Tang, Rothbart, et al., 2012).

Recent research has also sought to examine the attention network-related neural *changes* associated with mindfulness training. As mentioned previously, 5 days of IBMT increased brain activity in parts of the executive attention network, namely, the ACC, insula, and striatum (Tang et al., 2009). Using diffusion tensor imaging, several recent studies have shown that training results in changes in white-matter efficiency and integrity as measured by fractional anisotropy. For example, we found that 4 weeks of IBMT training improved fractional anisotropy in areas surrounding the ACC more than relaxation training (Tang et al., 2010), suggesting improved executive attention and self-regulation. We then explored the mechanisms explaining these white-matter changes. Specifically, we tested for reductions in *radial diffusivity* (RD), which has been interpreted as improved myelination, and reductions in *axial diffusivity* (AD), which reflects increased axonal density and other mechanisms (Tang et al., 2010). We found that after 4 weeks of IBMT, both RD and AD decreased in brain areas and accompanied increased fractional anisotropy. This suggested that the improved efficiency of white matter involved increased myelin and other axonal changes. However, after 2 weeks of IBMT, we found only reduced AD, not reduced RD (Tang, Lu, Fan, Yang, & Posner, 2012). This suggested that changes in axonal density occur prior to myelination. Furthermore, Tang, Lu, and colleagues (2012) also found a correlation between AD reduction and improved mood.

Our results demonstrate the time course of white-matter neuroplasticity in short-term meditation. This dynamic pattern of white-matter change involving the ACC, a part of the brain related to executive attention and self-regulation, is somewhat similar to the order of white-matter changes found during child development. Further studies of mindfulness training could provide a means to better understand developmental changes in executive attention, and perhaps lead to interventions to improve attention or prevent attention problems in children and adults (Tang, Lu, et al., 2012). Indeed, initial research suggests that mindfulness training interventions may decrease attention-deficit/ hyperactivity disorder symptomatology in at-risk adolescents (Zylowska et al., 2008).

Integration and Conclusions

In this chapter, we have discussed mindfulness training in terms of the brain's attention system. The training studies reviewed here point to meaningful changes in the executive attention network in particular. Mindfulness training using the IBMT model produced changes in executive attention behavioral performance and changes in activity in brain regions associated with executive attention, particularly in the ACC. Increased connectivity of the ACC to the striatum and other brain areas was also found, indicating that IBMT modulates ACC and striatal circuits. We also have reviewed initial evidence identifying changes in connectivity that may underlie improvements in executive attention associated with mindfulness training, namely, increased white-matter myelination and axonal density.

We also found that the meditative state, and the brain regions identified here, are associated with a dominance of parasympathetic over sympathetic activity in the autonomic nervous system. We believe that this change in autonomic system activity produced through training is critical to the beneficial effects on stress and immune system function that we and other researchers have found (Hölzel et al., 2011; Tang et al., 2007). Stress reduction is likely due, at least in part, to improved executive attention, as represented by more efficient ACC connectivity (Hölzel et al., 2011; Tang, Rothbart, et al., 2012) and to self-regulatory processes that depend on executive attentional control. Further studies may allow us to delineate the importance of various neural markers, including increased functional connectivity, improved axonal density, and increased myelination, for the various behavioral consequences of mindfulness training, including higher alertness, reduced stress, better endocrine and immune responses, and healthy mood profiles, such as reduced negative mood, increased positive mood (Tang, Lu, et al., 2012).

Further investigation of mindfulness training may also be aided by considering it in similar terms to other forms of expertise. For example, it will be useful to understand individual differences in meditative practice and the training-related benefits associated with those differences. One study found that the amount of time participants spent meditating each day, rather than the total number of hours of meditative practice accumulated, was correlated with attention performance as measured by Stroop task (Chan & Woollacott, 2007). Capacities for meditative expertise may also differ between individuals. These differences may be due in part to genetic variations known to influence attention (Posner, Rothbart, & Sheese, 2007). Future studies should be directed toward understanding how a variety of individual differences translate into capacities for mindful attention and the benefits accruing from those capacities.

ACKNOWLEDGMENTS

We are grateful for support by National Institues of Health Grant No. R21DA030066 and the Office of Naval Research Grant No. N000141110034. We thank Rongxiang Tang for manuscript preparation.

REFERENCES

Berger, A., Tzur, G., & Posner, M. I. (2006). Infant babies detect arithmetic error. *Proceedings of the National Academy of Sciences, 103*, 12649–12553.

Brefczynski-Lewis, J. A., Lutz, A., Schaefer, H. S., Levinson, D. B., & Davidson, R. J. (2007). Neural correlates of attentional expertise in long-term meditation practitioners. *Proceedings of the National Academy of Sciences, 104*, 11483–11488.

Bush, G., Luu, P., & Posner, M. I. (2000). Cognitive and emotional influences in the anterior cingulate cortex. *Trends in Cognitive Science, 6*, 215–222.

Carver, C. S., & Scheier, M. F. (2011). Self-regulation of action and affect. In K. D. Vohs & R. F. Baumeister (Eds.), *Handbook of self-regulation: Research, theory, and applications* (2nd ed., pp. 3–21). New York: Guilford Press.

Chambers, R., Gullone, E., & Allen, N. B. (2009). Mindful emotion regulation: An integrative review. *Clinical Psychology Review, 29*, 560–572.

Chan, D., & Woollacott, M. (2007). Effects of level of meditation experience on attentional focus: Is the orientation of executive or orientation networks improved? *Journal of Alternative and Complementary Medicine, 13*, 651–657.

Fair, D. A., Dosenbach, N. U., Church, J. A., Cohen, A. L., Brahmbhatt, S., Miezin, F. M., et al. (2007). Development of distinct control networks through segregation and integration. *Proceedings of the National Academy of Sciences, 104*, 13507–13512.

Fan, J., McCandliss, B. D., Fossella, J., Flombaum, J. I., & Posner, M. I. (2005). The activation of attentional networks. *NeuroImage, 26,* 471–479.

Fan, J., McCandliss, B. D., Sommer, T., Raz, M., & Posner, M. I. (2002). Testing the efficiency and independence of attentional networks. *Journal of Cognitive Neuroscience, 3,* 340–347.

Fan, J., & Posner, M. I. (2004). Human attentional networks. *Psychiatrische Praxis, 31,* S210–S214.

Farb, N. A., Segal, Z. V., & Anderson, A. K. (2013). Mindfulness meditation training alterscortical representations of interoceptive attention. *Social Cognitive and Affective Neuroscience, 8,* 15–26.

Farb, N. A. S., Segal, Z. V., Mayberg, H., Bean, J., McKeon, D., Fatima, Z., et al. (2007). Attending to the present: Mindfulness meditation reveals distinct neural modes of self-reference. *Social Cognitive and Affective Neuroscience, 2,* 313–322.

Hölzel, B. K., Lazar, S. W., Gard, T., Schuman-Olivier, Z., Vago, D. R., & Ott, U. (2011). How does mindfulness meditation work?: Proposing mechanisms of action from a conceptual and neural perspective. *Perspectives on Psychological Science, 6,* 537–559.

Jensen, C. G., Vangkilde, S., Frokjaer, V., & Hasselbalch, S. G. (2012). Mindfulness training affects attention—or is it attentional effort? *Journal of Experimental Psychology: General, 141,* 106–123.

Jha, A. P., Krompinger, J., & Baime, M. J. (2007). Mindfulness training modifies subsystems of attention. *Cognitive, Affective, and Behavioral Neuroscience, 7,* 109–119.

Kabat-Zinn, J. (1990). *Full catastrophe living.* New York: Delta.

Lutz, A., Slagter, H. A., Dunne, J. D., & Davidson, R. J. (2008). Attention regulation and monitoring in meditation. *Trends Cognitive Sciences, 12,* 163–169.

Matthias, E., Schandry, R., Duschek, S., & Pollatos, O. (2009). On the relationship between interoceptive awareness and the attentional processing of visual stimuli. *International Journal of Psychophysiology, 72*(2), 154–159.

Petersen, S. E., & Posner, M. I. (2012). The attention system of the human brain: 20 years after. *Annual Review of Neuroscience, 35,* 73–89.

Petersen, S. E., van Mier, H., Fiez, J. A., & Raichle, M. E. (1998). The effects of practice on the functional anatomy of task performance. *Proceedings of the National Academy of Science, 95,* 853–860.

Posner, M. I. (1980). Orienting of attention. *Quarterly Journal of Experimental Psychology, 32,* 3–25.

Posner, M. I. (2012). Imaging attention networks. *NeuroImage, 61,* 450–456.

Posner, M. I., & Rothbart, M. K. (2007). *Educating the human brain.* Washington, DC: American Psychological Association.

Posner, M. I., Rothbart, M. K., Rueda, M. R., & Tang, Y. Y. (2010). Training effortless attention. In B. Bruya (Ed.), *Effortless attention: A new perspective in the cognitive science of attention and action* (pp. 410–424). Cambridge, MA: MIT Press.

Posner, M. I., Rothbart, M. K., & Sheese, B. E. (2007). Attention genes. *Developmental Science, 10,* 24–29.

Posner, M. I., Rothbart, M. K., Sheese, B. E., & Tang, Y. (2007). The anterior cingulate gyrus and the mechanisms of self regulation. *Cognitive, Affective, and Behavioral Neuroscience, 7,* 391–395.

Posner, M. I., Rothbart, M. K., Sheese, B. E., & Voelker, P. (2012). Control networks and neuromodulators of early development. *Developmental Psychology, 48,* 827–835.

Rothbart, M. K. (2011). *Becoming who we are: Temperament and personality in development.* New York: Guilford Press.

Rueda, M. R., Checa, P., & Cómbita, L. M. (2012). Enhanced efficiency of the executive attention network after training in preschool children: Immediate changes and effects after two months. *Developmental Cognitive Neuroscience, 2*, S192–S204.

Rueda, M. R., Rothbart, M. K., McCandliss, B. D., Saccamanno, L., & Posner, M. I. (2005). Training, maturation and genetic influences on the development of executive attention. *Proceedings of the National Academy of Sciences, 102*, 14931–14936.

Shacham, S. (1983). A shortened version of the Profile of Mood States. *Journal of Personality Assessment, 47*, 305–306.

Tang, Y. Y., Lu, Q., Fan, M., Yang, Y., & Posner, M. I. (2012). Mechanisms of white matter changes induced by meditation. *Proceedings of the National Academy of Sciences, 109*, 10570–10574.

Tang, Y. Y., Lu, Q., Geng, X., Stein, E. A., Yang, Y., & Posner, M. I. (2010). Short-term meditation induces white matter changes in the anterior cingulate. *Proceedings of the National Academy of Sciences, 107*, 15649–15652.

Tang, Y. Y., Ma, Y., Fan, Y., Feng, H., Wang, J., Feng, S., et al. (2009). Central and autonomic nervous system interaction is altered by short-term meditation. *Proceedings of the National Academy of Sciences, 106*, 8865–8870.

Tang, Y. Y., Ma, Y., Wang, J., Fan, Y., Feng, S., Lu, Q., et al. (2007). Short-term meditation training improves attention and self-regulation. *Proceedings of the National Academy of Sciences, 104*, 17152–17156.

Tang, Y. Y., & Posner, M. I. (2009). Attention training and attention state training. *Trends in Cognitive Sciences, 13*, 222–227.

Tang, Y. Y., Rothbart, M. K., & Posner, M. I. (2012). Neural correlates of establishing, maintaining and switching brain states. *Trends in Cognitive Sciences, 16*, 330–337.

Wadlinger, H. A., & Isaacowitz, D. M. (2011). Fixing our focus: Training attention to regulate emotion. *Personality and Social Psychology Review, 15*, 75–102.

Zeidan, F., Johnson, S. K., Diamond, B. J., David, Z., & Goolkasian, P. (2010). Mindfulness meditation improves cognition: evidence of brief mental training. *Consciousness and Cognition, 19*, 597–605.

Zylowska, L., Ackerman, D. L., Yang, M. H., Futrell, J. L., Horton, N. L., Hale, T. S., et al. (2008). Mindfulness meditation training in adults and adolescents with ADHD: A feasibility study. *Journal of Attention Disorders, 11*(6), 737–746.

CHAPTER 6

Mindfulness in the Context of Processing Mode Theory

Edward R. Watkins

Mindfulness can be broadly defined as the intentional and deliberate allocation of nonjudgemental awareness to experience in the present moment (see definitions and discussion in Gethin [Chapter 2], Davis & Thompson [Chapter 3], and Quaglia, Brown, Lindsay, Creswell, & Goodman [Chapter 9], this volume). It has been found to have beneficial effects on well-being and to reduce psychological distress and stress-related symptoms, and to improve physical health (see Parts IV and V, this volume). In recent years, there has been a growing interest in determining the possible mechanisms by which mindfulness and training in it may engender these benefits, with a range of putative mediators proposed, including improved attentional control (see Tang & Posner [Chapter 5], this volume), enhanced emotion regulation (see Arch & Landy [Chapter 12] and Lynch, Lazarus, & Cheavens [Chapter 18], this volume), greater self-compassion (Kuyken et al., 2010), and change in perspective on the self—in particular, an ability to step back from thoughts and feelings in a decentered way (see Szabo, Long, Villatte, & Hayes [Chapter 8] and Irving, Farb, & Segal [Chapter 19], this volume). In this chapter I propose an additional and complementary mechanism by which mindfulness and mindfulness training (MT) may exert their effects: a shift in the processing mode adopted during processing of personally relevant information, away from a conceptual and abstract mode, toward an experiential and concrete mode of processing. *Processing mode* refers to the manner or style in which an individual tends to process information, here differentiating between representing events and actions in either an abstract or a concrete way.

This account is framed within recent accounts of psychopathology, most notably interacting cognitive subsystems (ICS; Teasdale & Barnard, 1993; Teasdale, Segal, & Williams, 1999) and processing mode theory (Watkins, 2008, 2011), itself located within a control theory framework (Carver & Scheier, 1982, 1990, 1998). These

90

approaches have principally been developed in the context of understanding and treating depression and rumination, and are therefore the main focus of this chapter. Indeed, the conceptualization of distinct processing modes is a key theoretical underpinning for the development of mindfulness-based cognitive therapy (MBCT) as a relapse prevention treatment for depression (Segal, Williams, & Teasdale, 2002). In this chapter I first review the ICS and processing mode theoretical accounts, before summarizing the relevant evidence regarding the role of processing mode in mediating the effects of mindfulness and MT.

Depressive Relapse and Patterns of Information Processing

Processing mode accounts originally derive from consideration of (1) the chronically relapsing nature of depression and (2) the characteristic patterns of depressogenic cognitive processing (Teasdale, 1999; Teasdale & Barnard, 1993; Teasdale et al., 1995). Rates of relapse and recurrence in those who have had at least one previous episode of depression are at least 50% (Judd, 1997), with even those who have had successful treatment likely to experience a relapse or recurrence (Hollon, Stewart, & Strunk, 2006). A robust finding from examinations of risk of relapse in depression is that those more prone to further episodes of depression show increased activation of maladaptive negative thinking in response to mild changes in mood, relative to those less prone to future episodes (known as *cognitive reactivity*; e.g., Segal et al., 2006). In other words, relative to those less at risk, among those prone to depression, mild sadness is more likely to reinstate more global and extreme patterns of negative thinking and feeling, such as hopelessness about recovery, characterological self-blame, and "depression about depression" (i.e., to activate a depressogenic mode of processing; Teasdale, 1983, 1988).

Rumination

Foremost among these patterns of information processing is the tendency toward depressive rumination and ruminative self-focus (Ingram, 1990). *Rumination* is defined as "behaviours and thoughts that focus one's attention on one's depressive symptoms and on the implications of those symptoms" (Nolen-Hoeksema, 1991, p. 569). Both prospective longitudinal and experimental studies have confirmed that rumination plays an important causal role in the onset, maintenance, and recurrence of depression. Rumination prospectively predicts the onset of major depressive episodes, the severity of depressive symptoms in nondepressed and currently depressed individuals, and mediates the effects of other risk factors on depression (e.g., Nolen-Hoeksema, 2000; Spasojevic & Alloy, 2001; see meta-analysis by Mor & Winquist, 2002; and reviews by Nolen-Hoeksema, Wisco, & Lyubomirsky, 2008; Watkins, 2008).

Moreover, there is extensive experimental evidence that manipulating rumination causally exacerbates existing negative affect and increases negative cognition;

that is, it is a key driver in the activation of those maladaptive patterns of information processing associated with an episode of depression. Researchers have used a standardized rumination induction, in which participants are instructed to spend 8 minutes concentrating on a series of sentences that involve rumination about themselves, their current feelings and physical state, and the causes and consequences of their feelings (e.g., "Think about the way you feel inside"; Lyubomirsky & Nolen-Hoeksema, 1995). As a control condition, a distraction induction is typically used, in which participants are instructed to spend 8 minutes concentrating on a series of sentences that involve imagining visual scenes that are unrelated to the self or to current feelings (e.g., "Think about a fire darting round a log in a fireplace"). Compared to the distraction induction, the rumination induction is reliably found to have negative consequences on mood and cognition, but only when participants are already in a negative rather than a neutral mood (e.g., selected dysphoric or depressed participants, or following a sad mood induction) before the manipulations. Thus, for participants in a sad mood, compared to distraction, rumination exacerbates negative mood, increases negative thinking about the self, increases negative autobiographical memory recall, reduces the specificity of autobiographical memory retrieval, increases negative thinking about the future, impairs concentration and central executive functioning, and impairs social problem solving (e.g., Lyubomirsky & Nolen-Hoeksema, 1995; Rimes & Watkins, 2005; Watkins & Brown, 2002; Watkins & Teasdale, 2001; see a review in Watkins, 2008).

This convergent evidence indicates the importance of rumination in depression, of understanding the mechanisms underpinning rumination, and of deriving tractable theoretical accounts of rumination. To anticipate findings summarized in more detail later, experimental attempts to disentangle the mechanisms of rumination revealed that there are distinct modes of processing within rumination with distinct functional effects (adaptive vs. maladaptive; e.g., Watkins & Moulds, 2005; Watkins & Teasdale, 2001, 2004), leading to the elaboration of a processing mode theory (Watkins, 2008). In parallel to this empirical development, attempts to understand patterns of cognition and emotion in depression led to the development of theoretical accounts of rumination that hypothesized distinct modes of processing, in particular the ICS model (Teasdale & Barnard, 1993).

Interacting Cognitive Subsystems (ICS)

In response to a number of clinical and experimental findings that were hard to explain within theories that posited a single level of meaning representation, Teasdale and Barnard (1993) developed the ICS framework (see Figure 6.1). Within ICS, different aspects of experience are represented in patterns of qualitatively different kinds of information, or mental codes, which interact with each other, with the output code from one subsystem providing the input into another subsystem. The levels of representation build up from sensory codes representing basic features of sensory input (visual, acoustic, and body state input). In turn, recurring regular patterns within these codes are represented in higher-level codes that reflect the abstraction of the

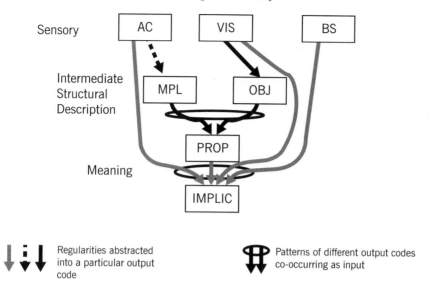

FIGURE 6.1. Interacting cognitive subsystems (ICS): The relationship between sensory, inter-mediate, and meaning codes. AC, acoustic; VIS, visual; BS, body state; MPL, morphonolexical; OBJ, object; PROP, propositional; IMPLIC, implicational. From Teasdale, Segal, and Williams (1995). Copyright 1994. Reprinted with permission from Elsevier.

repeated co-occurrence across and within the sensory codes (e.g., the morphonolexical code is a speech-level code capturing regularities common to the sounds of words across different sensory presentations, such as the elements of the sound of the word *ball* that are common across different accents, different tones, and different speakers ; the object code represents common patterns occurring to similar objects seen in different lights and from different orientations, such as the shape of a ball).

Implicational versus Propositional Meaning

Key to the theory is the proposal of two qualitatively different subsystems representing different levels of meaning that emerge from co-occurring regularities in lower-level codes: *propositional* versus *implicational* meaning. The propositional level encodes explicit specific and conceptual meanings that can be represented in language (regularities integrated across morphonolexical and object codes, e.g., the visual pattern of the shape of a ball occurring with the sound "ball"). The implicational level encodes higher-order implicit meanings in the form of schematic mental models, representing recurring patterns and themes that are built up from all aspects of experience, including direct sensory information and specific meanings (i.e., recurring patterns integrated from both the basic sensory and propositional subsystems).

Propositional information can easily be expressed in single sentences, whereas implicational knowledge is hard to express in words because it reflects more generic, holistic information, such as might reflect "gut feelings" or an intuitive "felt sense." Thus, when a person is speaking to you, your propositional system would be encoding the conceptual meaning of what is said, whereas your implicational system would combine this with information about the person's facial expression, tone, and volume of voice, and with your internal state regarding posture, arousal, tension, and energy, which could convey a very different overall meaning. A good example of the value of these two levels of meaning is that they capture the important distinction between "intellectual," "rational," "cold" knowledge and "emotional," "gut-level," and "hot" knowledge, such when in cognitive therapy, a patient reports that he or she intellectually understands how his or her thinking may be disproportionately negative and not fit the actual evidence, but he or she remains emotionally unconvinced by this knowledge.

Interaction between Implicational and Propositional Meanings

ICS hypothesizes dynamic feedback between implicational and propositional levels of self-representation in which information can be represented in each of the different processing modes, and is transformed as it is transferred from one to the other mode, potentially in a reciprocal loop (Teasdale, 1999; Teasdale & Barnard, 1993; Teasdale et al., 1995; Williams, 2008). Critically, and as Figure 6.2 illustrates, only implicational schematic models are involved in the generation and experience of emotion because they can integrate specific meaning with external and internal sensory input, whereas specific-level meanings derived from propositional information cannot. The maintenance of a particular emotional state is dependent on the dynamic maintenance of the relevant implicational schematic mental model. For example, a depressed emotional state results from the generation of a schematic model encoding generic themes such as "globally negative view of self" and/or "hopeless situation that cannot improve" comprising patterns of specific propositional meanings relating to episodes of failure and/or criticism (e.g., "I am no good") and of associated sensory codes (e.g., visual images of others' hostile expressions; sarcastic tone of voice; internal feelings of fatigue; slumped and submissive posture), built up from co-occurring commonalities that are prototypical of previous depressive experiences. This schematic model can be maintained by input from specific propositional meanings and/or sensory codes (see Figure 6.2) that are sufficiently consistent with the overall pattern to facilitate the resynthesis of the full depressogenic pattern. ICS therefore proposes that ongoing depression results from the formation of self-perpetuating processing configurations that regenerate the depressive schematic model—a mechanism called "depressive interlock."

Maintenance of Depression

As well as the other codes inputting into the implicational subsystem, ICS proposes that the implicational subsystem feeds back into the propositional system and the body state system, which encodes proprioceptive and interoceptive sensory input (e.g., tension in body, posture). The former output reflects the property that specific, explicit meanings, such as predictions, attributions, and appraisals, can be derived from holistic, generic, and implicit meanings that capture regularities across past

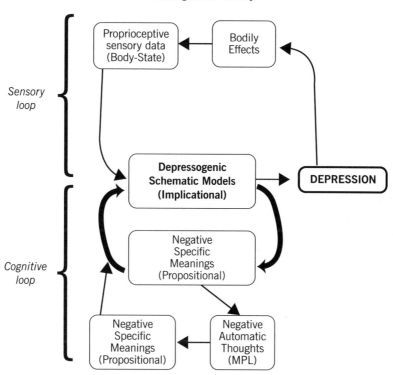

FIGURE 6.2. The "internal" maintenance of depression by a self-perpetuating "depressive interlock" processing configuration. The "central engine" of cognition (the *implicational–propositional–implicational* loop) is shown as broad, hatched arrows. From Teasdale, Segal, and Williams (1995). Copyright 1994. Reprinted with permission from Elsevier.

experiences. For example, when driving, an implicit schematic model ["unpredictable"] may be activated by the combination of meanings and sensory cues [car type, road conditions, car movements] based on past experience, and thereby derive the propositional prediction that another driver will pull out without signaling. Because the propositional subsystem generates an input back into the implicational subsystem, there is potential for a cognitive loop (implicational–propositional–implicational) to develop where the propositional output arising from the implicational level serves to contribute to the continued regeneration of the implicational schematic model (see Figure 6.2). Thus, in depression, the implicational system-derived ["globally negative view of self"] schematic model would generate specific cognitive products (e.g., negative memories, negative judgments) that contribute to the regeneration of the same negative model, assuming that sufficient elements within the overall pattern are activated. Teasdale and Barnard (1993) described this cognitive loop as the "central engine" of cognition. As Teasdale and colleagues (1995, p. 30) noted, this analysis suggests that "in the depressive interlock configuration, 'central engine' resources are devoted to repetitive, 'ruminative,' information processing cycles motivated to the attainment of central personal goals, or intentions, that can neither be attained nor relinquished." Thus, ruminative processing is at the heart of the ICS analysis of depression and a key component within depressive interlock. Similarly, in the sensory loop (implicational–body state–implicational), the schematic models generate outputs reflecting emotional reaction such as reduced activation, submissive posture, and sad facial expression that lead to body state elements that can then feed back into the implicational system and potentially maintain the schematic model.

Thus, ICS predicts that changes in affect-related implicational schematic mental models are necessary in order to change emotional state, including ameliorating depression, and that interventions that disrupt the self-perpetuating processing configurations (cognitive and sensory loops) are essential to produce such therapeutic change. More specifically, reflecting the cognitive reactivity literature, Teasdale and colleagues (1995, p. 30) proposed that "vulnerability to relapse depends on the ease with which the depressive interlock configurations that have maintained an episode of depression can be reinstated, subsequently, in situations of mild negative affect."

Multiple Modes of Processing

ICS further proposes that an individual can only consciously focus on information within one level of meaning at any one moment in time, such that at any one moment, the meaning of events is consciously processed predominantly at either an implicational or a propositional level. This assumption predicts three incompatible modes in which meanings can be consciously processed (Teasdale, 1999): within the implicational mode (labeled "mindful experiencing"), within the propositional mode (labeled "conceptualizing/doing"), or within a third mode characterized by not consciously attending to either level of meaning but focusing directly on sensory information ("mindless emoting"), which would be experienced as complete absorption in an emotional reaction (Teasdale, 1999).

In effect, these assumptions within ICS predict the existence of distinct modes of self-focused attention with distinct functional properties (Teasdale, 1999; Teasdale & Barnard, 1993; Teasdale & Chaskalson, 2011). Within ICS, processing self-related information predominantly at the propositional level would be characterized by conceptual, analytical, evaluative, "thinking about" the self, focusing on discrepancies between current and wanted outcomes (sometimes referred to as a conceptual–evaluative mode and a discrepancy-based, or "doing," mode; Williams, 2008). This mode is not necessarily maladaptive, since such discrepancy-based processing is a core element within problem solving and planning. However, when this conceptual discrepancy-focused mode is applied to internal states such as negative feelings and negative aspects of the self, it overlaps considerably with the phenomenology characteristic of ruminative processing: Both involve judging, comparing, evaluating, and analyzing negative self-relevant information; are potentially maladaptive by making such difficulties more salient in awareness without being able to reduce them; move away from direct experience; and tend to involve considerable focus on the past and future.

In contrast, self-focused attention predominantly at the implicational level would be characterized by a nonevaluative, intuitive, direct experiential awareness of experience in the moment (henceforward referred to as an *experiential mode*). Such a processing mode overlaps with the phenomenology characteristic of mindfulness. Based on this analysis, the experiential mode would be characterized by attentional focus on present-moment sensory experience; nonconceptual, intuitive processing; and disengagement from comparisons and judgments.

Moreover, Teasdale (1999) proposed that change in schematic mental models would be facilitated by processing at the implicational level (within experiential mode) where these models would be accessed and modified more directly, but hindered by processing at the propositional level (within conceptual–evaluative mode), which enhances the likelihood of depressive interlock. Thus, ICS predicts that self-focused processing of emotional material would be adaptive and facilitate emotional processing in the experiential mode but would be maladaptive and prevent effective emotional processing in the conceptual–evaluative mode. Thus, Teasdale contrasted ruminative self-focus and mindful self-awareness as distinct and incompatible modes of mind, the former focusing on analytical, "thinking about" experience, and the latter focusing on direct, intuitive, experiential awareness of experience in the moment.

In summary, ICS characterizes maladaptive rumination as involving the adoption of an analytical, evaluative propositionally based processing mode in the context of a generic and negative implicational schematic model of the self. When coupled with such a schematic model of the self, this mode of processing is hypothesized to contribute to the state of "depressive interlock" outlined earlier. That is, the combination of an analytical conceptual processing mode focused on self-related propositional meanings and negative schematic models of the self are the setting conditions for both pathological rumination and for the onset and maintenance of depression. In contrast, shifting into an experiential processing mode and away from ruminative thinking about one's difficulties and their implications should reduce the tendency to become stuck in depressive interlock, and thereby reduce the risk of depressive relapse.

For these reasons (among others), Teasdale and colleagues (1995) suggested that recovered recurrently depressed patients should be trained in mindful self-awareness as a way to counter rumination and so reduce risk of future relapse and recurrence. This provided the theoretical foundations for the development of MBCT (Segal et al., 2002), a psychosocial, group-based relapse prevention program that incorporates mindfulness meditation practice within the framework of cognitive-behavioral therapy (CBT) principles as a means to increase resilience against depression (see Irving et al., Chapter 19, this volume).

A key element of the intervention is mindfulness practice in which participants learn experientially to maintain their attention to their breath, thoughts, and feelings, and to hold such experiences in awareness, in a nonjudgmental and accepting way. These mindfulness skills are proposed to enable individuals to develop alternative responses to negative thoughts and feelings, and thereby to step out of habitual patterns of rumination at times of potential relapse.

Evidence for Distinct Processing Modes: Conceptual–Evaluative versus Experiential

Several experiments provide support for Teasdale's (1999) conceptualization of conceptual–evaluative self-focus and experiential self-awareness as functionally distinct modes of ruminative self-focus, with differing consequences for depresso-genic processes. Watkins and Teasdale (2001, 2004) developed versions of a standard rumination induction that are equivalent in focus on mood, symptoms, and self, but that differ in the mode of thinking, either encouraging an analytical, conceptual, eval-uative orientation ("Think about the causes, meanings, and consequences of . . .") or an experiential orientation ("Focus your attention on your experience of . . .") toward the same self-related items. These two manipulations have distinct functional effects on overgeneral autobiographical memory recall in depressed patients: Conceptual–evaluative self-focus maintains overgeneral memory, whereas experiential self-focus reduces overgeneral memory (Watkins & Teasdale, 2001, 2004). Overgeneral auto-biographical memory (Williams et al., 2007) is the recall of categorical summaries of repeated events (e.g., "playing golf every week") even when asked to recall specific memories located at a particular place and time (e.g., "beating my friend Paul at golf last Saturday"). Overgeneral memory recall is clinically important because it (1) is elevated in depressed patients compared to controls and (2) predicts poorer long-term outcome in depression (see Williams et al., 2007, for a review).

Watkins and Moulds (2005) further extended the distinct effects of these manipulations to social problem solving. In patients with major depression, rela-tive to conceptual–evaluative self-focus, experiential self-focus improved subsequent social problem solving. Similarly, Rimes and Watkins (2005) found that in depressed patients, experiential rumination reduced negative global self-judgments, such as "I am worthless," relative to analytical rumination.

Watkins (2004) explicitly tested the prediction from Teasdale (1999) that an experiential mode of self-focused attention would facilitate recovery from an upset-ting event in comparison to a conceptual–evaluative mode of self-focused atten-tion. Participants wrote about an induced failure experience in either a conceptual–evaluative condition (e.g., "Why did you feel this way?"), or an experiential condition ("How did you feel moment by moment?"). Consistent with the hypothesis, in the conceptual–evaluative condition, but not in the experiential condition, higher levels of the self-reported disposition to ruminate were associated with relatively greater increases in negative mood 12 hours after the failure. Furthermore, the conceptual–evaluative condition resulted in more cognitive intrusions about the failure than the experiential condition, supporting the differentiation of rumination into distinct modes of self-focused attention with distinct functional effects. Thus, there is grow-ing evidence consistent with the suggested distinction derived from ICS between a conceptual–evaluative mode and an experiential mode of self-focused attention, with the former unhelpful and the latter helpful.

Processing Mode Theory within Control Theory

Paralleling ICS is a complementary account, called *processing mode theory* (Wat-kins, 2008), which shares with ICS an emphasis on (1) self-related discrepancies driv-ing rumination and (2) different levels of processing and mental representation, albeit within control theory and without making the ICS assumptions about specific mental codes and their interactions. Watkins developed an elaborated version of control theory (Carver & Scheier, 1982) in order to account for the aforementioned evidence that there are distinct processing modes within rumination.

Control theory proposes that all behavior, including mental activities, reflect a process of feedback control. Individuals perceive their current state and behavior, and then compare these perceptions with salient reference values such as their goals, standards, or desired outcomes. If the comparison indicates a discrepancy between perceived state and reference value, such as an unresolved goal, behavior will be adjusted in order to bring the perceived state closer to the reference value (Carver & Scheier, 1982, 1998). In particular, discrepancies between expected rates of progress toward goals are hypothesized to influence behavior and affect. This discrepancy-focused element within control theory had already been proposed to explain the onset and maintenance of rumination: Martin and Tesser (1989, 1996) hypothesized that rumination occurs in response to an unattained or unresolved goal and persists until the goal is attained or abandoned, with the thought content depending on the unresolved goal.

Following a systematic review of repetitive thought, including worry and rumination, Watkins (2008) proposed a further elaboration of control theory to account for the evidence that there are distinct constructive and unconstructive forms of rumination. Within control theory, representations of events, behaviors, or goals can be arranged in a hierarchy of means and ends, represented at different levels of abstraction, in which subordinate, concrete goals, or means, serve to achieve the more abstract, superordinate goals or ends, which in turn guide and inform the subordinate goals. Within this hierarchy, a more abstract level of representation involves general, superordinate, and decontextualized mental representations that convey the essential meaning of goals, events, and actions that denote the "why" aspects of an action, including the ends that are consequential to it. In contrast, a more concrete level of representation involves subordinate, contextual, and specific details of goal, events, and actions that denote the feasibility, mechanics, and means of "how" to do the action.

A particular level in the hierarchy may be functionally and operationally superordinate at any moment in time, reflecting whether the individual is focusing attention and awareness on a more abstract or concrete level, and thereby representing reference values (goals, expectations) and perceptual signals (e.g., events and actions in the world) in a more abstract or concrete manner (Carver & Scheier, 1982; Vallacher & Wegner, 1987; Watkins, 2008). Thus, in this account, depressive rumination would be conceptualized as processing of negative self-referent material at an abstract level (focused on meanings, implications, and why, and distanced from perceptual details), whereas processing of negative self-referent material at a concrete level (specific, contextual details, in the moment) would be an incompatible alternative to rumination.

Effective self-regulation is argued to require flexible and balanced coordination between the different levels within the goal hierarchy, such that the superordinate level of control adaptively varies in response to situational and task demands (Watkins, 2011). Depending on context, a level of control that is too abstract, too concrete, or that fails to link abstract levels to concrete levels is hypothesized to be detrimental (Carver & Scheier, 1998).

The processing mode account (Watkins, 2008) proposes that the consequences of abstract versus concrete processing are determined by their relative sensitivity to contextual and situational detail. Within control theory, relative to concrete processing, abstract processing (1) insulates an individual from the specific context; (2) generates inferences across different situations beyond available data, such that transfer of learning from one situation to another is enabled; and (3) represents events and actions in terms of their implications for more abstract goals (i.e., more personally meaningful ends). When there is extensive, relevant procedural knowledge that specifies the links between the abstract ends and the concrete means necessary to achieve them (e.g., when an activity or situation is familiar), these effects make abstract processing more adaptive because they make the individual less distractible and impulsive, they enable consistency and stability of goal pursuit across time, and they afford useful generalizations about the world, along with effective action.

However, the abstract mode can also make the individual less responsive to the environment and to any situational change, and provides fewer specific guides to action and problem solving because of its distance from the mechanics of action (see Watkins, 2008, 2011). Thus, abstract processing will be unconstructive when there is no extensive procedural knowledge, such as during unexpected, difficult, or stressful circumstances. In these circumstances, a concrete processing mode will be adaptive relative to an abstract processing mode because it will result in (1) improved self-regulation focused on the immediate demands of the situation rather than its evaluative implications (Leary, Adams, & Tate, 2006); (2) reduced negative overgeneralizations to emotional events, wherein a single failure is explained in terms of a global personal inadequacy, which is implicated in increased emotional reactivity (Carver & Scheier, 1982) and vulnerability to depression (Carver, 1998); (3) more effective problem solving by providing more elaborated and contextual detail about the specific means and actions by which to best proceed when faced with difficult, novel, or complex situations; (4) because abstract representations are linked to personal identity, goals represented at a concrete level will be easier to relinquish when progress is difficult, reducing the risk of being trapped in chronic, unhelpful rumination.

Evidence for Distinct Processing Modes: Abstract versus Concrete

Experimental studies have demonstrated that manipulation of processing mode influences the consequences of rumination, consistent with processing mode theory. First, the experimental studies noted earlier comparing conceptual and experiential modes of processing are consistent with the concrete versus abstract distinction, which is an alternative operationalization of these processing configurations. Second, experimental studies have also investigated whether alternative means to manipulate processing mode, via asking participants to think about why an event happened (abstract) or how it happened (concrete) influences problem solving and the emotional response to analogue loss and trauma events. Watkins and Baracaia (2002) found that questions inducing an abstract mode characteristic of depressive rumination (e.g., "Why do I have this problem?") significantly impaired concurrent social problem solving in recovered depressed patients compared to questions increasing concrete processing (e.g., "How am I deciding what to do next?"). The concrete questions significantly improved problem solving in currently depressed patients compared to the abstract questions and a no-question control condition. Relative to manipulations to engage in abstract rumination, manipulations that instructed participants to engage in concrete rumination produced faster recovery from negative affect and reduced intrusions after a previous negative induction (Ehring, Szeimies, & Schaffrick, 2009; Watkins, 2004).

Further studies have trained participants to think in an abstract or a concrete way, through repeated practice at either abstractly evaluating the causes, meanings, and implications of emotional scenarios, or imagining the concrete details of how an event is occurring, prior to an unanticipated failure. Individuals trained to think about emotional events in a concrete way had reduced emotional reactivity to a subsequent experimental stressor relative to those who trained to be abstract (Moberly & Watkins, 2006; Watkins, Moberly, & Moulds, 2008).

Consistent with the hypothesis that abstract rumination reduces responsiveness to the environment, inducing preoccupation about everyday concerns in individuals prone to such rumination reduced the processing of interpersonal information, as indexed by the ability to recall emotion-related details from a previously watched video of a family interaction, in individuals prone to preoccupation (Lehtonen et al., 2009). Such reduced responsiveness to the environment could lead to less contact with positive reinforcers and less awareness of positive contingency, contributing to anhedonia: Specifically, rumination is associated with melancholia, which is characterized by less responsiveness to the environment and increased anhedonia (Nelson & Mazure, 1985).

Thus, the processing mode theory hypothesizes that it is possible to shift from a maladaptive form of ruminative self-focus to a more adaptive form of self-focus by shifting processing mode from being abstractly focused on general meanings and implications (i.e., "Why?") into a more concrete mode focused on specific contextual details and the process of *how* things happen. Consistent with a causal relationship between processing mode and individual differences in rumination, a proof-of-principle randomized controlled treatment intervention trial found that training dysphoric individuals to be more concrete when faced with difficulties reduced depression, anxiety, and rumination relative to a no-treatment control (Watkins, Baeyens, & Read, 2009). The concreteness training involved repeated practice at asking "How?" and focusing on specific details when thinking about recent difficulties. In a Phase II randomized controlled trial, an elaborated guided self-help variant of this concreteness training was found to be superior to treatment as usual (as provided by general practitioners, in which 50% received antidepressant medication) in reducing rumination, worry, and depression in patients with major depression recruited in a primary care setting (Watkins et al., 2012). Thus, shifting depressed patients into a more concrete processing mode reduced rumination and symptoms of depression and anxiety, consistent with the adaptive self-focus hypothesis described earlier.

Given that mindfulness meditation explicitly encourages awareness of thoughts, feelings, and sensation in the present moment, with a focus on attending to process and noticing the specific context, it is plausible to hypothesize that mindfulness and MT would engender a more concrete mode of processing (along with any other putative effects; e.g., increased attentional control, decentering from mental events, and increased compassion). Given that concreteness training alone has been shown to reduce rumination, emotional reactivity, and depression, then increased concreteness could be one mechanism by which MT has its beneficial effects.

Evidence for Processing Mode as a Mechanism within Mindfulness and MT

The ICS and processing mode theories both hypothesize that shifts in processing mode (conceptual–abstract versus experiential–concrete) may be an important element within mindfulness and MT, and causally contribute to its observed effects. Although processing mode has not often been evaluated directly in the context of MT (for one exception, see Farb et al., 2007), there is growing evidence that is consistent with specific predictions arising from the ICS and processing mode accounts. Specifically, both accounts predict that inducing a concrete–experiential processing mode (relative to an abstract–analytical processing mode) will result in (1) reduced depressive rumination; (2) more specific and contextual representations of emotional and personally relevant information (e.g., increased recall of specific autobiographical memories; Williams et al., 2007); and (3) greater engagement with the environment and thereby a greater chance of benefiting from positive events. If mindfulness involves the adoption of a concrete processing mode as hypothesized, then mindfulness would be expected to influence each of these dependent variables. Thus, processing mode can be conceived as both a potential element within the state of mindfulness (being in the here-and-now context) and a putative mediator of MT effects on depression. In the next section I review evidence relevant to these predictions, with evidence from experimental studies, analogue studies using mindfulness interventions in nonclinical groups, and clinical treatment trials.

Direct Experimental Investigation of Processing Mode in Mindfulness

The original manipulations used by Watkins and colleagues (Rimes & Watkins, 2005; Watkins & Moulds, 2005; Watkins & Teasdale, 2001, 2004) have been conceptualized as a close experimental analogue to components of MT, with the instruction to "focus your attention on your experience" of internal states, having good face validity, with the operationalization of mindfulness as nonjudgmental awareness to experience in the present moment, albeit without capturing all the complexity of mindfulness meditation (Teasdale & Chaskalson, 2011; Williams, 2010). Thus, these manipulations are arguably inducing some elements of the mindful state. Moreover, the differential effects of these experiential versus analytical manipulations have been replicated by other research teams.

Crane, Barnhofer, Visser, Nightingale, and Williams (2007) found that the analytical condition reduced autobiographical memory specificity pre- to postmanipulation relative to the experiential manipulation in patients with a history of depression and high levels of trait rumination. Lo, Ho, and Hollon (2010) found a stronger positive relationship between negative attributional style and level of depressive symptoms for participants in the analytical condition, relative to experiential and distraction conditions, indicating that processing mode during rumination moderated the relationship between depressive symptoms and negative attributional style. Rawal, Williams, and Park (2011) compared the experiential versus the analytical conditions prior to the stressor of imagining eating a large meal in (1) students high in eating disorder psychopathology and (2) patients with anorexia nervosa, and found lower post-stressor estimates of weight and shape change and less attempt to neutralize (e.g., to imagine exercising) in the experiential condition relative to the analytical condition. Sanders and Lam (2010) examined social problem solving in dysphoric participants before and after the experiential versus the analytical conditions, and found that for participants with high trait rumination, the experiential condition significantly improved social problem solving.

The success of this simple manipulation to influence the specificity of memory, the nature of self-judgments, and social problem solving is preliminary evidence that MT could have similar effects, assuming that this simple experiential focus still exerts these effects when it is one element within more complex mindfulness interventions. Furthermore, such effects on problem solving and cognition resulting from a shift in processing mode may be one potential means by which MBCT reduces depressive relapse.

Recent neuroimaging studies using variants on these experimental manipulations in individuals undergoing mindfulness practice suggest that the previous assumption is a reasonable one. Farb and colleagues (2007) used functional neuroimaging to examine brain activation in response to a narrative–conceptual focus condition involving focus on the meanings and implications of trait-related adjectives versus an experiential focus condition that involved noticing the experience of reading the same trait-related adjectives (adapted from Watkins & Teasdale, 2001). Two groups were studied: a novice group awaiting an intensive 8-week mindfulness-based stress reduction (MBSR) program and a mindfulness group that had completed the MBSR program. In the novice group, relative to narrative self-focus, experiential self-focus was associated with reductions in several discrete regions along the cortical midline implicated in self-referential and conceptual processing, such as the medial prefrontal cortex (mPFC). In the mindfulness group, there were greater and more pervasive reductions in mPFC activation in the experiential self-focus condition relative to the narrative self-focus condition. Furthermore, in the mindfulness group, experiential self-focus also resulted in increased recruitment of right lateralized prefrontal cortical and paralimbic structures such as the insula, implicated in awareness of viscerosomatic representations (i.e., awareness of body state).

Functional connectivity analyses demonstrated a strong coupling between activity in the right insula and the mPFC in novices, suggesting that it may be difficult for them to dissociate the experiential versus conceptual modes. However, this coupling was not present in the mindfulness group, suggesting that MT may make it easier to access the experiential processing mode. Thus, these findings provide a replication of the Watkins and Teasdale (2001) effect, but with brain activation as the dependent variable, and indicate that the effects of these manipulations are moderated by mindfulness practice, with MT associated with a greater effect of experiential self-focus. Therefore, this is evidence that mindfulness may enhance the ability to adopt an experiential processing mode that involves the engagement of viscerosomatic processing and reduces conceptual processing. However, a key limitation of this study is that there was no pre- and posttraining assessment to confirm whether MT was responsible for the change in patterns of neural activation.

Farb and colleagues (2010) further examined neural activity in response to experimentally induced sadness, provoked by watching sad film clips, versus a neutral mood condition, again in a group awaiting MBSR versus a group that had completed MBSR. Although the sadness provocation produced a similar increase in self-reported sadness in both groups, there was a differential pattern of neural activation consistent with Farb and colleagues (2007). Relative to the neutral condition, the sadness condition activated the same regions along the cortical midline involved in self-referential and conceptual processing as the narrative self-focus condition. Moreover, for the MBSR condition, there was reduced activation of these areas and increased activation of right lateralized prefrontal cortical areas and insula, indicating a shift from activation in brain regions linked to conceptual processing to activation in brain regions associated with interoceptive awareness and viscerosomatic processing.

The Effects of Mindfulness Training: Tests of Processing Mode Predictions

Mindfulness Training Prevents Depressive Relapse

The first and key prediction of the ICS approach to mindfulness is that MT would be an effective relapse prevention treatment in depression for those with a history of recurrent depression (Teasdale et al., 1995). MBCT has been demonstrated to be an effective relapse prevention treatment for individuals with three or more episodes of depression in a number of randomized trials (see meta-analysis by Piet & Hougaard, 2011). Two randomized clinical trials (Ma & Teasdale, 2004; Teasdale et al., 2000) have shown that, compared with treatment as usual, MBCT halved relapse rates for patients with three or more previous episodes of major depression. Kuyken and colleagues (2008) demonstrated that MBCT had similar rates of relapse over 1-year follow-up to continuation antidepressant medication for patients with recurrent depression. The effectiveness of MBCT is consistent with the underlying hypothesis that experiential (mindful) self-awareness and analytical rumination are functionally distinct modes of self-attention, and that the former is adaptive, whereas the latter is maladaptive. However, without specific investigation of processing mode as the mediator for this relapse prevention effect, we cannot rule out other plausible mechanisms for the effects of MBCT.

Mindfulness Training Reduces Rumination

Both ICS and processing mode accounts predict that mindfulness would reduce rumination, with this underlying the proposal that MBCT would be an effective relapse prevention treatment. Consistent with this prediction, MT approaches have been found to reduce rumination. In an experimental analogue study, Feldman, Greeson, and Senville (2010) compared mindful breathing, progressive muscle relaxation, and loving-kindness meditation on decentering and negative reactions to repetitive thoughts in undergraduates, and found that the association between frequency of repetitive thoughts and degree of negative reaction to thoughts was significantly less in the mindful breathing condition relative to the other two, suggesting that mindfulness reduced the impact of rumination. Two studies comparing pre- to postchange in rumination in MT (MBSR: Ramel, Goldin, Carmona, & McQuaid, 2004; mindfulness meditation: Chambers, Lo, & Allen, 2010) versus a matched waiting-list control demonstrated a reduction in rumination, particularly reflective pondering (one subtype assessed on the standard measure of depressive rumination), in the treatment group, although neither study randomized to condition. A randomized trial of mindfulness mediation versus relaxation in a nonclinical sample demonstrated a reduction in rumination (Jain et al., 2007). In another randomized controlled trial, Geschwind, Peeters, Drukker, van Os, and Wichers (2011) found that MBCT reduced self-reported rumination pre- to postintervention relative to waiting-list control in patients with a history of major depression and current residual symptoms. However, Kuyken and colleagues (2008, 2010) failed to find that MBCT reduced rumination more than continuation antidepressant medication in patients with a history of recurrent depression.

Mindfulness Training Increases Concrete and Specific Processing

A key prediction of both theoretical accounts is that mindfulness would increase the specificity and concreteness of cognitive products and representations if it involves the adoption of a concrete–experiential processing mode. Consistent with this prediction, MBCT has been found to (1) reduce overgeneral autobiographical memory in patients with a history of depression relative to treatment as usual (Williams, Teasdale, Segal, & Soulsby, 2000); (2) maintain the specificity of descriptions of previous warning signs for suicidal crises in patients with major depression and a history of suicidal attempts pre- to postintervention, whereas the specificity of descriptions decreased during treatment as usual (Hargus, Crane, Barnhofer, & Williams, 2010); and (3) increase the specificity of the description of positive future personal goals and plans in patients with current depression and a history of suicidal ideation relative to treatment as usual (Crane, Winder, Hargus, Amarsinghe, & Barnhofer, 2012). Together, this convergent evidence suggests that MBCT involves concrete processing relative to treatment as usual in depressed patients because specificity is increased across three different cognitive products (memories, goals, descriptions of warning signs). However, in the absence of a treatment control or the examination of other forms of mindfulness or other samples, it remains to be determined whether these effects are unique to MBCT, generalize to other mindfulness interventions, or even are a generic effect of effective interventions in depression.

Mindfulness Training Increases Responsiveness to Positive Events

The processing mode theory predicts that increased concrete processing would facilitate the ability to benefit from positive events because an individual would then be more directly connected with experience. In a recent study, Geschwind and colleagues (2011) used an experience-sampling methodology to measure momentary positive emotions, the appraisal of pleasant activities, and the effect of pleasant experiences on positive affect in daily life, for 6 days pre- and postintervention for patients with a history of major depression and current residual symptoms randomly allocated to MBCT or waiting-list control. Momentary positive affect, appraisal of pleasant activities, and the effect of pleasant experiences on positive affect (the index of an individual's sensitivity to reward), all significantly increased pre to postintervention in MBCT relative to waiting-list control, even after researchers controlled for change in depressive symptoms. Thus, as predicted by the processing mode account, MT resulted in greater ability to benefit from positive events.

In summary, there is convergent evidence consistent with the hypothesis that mindfulness involves a concrete–experiential processing mode: MT has effects paralleling those of the concrete–experiential experimental condition on autobiographical memory, reduces rumination just as concreteness training does, enhances the effects of the experiential manipulation, and increases specificity of processing. However, there are limitations to this evidence. First, only Farb and colleagues (2007) directly manipulated processing mode and examine the effects of MT on response to these modes. There is scope to examine whether MT moderates the effects of manipulated processing mode on other observed effects, such as negative thinking, problem solving, and emotional reactivity. Second, whereas a number of these studies indicate that MT acts in a way that is consistent with shifting into a concrete processing mode, few directly assess whether MT increases concrete processing (e.g., Watkins et al., 2009), although the studies indicating increased specificity of mental representations are good evidence for this.

Third, none of the studies directly test whether the adoption of processing mode is a mediator of the benefits of MT. This is a necessary next step for investigation, in which indices of processing mode are completed before (T1), during (T2) and after MT (T3), and change in processing mode (T1–T2) is examined as a predictor of subsequent symptom improvement (T2–T3), controlling for any prior symptom improvement (T1-T2), in line with Kraemer, Wilson, Fairburn, and Agras's (2002) recommendations. Critically, these criteria require that change in the putative mediator temporally precede the outcome variable to rule out reverse causality. A fourth limitation on the mindfulness–concrete processing mode linkage, as noted earlier, is that the processing mode account has been principally developed in the context of depression, and this evidence base is mainly from studies of patients with a history of depression and using MBCT. The generalizability of these effects to other mental and physical disorders, and other variants of MT remain to be determined.

Future Directions

There is nonetheless sufficient evidence to consider that the processing mode account might usefully add to our understanding of the mechanisms of mindfulness and MT, and therefore deserves further evaluation. As noted earlier, it is now necessary to assess more directly processing mode during mindfulness interventions and to design studies to examine its potential role as a mediator of outcomes. The processing mode account also needs to be examined in mental health conditions other than depression.

Another important area for future research is to unpack the relationship between processing mode and other putative mechanisms of mindfulness and MT. For example, how is a shift into an experiential mode related to the ability to decenter from thoughts and feelings and see them as mental events? Or how is increased concreteness related to becoming self-compassionate? Teasdale and colleagues (1999) describe both the experiential mode and decentering as potential benefits of mindfulness meditation in depression. Moreover, the ICS account proposes that adopting an implicational mode would facilitate both decentering and an experiential mode (see Teasdale & Chaskalson, 2011). It certainly seems unlikely that these mechanisms would be completely independent: For example, the analytical mode tends to be more judgmental, which puts it at odds with being more compassionate. Resolving their interrelationships is an important focus within understanding mindfulness. One of the reasons MT is potentially such a potent intervention may be because it can harness a constellation of these different effects.

A further area for theoretical work is in comparing the ICS and processing mode theory accounts. As this chapter has made clear, there is considerable overlap between them in key assumptions (multiple levels of representation; discrepancy processing; only a single mode active at any moment in time) and, as such, they make very similar predictions. Essentially, in most respects, they are highly complementary, describing the same phenomena but at different levels of description. In ICS there are a number of independent mental codes hypothesized to reflect information from particular sources; in processing mode theory, information in general is represented at different levels of abstraction. Nonetheless, it would be useful to determine whether and where these accounts may differ in their predictions to further refine the processing mode approach. Two potential points of divergence are apparent. First, ICS emphasizes the role of schematic mental models in a way that the processing mode account does not. Second, the models differ in their emphasis on the importance of moving away from discrepancy-based processing: ICS argues that a key benefit of the experiential mode is that it reduces such goal-based striving, whereas processing mode theory proposes that, depending on circumstances, different modes are more adaptive means to focus on such discrepancies. Further work is required to determine whether tractable and empirically testable predictions emerge from these differences.

Conclusion

This chapter has proposed an additional mechanism by which mindfulness and MT may exert their effects: a shift in the processing mode adopted during the processing of personally relevant information, away from a conceptual and abstract mode, toward an experiential and concrete mode of processing. This hypothesis is consistent with two theoretical models—the ICS model (Teasdale & Barnard, 1993) and an elaborated control theory account of rumination, namely, processing mode theory (Watkins, 2008). Although by no means proven, there is sufficient preliminary evidence, at least in the context of depression, for this hypothesis to be further systematically investigated.

REFERENCES

Carver, C. S. (1998). Generalization, adverse events, and development of depressive symptoms. *Journal of Personality, 66,* 607–619.

Carver, C. S., & Scheier, M. F. (1982). Control theory: A useful conceptual framework for personality–social, clinical, and health psychology. *Psychological Bulletin, 92,* 111–135.

Carver, C. S., & Scheier, M. F. (1990). Origins and functions of positive and negative affect: A control-process view. *Psychological Review, 97,* 19–35.

Carver, C. S., & Scheier, M. F. (1998). *On the self-regulation of behavior.* Cambridge, UK: Cambridge University Press.

Chambers, R., Lo, B. C. Y., & Allen, N. B. (2010). The impact of intensive mindfulness training on attentional control, cognitive style and affect. *Cognitive Therapy and Research, 32,* 303–322.

Crane, C., Barnhofer, T., Visser, C., Nightingale, H., & Williams, J. M. G. (2007). The effects of analytical and experiential rumination on autobiographical memory specificity in individuals with a history of depression. *Behaviour Research and Therapy, 45,* 3077–3087.

Crane, C., Winder, R., Hargus, E., Amarsinghe, M., & Barnhofer, T. (2012). Effects of mindfulness-based cognitive therapy on specificity of life goals. *Cognitive Therapy and Research, 36*(3), 182–189.

Ehring, T. A., Szeimies, A. K., & Schaffrick, C. (2009). An experimental analogue study into the role of abstract thinking in trauma-related rumination. *Behaviour Research and Therapy, 47,* 285–293.

Farb, N. A. S., Anderson, A. K., Mayberg, H., Bean, J., McKeon, D., & Segal, Z. V. (2010). Minding one's emotions: Mindfulness training alters the neural expression of sadness. *Emotion, 10,* 25–33.

Farb, N. A. S., Segal, Z. V., Mayberg, H., Bean, J., McKeon, D., Fatima, Z., et al. (2007). Attending to the present: Mindfulness meditation reveals distinct neural modes of self-reference. *Social Cognitive and Affective Neuroscience, 2,* 313–322.

Feldman, G., Greeson, J., & Senville, J. (2010). Differential effects of mindful breathing, progressive muscle relaxation, and loving-kindness meditation on decentering and negative reactions to repetitive thoughts. *Behaviour Research and Therapy, 48,* 1002–1011.

Geschwind, N., Peeters, F., Drukker, M., van Os, J., & Wichers, M. (2011). Mindfulness training increases momentary positive emotions and reward experience in adults vulnerable to depression: A randomized controlled trial. *Journal of Consulting and Clinical Psychology, 79,* 618–628.

Hargus, E., Crane, C., Barnhofer, T., & Williams, J. M. G. (2010). Effects of mindfulness on meta-awareness and specificity of describing prodromal symptoms in suicidal depression. *Emotion, 10,* 34–42.

Hollon, S. D., Stewart, M. O., & Strunk, D. (2006). Enduring effects for cognitive behavior therapy in the treatment of depression and anxiety. *Annual Review of Psychology, 57,* 285–315.

Ingram, R. E. (1990). Self-focused attention in clinical disorders: Review and a conceptual model. *Psychological Bulletin, 107,* 156–176.

Jain, S., Shapiro, S. L., Swanick, S., Roesch, S. C., Mills, P. J., Bell, I., et al. (2007). A randomized controlled trial of mindfulness meditation versus relaxation training: Effects on distress, positive states of mind, rumination, and distraction. *Annals of Behavioral Medicine, 33,* 11–21.

Judd, L. L. (1997). The clinical course of unipolar major depressive disorder. *Archives of General Psychiatry, 54,* 989–991.

Kraemer, H. C., Wilson, G. T., Fairburn, C. G., & Agras, W. S. (2002). Mediators and moderators of treatment effects in randomized clinical trials. *Archives of General Psychiatry, 59,* 877–883.

Kuyken, W., Byford, S., Taylor, R. S., Watkins, E. R., Holden, E., White, K., et al. (2008). Mindfulness-based cognitive therapy to prevent relapse in recurrent depression. *Journal of Consulting and Clinical Psychology, 76,* 966–978.

Kuyken, W., Watkins, E. R., Holden, E., White, K., Taylor, R. S., Byford, S., et al. (2010). How does mindfulness-based cognitive therapy work? *Behaviour Research and Therapy, 48,* 1105–1112.

Leary, M. R., Adams, C. E., & Tate, E. B. (2006). Hypo-egoic self-regulation: Exercising self-control by diminishing the influence of the self. *Journal of Personality, 74,* 1803–1831.

Lehtonen, A., Jakub, N., Craske, M., Doll, H., Harvey, A., & Stein, A. (2009). Effects of preoccupation on interpersonal recall: A pilot study. *Depression and Anxiety, 26,* 1–6.

Lo, C. S. L., Ho, S. M. Y., & Hollon, S. D. (2010). The effects of rumination and depressive symptoms on the prediction of negative attributional style among college students. *Cognitive Therapy and Research, 34,* 116–123.

Lyubomirsky, S., & Nolen-Hoeksema, S. (1995). Effects of self-focused rumination on negative thinking and interpersonal problem-solving. *Journal of Personality and Social Psychology, 69,* 176–190.

Ma, S. H., & Teasdale, J. D. (2004). Mindfulness-based cognitive therapy for depression: Replication and exploration of differential relapse prevention effects. *Journal of Consulting and Clinical Psychology, 72,* 30–40.

Martin, L. L., & Tesser, A. (1989). Toward a motivational and structural theory of ruminative thought. In J. S. Uleman & J. A. Bargh (Eds.), *Unintended thought* (pp. 306–326). New York: Guilford Press.

Martin, L. L., & Tesser, A. (1996). Some ruminative thoughts. In R. S. Wyer, Jr. (Ed.), *Advances in social cognition* (Vol. 9, pp. 1–47). Hillsdale, NJ: Erlbaum.

Moberly, N. J., & Watkins, E. (2006). Processing mode influences the relationship between trait rumination and emotional vulnerability. *Behavior Therapy, 37,* 281–291.

Mor, N., & Winquist, J. (2002). Self-focused attention and negative affect: A meta-analysis. *Psychological Bulletin, 128,* 638–662.

Nelson, J. C., & Mazure, C. (1985). Ruminative thinking: A distinctive sign of melancholia. *Journal of Affective Disorders, 9,* 41–46.

Nolen-Hoeksema, S. (1991). Responses to depression and their effects on the duration of depressive episodes. *Journal of Abnormal Psychology, 100,* 569–582.

Nolen-Hoeksema, S. (2000). The role of rumination in depressive disorders and mixed anxiety/depressive symptoms. *Journal of Abnormal Psychology, 109,* 504–511.

Nolen-Hoeksema, S., Wisco, B. E., & Lyubomirsky, S. (2008). Rethinking rumination. *Perspectives on Psychological Science, 3,* 400–424.

Piet, J., & Hougaard, E. (2011). The effect of mindfulness-based cognitive therapy for prevention of relapse in recurrent major depressive disorder: A systematic review and meta-analysis. *Clinical Psychology Review, 31,* 1032–1040.

Ramel, W., Goldin, P. R., Carmona, P. E., & McQuaid, J. R. (2004). The effects of mindfulness meditation on cognitive processes and affect in patients with past depression. *Cognitive Therapy and Research, 28,* 433–455.

Rawal, A., Williams, J. M. G., & Park, R. J. (2011). Effects of analytical and experiential self-focus on stress-induced cognitive reactivity in eating disorder psychopathology. *Behaviour Research and Therapy, 49,* 635–645.

Rimes, K. A., & Watkins, E. (2005). The effects of self-focused rumination on global negative self-judgements in depression. *Behaviour Research and Therapy, 43,* 1673–1681.

Sanders, W. A., & Lam, D. H. (2010). Ruminative and mindful self-focused processing modes and their impact on problem-solving in dysphoric individuals. *Behaviour Research and Therapy, 48,* 747–753.

Segal, Z. V., Kennedy, S., Gemar, M., Hood, K., Pedersen, R., & Buis, T. (2006). Cognitive reactivity to sad mood provocation and the prediction of depressive relapse. *Archives of General Psychiatry, 63,* 749–755.

Segal, Z. V., Williams, J. M. G., & Teasdale, J. D. (2002). *Mindfulness-based cognitive therapy for depression: A new approach to preventing relapse.* New York: Guilford Press.

Spasojevic, J., & Alloy, L. B. (2001). Rumination as a common mechanism relating depressive risk factors to depression. *Emotion, 1,* 25–37.

Teasdale, J. D. (1983). Negative thinking in depression: Cause, effect, or reciprocal relationship? *Advances in Behaviour Research and Therapy, 5,* 3–25.

Teasdale, J. D. (1988). Cognitive vulnerability to persistent depression. *Cognition and Emotion, 2,* 247–274.

Teasdale, J. D. (1999). Emotional processing, three modes of mind and the prevention of relapse in depression. *Behaviour Research and Therapy, 37,* S53–S77.

Teasdale, J. D., & Barnard, P. J. (1993). *Affect, cognition and change.* London: Erlbaum.

Teasdale, J. D., & Chaskalson, M. (2011). How does mindfulness transform suffering?: II. The transformation of dukkha. *Contemporary Buddhism, 12,* 103–124.

Teasdale, J. D., Segal, Z., & Williams, J. M. G. (1995). How does cognitive therapy prevent depressive relapse and why should attentional control (mindfulness) training help. *Behaviour Research and Therapy, 33,* 25–39.

Teasdale, J. D., Segal, Z. V., Williams, J. M. G., Ridgeway, V. A., Soulsby, J. M., & Lau, M. A. (2000). Prevention of relapse/recurrence in major depression by mindfulness-based cognitive therapy. *Journal of Consulting and Clinical Psychology, 68,* 615–623.

Vallacher, R. R., & Wegner, D. M. (1987). What do people think they're doing?: Action identification and human behavior. *Psychological Review, 94,* 3–15.

Watkins, E. (2004). Adaptive and maladaptive ruminative self-focus during emotional processing. *Behaviour Research and Therapy, 42,* 1037–1052.

Watkins, E., & Baracaia, S. (2002). Rumination and social problem-solving in depression. *Behaviour Research and Therapy, 40,* 1179–1189.

Watkins, E., & Brown, R. G. (2002). Rumination and executive function in depression: An experimental study. *Journal of Neurology Neurosurgery and Psychiatry, 72,* 400–402.

Watkins, E., & Moulds, M. (2005). Distinct modes of ruminative self-focus: Impact of abstract versus concrete rumination on problem solving in depression. *Emotion, 5,* 319–328.

Watkins, E., & Teasdale, J. D. (2001). Rumination and overgeneral memory in depression: Effects of self-focus and analytic thinking. *Journal of Abnormal Psychology, 110,* 353–357.

Watkins, E. R. (2008). Constructive and unconstructive repetitive thought. *Psychological Bulletin, 134,* 163–206.

Watkins, E. R. (2011). Dysregulation in level of goal and action identification across psychological disorders. *Clinical Psychology Review, 31,* 260–278.

Watkins, E. R., Baeyens, C. B., & Read, R. (2009). Concreteness training reduces dysphoria: Proof-of-principle for repeated cognitive bias modification in depression. *Journal of Abnormal Psychology, 118,* 55–64.

Watkins, E. R., Moberly, N. J., & Moulds, M. (2008). Processing mode causally influences emotional reactivity: Distinct effects of abstract versus concrete construal on emotional response. *Emotion, 8,* 364–378.

Watkins, E. R., Taylor, R. S., Byng, R., Baeyens, C. B., Read, R., Pearson, K., et al. (2012). Guided self-help concreteness training as an intervention for major depression in primary care: A randomized controlled trial. *Psychological Medicine, 42*(7), 1359–1371.

Watkins, E. R., & Teasdale, J. D. (2004). Adaptive and maladaptive self-focus in depression. *Journal of Affective Disorders, 82,* 1–8.

Williams, J. M. G. (2008). Mindfulness, depression and modes of mind. *Cognitive Therapy and Research, 32,* 721–733.

Williams, J. M. G. (2010). Mindfulness and psychological process. *Emotion, 10,* 1–7.

Williams, J. M. G., Barnhofer, T., Crane, C., Hermans, D., Raes, F., Watkins, E., et al. (2007). Autobiographical memory specificity and emotional disorder. *Psychological Bulletin, 133,* 122–148.

Williams, J. M. G., Teasdale, J. D., Segal, Z. V., & Soulsby, J. (2000). Mindfulness-based cognitive therapy reduces overgeneral autobiographical memory in formerly depressed patients. *Journal of Abnormal Psychology, 109,* 150–155.

CHAPTER 7

Being Aware and Functioning Fully

Mindfulness and Interest Taking within Self-Determination Theory

Edward L. Deci, Richard M. Ryan, Patricia P. Schultz, and Christopher P. Niemiec

To be *autonomous* is to act with a full sense of volition, willingness, and choice (e.g., Deci & Ryan, 2000). When autonomous, people are authentic, congruent, and integrated in their actions, they tend to be more prosocial and responsive to others, and, when acting, they are more wholeheartedly effortful, persistent, and creative. Yet autonomy is a human *capacity*, a potential that is by no means automatic, and as such it is founded in specific processes and functions.

According to *self-determination theory* (SDT; Ryan & Deci, 2000), among the functions essential for autonomy is *awareness*. We conceptualize awareness as the clear perception and insightful understanding of events, with the fullest or most optimal forms of awareness being those described by a *relaxed attention and interest* in what is occurring (Deci & Ryan, 1985; Ryan & Deci, 2008a). To be aware—that is, to be open and receptive to both internal states and external conditions—promotes autonomy or true self-regulation. Such high-quality awareness puts people in better touch with their needs, feelings, interests, and values, as well as external conditions, helping them better select goals and activities that leave them feeling more efficacious, related and connected to others, and congruent and authentic in their behaviors. All of this conduces toward greater individual and relational wellness.

The role of awareness in supporting healthy self-regulation has been understood and researched within SDT through two important and closely related constructs. The first is *mindfulness*, which we, following Brown and Ryan (2003), define as an *open and receptive attention to what is occurring in the present.* As such, mindfulness represents an "allowing" form of awareness; one merely observes rather than resists, blocks, manipulates, or latches onto what is occurring. Mindfulness, when so understood is neither selective nor active in the sense of focusing one's attention on specific goals or objects with the intent of making something happen, but instead entails a full acceptance of whatever is. The second, related component of awareness is described in SDT as *interest taking* (Ryan & Deci, 2008a; Weinstein, Przybylski, & Ryan, 2012). Like mindfulness, interest taking is open and receptive, but it takes the form of attention to specific phenomena that are salient in the individual's experience—it is a focused receptivity. Through mindfulness, people allow awareness to unfold; through interest taking, people actively bring to bear interest and receptive attention on inner or outer events, engaging them with curiosity. Both mindfulness and interest taking promote autonomous regulation.

SDT recognizes that there are many barriers to both of these forms of open and receptive awareness. People frequently encounter environments structured in ways that distract or fracture experience, or that pressure them to experience only certain feelings or ideas. For example, parents frequently treat children in ways that interfere with children's awareness of needs and feelings in order to focus them on what the parents think they should do; peers often pressure friends to express opinions that may not be authentic; and bosses can prompt employees to act against their values. As well, consumers are faced with a multibillion dollar advertising industry that attempts to influence them to want specific things and to act, not in accord with their true needs, but rather in accord with these engendered desires. In short, forces against awareness are pervasive. Within SDT these forces are understood as *controlling;* in contrast, autonomy support is the characteristic of social contexts that allows individuals to experience events freely and therefore is conducive to mindfulness and interest taking.

Substantial research accumulated over more than three decades has confirmed that when people are mindful and take interest, they are more likely to be autonomously motivated. As well, they tend to live in fuller, more deeply satisfying ways— that is, they tend to experience *eudaimonic* well-being (Ryan, Huta, & Deci, 2008). In contrast, succumbing to controlling forces and blocks to mindful attention can have myriad negative consequences across life domains. It is these interconnections among awareness (i.e., mindfulness and interest taking), autonomous self-regulation, and a life of values and wellness that we describe in this chapter. Before examining these interconnections we begin by describing the core motivational concepts of SDT that are important for understanding the role of awareness in fostering self-regulation and well-being.

Self-Determination Theory

SDT is a macrotheory of human motivation that has been built around the differentiation of motivational concepts. Within SDT, motivation is understood not primarily in terms of how much motivation a person has but in terms of what kinds of motivation are operative (Deci & Ryan, 1985; Ryan & Deci, 2008b). The primary motivational distinction is between *autonomous motivation* and *controlled motivation*, and together these two types of motivation stand in contrast to *amotivation*, which means to have no motivation—that is, to have no intention to pursue a goal or engage in a behavior. Many studies have shown that, when autonomously motivated, people learn in a deeper way, perform better at heuristic tasks, persist longer at activities, experience more positive affect, display greater psychological well-being, and experience higher-quality relationships than when they are controlled or amotivated (Deci & Ryan, 2012). These different types of motivation are also associated with people experiencing differing degrees of satisfaction of their basic psychological needs.

SDT's Basic Psychological Needs

Needs is a motivational concept that explains the energy for action. People require certain nutrients or experiences to be healthy and effective; they are typically energized to engage in behaviors that are likely to yield those required entities. These nutrients are appropriately called *needs*, in the sense that people *need* these nutrients, so they engage in behaviors that are likely to satisfy them. Needs satisfaction, in turn, yields well-being and full functioning, whereas need frustration contributes to control, amotivation, and ill-being (Ryan, Deci, Grolnick, & La Guardia, 2006). SDT research has consistently highlighted three fundamental or basic psychological needs—competence, autonomy, and relatedness.

The concept of *basic psychological needs* emerged from attempts to interpret various phenomena related to intrinsic and extrinsic motivations. Subsequent to being posited, satisfaction of the three basic needs was assessed in numerous populations across multiple cultures, and it consistently predicted wellness and optimal functioning. For example, despite different economic and political systems, individuals in both Bulgaria and the United States who experienced greater satisfaction of competence, relatedness, and autonomy needs at work evidenced more engagement and better psychological health (Deci et al., 2001). Chirkov, Ryan, and Willness (2005) found that students in Brazil and Canada who experienced support for competence, autonomy, and relatedness needs reported greater psychological wellness and less cultural alienation. Jang, Reeve, Ryan, and Kim (2009) showed that basic needs satisfactions predicted Korean high school students' motivation, performance, and wellness. Such studies are illustrative of an increasingly expansive cross-cultural literature on this topic.

One of the most important functions served by the construct of basic psychological needs is that it specifies what conditions support human flourishing. Recognizing that satisfaction of basic psychological needs universally enhances autonomy and well-being highlights many opportunities to create facilitative conditions in homes, classrooms, workplaces, and clinics. As an example, knowing that people need to feel competent allows individuals to predict that positive feedback will enhance motivation and wellness; knowing that people need relatedness leads to the expectation that treating people with respect will similarly yield positive outcomes; and knowing that people need to feel autonomous provides the basis for predicting that coercion and pressure will diminish motivation, engagement, and well-being. Indeed, hundreds of studies support the view that basic psychological needs satisfaction promotes positive consequences.

Intrinsic Motivation

The prototype of autonomous motivation is *intrinsic motivation*, which concerns people's engagement in an activity because they find it interesting and enjoyable. Intrinsic motivation is a natural manifestation of the inherent human tendency to be curious and engaged, which is exemplified in children's play. No one has to motivate them; it is in their nature to experience delight as they manipulate objects, explore surroundings, and in the process learn and assimilate. Adults, too, experience intrinsic motivation in leisure activities and, when fortunate, may also experience intrinsic motivation at work.

When people are intrinsically motivated, they tend to be open to experience and to be aware of themselves and the activity as they engage it. This does not mean being *aware* in the sense of being publicly self-conscious or focused on themselves (Fenigstein, Scheier, & Buss, 1975) but rather in the sense of being open, vital, fully engaged, and interested in the activity. Csikszentmihalyi (1990) referred to this state as "flow." Such intrinsically motivated actions are volitional and experienced as congruent and self-endorsed.

The concept of intrinsic motivation was introduced to the literature by Harlow (1950), then elaborated by White (1959). In his discussion, White proposed a new type of motivation that is not based in drives but has to do with people's ongoing interactions with the environment as they develop their competencies and feel a sense of efficacy. Thus, the core concept in his new approach to motivation was that of *competence*. Later, de Charms (1968) suggested that people need to experience *personal causation*. Deci and Ryan (1980), building on the work of White, de Charms, and their own early empirical findings, proposed that underlying intrinsic motivation are basic psychological needs for *competence* and *autonomy*. They argued that although intrinsic motivation is a natural or evolved propensity, for it to be enhanced or maintained requires the person to experience competence and autonomy satisfactions.

Intrinsic Motivation Research

Research on intrinsic motivation has explored how specific aspects of social environments affect people's intrinsic motivation by impacting feelings of autonomy or competence. For example, a meta-analysis of more than 100 experiments confirmed that using tangible rewards to enhance intrinsic motivation has a paradoxical undermining effect because it thwarts people's need for autonomy (Deci, Koestner, & Ryan, 1999). Similarly, other interpersonal events that tend to be experienced as controlling (or autonomy thwarting), such as deadlines, evaluations, and competitive pressures, also undermine intrinsic motivation, as do events such as negative feedback that decrease perceived competence.

External events can also support autonomy and competence and therefore enhance intrinsic motivation. Research has shown, for example, that when people experience choice about their behavior, it enhances intrinsic motivation (see meta-analysis by Patall, Cooper, & Robinson, 2008). Studies have also shown that taking others' perspectives and acknowledging their feelings tend to enhance autonomy and can, for example, increase intrinsic motivation (e.g., Koestner, Ryan, Bernieri, & Holt, 1984). In summary, events that affect people's basic psychological needs can either diminish or enhance intrinsic motivation.

Extrinsic Motivation

The concept of extrinsic motivation conveys that one engages in an activity because it is instrumental to some separable consequence. The classic examples are behaving to attain a reward or avoid a punishment, rather than doing the activity because it is interesting in its own right. Within SDT, however, extrinsic motivation is seen as a broad category with varied motives that can be organized in terms of a continuum of autonomy. More specifically, SDT proposes four types of extrinsic motivation that differ in the degree to which they have been internalized and integrated—that is, in their *relative autonomy* (Deci & Ryan, 2000; Ryan & Connell, 1989).

External regulation, which is the classic type of extrinsic motivation, involves people being controlled by external contingencies and their behavior being dependent on the continued power of those contingencies. People lack autonomy in their actions and therefore often do the minimum required to obtain outcomes, so that engagement is of low quality. It is also the case that when people are motivated by external factors such as the seduction of rewards or the coercion of threatened punishments, their levels of awareness tend to be very low because they are distracted by their focus on future outcomes or self-evaluations rather than being fully present in the moment for what is occurring. Recent experiments have shown this in detailed ways. For example, Legault and Inzlicht (2013) found that when people are more externally regulated, they are less likely to process error-related information deeply, thus diminishing their performance compared to more autonomously motivated individuals. That is, they have poorer quality awareness with respect to negative events that occur.

Extrinsic motivation also takes the form of *introjected regulation*, in which the individual is motivated by either avoidance of guilt and anxiety or the attainment of pride and self-aggrandizement. Introjection is classically illustrated by the phenomenon of *ego-involvement*, in which people are driven to maintain self-esteem (Ryan & Brown, 2003). Interestingly, although this is somewhat more autonomous than external regulation, introjected regulation is accompanied by experiences and consequences associated with its controlling nature, such as pressure, tension, and more volatility of self-related experiences. As we shall review, the ego-involvement and self-esteem-preoccupation associated with introjection is specifically contrary to the open and receptive awareness entailed in mindfulness (Niemiec, Ryan, & Brown, 2008).

A still more autonomous form of extrinsic motivation is referred to as *identified regulation*, in which people identify with the value of the activity for themselves and accept its regulation as their own. This type of regulation, which is accompanied by more positive experiences and consequences than is introjected regulation (e.g., Ryan, Rigby, & King, 1993), is based on the person's endorsement of the values underlying an action. Finally, when people have integrated an identification with other aspects of their interests, values, and needs, the extrinsic motivation is referred to as *integrated regulation*. Although integrated regulation, like intrinsic motivation, is characterized by high autonomy, intrinsic and integrated motivations are distinct, for intrinsic motivation is based in one's interest in an activity itself, whereas integrated extrinsic motivation is based in a wholehearted valuing of the activity's utility. For example, with integrated regulation, people might willingly engage in physical exercise because they congruently value it for their long-term health, yet the exercise is still extrinsically motivated because it is instrumental. As we shall see, integration is dependent on a high level of awareness in which values can be weighed within a truly open consideration of one's actions.

Need Satisfaction, Relative Autonomy, and Wellness

The processes of internalization and integration are central in psychosocial development. Children naturally internalize and integrate, and as they do, they become more autonomously self-regulating. Yet, as with intrinsic motivation, internalization and integration require nutrients to operate effectively. Considerable research has now shown that when people experience greater satisfaction of the needs for competence, relatedness, and autonomy in relation to some new behavior, they are more likely to internalize and integrate regulation of the behavior (see Deci & Ryan, 2012).

For example, a recent meta-analysis of physical activity and health behaviors (Ng et al., 2012) reviewed dozens of studies confirming relations of needs satisfaction to internalization and integration of health behaviors—that is, to more autonomous regulation. In turn, as people became more autonomous in enacting behaviors, they also evidenced greater well-being. This relation of autonomous motivation to psychological wellness has been found in many domains. For example, Chirkov, Ryan, Kim, and Kaplan (2003) found that people in Korea, Russia, Turkey, and the United States who behaved more autonomously when enacting their own ambient cultural values evidenced greater psychological wellness than did those who acted with less autonomy.

Extrinsic Motivation and Awareness

We mentioned earlier that with the classic type of extrinsic motivation—namely, rewards and punishments—people's awareness tends to be low because they are focused on the external contingencies and pressures. However, as the motivation is internalized and people's autonomy for the behavior increases, so, too, does their awareness. That is, as they become more autonomous by identifying with and integrating an extrinsic motivation, they also become more aware of themselves and the relevant behavior in an open and interested way. Moreover, their desires can be more reflectively considered for their compatibility with abiding values and needs, which is an essential element of more fully integrated regulation. That is, when people are aware of what is truly occurring internally and externally, they are more able to make choices and engage in behaviors that are compatible and authentic (Ryan, Legate, Niemiec, & Deci, 2012).

Studies on Mindfulness and Autonomous Motivation

Research has shown, for example, that both autonomous self-regulation and satisfaction of the basic psychological needs are correlated with greater mindfulness (Brown & Ryan, 2003). This research examined mindfulness as both a general individual difference and a state. In the latter case, using ecological momentary assessments (i.e., experience sampling) in both student and community samples, greater mindfulness at both between- and within-person levels predicted more autonomy in daily activities and less unpleasant affect. The relations of mindfulness to autonomy at the two levels were independent, indicating that even short-term experiences of mindfulness can promote more autonomous motivation and affective well-being in people's daily lives.

Mindful awareness can promote autonomous self-regulation and well-being in part by helping people free themselves from external and internal controlling forces (Brown, Ryan, & Creswell, 2007b) that are extraneous to their true selves. Particularly relevant are internal pressures such as ego-involvements and introjects, as well as the stress and defense associated with them. For example, studies have shown that ego-involvement is associated with less autonomy and vitality, as well as higher levels of pressure and tension (e.g., Ryan, 1982). In contrast, evidence underscores the association of mindfulness with more autonomy and less defensiveness, for it promotes more openness toward both pleasant and unpleasant experiences (Weinstein, Brown, & Ryan, 2009). This is important because both unpleasant and pleasant experiences hold important information, and people's confrontation and integration of negative experiences into their sense of self are important for autonomous motivation and psychological wellness (Weinstein, Deci, & Ryan, 2011).

Motivations: In Summary

We have discussed both intrinsic motivation and extrinsic motivation, pointing out that intrinsic motivation is prototypically autonomous, whereas the classic extrinsic motivation of behaving to gain rewards or avoid punishments is more controlled. However, we also have discussed how extrinsic motivation can be internalized, and as it becomes more fully integrated, people are more autonomous in their actions. We have pointed out that the two types of extrinsic motivation that are least internalized—namely, external and introjected regulation—comprise the category of controlled motivation; whereas intrinsic motivation, and identified and integrated forms of extrinsic motivation, make up the category of autonomous motivation. Research has shown that these more autonomous forms of motivation facilitate well-being and performance, especially on complex or heuristic tasks (e.g., Deci & Ryan, 2012; Ryan et al., 2008). Moreover, when people are autonomous, they tend to be more aware, open to experience, and interested, allowing increased access to their needs, values, and circumstances as they regulate actions.

Aspirations and Life Goals

Among the most common motivational concepts in today's psychological science is that of *goals*. Goals are important for behavioral regulation because people use goals to direct and guide their behavior toward desired outcomes. However, although "goals" are useful in specifying the direction of behavior, SDT argues that not all goals are created equal. Some goals are likely to fulfill basic psychological needs, whereas others may fail to satisfy these needs or even thwart their satisfaction. Thus, research within the SDT tradition has examined the importance people place on various long-term goals and the impact of that on wellness.

Kasser and Ryan (1996), for example, found that the goals of amassing wealth, becoming popular, and having an attractive image loaded together on a factor they labeled *extrinsic aspirations*, whereas attaining personal growth, meaningful relationships, and community contributions loaded on a factor they called *intrinsic aspirations*. They found that the more people rated the extrinsic goals as important relative to intrinsic goals, the lower their wellness. People strongly invested in extrinsic life goals evidenced higher anxiety, depression, and narcissism, and lower self-esteem and self-actualization.

Goals and Motivations

Goals can be thought of as the content of the outcomes toward which people's motivated actions are directed, whereas *motivation* concerns whether the actions directed toward those goal contents are autonomous or controlled. Research has shown that when people pursue extrinsic life goals, they tend to do so in a controlled way, and when they pursue intrinsic life goals, they tend to do so in an autonomous way (Kasser & Ryan, 1996). Yet the autonomous versus controlled motives for goal pursuits and the intrinsic versus extrinsic goal contents of them each explain significant, and independent, variance in psychological wellness (e.g., Sheldon, Ryan, Deci, & Kasser, 2004).

Other research has examined not the pursuit of intrinsic and extrinsic aspirations but the actual attainment of those life goals. For example, Niemiec, Ryan, and Deci (2009) followed young adults over a 1-year period, beginning a year after they graduated from college, with many of them in early career jobs. The research showed that the degree to which people attained intrinsic goals over that year predicted increases in well-being and decreases in ill-being. In contrast, the degree to which they attained extrinsic goals over the year was unrelated to change in well-being, but it did predict an increase in symptoms of ill-being.

Within SDT, the reason that intrinsic goals are more advantageous and healthful than extrinsic ones is that the intrinsic goals are more directly linked to satisfaction of the basic psychological needs, whereas the extrinsic aspirations are only indirectly linked and may even be antagonistic to basic needs satisfaction. For example, someone who is very strongly oriented toward pursuing wealth and fame might, in doing so, fail to spend time seeking satisfaction of the relatedness and autonomy needs. In fact, in the Niemiec and colleagues (2009) research, basic needs satisfaction fully mediated the relations between intrinsic and extrinsic goal attainments and, respectively, the well-being and ill-being outcomes that followed.

Mindfulness and Intrinsic Aspirations

Mindfulness has been empirically linked to a stronger focus on intrinsic aspirations. For example, Brown and Kasser (2005) reported positive relations between mindfulness and intrinsic life goals and, as we see later in the chapter, other studies have shown that people higher in mindfulness behaved in ways congruent with intrinsic aspirations (e.g., Barnes, Brown, Krusemark, Campbell, & Rogge, 2007).

Awareness in SDT

As noted, awareness is foundational to autonomy, supplying its informational basis. For example, Ryan and Deci (2008a) stated that "awareness refers to a state in which people experience a relaxed interest, free in the moment from introjected agendas and ego-involvements" (p. 189). Awareness allows people to be more in touch with their emotions, introjects, and suppressed experiences. Awareness therefore enhances autonomy by fostering fuller access to varied parts of personality, so they can become more integrated.

Indeed, awareness facilitates autonomous motivation, for being autonomous requires people to be in touch with themselves and their world, so they can concur with their actions, behave in volitional ways, and guide their actions in accord with intrinsic aspirations, deeply held values, and basic psychological needs (Hodgins & Knee, 2002). Without awareness people are more likely to behave automatically, responding to stimuli without reference to whether the responses are aligned with their values and interests, or whether they are likely to satisfy needs for competence, autonomy, and relatedness. As such, their behaviors are more susceptible to ego-involvements, as well as external pressures and seductions. Part of the function of awareness is therefore to quiet appetites, habits, and ego-involvements that interfere with autonomous self-regulation and needs satisfaction (Niemiec et al., 2008; Schultz & Ryan, in press). We therefore turn to SDT research on two forms of awareness, namely, mindfulness and interest taking.

Mindfulness

Research assessing mindfulness has supplied an important inroad for exploring awareness and its relations with autonomy. As noted, we define *mindfulness* as a state of allowing, relaxed, and receptive attention to oneself and one's surroundings in the present moment (e.g., Brown & Ryan, 2003; Kabat-Zinn, 2003). Some other researchers have used alternative definitions of mindfulness by including additional qualities, such as acceptance (Bishop et al., 2004), and the presence of a set of supportive skills (Baer, Smith, Hopkins, Krietemeyer, & Toney, 2006). Brown and colleagues (2007a, 2007b) argued that these added characteristics are best thought of as not being part of mindfulness per se but as characteristics that often result when people are mindful. Brown and colleagues (2007b) therefore suggested keeping the definition of mindfulness more parsimonious.

In addition to mindfulness, within SDT, we also use the concept of *interest taking*, which is the process of being open and receptively curious and inquisitive about specific events that one perceives and experiences. Interest taking thus supplements mindfulness as another aspect of awareness. As such, mindfulness concerns being openly receptive to all that occurs, whereas interest taking involves a more focused receptivity and relaxed or disinvested interest in specific phenomenal events and personal actions. We have regarded interest taking as central to autonomous functioning from the beginning of the development of SDT (Deci & Ryan, 1980), but it can also be related to the active, interested type of mindfulness described by Langer (1989).

Central to mindfulness is the idea of *allowing* rather than deliberately manipulating experience, which includes allowing inner chatter and demands, without attaching to or indulging them. This entails a kind of ego-detachment, which helps facilitate autonomous motivation, because behavior can be informed by a nonjudgmental awareness instead of the distorted self-cognitions associated with pressures and ego-involvements. This "detachment" is not to be confused with aloofness, lack of interest, or disconnection with the world; to the contrary, it is an ever more "alert participation in the ongoing process of living" (Gunaratana, 2002, p. 142).

To illustrate, Brown and Ryan (2003), using an instrument they developed called the Mindful Attention Awareness Scale (MAAS), reported that mindfulness is positively related to the "Big Five" concept of Openness to Experience (Costa & McCrae, 1992), but, importantly, it was negatively related to forms of reflexive self-awareness, such as public self-consciousness (Fenigstein et al., 1975) and neurotic self-consciousness (Costa & McCrae, 1992), and it was unrelated to self-monitoring (Snyder & Gangestad, 1986). These latter traits involve an evaluation or filtering of experiences with reference to the self. Thus, mindfulness means being open to perceptions without being directed by ego-involvements, introjects, or pressures.

Research on Mindfulness and SDT

Now that we have presented some central components of SDT and discussed how the concept of mindfulness relates to important aspects of the theory, we examine in detail research on how mindfulness relates positively to autonomous motivation and intrinsic aspirations. The openness inherent to mindfulness is thought to foster an accurate perception of reality without distortion or avoidance, including a greater ability to "encounter experience without being threatened or defending against it" (Hodgins & Knee, 2002, pp. 88–89). Thus, we also examine how mindfulness promotes adaptive stress appraisals and lower defense responses.

MINDFULNESS AND AUTONOMOUS MOTIVATION

As noted, mindfulness facilitates the self-insight necessary for people to behave in accord with their values and needs, which in turn supports the synthesis (i.e., integration) of that behavior with other aspects of self—that being a defining element of autonomy (Deci & Ryan, 1985). As people become more autonomous, they are also more likely to pursue intrinsic life goals, to experience satisfaction of the basic psychological needs, and to live in a fuller, more eudaimonic way. Indeed, Brown and Ryan (2003) reported that mindfulness is strongly related to autonomous motivation, to satisfaction of the three basic psychological needs, and to indicators of well-being, such as vitality and self-actualization.

Mindfulness, through its openness to reality "as it is," attenuates reactivity to stressful situations (Weinstein et al., 2009). Across several studies, these researchers showed that people higher in trait mindfulness experienced less stress, were less likely to experience demanding situations as stressful and threatening, and were more likely to cope with stress in active, adaptive ways.

MINDFULNESS, AUTONOMY, AND MODERATION OF DEFENSE

Researchers have also examined whether mindfulness moderates defensive processes commonly active in social relations. For example, Brown and Ryan (2003) found that people higher in mindfulness showed significant concordance between implicit and explicit measures of affect, whereas people low in mindfulness did not. This is important because it has been commonly accepted that implicit and explicit measures of various psychological variables are uncorrelated, but the Brown and Ryan research indicated that that is true only for people low in mindfulness. That is, people who are not aware of themselves with the relaxed attentiveness characteristic of mindfulness did not make contact with their nonconscious affective states in order to bring their conscious, self-reported feelings into line with the deeper affect. This dissociation between implicit and explicit affective states would seem to reflect a defensive process in which people do not access nonconscious affect (e.g., Weinstein, W. S. Ryan, et al., 2012); however, mindfulness seems to allow them to overcome this.

In a different line of research, Niemiec and colleagues (2010) explored the role of mindfulness in moderating defensive responding in the face of existential threat. They used a paradigm derived from *terror management theory* (TMT; Greenberg, Solomon, & Pyszczynski, 1997), in which people's mortality (i.e., their eventual death) is made salient. Studies have commonly indicated that people typically respond defensively by suppressing the death thoughts, derogating outgroup members, or striving for self-esteem. The idea is that the death reminder stimulates existential anxiety against which individuals will defend, and this typically happens when they turn their attention away from the mortality cues. Because the defense responses occur when people are less directly aware of the mortality prompts, it seems that these phenomena would be most likely to occur for people lower in mindfulness, who are likely to be less directly attentive to the threat of mortality. For people higher in mindfulness, these thoughts may be more accessible to awareness, allowing those individuals to process the experience, then act in less defensive ways.

In the Niemiec and colleagues (2010) research, the investigators assessed trait mindfulness with the MAAS, then randomized participants to mortality salience (MS) or control inductions. In one experiment, participants read a legal case and were asked to indicate the level of guilt of the defendant and to assign a jail term to that person. Those in the MS group who were lower in mindfulness displayed substantial worldview defense by being much harsher when the defendant was a member of a different race than their own, whereas the more mindful participants in the MS condition did not show a difference in judgments as a function of race.

In another experiment, Niemiec and colleagues (2010) found that less mindful participants in the MS condition tended to defend against their death anxiety by striving to boost their self-esteem in order to feel more secure, but more mindful people did not respond in this self-defensive way. Still another experiment examined death thought accessibility. Past studies had shown that, in general, people tend to suppress threatening thoughts related to death immediately after being reminded of it through an MS induction, then gradually, over several minutes, those thoughts creep to the fringes of consciousness. Typically, then, there is low death thought accessibility right after the MS induction but higher accessibility after a delay. It is these accessible, yet nonconscious, death thoughts that are theorized to lead to worldview and other social defenses. Niemiec and colleagues predicted that this defensive phenomenon of initial suppression of the death thoughts would occur for people lower in mindfulness, but that people higher in mindfulness would be less likely to suppress the thoughts, instead initially processing them quite openly and actively and then be done dealing with them. In fact, more mindful participants showed higher death thought accessibility immediately after the MS manipulation and lower access after the delay. Thus, people higher in mindfulness tended to be more open and attentive to their experience, when it occurred, then later show lower levels of defense.

MINDFULNESS, ASPIRATIONS, AND LIFE GOALS

As elaborated earlier in the chapter, SDT is also concerned with the content of the goals people pursue and attain, as well as the relation of those goals to well-being and ill-being consequences, and we noted positive associations between mindfulness and intrinsic aspirations (e.g., Brown & Kasser, 2005). There is now growing evidence that mindfulness supports the development of intrinsic goals or aspirations, such as close relationships, personal growth, and community involvement, relative to extrinsic goals such as wealth, fame, and image. For example, Brown and Kasser reported that people higher in mindfulness behaved in ways that were more ecologically responsible, which is congruent with the intrinsic aspiration of community contribution. In addition, Brown, Kasser, Ryan, Linley, and Orzech (2009) found that people higher in mindfulness were also less susceptible to consumerist messages, more likely to savor experiences, and more accepting of themselves and their material circumstances. Mindfulness is also important with respect to close relationships, which is another intrinsic goal. For example, Barnes and colleagues (2007) found that the MAAS predicted greater relationship satisfaction and investment. After discussion of a conflict, partners higher in mindfulness showed less anger, hostility, anxiety, negativity, and withdrawal. MAAS scores also predicted more love, commitment, and support for the partner postdiscussion, outcomes interpreted as resulting from being more present for him or her.

Others have reported that mindfulness is related to higher compassion and empathy (e.g., Beitel, Ferrer, & Cecero, 2005; Brown et al., 2007b). In a study involving medical students who underwent mindfulness training, Shapiro, Schwartz, and

Bonner (1998) found that these students displayed higher empathy when compared to a control group. While these studies emphasize the relations among mindfulness, intrinsic aspirations, and well-being, SDT evidence indicates that these salutary effects stem from the fact that intrinsic aspirations are closely related to satisfaction of the basic psychological needs (Niemiec et al., 2009), which is also related to higher autonomous motivation. It therefore seems that this open receptiveness to internal and external cues, which defines mindfulness, may act as a buffer to reduce the susceptibility to seductive extrinsic goals. That is, it may be that people higher in mindfulness are more likely to see material goods, displays of wealth, and social recognition as being distant from their basic psychological needs and from behaviors that would fulfill those needs, so holding these goals strongly is associated with poorer well-being. The research reviewed herein indicates that mindfulness supports basic needs satisfaction through intrinsic goal pursuits, resulting in more autonomous regulation and eudaimonic well-being (e.g., Brown et al., 2009).

Interest Taking

Whereas mindfulness involves being open and receptive to whatever is occurring in the present, *interest taking*, which is the other aspect of awareness discussed within SDT, represents a form of inquiry that can lead to insight—for example, attending to an inner tension to learn more about it. The concept of interest taking within SDT has been highlighted by discussions of psychotherapy (Deci & Ryan, 1985; Ryan & Deci, 2008a) in which an autonomy-supportive therapist helps patients be open and receptive by taking interest in particular events—be they emotions, memories, or responses—in order to facilitate patients' insight. The therapist's interest is wholly nonjudgmental and curious, and he or she works to facilitate that orientation in the patient as part of a collaborative process of discovering what is significant within an event. This aspect of awareness has been part of both psychodynamic (e.g., Perls, 1973) and humanistic (e.g., Rogers, 1951) traditions of therapy and is theorized to result in lower defensiveness, greater access to experience, and more insight.

As an individual difference variable, propensities toward interest-taking have been found to be associated with more basic psychological need satisfaction and more autonomous self-regulation (Deci & Ryan, 1985; Weinstein, Przybylski, et al., 2012). Weinstein and colleagues, reporting on their newly developed individual-differences measure of interest taking, found that among its highest correlates was trait mindfulness, which in SDT is the other component of awareness. According to SDT, bringing an interested focus to an event facilitates learning from it. For example, as one is snacking, taking interest in the eating might lead the person to align current behaviors with actual needs and values. If sated, taking interest in the feeling of fullness may lead to stopping. Similarly, when one feels threatened by another person, interest taking may lead to less defensive responding as one becomes aware that the threat is primarily left over from earlier, unresolved experiences with significant others.

Empirical work by Weinstein (2010) experimentally manipulated interest taking, comparing it to a suppression condition and an expression condition. In each condition, participants were led to believe that another participant had rejected them, and they were subsequently asked to spend 7 minutes writing an essay. In the *suppression condition*, they were asked to describe in detail what they had done since they got up that morning, being specific about events but ignoring any feelings or emotions. In the *expression condition*, they were asked to write about current thoughts and feelings, positive or negative, regarding the rejection they had experienced from the other "participant." Finally, in the *interest-taking condition*, participants were also asked to write about their positive or negative thoughts and feelings regarding the feedback from the other "participant" and, as they were doing so, to "take interest" in those feelings and their sources. Subsequently, all participants watched two brief videos: One was of the person who had rejected them and the other was of another, neutral person. The participants then rated each of these people on their likability and intelligence.

As expected, participants in all three groups rated the rejecter negatively. More interesting, however, is how the participants rated the neutral person. Those in the suppression and expression conditions also rated the neutral person negatively, whereas those in the interest-taking condition rated the neutral person significantly more positively. That is, participants in the suppression and expression conditions *displaced* some aggression prompted by the rejecter onto the neutral person, whereas participants in the interest-taking condition, having been made more aware by the interest-taking induction, did not engage in displacement. Finally, at the end of the experimental session, participants in the interest-taking condition reported more prosocial affect and less anger and feelings of rejection than participants in the other conditions. Therefore, we see that interest taking promotes greater awareness and less defense. As well, it facilitates autonomous behavior. For example, it is closely related to acting self-congruently and with less susceptibility to controlling forces (Weinstein, Przybylski, et al., 2012).

Interest Taking and Emotion Regulation

Interest taking is particularly important with respect to emotion regulation. Within SDT, investigators have studied three types of emotion regulation, namely, integrated regulation, suppressive regulation, and dysregulation (Roth, Assor, Niemiec, Ryan, & Deci, 2009). *Integrated emotion regulation* involves people being aware of their feelings, understanding that the proximal cause of the feelings is their interpretations of stimuli or events, and choosing whether and how to express the feelings. In the Weinstein (2010) experiment, people who were asked to "suppress" their feelings toward a perpetrator nonetheless tended to be angry with the perpetrator and also displace anger onto another innocent individual. Furthermore, those asked to express their feelings did not become more integrated, for they still displaced their anger and were resentful. Only when people were asked to take interest in the internal processes related to their feelings were they able to integrate the feelings, refrain from displacing them, and be more prosocial.

Within SDT, emotions are viewed as sources of information that can help guide people toward effective behavior and growth (Ryan et al., 2006). To take interest in this information puts individuals in a better position to cope effectively with either distress or excitement. In interest taking, the informational value of emotions is salient, largely because the ego is quiescent and the integrative self is more engaged (Brown, Ryan, Creswell, & Niemiec, 2008).

Summary and Conclusions

In this chapter we have discussed the role of awareness within SDT, paying particular attention to mindfulness and interest taking as two states of being attentive, in the moment, in an interested, relaxed, and receptive way. In mindfulness, people attend to their experiences openly, without evaluating or holding on to them. In interest taking, they also bring an open, inquisitive attention to specific foci, with the intent of understanding their meaning and significance. We have argued that both of these states of awareness support autonomous regulation, and that people who are more aware in these ways are also more likely to orient toward intrinsic aspirations such as personal growth, intimate relationships, and contributing to community than toward the extrinsic goals of gaining wealth, fame, and a favorable image. In addition, research suggests that people who are higher in mindfulness or interest taking tend to respond less defensively in social situations.

In conclusion, we reiterate that mindfulness and interest taking are important for living a fuller and more satisfying life, in part because they help people more easily satisfy their basic psychological needs for competence, autonomy, and relatedness. Mindfulness is, in this regard, ever more important in the increasingly rushed pace of modern societies, in which an excess of distractions (e.g., commercial, social, and political messages) can leave little space for people to be present for their moment-to-moment lived experiences. While the research is still nascent, interest taking appears to help people understand and volitionally respond to significant events, allowing them to reflect openly on, process, and understand what has occurred. Both mindfulness and interest taking are conducive to greater autonomy and integrity in action.

REFERENCES

Baer, R. A., Smith, G. T., Hopkins, J., Krietemeyer, J., & Toney, L. (2006). Using self-report assessment methods to explore facets of mindfulness. *Assessment, 13,* 27–45.

Barnes, S., Brown, K. W., Krusemark, E., Campbell, W. K., & Rogge, R. D. (2007). The role of mindfulness in romantic relationship satisfaction and responses to relationship stress. *Journal of Marital and Family Therapy, 33,* 482–500.

Beitel, M., Ferrer, E., & Cecero, J. J. (2005). Psychological mindedness and awareness of self and others. *Journal of Clinical Psychology, 61,* 739–750.

Bishop, S. R., Lau, M., Shapiro, S., Carlson, L., Anderson, N. D., Carmody, J., et al. (2004). Mindfulness: A proposed operational definition. *Clinical Psychology: Science and Practice, 11,* 230–241.

Brown, K. W., & Kasser, T. (2005). Are psychological and ecological well-being compatible?: The role of values, mindfulness, and lifestyle. *Social Indicators Research, 74,* 349–368.

Brown, K. W., Kasser, T., Ryan, R. M., Linley, P. A., & Orzech, K. (2009). When what one has is enough: Mindfulness, financial desire discrepancy, and subjective well-being. *Journal of Research in Personality, 43,* 727–736.

Brown, K. W., & Ryan, R. M. (2003). The benefits of being present: Mindfulness and its role in psychological well-being. *Journal of Personality and Social Psychology, 84,* 822–848.

Brown, K. W., Ryan, R. M., & Creswell, J. D. (2007a). Addressing fundamental questions about mindfulness. *Psychological Inquiry, 18,* 272–281.

Brown, K. W., Ryan, R. M., & Creswell, J. D. (2007b). Mindfulness: Theoretical foundations and evidence for its salutary effects. *Psychological Inquiry, 18*, 211–237.

Brown, K. W., Ryan, R. M., Creswell, J. D., & Niemiec, C. P. (2008). Beyond me: Mindful responses to social threat. In H. A. Wayment & J. J. Bauer (Eds.), *Transcending self-interest: Psychological explorations of the quiet ego* (pp. 75–84). Washington, DC: American Psychological Association.

Chirkov, V., Ryan, R. M., Kim, Y., & Kaplan, U. (2003). Differentiating autonomy from individualism and independence: A self-determination theory perspective on internalization of cultural orientations and well-being. *Journal of Personality and Social Psychology. 84*, 97–110.

Chirkov, V. I., Ryan, R. M., & Willness, C. (2005). Cultural context and psychological needs in Canada and Brazil: Testing a self-determination approach to internalization of cultural practices, identity and well-being. *Journal of Cross-Cultural Psychology, 36*, 423–443.

Costa, P. T., Jr., & McCrae, R. R. (1992). *Revised NEO Personality Inventory (NEO PI-R) and NEO Five-Factor Inventory (NEO-FFI): Professional manual.* Odessa, FL: Psychological Assessment Resources.

Csikszentmihalyi, M. (1990). *Flow: The psychology of optimal experience.* New York: Harper & Row.

de Charms, R. (1968). *Personal causation: The internal affective determinants of behavior.* New York: Academic Press.

Deci, E. L., Koestner, R., & Ryan, R. M. (1999). A meta-analytic review of experiments examining the effects of extrinsic rewards on intrinsic motivation. *Psychological Bulletin, 125*, 627–668.

Deci, E. L., & Ryan, R. M. (1980). The empirical exploration of intrinsic motivational processes. In L. Berkowitz (Ed.), *Advances in experimental social psychology* (Vol. 13, pp. 39–80). New York: Academic Press.

Deci, E. L., & Ryan, R. M. (1985). *Intrinsic motivation and self-determination in human behavior.* New York: Plenum Press.

Deci, E. L., & Ryan, R. M. (2000). The "what" and "why" of goal pursuits: Human needs and the self-determination of behavior. *Psychological Inquiry, 11*, 227–268.

Deci, E. L., & Ryan, R. M. (2012). Self-determination theory. In P. A. M. Van Lange, A. W. Kruglanski, & E. T. Higgins (Eds.), *Handbook of theories of social psychology* (Vol. 1, pp. 416–437). Thousand Oaks, CA: Sage.

Deci, E. L., Ryan, R. M., Gagné, M., Leone, D. R., Usunov, J., & Kornazheva, B. P. (2001). Need satisfaction, motivation, and well-being in the work organizations of a former Eastern Bloc country. *Personality and Social Psychology Bulletin, 27*, 930–942.

Fenigstein, A., Scheier, M. F., & Buss, A. H. (1975). Public and private self-consciousness: Assessment and theory. *Journal of Consulting and Clinical Psychology, 43*, 522–527.

Greenberg, J., Solomon, S., & Pyszczynski, T. (1997). Terror management theory of self-esteem and social behavior: Empirical assessments and conceptual refinements. In M. P. Zanna (Ed.), *Advances in experimental social psychology* (Vol. 29, pp. 61–139). San Diego, CA: Academic Press.

Gunaratana, B. H. (2002). *Mindfulness in plain English.* Boston: Wisdom.

Harlow, H. F. (1950). Learning and satiation of response in intrinsically motivated complex puzzle performance by monkeys. *Journal of Comparative and Physiological Psychology, 43*, 289–294.

Hodgins, H. S., & Knee, C. R. (2002). The integrating self and conscious experience. In E. L. Deci & R. M. Ryan (Eds.), *Handbook of self-determination research* (pp. 87–100). Rochester, NY: University of Rochester Press.

Jang, H., Reeve, J., Ryan, R. M., & Kim, A. (2009). Can self-determination theory explain what underlies the productive, satisfying learning experiences of collectivistically oriented Korean students? *Journal of Educational Psychology, 101,* 644–661.

Kabat-Zinn, J. (2003). Mindfulness-based interventions in context: Past, present, and future. *Clinical Psychology: Science and Practice, 10,* 144–156.

Kasser, T., & Ryan, R. M. (1996). Further examining the American dream: Differential correlates of intrinsic and extrinsic goals. *Personality and Social Psychology Bulletin, 22,* 280–287.

Koestner, R., Ryan, R. M., Bernieri, F., & Holt, K. (1984). Setting limits on children's behavior: The differential effects of controlling versus informational styles on intrinsic motivation and creativity. *Journal of Personality, 52,* 233–248.

Langer, E. J. (1989). *Mindfulness.* Reading, MA: Addison-Wesley.

Leary, M. R., & Tate, E. B. (2007). The multi-faceted nature of mindfulness. *Psychological Inquiry, 18,* 251–255.

Legault, L., & Inzlicht, M. (2013). Self-determination, self-regulation, and the brain: Autonomy improves performance by enhancing neuroaffective responsiveness to self-regulation failure. *Journal of Personality and Social Psychology, 105*(1), 123–138.

Ng, J. Y. Y., Ntoumanis, N., Thøgersen-Ntoumani, C., Deci, E. L., Ryan, R. M., Duda, J., et al. (2012). Self-determination theory applied to health contexts: A meta-analysis. *Perspectives on Psychological Science, 7,* 325–340.

Niemiec, C. P., Brown, K. W., Kashdan, T. B., Cozzolino, P. J., Breen, W. E., Levesque, C. S., et al. (2010). Being present in the face of existential threat: The role of trait mindfulness in reducing defensive responses to mortality salience. *Journal of Personality and Social Psychology, 99,* 344–365.

Niemiec, C. P., Ryan, R. M., & Brown, K. W. (2008). The role of awareness and autonomy in quieting the ego: A self-determination theory perspective. In H. A. Wayment & J. J. Bauer (Eds.), *Transcending self-interest: Psychological explorations of the quiet ego* (pp. 107–116). Washington, DC: American Psychological Association.

Niemiec, C. P., Ryan, R. M., & Deci, E. L. (2009). The path taken: Consequences of attaining intrinsic and extrinsic aspirations in post-college life. *Journal of Research in Personality, 43,* 291–306.

Patall, E. A., Cooper, H., & Robinson, J. C. (2008). The effects of choice on intrinsic motivation and related outcomes: A meta-analysis of research findings. *Psychological Bulletin, 134,* 270–300.

Perls, F. S. (1973). *The Gestalt approach and eyewitness to therapy.* Ben Lomond, CA: Science and Behavior Books.

Rogers, C. (1951). *Client centered therapy.* Boston: Houghton Mifflin.

Roth, G., Assor, A., Niemiec, C. P., Ryan, R. M., & Deci, E. L. (2009). The emotional and academic consequences of parental conditional regard: Comparing conditional positive regard, conditional negative regard, and autonomy support as parenting practices. *Developmental Psychology, 45,* 1119–1142.

Ryan, R. M. (1982). Control and information in the intrapersonal sphere: An extension of cognitive evaluation theory. *Journal of Personality and Social Psychology, 43,* 450–461.

Ryan, R. M., & Brown, K. W. (2003). Why we don't need self-esteem: Basic needs, mindfulness, and the authentic self. *Psychological Inquiry, 14,* 71–76.

Ryan, R. M., & Connell, J. P. (1989). Perceived locus of causality and internalization: Examining reasons for acting in two domains. *Journal of Personality and Social Psychology, 57,* 749–761.

Ryan, R. M., & Deci, E. L. (2000). Self-determination theory and the facilitation of intrinsic motivation, social development, and well-being. *American Psychologist, 55,* 68–78.

Ryan, R. M., & Deci, E. L. (2008a). A self-determination approach to psychotherapy: The motivational basis for effective change. *Canadian Psychology, 49,* 186–193.

Ryan, R. M., & Deci, E. L. (2008b). Self-determination theory and the role of basic psychological needs in personality and the organization of behavior. In O. P. John, R. W. Robbins, & L. A. Pervin (Eds.), *Handbook of personality: Theory and research* (pp. 654–678). New York: Guilford Press.

Ryan, R. M., Deci, E. L., Grolnick, W. S., & La Guardia, J. G. (2006). The significance of autonomy and autonomy support in psychological development and psychopathology. In D. Cicchetti & D. Cohen (Eds.), *Developmental psychopathology: Vol. 1. Theory and methods* (2nd ed., pp. 295–849). New York: Wiley.

Ryan, R. M., Huta, V., & Deci, E. L. (2008). Living well: A self-determination theory perspective on eudaimonia. *Journal of Happiness Studies, 9,* 139–170.

Ryan, R. M., Legate, N., Niemiec, C. P., & Deci, E. L. (2012). Beyond illusions and defense: Exploring the possibilities and limits of human autonomy and responsibility through self-determination theory. In P. R. Shaver & M. Mikulincer (Eds.), *Meaning, mortality, and choice* (pp. 215–233). Washington, DC: American Psychological Association.

Ryan, R. M., Rigby, S., & King, K. (1993). Two types of religious internalization and their relations to religious orientations and mental health. *Journal of Personality and Social Psychology, 65,* 586–596.

Schultz, P. P., & Ryan, R. M. (in press). The "why," "what," and "how" of healthy self-regulation: Mindfulness and well-being from a self-determination theory perspective. In B. D. Ostafin, M. D. Robinson, & B. P. Meier (Eds.), *Handbook of mindfulness and self-regulation.* New York: Springer.

Shapiro, S. L., Schwartz, G., & Bonner, G. (1998). Effects of mindfulness-based stress reduction on medical and premedical students. *Journal of Behavioral Medicine, 21,* 581–599.

Sheldon, K. M., Ryan, R. M., Deci, E. L., & Kasser, T. (2004). The independent effects of goal contents and motives on well-being: It's both what you pursue and why you pursue it. *Personality and Social Psychology Bulletin, 30,* 475–486.

Snyder, M., & Gangestad, S. (1986). The nature of self-monitoring. *Journal of Personality and Social Psychology, 51,* 125–129.

Weinstein, N. (2010). *Interest-taking and carry-over effects of incidental rejection emotions.* Unpublished doctoral dissertation, University of Rochester, Rochester, NY.

Weinstein, N., Brown, K. W., & Ryan, R. M. (2009). A multi-method examination of the effects of mindfulness on stress attribution, coping, and emotional well-being. *Journal of Research in Personality, 43,* 374–385.

Weinstein, N., Deci, E. L., & Ryan, R. M. (2011). Motivational determinants of integrating positive and negative past identities. *Journal of Personality and Social Psychology, 100,* 527–544.

Weinstein, N., Przybylski, A., & Ryan, R. M. (2012). The index of autonomous functioning: Development of a scale of human autonomy. *Journal of Research in Personality, 46,* 397–413.

Weinstein, N., Ryan, W. S., DeHaan, C. R., Przybylski, A. K., Legate, N. & Ryan, R. M. (2012). Parental autonomy support and discrepancies between implicit and explicit sexual identities: Dynamics of self-acceptance and defense. *Journal of Personality and Social Psychology, 102,* 815–832.

White, R. W. (1959). Motivation reconsidered: The concept of competence. *Psychological Review, 66,* 297–333.

CHAPTER 8

Mindfulness in Contextual Cognitive-Behavioral Models

Thomas G. Szabo, Douglas M. Long, Matthieu Villatte,
and Steven C. Hayes

In this chapter, we discuss mindfulness from the perspective of contextual cognitive-behavioral models, review relevant research findings, examine putative mechanisms that seem to underlie mindfulness, and suggest future directions. We place our discussion of the evidence for mindfulness and underlying mechanisms within the framework of learning processes, or the study of social and environmental conditions under which mindfulness occurs and improves. Our purpose is to aid in theoretical developments that help predict and influence human action so as to reduce suffering and increase well-being.

In the main, contextual cognitive-behavioral models of mindfulness have been tangibly practical. They have been developed in the clinical context, and are primarily used to guide therapists and clinical researchers in predicting and influencing client behaviors. But this clinical agenda creates some difficulty in our attempt to separate the concept of mindfulness from related but distinct clinical issues such as goals and values. Thus, in this chapter we touch briefly on other processes in specific clinical approaches that are necessary to understand how mindfulness is used to produce a practical impact.

Contextual perspectives in psychology trace their lineage back to William James (1907/2003) and, arguably, include such giants of behavioral thinking as B. F. Skinner (Hayes, Hayes, & Reese, 1988). While the contextualistic perspective has been applied to behavior therapy for some time (Hayes, Follette, & Follette, 1995; Jacobson, 1997), its influence has recently been felt more broadly across the cognitive-behavioral therapies (Hayes, 2004). This has been especially useful in understanding the development of contemporary psychotherapeutic perspectives on mindfulness (Hayes, Villatte, Levin, & Hildebrandt, 2011). Since the term *contextual cognitive-behavioral therapy* (contextual CBT) is relatively new, we begin here with a brief historical review of the approach, so that this perspective on mindfulness can be appreciated. Some of the assumptions, principles, and models of contextual CBT have arisen from distinct research communities, each with different methodological and terminological conventions; thus, aspects of this history are relevant to specific contextual approaches in CBT.

Contextual CBT

CBT emerged as an extension of behavior therapy, which conceptualized client difficulties using principles such as operant and respondent conditioning principles that had been developed in animal learning laboratories (Wilson, 1997). Behavioral psychology has always included both a relatively mechanistic or elemental realist wing, affiliated with the associationism of stimulus–response (S-R) learning theory, and a more functional analytic wing affiliated with behavior analysis; thus, the contextualistic qualities of behavior therapy vary considerably. Basing clinical work on case conceptualizations using behavioral principles proved to be quite useful, and many of the best validated clinical methods today emerged from that work. But this approach encountered difficulty when dealing with cognitive phenomena that seemed central to the therapy process. Therapy often takes place through verbal exchanges, and many clinical difficulties seem to involve cognitive processes that cannot be tested in animal learning laboratories. Thus, in the mid-1970s, behavioral models of clinical change shifted to emphasize concepts such as dysfunctional beliefs, automatic thoughts, and cognitive schemas (e.g., Mahoney, 1974).

Similar to behavior therapy, which sought to change the form of problem behaviors, these cognitive-behavioral approaches sought to alter the occurrence or form of problematic thoughts, an approach that is still central to CBT in the modern era (e.g., Beck, 1993). Most empirically validated methods in clinical psychology reside under the CBT label (O'Donohue, Fisher, & Hayes, 2003).

Although CBT's utility for treating a wide variety of disorders has been repeatedly demonstrated, controversy remains with respect to the processes by which CBT has its effects (Longmore & Worrell, 2007). Some argue that changes in the logical and semantic content of thoughts are necessary for therapeutic change to occur. In contrast, others argue that while thought content change may be beneficial, this constitutes neither a necessary nor sufficient condition for therapeutic growth. Instead, it is suggested that contextual changes can alter cognition's impact or function even if its semantic and logical content remains formally unchanged. This debate fueled by not only philosophical differences but also a series of empirical findings (e.g., Dimidjian et al., 2006; Gortner, Gollan, Dobson, & Jacobson, 1998; Jacobson et al., 1996), and by the rise of acceptance- and mindfulness-based interventions (Hayes, Follette, & Linehan, 2004).

Hayes (2004) described these trends as indicative of an emerging "third wave" or "third generation" of behavior therapies, and in the interest of abandoning these temporally limited terms, has more recently emphasized the shared features of a family of contextual CBTs (Hayes et al., 2011). We focus on the following four models[1] in this review: mindfulness-based cognitive therapy (MBCT), metacognitive therapy (MCT), acceptance and commitment therapy (ACT), and dialectical behavior therapy (DBT). The four we review have all focused on mindfulness in the service of achieving greater psychological *openness* to unwanted thoughts, feelings, memories, and sensations; improved flexible *awareness* of the present moment—including physical surroundings, as well as the perspectives of others; and enhanced *activation* toward valued ends and desired changes (Hayes et al., 2011). Furthermore, these models share more general features (Hayes, 2004), including a focus on changing the context and function of cognition rather than its form or content, a focus on building broad and flexible repertoires rather than eliminating symptoms, attention to more complex issues (e.g., spirituality) than in earlier forms of CBT, applications to clinicians in addition to their clients, and continuity with previously developed strands of CBT.

The developers of these four methods do not necessarily adopt contextualism in a philosophical sense (e.g., Hayes, Hayes, Reese, & Sarbin, 1993) but all are clear in their focus on context and function. The developers of MBCT, Segal, Williams, and Teasdale (2002), have stated that "unlike CBT, there is little emphasis in MBCT on changing the content of thoughts; rather, the emphasis is on changing awareness of and relationship to thoughts" (p. 54). The developer of MCT has emphasized that "MCT does not advocate challenging of negative automatic thoughts or traditional schemas" (Wells, 2008, p. 651), adding that while "CBT is concerned with testing the validity of thoughts. . . . MCT is primarily concerned with modifying the way in which thoughts are experienced and regulated" (p. 652). The developers of ACT state that "the ACT model points to the context of verbal activity as the key element, rather than the verbal content. It is not that people are thinking the wrong thing— the problem is . . . how the verbal community supports [thought's] excessive use as a mode of behavioral regulation" (Hayes, Strosahl, & Wilson, 1999, p. 49). Finally, Linehan, developer of DBT, notes that "focusing primarily on changing how the individual thinks . . . is frequently too similar to the invalidating environment" (1993, p. 369), and as an alternative advocates a dialectical approach that shares many characteristics with "recent advances in radical behaviorism and contextual theories [of] behavior therapy" (1993, p. 21).

In what follows we first briefly review the concept of mindfulness from the points of view of MBCT, MCT, ACT, and DBT. When referring to contextual CBT in the rest of the chapter, we focus on these four as a set, even though it is a much larger tradition.

Mindfulness-Based Cognitive Therapy

MBCT was developed by Segal, Williams, and Teasdale (2002) as part of research aimed at extending cognitive therapy (CT; Beck, 1993) into a depression relapse prevention program. In their analysis of CT's effectiveness, they emphasized the concept of *decentering*, which refers to a shift in one's relationship to thoughts. Previous explanations of CT have treated decentering as a step along the path to changes in thought content. However, MBCT emphasizes the development of a decentered perspective itself as the more central therapy process. From a decentered perspective, thoughts and feelings are experienced merely as passing events rather than as reflections of reality, and do not need to be evaluated as true or false. In their efforts to utilize the decentered perspective, the developers of MBCT were heavily influenced by Jon Kabat-Zinn's mindfulness-based stress reduction (MBSR; Kabat-Zinn, 1990), which involves the secular application of Buddhist principles and mindfulness practices in a stress reduction context to serve clients with diverse ailments.

Jon Kabat-Zinn (1994) provides perhaps the best-known definition of *mindfulness*: "Mindfulness means paying attention in a particular way: on purpose, in the present moment, and non-judgmentally" (p. 4). This definition, along with many practical principles and techniques, has been carried forward into MBCT. Regular mindfulness meditation practices are used to instill a particular kind of awareness, one colored by curiosity and gentleness. The training of mindfulness begins with a focus on breath and bodily sensations, so as to build attentional flexibility, and is then extended to moods and cognition. Importantly, in the practice of mindfulness, there is no "right" or "wrong" experience to be had. If one feels bored, tired, or anxious while being mindful, this does not indicate "failure." Instead, these experiences provide more sensations to notice in a curious and nonjudgmental manner.

Because of its focus on depression relapse prevention, MBCT trains recognition of and disengagement from mind states characterized by spiraling patterns of ruminative, negative thought. For example, clients are taught about "doing" mode, wherein the mind has a problem-solving focus and analyzes possible ways of reducing discrepancies between desired and current events. Clients are trained to shift deliberately from the "doing" to the "being" mode. "Being" mode is dedicated to awareness of one's moment-to-moment experience in a direct and intimate manner. While in the "being" mode, negative cognitive and emotion patterns may still occur, but they are experienced from a decentered perspective—as objects of awareness that rise and pass naturally, rather than as problems to be solved. Importantly, "being" and "doing" modes are not identified with any particular type of feeling or action. One can be in the "being" mode while doing laundry, giving a speech, or exercising, for example. Likewise, one can be in "doing" mode while meditating.

Metacognitive Therapy

MCT (Fisher & Wells, 2009; Wells, 2000) extends and elaborates on the traditional cognitive-behavioral approaches by building its theory on a multilevel information-processing model. MCT's particular information-processing model is known as the self-regulatory executive function model (S-REF; Wells & Matthews, 1994). This model holds that an inflexible cognitive style, called the cognitive attentional syndrome (CAS), is a common cause of human suffering by prolonging and intensifying distress through threat monitoring, worry, rumination, and maladaptive coping behaviors. The CAS is maintained by metacognitive beliefs that are either positive (e.g., "Worry is useful for avoiding danger") or negative (e.g., "If I keep thinking like this, it will ruin me"), with the particular beliefs giving rise to different disorders. Unfortunately, such metacognitive beliefs can often be self-defeating and may lead to maladaptive coping behaviors. The goal of MCT is therefore to develop better cognitive control through experiential exercises aimed at increased attentional and behavioral flexibility when old thinking patterns arise.

To enhance cognitive control and response flexibility, a metacognitive mode is instilled through training in a "detached mindfulness" (DM) form of processing. Here, *mindfulness* refers to the awareness of a thought or belief; *detachment* refers to the separation of self from thought, as well as the suspension of CAS coping strategies. In contrast to other forms of mindfulness, DM can be very brief, can target responses to specific events, and avoids self-attention that could serve to evoke CAS self-focused processes. Common DM exercises include free association and bringing to mind an image without trying to influence it. Additionally, flexibility and executive control are promoted using attention training techniques (discrete sessions using multiple auditory stimuli to practice selective attention, attention switching, and divided attention). Situational attentional refocusing is sometimes also used, and involves the focused redirection of attention to anxiety-provoking situations so as to facilitate the acquisition of more accurate beliefs. Through all of these MCT methods, it is hoped that a client learns that thoughts are merely internal events that do not need to be responded to with other thoughts. Additionally, repeated practice of MCT should allow clients to replace the CAS with a new metacognitive coping plan involving the above methods.

Acceptance and Commitment Therapy

ACT (said as a word; Hayes et al., 1999) seeks to promote psychological flexibility—the ability to consciously contact the present, internally or externally, and change or persist in one's behavior in a manner that effectively furthers one's chosen goals and values. The ACT model is embedded in a larger scientific agenda, which seeks to guide ACT with principles from relational frame theory (RFT; Hayes, Barnes-Holmes, & Roche, 2001)—a modern functional–contextual analysis of cognition. Some aspects of RFT are familiar to the behavior analytic tradition, including the idea that cognitive phenomena are considered socially shaped behaviors. Unique to RFT is the approach to cognition as operant behavior. That is, in RFT, cognition is seen as the ability to relate to events independently of their formal characteristics. In this view, humans build, derive, and understand relations that lead to a transformation of function, or meaning, of events composing the environment.

RFT research has demonstrated a large variety of learned relations (called *frames*) that can be quite useful to everyday functioning. Unfortunately, such frames can easily be overextended and misapplied. For example, we may be told as children that we should not run with scissors because doing so could result in pain, and that would be bad. The cognitive frame between *pain* and *bad* can help us avoid unsafe behaviors but it can be overextended to emotional pain that comes naturally as a result of being a caring human being. As a result, we could, say, avoid interpersonal closeness in relationships—knowing that intimacy can eventually lead to "bad" feelings of emotional pain. Such overextension is supported by a social context that reinforces the consistency of relational networks—that is, being right over other, perhaps more adaptive responses. One result of this can be psychological rigidity—dominant behavioral repertoires that are artificially narrowed by aversive control and excessive rule governance, and are linked for their development to avoidant or compliant verbal contexts.

Psychological rigidity is targeted in ACT through six processes: defusion, acceptance, self as perspective, flexible contact with the present moment, values, and committed action. The last four are considered to be commitment and behavioral activation strategies; the first four are acceptance and mindfulness strategies, and we discuss this latter set of processes here. *Mindfulness* is defined as "the defused, accepting, open contact with the present moment and the private events it contains as a conscious human being experientially distinct from the content being noticed" (Fletcher & Hayes, 2005, p. 322).

Defusion

Defusion seeks to alter and broaden the functions served by cognition by changing the social–verbal context in which it occurs from one of literal meaning, problem solving, or reason giving, to a context of observation and workability. Defusion methods help people notice the process and impact of thinking instead of merely the world structured by thinking. For example, a word may be repeated over and over again, until it loses its meaning and behavioral impact; or a difficult thought may be watched as it on a leaf floating by in a stream.

Acceptance

Acceptance is a process of fully embracing experience in any given moment—welcoming what feelings and thoughts life has presented with openness, kindness, and curiosity. This can be practiced clinically, for example, by deliberately noticing where in one's body feelings occur as difficult emotions are discussed.

Self as Perspective

Stories about the self can be especially resistant to change, in the absence of awareness of the "I/here/now"-ness of perspective taking. This alternative sense of self is established by adopting a habit of noticing the distinction between the content of awareness on the one hand, and conscious awareness as the context for that knowledge on the other. For example, when dealing with a difficult bit of emotional content, a therapist might unexpectedly insert the question, "And who is noticing that?" Shifts in perspective are employed in this pursuit, such as in imagination moving forward in time, examining current suffering from that distant future, then writing a note to the present about how to engage with the present difficulties.

Flexible Contact

The present moment is where new learning occurs, and flexible attentional contact with events in the present is a focus of ACT. Traditional mindfulness meditations involving either the deliberate shifting of attention between different stimuli, or narrowed focusing on a single stimulus, may be used to promote attentional flexibility. The purpose of such exercises is to help clients learn to broaden or narrow their attentional focus contingently according to what is most useful in any given moment.

Dialectical Behavior Therapy

DBT (Linehan, 1993) was developed as an eclectic approach to the treatment of individuals with severe emotion dysregulation difficulties and seeks to provide them with a safe, stable, and meaningful life. Built from a biosocial and transactional model, DBT integrates practices and principles from Zen Buddhism, dialectical philosophy, behavior analysis, CT, and social psychology. DBT emphasizes the didactic and experiential training of multiple behavioral skills sets designed for effective coping with and enjoyment of life—such as validation, emotion regulation, interpersonal effectiveness, and others. The many different techniques employed in DBT are unified in their promotion of dialectical thinking, wherein apparently polarized opposites are synthesized and a "middle path" is found. For example, one of the primary tensions used in DBT is that between acceptance and change. Clients are taught both to embrace their emotions openly and to distract from them. A middle path can be found in this case by noticing that both approaches can be effective depending on one's goals in a particular context.

Of the many skills taught in DBT, mindfulness is considered to be foundational and is said to involve both "what" and "how" skills. The "what" skills are observation, description, and participation. The observation skills involve simple nonverbal discriminations between stimuli. In order to observe, one simply notices one's experiences and environment. This may be practiced, for example, by listening intently to the fluctuations in sound emanating from a ringing bell. Description skills involve the process of putting words upon what one observes, such as would be practiced with a statement such as "I notice that there are waves of intensity in the bell's ringing—they grow and fade over time." Observe and describe skills are differentiated from one another so as to highlight the distinction between direct experience and cognitive interpretation. Use of the participation skills involves deliberately immersing oneself in an activity so that one experiences a sense of nonverbal fluidity in one's actions—such as might be felt when a dancer executes a well-practiced routine. The "how" skills refer to the ways in which each of the preceding "what" skills is to be practiced. They are to be practiced nonjudgmentally (without evaluation), one-mindfully (focusing on one thing at a time), and effectively (in a way that serves one's goals). It is hoped that by repeated practice of the mindfulness skills, clients will more easily be able to bring themselves to a centered and calm state of "wise mind." Wise mind is described as the synthesis of both emotional and rational modes of being wherein clients are able to gain perspective on their difficulties and make wise decisions.

Researching Mindfulness
from a Contextual Behavior Science Perspective

The mindfulness construct originated in the spiritual and religious sphere, not in behavioral science. Mindfulness concepts and practices are linked to spiritual traditions that are thousands of years old, and distinctions between various perspectives on mindfulness and its effective promotion have been the focus of struggle for millennia.

That historical context sheds light on some of the difficulties inherent in establishing a thoroughgoing theory and progressive investigative strategy to address these concepts and practices in psychology. Contemporary researchers are challenged to use the term in ways that help them to ask meaningful questions and gain interpretable results, but it is easy to lose sight of that goal and instead try to force the proper definition before research can help us pull this concept at its joints. Researchers and clinicians are unlikely to be any more effective than Buddhist monks and scholars in definitively describing the concept.

It is worth noting that researchers and treatment developers in the contextual wing of CBT have attempted to state their assumptions, to define their terms, to specify component processes, to link intervention procedures to these processes, and to measure the processes of change and outcomes of these procedures. That, in and of itself, is an enormous achievement and it sets the occasion for additional progress to be made. The goal is to develop concepts that are precise enough to explain single events in their context, broad enough in scope to cover a wide range of phenomena, and deep enough to integrate findings across levels of analysis (e.g., across the behavioral and neurobiological level). It is important to distinguish times when *mindfulness* is being used as a term to describe a technique or method, times when it is being referred to as a psychological process, and times when it is being discussed as an outcome of a method or process (Fletcher, Schoendorff, & Hayes, 2010).

One issue that is difficult to overcome is that deep theoretical and philosophical divisions exist in the behavioral sciences. When referring to *processes*, cognitive science holds that these are internal mental mechanisms operating upon and influenced by the environment, but existing as independent entities within the organism. In contrast, from a behavioral perspective, *processes* are seen as either verbal or nonverbal, but they are not things to be found on the inside; instead, they are seen as naturally selected patterns of responding to environmental situations. Such differences in both orientation and terminology have posed difficulties for those who would operationalize mindfulness for research purposes. However, using mindfulness in a clinical context helps restrict these differences in a useful way. For the term *mindfulness* to matter to clinicians, it has to orient researchers and practitioners toward manipulable processes that can be changed to produce better clinical outcomes (Fletcher et al., 2010). That is one reason that a science of mindfulness has taken particular root within the contextual CBT traditions.

To illustrate the advances that have been made in these traditions, we discuss in the next section measures, mediators, and moderators that have shown promise. We also suggest avenues of further research that may be useful.

Mindfulness Measurement

A robust appreciation of how treatments work demands that the hypothesized processes of change be measured. Toward this end, consensus in the field to date has been to focus on the generation of mindfulness self-report scales. They are efficient and convenient to administer, systematic, and permit both within- and between-subject comparisons (Baer, 2011). Additionally, anonymous administration environments have been shown to reduce the problem of self-representation bias (Costa & McCrae, 1992). However, designing an internally consistent, valid, reliable, comprehensive, yet nonredundant measure of mindfulness has proven to be a significant challenge. We briefly list the most well known and well studied of these scales, then evaluate the challenges ahead from a contextual CBT perspective.

The Cognitive and Affective Mindfulness Scale—Revised (CAMS-R; Feldman, Hayes, Kumar, Greeson, & Laurenceau, 2007) is a 12-item measure of four constructs related to mindfulness: attention, awareness, present focus, and acceptance. The Freiburg Mindfulness Inventory, (FMI; Buchheld, Grossman, & Walach, 2001) assesses nonjudgmental present-moment observation and openness to negative experience in 30 items. The Five Facet Mindfulness Questionnaire (FFMQ; Baer, Smith, Hopkins, Krietemeyer, & Toney, 2006) is a 39-item questionnaire that captures observing, describing, acting with awareness, nonjudgment of experience, and nonreactivity to inner experience. The Kentucky Inventory of Mindfulness Skills (KIMS; Baer, Smith, & Allen, 2004) is a 39-item inventory that measures observing present-moment experiences, applying verbal labels, acting with awareness, and accepting present-moment experiences without judgment. The Mindful Attention Awareness Scale (MAAS; Brown & Ryan, 2003) is a 15-item scale that evaluates attention to and awareness of present-moment experience in daily life. The Philadelphia Mindfulness Scale (PHLMS; Cardaciotto, Herbert, Forman, Moitra, & Farrow, 2008) is a 20-item instrument that measures awareness and acceptance. All of these scale measure mindfulness as a trait or disposition, whereas the Toronto Mindfulness Scale (TMS; Lau et al., 2006) measures curiosity about (or interest in) inner experiences and decentering from experiences at a state level—that is, in reference to an immediately prior event or experience (e.g., meditation; see also the state version of the Mindfulness Attention Awareness Scale [MAAS]; Brown & Ryan, 2003).[2]

Mindfulness within the ACT tradition is a composite concept that involves defusion, acceptance, self as perspective, and present-moment awareness (flexible contact). Numerous scales and behavioral assessment tools that have been developed tap into these concepts. The best known is the Acceptance and Action Questionnaire (AAQ; Bond et al., 2011; Hayes et al., 2004) and its many variants for specific problem areas (e.g., weight issues: Lillis & Hayes, 2008; diabetes: Gregg, Callaghan, Hayes, & Glenn-Lawson, 2007; and several others). Although "mindfulness" in not in the name of these scales, it is worth noting that all mindfulness measures explicitly or implicitly include elements of acceptance.

This is shown in the results of a series of meetings held by Bishop and colleagues with other researchers in an attempt to consolidate and filter out unnecessary terms. The meeting resulted in a consensus agreement to adopt a two-factor approach to mindfulness, including sustained attention to present experience and an attitude of openness, curiosity, and acceptance (Bishop et al., 2004). Despite the apparent consensus, new scales with new items have continued to emerge, and there is no indication that this is coming to end. There is a simple reason for this: Mindfulness means different things to different people, and it always has because of differences in theory and philosophy. That is as true in science as it is in religion: The difference is that in science, data can be used to evaluate the utility and coherence of particular mindfulness constructs.

A second issue with respect to the existing scales is that many of these contain items that do not adequately ask respondents to examine the context in which they experience mindfulness. For example, the CAMS-R uses generic statements, such as "I am able to focus on the present moment" and "I am preoccupied with the past." These items lack the sense of a situated act in context, and may therefore be less useful at identifying learning processes that are engaged during mindful activity. Such items are also less useful in that they appear to measure only attitudes and fail to examine overt behavior. In contrast, items on the KIMS, such as, "When I'm walking, I deliberately notice the sensations of my body moving," and, "When I do things, my mind wanders off and I'm easily distracted" ask respondents to consider both overt and covert behavior in a recognizable context. From a contextual CBT perspective, more scales that measure action in context are needed.

Mindfulness as Mediator and Moderator of Contextual CBT Effects

Tests of mediation and moderation are currently generating excitement in the analysis of treatment effect in psychotherapy because they allow us to explain those effects. Mediators explain how or why the treatment variable is exerting influence, and moderators predict circumstances under which the treatment will increase or diminish in effect. Although the basic approach has been used since the mid-20th century (cf. MacCorquodale & Meehl, 1948), only in the last two decades has causal modeling been incorporated into the study of mindfulness. In their many forms, these statistical tools make up what today is known as process analysis and help us to understand the variables that predict treatment outcome. In what follows, we consider the degree to which mindfulness or its elements are known to mediate or moderate contextual CBT effects.

Mindfulness as Mediator

Mediators are generally considered process variables or ingredients that are responsible for an outcome. Many of the mediation studies within contextual CBT have not tested the role of mindfulness or any of its elements as a mediator of treatment effects. One exception, by Hill (2009) compared an Appetite Focused DBT treatment to traditional CBT and found that restraint and appetite awareness mediated purge reduction in the DBT group. Roussis and Wells (2006) came closer, finding that thought control strategies and positive and negative metacognitions in MCT mediated the impact of the treatment on stress symptoms. Unfortunately, while some of these processes may arguably be related to mindfulness, they are not the same as showing that the concept of "detached mindfulness" in MCT acts as a mediator.

There is growing evidence for mindfulness or its elements mediating important psychological change processes in the other contextual CBTs, however. This is true for MBCT (e.g., Shahar, Britton, Sbarra, Figueredo, & Bootzin, 2010), and particularly so for ACT, with over 20 studies showing mediation by the AAQ, by a measure of cognitive defusion, or by related measures (e.g., Bond & Bunce, 2000; Forman et al., 2012; Zettle, Rains, & Hayes, 2011).

Mindfulness as Moderator

Moderators are most often viewed as baseline characteristics or population groups that interact with treatment in predictable ways. Traditionally, these characteristics have been evaluated for their attenuating effect upon treatment outcome. The four treatment modes that serve as our exemplars in this chapter have been evaluated for moderation, but only a few studies have shown that mindfulness elements function as moderators for contextual CBT. For example, Masuda and colleagues (2007) reported that ACT is relatively more effective for participants who are highly experientially avoidant, while Rusch and colleagues (2008) found that dropout rates from DBT are particularly high in patients with high levels of experiential avoidance and anxiety. Thus, more research is needed to see whether baseline levels of mindfulness moderate the impact of contextual CBT procedures (cf. Shapiro, Brown, Thoresen, & Plante, 2011).

The evidence of other moderators for contextual CBT reveals conditions under which it may be less effective. For example, MBCT has been shown to be less effective for those with a depression history of less than three episodes (Teasdale et al., 2000), and Muto, Hayes, and Jeffcoat (2011) showed that ACT is more effective for persons with more severe problems. It is not yet known why these effects occur, but it seems possible that mindfulness-based procedures can be somewhat dysregulating and would be less welcome, or at least less useful, for those who have less severe difficulties.

We have indicated in the preceding sections that a variety of specific definitions of mindfulness have been applied in contextual CBT, that the treatment models that have emerged have been quite useful, and that there is some evidence that mindfulness processes both mediate and moderate the impact of the contextual CBTs. We now turn our attention to a discussion of its depth. Specifically, we discuss how contextual approaches to mindfulness may alter other psychological processes.

The Behavioral Implications of Mindfulness

The first aim of mindfulness in contextual CBTs is to help clients become more aware of their behavior and its workability. In other words, mindfulness enhances the ability of clients and therapists to track experiences and to note relationships between things that have no physical similarity. For example, a client invited to observe her bodily sensations may notice that she has judgmental thoughts as soon as she brings her attention to a painful part or her body (e.g., "This sensation is unbearable"). She may notice that what comes next is an urge to bring her attention to a more neutral part of her body, and that she feels better when she does so, but only briefly. This sequence of observations helps both client and therapist notice that painful sensations are avoided, with success in the short term but not in the long term. By repeating this type of exercise, the client becomes more aware of her urges to avoid painful bodily sensations and of the consequences that will occur if she responds to these urges.

Being aware of the ineffectiveness of a behavior constitutes only a first step toward changing it. Thus, the second aim of mindfulness is to help clients be more flexible in their ability to detect and manage the variables that control their behaviors. Two main classes of variables seem relevant: direct contingencies and verbal–cognitive contingencies. The former category corresponds to the processes that behavior therapy traditionally targets, such as antecedent and consequential control. In particular, problematic behaviors are often maintained by short-term consequences even though their long-term consequences are actually detrimental. Variable reinforcement can maintain a behavior despite a low rate of success if one is not fully aware of these consequences. For example, a client who withdraws and pouts to get more attention from friends may feel closer to them if they inquire about his feelings. Even if this strategy works only from time to time, it can be sufficient to maintain the illusion of efficacy. Antecedents need also to be watched, since they set the context in which problematic behaviors occur. For example, a client suffering from addiction to alcohol may think that his urges to drink happen only in stressful situations related to work. In fact, closer attention to the antecedents may reveal that intense emotions in general (e.g., anger, excitement) all trigger urges and are to be considered in order to effectively change the client's response.

The second category of variables involved in the development and maintenance of problematic behaviors corresponds to the processes that cognitive therapy traditionally targets, namely, thought processes. Of particular interest, rules specifying the consequences of a given action can lead to persisting in ineffective behaviors, since one becomes more attached to the rule than to the actual consequences. For example, a depressed client might think, "I can't see anybody when I feel like this. I'd better wait until I get better." The client therefore waits for her mood to improve even though it only makes things worse because she is now more sensitive to the consequences stated by the rule than to the actual consequences of her behavior (Törneke, Luciano, & Valdivia-Salas, 2008). Mindfulness helps the person step back and become more aware of how automatic patterns of responding, regulated by both of these classes of contingencies, can lead to desirable or undesirable outcomes.

A third aim of using mindfulness in contextual CBTs builds on the increased awareness of reactions and contingencies: helping people respond less to deleterious contingencies and more to useful contingencies. In particular, clients are trained to let go of rigid thoughts or urges and to engage in actions that increase the probability of contacting greater satisfaction in the long term. For example, one technique consists of repeating a word or a thought over and over again in order to decrease the control exerted by its meaning on the client's behavior; as a result, the client becomes able to engage in desynchronized actions—that is, to do something different than what a thought says (Masuda, Hayes, Sackett, & Twohig, 2004; Wells, 2006). Similarly, the therapist can formulate a series of evaluations, comments, and suggestions to act in a certain way while engaging with the client. On his or her side, the client practices behaving in a way that does not match the thoughts indicated by what the therapist says; for example, the therapist tells the client to sit down and the client keeps walking (Hayes et al., 1999). This exercise also increases the capacity of the client to notice problematic contingencies and to evaluate whether or not to act on more immediate psychological experiences.

Other mindfulness techniques target more specifically avoidant responses to painful emotions and sensations. For example, a therapist can invite the client to describe as precisely as possible how she is feeling now, while a painful memory is recalled. If the client changes the topic of their conversation to avoid feeling sad, the therapist encourages her to return to observing sensations associated with this emotion. This blocks avoidance and improves the client's skill at managing difficult experiences. With time and practice, she learns that emotions do not constitute absolute barriers to action. For example, she may decide to go out at night again to enjoy being with her friends, even if it triggers painful memories.

Finally, mindfulness techniques help clients contact powerful but distal reinforcers that increase motivation to engage in strategies that are more workable in the long term. For example, the sweet spot exercise (Wilson & DuFrene, 2009) consists of asking a client to describe the emotions and sensations linked to a meaningful memory. By doing so, the client develops a better sense of what matters in his life and can start choosing actions more consistent with his identified values.

Future Directions

A number of contextual CBT models using mindfulness have been developed over the past two decades. Some models were developed to improve the treatment of a specific population (e.g., MBCT for depression, DBT for borderline personality disorder). Others (ACT and MCT) resulted from new evidence allowing the revision of certain assumptions of traditional behavioral and cognitive therapies. There is a degree of conceptual redundancy across these models. For example, nonjudgmental acceptance appears to be a common thread in all four of the approaches reviewed herein. Moving forward, two avenues seem promising.

First, framing the effects of mindfulness techniques in terms of basic principles makes possible a precise identification of the functions these strategies target. This is pragmatic for a number of reasons. Identifying the meaning of various process terms developed in different camps is facilitated when they are categorized by function. For example, acceptance as a process may be used to transform an individual's relationship to an event or merely to help an individual learn to describe important psychological events nonjudgmentally. Categorizing the meaning of acceptance by its function makes analysis across camps more feasible. Since the function of a technique may differ depending on the context, this should be useful to clinicians who need to select appropriate interventions, independent of particular models but with fidelity to the science underlying their practice (see Carmody, Chapter 4, this volume). Understanding mindfulness in terms of basic principles such as reinforcement and extinction will also be useful to clinical researchers whose aim is to evaluate the mechanisms underlying effective treatment. Indeed, understanding how therapeutic techniques work at the level of basic principles allows the building of bridges among clinical models and adaptations to the specifics of each client case. Since contextual CBT models come from different traditions (behavioral psychology for ACT and DBT, and cognitive psychology for MCT and MBCT), elaborating a common theoretical perspective will require further effort. In this regard, the willingness of behavioral psychologists to study cognition (cf. Törneke, 2010) fosters this commonality, as does the functional perspective taken by some cognitive psychologists (e.g., De Houwer, 2011).

Second, measuring mindfulness processes in clinical interventions and empirical research will allow identification of the most effective components of treatment, irrespective of the package. For example, it has been proposed that mindfulness is a common core psychotherapy process across both psychodynamic and CBT therapies (Martin, 1997). Whether or not this is so, measuring mindfulness processes has been used in ACT research almost from the beginning, and it is present in other forms of CBT as well (e.g., Arch et al., 2012). It seems important to continue to study a variety of mindfulness techniques and to examine when particular methods are most useful. The very goal of mindfulness is to improve flexible repertoires in contexts that have in the past been discriminative for lockstep behavior. In a parallel way it is useful to increase the number of techniques available to contextual therapists.

Conclusion

In this chapter, we have presented mindfulness from the perspective of contextual CBT, reviewed relevant research findings, and discussed behavioral mechanisms by which these techniques appear to function. We have suggested that future conceptual and terminological refinements would be useful, for example, regarding the meaning and measurement of mindfulness. Moreover, we have proposed that dialogue among theorists, researchers, and practitioners from different traditions might be fruitful provided we share a common purpose. One common aim that is universal is a dedication to the alleviation of human suffering and the promotion of well-being. There is a growing body of evidence that mindfulness methods have a role to play in fostering that purpose, and contextual CBT is positioned to be at the forefront of the empirical analysis of how best to do so.

NOTES

1. To conserve space, we exclude other important therapeutic methods that involve mindfulness, such as compassionate mind therapy (Gilbert, 2009), Lojong meditation (Pace et al.,

2009), mindfulness-based relapse prevention (Witkiewitz, Marlatt, & Walker, 2005), and loving-kindness meditation (e.g., Carson et al., 2005).

2. See Quaglia, Brown, Lindsay, Creswell, and Goodman (Chapter 9, this volume) for more detailed descriptions of mindfulness measures and research that addresses their validity.

REFERENCES

Arch, J., Eifert, G. H., Davies, C., Plumb-Vilardaga, J. C., Rose, R. D., & Craske, M. (2012). Randomized clinical trial of cognitive behavioral therapy (CBT) versus acceptance and commitment therapy (ACT) for mixed anxiety disorders. *Journal of Clinical and Consulting Psychology, 80*(5), 750–765.

Baer, R. (2011). Measuring mindfulness. *Contemporary Buddhism, 12*, 241–261.

Baer, R., Smith, G. T., & Allen, K. B. (2004). Assessment of mindfulness by self-report: The Kentucky Mindfulness Questionnaire of Mindfulness Skills. *Assessment, 11*, 191–206.

Baer, R., Smith, G. T., Hopkins, J., Krietemeyer, J., & Toney, L. (2006). Using self-report assessment methods to explore facets of mindfulness. *Assessment, 13*, 27–45.

Beck, A. T. (1993). Cognitive therapy: Past, present, and future. *Journal of Consulting and Clinical Psychology, 61*, 194–198.

Bishop, S. R., Lau, M., Shapiro, S., Carlson, L., Anderson, N. C., Carmody, J., et. al. (2004). Mindfulness: A proposed operational definition. *Clinical Psychology: Science and Practice, 11*, 230–241.

Bond, F. W., & Bunce, D. (2000). Mediators of change in emotion-focused and problem-focused worksite stress management interventions. *Journal of Occupational Health Psychology, 5*, 156–163.

Bond, F. W., Hayes, S. C., Baer, R. A., Carpenter, K. M., Guenole, N., Orcutt, H. K., et al. (2011). Preliminary psychometric properties of the Acceptance and Action Questionnaire–II: A revised measure of psychological inflexibility and experiential avoidance. *Behavior Therapy, 42*, 676–688.

Brown, K. W., & Ryan, R. M. (2003). The benefits of being present: Mindfulness and its role in psychological well-being. *Journal of Personality and Social Psychology, 84*, 822–848.

Buchheld, N., Grossman, P., & Walach, H. (2001). Measuring mindfulness in insight meditation and meditation-based psychotherapy: The development of the Freiburg Mindfulness Inventory (FMI). *Journal for Meditation Research, 1*, 11–34.

Cardaciotto, L., Herbert, J. D., Forman, E. M., Moitra, E., & Farrow, V. (2008). The assessment of present-moment awareness and acceptance: The Philadelphia Mindfulness Scale. *Assessment, 15*, 204–223.

Carson, J. W., Keefe, F. J., Lynch, T. R., Carson, K. M., Goli, V., Fras, A. M., et al. (2005). Loving-kindness meditation for chronic low back pain: Results from a pilot trial. *Journal of Holistic Nursing, 23*, 287–304.

Costa, P. T., & McCrae, R. R. (1992). Normal personality assessment in clinical practice: The NEO Personality Inventory. *Psychological Assessment, 4*, 5–15.

De Houwer, J. (2011). Why the cognitive approach in psychology would profit from a functional approach and vice versa. *Perspectives on Psychological Science, 6*(2), 202–209.

Dimidjian, S., Hollon, S. D., Dobson, K. S., Schmaling, K. B., Kohlenberg, R. J., Addis, M. E., et al. (2006). Randomized trial of behavioral activation, cognitive therapy, and antidepressant medication in the acute treatment of adults with major depression. *Journal of Consulting and Clinical Psychology, 74*, 658–670.

Feldman, G. C., Hayes, A. M., Kumar, S. M., Greeson, J. G., & Laurenceau, J. P. (2007). Mindfulness and emotion regulation: The development and initial validation of the Cognitive and Affective Mindfulness Scale—Revised (CAMS-R). *Journal of Psychopathology and Behavioral Assessment, 29*, 177–190.

Fisher, P., & Wells, A. (2009). *Metacognitive therapy: Distinctive features.* New York: Routledge.

Fletcher, L., & Hayes, S. C. (2005). Relational frame theory, acceptance and commitment therapy, and a functional analytic definition of mindfulness. *Journal of Rational Emotive and Cognitive Behavioral Therapy, 23*, 315–336.

Fletcher, L. B., Schoendorff, B., & Hayes, S. C. (2010). Searching for mindfulness in the brain: A process-oriented approach to examining the neural correlates of mindfulness. *Mindfulness, 1*, 41–63.

Forman, E. M., Chapman, J. E., Herbert, J. D., Goetter, E. M., Yuen, E. K., & Moitra, E. (2012). Using session-by-session measurement to compare mechanisms of action for acceptance and commitment therapy and cognitive therapy. *Behavior Therapy, 43*, 341–354.

Gilbert, P. (2009). Introducing compassion-focused therapy. *Advances in Psychiatric Treatment, 15*, 199–208.

Gortner, E. T., Gollan, J. K., Dobson, K. S., & Jacobson, N. S. (1998). Cognitive-behavioral treatment for depression: Relapse prevention. *Journal of Consulting and Clinical Psychology, 66*, 377–384.

Gregg, J. A., Callaghan, G. M., Hayes, S. C., & Glenn-Lawson, J. L. (2007). Improving diabetes self-management through acceptance, mindfulness, and values: A randomized controlled trial. *Journal of Consulting and Clinical Psychology, 75*(2), 336–343.

Hayes, S. C. (2004). Acceptance and commitment therapy, relational frame theory, and the third wave of behavior therapy. *Behavior Therapy, 35*, 639–665.

Hayes, S. C., Barnes-Holmes, D., & Roche, B. (2001). *Relational frame theory: A post-Skinnerian account of human language and cognition.* New York: Plenum Press.

Hayes, S. C., Follette, W. C., & Follette, V. (1995). Behavior therapy: A contextual approach. In A. S. German & S. B. Messer (Eds.), *Essential psychotherapies: Theory and practice* (pp. 128–181). New York: Guilford Press.

Hayes, S. C., Hayes, L. J., & Reese, H. W. (1988). Finding the philosophical core: A review of Stephen C. Pepper's *World Hypotheses. Journal of Experimental Analysis of Behavior, 50*, 97–111.

Hayes, S. C., Hayes, L. J., Reese, H. W., & Sarbin, T. R. (Eds.). (1993). *Varieties of scientific contextualism.* Oakland, CA: Context Press/New Harbinger.

Hayes, S. C., Follette, V. M., & Linehan, M. M. (Eds.). (2004). *Mindfulness and acceptance: Expanding the cognitive-behavioral tradition.* New York: Guilford Press.

Hayes, S. C., Strosahl, K. D., & Wilson, K. G. (1999). *Acceptance and commitment therapy: An experiential approach to behavior change.* New York: Guilford Press.

Hayes, S. C., Strosahl, K. D., Wilson, K. G., Bissett, R. T., Pistorello, J., Toarmino, D., et al. (2004). Measuring experiential avoidance: A preliminary test of a working model. *Psychological Record, 54*, 553–578.

Hayes, S. C., Villatte, M., Levin, M., & Hildebrandt, M. (2011). Open, aware, and active: Contextual approaches as an emerging trend in the behavioral and cognitive therapies. *Annual Review of Clinical Psychology, 7*, 141–168.

Hill, D. M. (2009). *Appetite-focused dialectical behavior therapy for the treatment of binge eating with purging: A randomized controlled trial.* Retrieved from Proquest Digital Dissertations (AAT 3295214).

Jacobson, N. S. (1997). Can contextualism help? *Behavior Therapy, 28,* 435–443.

Jacobson, N. S., Dobson, K. S., Truax, P. A., Addis, M. E., Koerner, K., Gollan, J. K., et al. (1996). A component analysis of cognitive behavioral treatment for depression. *Journal of Consulting and Clinical Psychology, 64,* 295–304.

James, W. (2003). *Pragmatism: A new name for some old ways of thinking.* New York: Barnes & Noble. (Original work published 1907)

Kabat-Zinn, J. (1990). *Full catastrophe living: Using the wisdom of your body and mind to face stress, pain, and illness.* New York: Bantam Dell.

Kabat-Zinn, J. (1994). *Wherever you go there you are.* New York: Hyperion.

Lau, M., Bishop, S., Segal, Z., Buis, T., Anderson, N., Carlson, L., et al. (2006). The Toronto Mindfulness Scale: Development and validation. *Journal of Clinical Psychology, 62,* 1445–1467.

Lillis, J., & Hayes, S. C. (2008). Measuring avoidance and inflexibility in weight related problems. *International Journal of Behavioral Consultation and Therapy, 4,* 372–378.

Linehan, M. M. (1993). *Cognitive-behavioral treatment of borderline personality disorder.* New York: Guilford Press.

Longmore, R. J., & Worrell, M. (2007). Do we need to challenge thoughts in cognitive behavior therapy? *Clinical Psychology Review, 27,* 173–187.

MacCorquodale, K., & Meehl, P. E. (1948). On a distinction between hypothetical constructs and intervening variables. *Psychological Review, 55,* 95–107.

Mahoney, M. J. (1974). *Cognitive and behavior modification.* New York: Ballinger.

Martin, J. R. (1997). Mindfulness: A proposed common factor. *Journal of Psychotherapy Integration, 7,* 291–312.

Masuda, A., Hayes, S. C., Fletcher, L. B., Seignourel, P. J., Bunting, K., Herbst, S. A., et al. (2007). The impact of acceptance and commitment therapy versus education on stigma toward people with psychological disorders. *Behavior Research and Therapy, 45,* 27–64.

Masuda, A., Hayes, S. C., Sackett, C. F., & Twohig, M. P. (2004). Cognitive defusion and self-relevant negative thoughts: Examining the impact of a ninety year old technique. *Behaviour Research and Therapy, 42,* 477–485.

Muto, Y., Hayes, S., & Jeffcoat, T. (2011). The effectiveness of acceptance and commitment therapy bibliotherapy for enhancing the psychological health of Japanese college students living abroad. *Behavior Therapy, 42,* 323–335.

O'Donohue, W., Fisher, J. E., & Hayes, S. C. (2003). *Cognitive behavior therapy: Applying empirically supported techniques in your practice.* Hoboken, NJ: Wiley.

Pace, T. W. W., Negi, L. T., Adame, D. D., Cole, S. P., Sivilli, T. I., Brown, T. D., et al. (2009). Effect of compassion meditation on neuroendocrine, innate immune and behavioral responses to psychosocial stress. *Psychoneuroendocrinology, 34,* 87–98.

Roussis, P., & Wells, A. (2006). Post-traumatic stress symptoms: Tests of relationships with thought control strategies and beliefs as predicted by the metacognitive model. *Personality and Individual Differences, 40,* 11–122.

Rusch, N., Schiel, S., Corrigan, P. W., Leihener, F., Jacob, G. A., Olschewski, M., et al. (2008). Predictors of dropout from inpatient dialectical behavior therapy among women with borderline personality disorder. *Journal of Behavior Therapy and Experimental Psychiatry, 39,* 497–503.

Segal, Z. V., Williams, J. M. G., & Teasdale, J. D. (2002). *Mindfulness-based cognitive therapy for depression: A new approach to preventing relapse.* New York: Guilford Press.

Shahar, B., Britton, W. B., Sbarra, D. A., Figueredo, A. J., & Bootzin, R. R. (2010). Mechanisms of change in mindfulness-based cognitive therapy for depression: Preliminary evidence from a randomized controlled trial. *International Journal of Cognitive Therapy, 3,* 402–418.

Shapiro, S. L., Brown, K. W., Thoresen, C., & Plante, T. G. (2011) The moderation of mindfulness-based stress reduction effects by trait mindfulness: Results from a randomized controlled trial. *Journal of Clinical Psychology, 67,* 267–277.

Teasdale, J. D., Segal, Z. V., Williams, J. M. G., Ridgeway, V. A., Soulsby, J. M., & Lau, M. A. (2000). Prevention of relapse/recurrence in major depression by mindfulness-based cognitive therapy. *Journal of Consulting and Clinical Psychology, 68,* 615–623.

Törneke, N. (2010). *Learning RFT: An introduction to relational frame theory and its clinical applications.* Oakland, CA: New Harbinger.

Törneke, N., Luciano, C., & Valdivia Salas, S. (2008). Rule-governed behavior and psychological problems. *International Journal of Psychology and Psychological Therapy, 8*(2), 141–156.

Wells, A. (2000). *Emotional disorders and metacognition: Innovative cognitive therapy.* Chichester, UK: Wiley.

Wells, A. (2006). Detached mindfulness in cognitive therapy: A metacognitive analysis and ten techniques. *Journal of Rational-Emotive Cognitive-Behavior Therapy, 23,* 337–355.

Wells, A. (2008). Metacognitive therapy: Cognition applied to regulating cognition. *Behavioral and Cognitive Psychotherapy, 36,* 651–658.

Wells, A., & Matthews, G. (1994). *Attention and emotion: A clinical perspective.* Hove, UK: Erlbaum.

Wilson, K. G. (1997). Science and treatment development: Lessons from the history of behavior therapy. *Behavior Therapy, 28,* 547–558.

Wilson, K. G., & DuFrene, T. (2009). *Mindfulness for two: An acceptance and commitment therapy approach to mindfulness in psychotherapy.* Oakland, CA: New Harbinger.

Witkiewitz, K., Marlatt, G. A., & Walker, D. D. (2005). Mindfulness-based relapse prevention for alcohol use disorders: The meditative tortoise wins the race. *Journal of Cognitive Psychotherapy, 19,* 211–228.

Zettle, R. D., Rains, J. C., & Hayes, S. C. (2011). Do acceptance and commitment therapy and cognitive therapy for depression work via the same process?: A reanalysis of Zettle and Rains, 1989. *Behavior Modification, 35,* 265–283.

PART III

THE BASIC SCIENCE OF MINDFULNESS

CHAPTER 9

From Conceptualization to Operationalization of Mindfulness

Jordan T. Quaglia, Kirk Warren Brown, Emily K. Lindsay,
J. David Creswell, and Robert J. Goodman

To study a phenomenon scientifically, it must be appropriately described and measured. How mindfulness is conceptualized and assessed has considerable importance for mindfulness science, and perhaps in part because of this, these two issues have been among the most contentious in the field. In recognition of the growing scientific and clinical interest in mindfulness, a number of textual scholars of mindfulness have in recent years made efforts to describe and explain the meaning of mindfulness within one or more Buddhist traditions (e.g., Bhikkhu Bodhi, 2011; Dreyfus, 2011; Dunne, 2011; Gethin, 2011, Chapter 2, this volume). This chapter addresses the other key contentious feature of mindfulness science noted earlier, the *operationalization* of mindfulness. Herein we offer a critical analysis of mindfulness operationalizations, which predominantly take the form of subjective, or self-report, methods. Mindfulness scales are used extensively in both basic and applied psychological research, and a number of questions about their use have arisen in recent years. We address several major questions in this chapter that center on the capacity of these measures to assess mindfulness validly.

How a construct is operationalized, from the items and dimensions used to represent it to the structure of the scale, is crucially dependent on the way it is conceptualized. Therefore, we begin with a brief discussion of classical scholarly and scientific conceptualizations of mindfulness, with particular attention to points of agreement and disagreement between mindfulness scholars and researchers. We subsequently review published self-report measures of mindfulness and some of the debates currently surrounding them. We then briefly discuss efforts to develop behavioral

151

measures of mindfulness and close with recommendations for further theoretical and empirical development in the assessment of mindfulness.

Conceptualizing Mindfulness

Classical Buddhist Scholarly Understandings

Scholarship on mindfulness offers an important interpretative lens through which to understand mindfulness as presented in Buddhist source texts. Buddhist scholarship, at its best, is built on a deep familiarity with such texts, the challenges stemming from their translations, and the difficulties inherent in changing word usage over the centuries (see Gethin, Chapter 2, this volume). From the outset of this discussion, it is important to convey that there is no single meaning of mindfulness to be found in Buddhism, and no single authoritative account that trumps all others (Anālayo, 2013; Dreyfus, 2011); each definition of mindfulness is rooted in a particular scholastic and practice tradition and must be understood within that context. Thus, we can speak of classical mindfulness, non-dual mindfulness, Zen mindfulness, and so on (Anālayo, 2013). As Dreyfus (2011) notes, "Buddhism is a plural tradition that has evolved over centuries to include a large variety of views about mindfulness" (p. 42).

Limitations of space and certainly, expertise, do not permit a discussion of all of these various understandings of mindfulness. For our purposes here we offer a brief look at several representative contemporary scholarly accounts of mindfulness as understood from classical Buddhist source texts (see Table 9.1, upper portion). By *classical* texts—also termed *canonical*—we refer to the Pali Canon, the oldest surviving, complete collection of Buddhist texts, which offers rich descriptions of mindfulness that informed subsequent interpretations and is still widely used today.

While by no means exhaustive, the scholarly accounts presented in Table 9.1 highlight conceptions of mindfulness as close, clear-minded attention to, or awareness of, what is perceived in the present. Noteworthy, however, are several key features of these canonical descriptions of mindfulness that are not easily conveyed in brief quotations. First, the scholarly accounts differ in referring to attention in some texts, and awareness in others. Differing usage of the terms *attention* and *awareness* may stem from the fact that, outside of cognitive science, the terms are sometimes used interchangeably (e.g., Merikle & Joordens, 1997). Some scholars have used both to describe mindfulness (e.g., Bhikkhu Bodhi, 2011; Wallace & Bhikkhu Bodhi, 2006) and, in fact, both terms may be applicable for two reasons. There is a close interrelation between attention and awareness in daily life (e.g., Lamme, 2003); also, and more specifically, an integration of attention and meta-awareness helps to distinguish mindfulness from related states. For example, attention may be concentrated, but only when coupled with meta-awareness—an apprehension of the current state of the mind that serves to monitor that focused attentiveness—does it become mindful (Dreyfus, 2011).

A second key feature of the canonical accounts bears on the role of thought in the meaning and expression of mindfulness. The mindfulness research literature frequently highlights the nonconceptual nature of mindfulness, wherein a de-fusion

TABLE 9.1. Selected Definitions of Basic Mindfulness in Contemporary Scholarship on Classical Buddhism and in the Scientific Literature

Source	Definition
Canonical Buddhist scholarly sources	
Anālayo (2003, p. 60)	". . . an alert but receptive equanimous observation."
Bhikkhu Bodhi (2011, p. 21)	". . . watchfulness, the lucid awareness of each event that presents itself on the successive occasions of experience."
Dreyfus (2011, p. 47)	"The mind's ability to keep the object in the ken [focus] of attention without losing it."
Gethin (Chapter 2, this volume, p. 32)	"A kind of lucid sustaining of attention on the object of awareness, in which the mind is both aware of the object and, in some sense, aware that it is aware . . ."
Scientific sources	
Kabat-Zinn (1994, p. 4)	"Paying attention in a particular way: on purpose, in the present moment, and nonjudgmentally."
Bishop et al. (2004, p. 232)	"[A] kind of nonelaborative, nonjudgmental, present-centered awareness in which each thought, feeling, or sensation that arises in the attentional field is acknowledged and accepted as it is."
Brown & Ryan (2004, p. 245)	"Open or receptive attention to and awareness of ongoing events and experience."

or disidentification from discursive thought is typically considered key (e.g., Bishop et al., 2004). Yet canonical interpretations of mindfulness see an important role for thought. For example, Bhikkhu Bodhi (2011) argues that as awareness becomes more lucid, comprehension of the nature and qualities of the phenomena observed also develops (e.g., an understanding of how anger arises in the mind). In this way, mindful awareness and comprehension of what is encountered are intertwined processes in practice, the combination of which leads to insight, or understanding of the mind and behavior. Bhikkhu Bodhi notes that clarity of awareness runs through all expressions of mindfulness, but can take on "varying layers of conceptual content ranging from 'heavy' to 'light' to 'zero'" (p. 31). Dreyfus (2011) proposes that only the basic expression of mindfulness (which he termed "mindfulness proper") concerns a sustained attention to perceptual objects, and it serves as a basis for the development of insight that a conjoining with comprehension provides. It is in this "wise mindfulness" that the potential of mindfulness to lessen suffering is realized.

A third central, and related, aspect of canonical mindfulness concerns the role of evaluation. This represents another point of difference from scientific and clinical conceptions of mindfulness wherein there is, as already noted, a dis-identification from thought, evaluative and otherwise. Evaluation here concerns discrimination, a reflective consideration of what is healthy and unhealthy, and wise or unwise action, for example, that comes with the conjoining of sustained attentiveness and comprehension. Bhikkhu Bodhi (2011, p. 26) makes this clear: "The practitioner of mindfulness must at times evaluate mental qualities and intended deeds, make judgments about them, and engage in purposeful action." In this way, canonical mindfulness can be value-laden, bringing together capacities of attention and discerning thought to regulate mental states and behavior.

Thus, mindfulness as understood in canonical commentaries is not antithetical to active cognitive operations. In a state of sustained, receptive attentiveness, evaluations and judgments, memories, and other cognitive operations can be closely attended to, and actively engaged, by a mind that is aware of what is happening moment to moment. As we will see, it is relative to thought, and evaluative thought in particular, that mindfulness primarily differs between canonical and many science-based conceptualizations, a difference that is important to understanding the diverse operationalizations of mindfulness.

Scientific Understandings

Examples of definitions of mindfulness in the scientific literature span a wide range, several of which are presented in Table 9.1 (lower portion). An early definition of mindfulness that continues to influence how clinicians and researchers understand the construct is that of Kabat-Zinn (1994), who describes mindfulness as intentional, nonjudgmental attention. Similarly, Bishop and colleagues (2004) proposed a two-factor definition of mindfulness comprising a self-regulation of attention to maintain focus on present experience, and a purposive, attitudinal orientation toward the present moment that includes, among other features, curiosity and acceptance. In contrast to these approaches, Brown and Ryan (e.g., 2003) focus on the deployment of attention that also characterizes the canonical descriptions of basic mindfulness outlined earlier. Brown and Ryan (2004) agree with the other science-based definitions here that nonjudgment is part of mindfulness, but they argue that it is inherent in the receptive attention deployed rather than being a separate attitude. This perspective is concordant with that of Anālayo (2003, p. 60) in describing mindfulness as "see[ing] things just as they are, unadulterated by habitual reactions and projections" (see also Table 9.1).

Of particular relevance to both the conceptualization and operationalization of mindfulness is the "nonjudgmental" or "acceptance" feature emphasized in most of these scientific definitions and in mindfulness research more broadly. This feature, generally framed as an attitude, represents a departure from canonical mindfulness. Bhikkhu Bodhi (2011; see also Wallace & Bhikkhu Bodhi, 2006), for example, has explicitly stated that what is commonly called "acceptance" is not part of mindfulness, as it does not distinguish between wholesome and unwholesome states of mind (also see Dreyfus, 2011). Dunne (2011) suggests that the nonevaluative, nonjudgmental feature highlighted in the Kabat-Zinn and other definitions bears similarity to a non-dual conception of mindfulness that arose centuries after the original, canonical conception (also see Kabat-Zinn, 2011). Yet Dreyfus (2011) points out that while nonjudgmental awareness is not an adequate theoretical description of canonical mindfulness, it can be useful as practical instruction in developing mindfulness, to enable a disengagement from habitual mental discursivity and reactivity that inhibits sustained attentiveness and the formation of mature discriminative judgments. Thus, nonjudgmentality represents a "skillful means" to enhance mindfulness rather than the thing itself. In this regard, it bears noting that while Kabat-Zinn's framing of mindfulness as nonjudgmental attention has had considerable impact on how researchers and clinicians understand the concept, his aim in defining it in this way was in fact to serve practical instruction rather than conceptual precision (Kabat-Zinn, 2011).

We believe there is considerable opportunity for further interchange between Buddhist scholarship and Western science in seeking shared understandings of mindfulness that are sensitive to differences among traditions and trainee populations (see Gethin, Chapter 2, this volume). Western science may also foster new insights about how to conceptualize mindfulness (e.g., Davis & Thompson, Chapter 3, and Tang & Posner, Chapter 5, this volume). For example, cognitive science research indicates that attention and conscious awareness can be decoupled (Koch & Tsuchiya, 2012; Watanabe et al., 2011), such that attention can serve as a gate to conscious awareness. This work suggests the possibility that both attention and awareness are needed for mindfulness to arise, and that attention is a necessary precondition for awareness. Interestingly, this is consistent with classical Buddhist theory, wherein attention toward one's present-moment experience fosters conscious awareness of phenomenal experience. Such research may help to reveal how mindfulness operates on a moment-to-moment basis, and how best to teach it.

Operationalizations of Mindfulness

Reflecting the varied conceptualizations of mindfulness, there have been numerous efforts to operationalize mindfulness, and to date, all have been informed by classical and/or science-based conceptions. Most measures of trait and state mindfulness take the form of self-report–based scales, although there is recent interest in behavioral measurement. Arguably, the use of mindfulness measures has contributed to our understanding of the construct and has shown how mindfulness itself—apart from the multicomponent training programs designed to enhance it—is related to numerous outcomes at the neurobiological, subjective, and behavioral levels in a variety of normative and clinical populations.

Before discussing research results employing the various mindfulness scales, it is important to note briefly the controversial issues surrounding their use. Questions concerning mindfulness scale use include the following:

Do self-report–based instruments actually measure mindfulness?
Can the same scales be used for both mindfulness-naive and trained populations?
Does the interpretation of scale items depend on first-person experience with mindfulness?
Is it appropriate to trust the self-endorsement of mindfulness, or are responses inherently biased? Do we need self-report-based or other measures of

mindfulness or is it sufficient to build a science based on measured outcomes of mindfulness training?

There is insufficient space to address these questions in detail here, but recently published articles debate these and other mindfulness measurement issues (Brown, Ryan, Loverich, Biegel, & West, 2011; Goodman, Quaglia, & Brown, in press; Grossman, 2011). In the remainder of this chapter, we consider three central questions about the assessment of mindfulness:

Do self-report scales measure mindfulness?
Are these measures valid predictors of theoretically meaningful outcomes?
How can mindfulness assessment be improved?

There are currently eight published self-report measures of trait or dispositional mindfulness for adults and two such scales for adolescents and children. Two additional scales measure state mindfulness in adults. *State mindfulness* concerns the quality of mindful presence at a given moment, or within a narrow window of time (e.g., the past 5 minutes). Measures of *trait* or *dispositional mindfulness* typically concern the general, cross-situational frequency of mindful states over time. Individual differences in trait mindfulness are thought to stem from two sources. First, many scholars and researchers agree that training in mindfulness techniques can lead to higher levels of dispositional mindfulness. Second, individuals may vary naturally in this trait, perhaps due to genetic predisposition, socialization, attention-intensive training, or other factors. Most measures of trait mindfulness were developed with this *innateist* (Dunne, 2011; also see Dreyfus, 2011) view in mind. Two trait scales were developed for use with mindfulness trainees (the Freiburg Mindfulness Inventory [FMI]: Walach, Buchheld, Buttenmuller, Kleinknecht, & Schmidt, 2006; the Toronto Mindfulness Scale [TMS]: Lau, Bishop, & Segal, 2006), thereby implicitly or explicitly taking a *constructivist* or training-dependent (Dunne, 2011) position on the development of the disposition. Yet several scales (e.g., the Five Facet Mindfulness Questionnaire [FFMQ]: Baer, Smith, Hopkins, Krietemeyer, & Toney, 2006; the Mindful Attention Awareness Scale [MAAS]: Brown & Ryan, 2003) have demonstrated reliability and validity in both general (nontrainee) and mindfulness trainee populations, as well as sensitivity to scale score changes coinciding with mindfulness training. Table 9.2 presents these scales: their primary conceptual origins, factor structures, and other psychometric properties; the populations in which each has been validated; evidence for the reliability and construct validity of each scale; and the types of outcomes to which each scale has been applied.

Do Self-Report Scales Measure Mindfulness?

Whether the extant scales actually measure mindfulness is a question prompted by recognition of the complex, subtle nature of mindfulness, the diversity of operationalizations of the construct, and the apparent similarity of some scales (and subscales) to other forms of attention. We address each issue in turn.

TABLE 9.2. Psychometric Characteristics of Self-Report Mindfulness Scales

Scale name/authors	No. of items	Primary conceptual origin	Factor(s)	Population(s) of application	Reliability	Validity	Outcome methods	Outcome domain
Trait scales for adults								
Cognitive and Affective Mindfulness Scale—Revised (CAMS-R; Feldman et al., 2007)	12	Clinical	Attention, Present-focus, Awareness, Acceptance	Undergraduate	Internal consistency	Convergent, discriminant, concurrent	SR, Task	CF, MH
Five Factor Mindfulness Questionnaire (FFMQ; Baer et al., 2006)	39	Clinical (DBT)	Observe, Describe, Act with awareness, Nonjudge, Nonreact	Undergraduate, experienced meditator, community adult, clinical	Internal consistency	Convergent, discriminant, concurrent	SR, EMA, Neuro, Task	CF, BR, ER, MH, PH
Freiburg Mindfulness Inventory (FMI; Walach et al., 2006)	30	Theravādan Buddhist (scholarly, popular), clinical	Mindfulness	Subclinical, diverse clinical, experienced meditator	Internal consistency	Convergent, discriminant, concurrent	SR	BR, MH
Kentucky Inventory of Mindfulness Skills (KIMS; Baer et al., 2004)	39	Clinical (DBT)	Observe, Describe, Act with awareness, Accept without judgment	Undergraduate, clinical	Internal consistency, test–retest	Convergent, discriminant, concurrent, predictive	SR, Neuro, Task	CF, ER, MH

(continued)

TABLE 9.2. (continued)

Scale name/authors	No. of items	Primary conceptual origin	Factor(s)	Population(s) of application	Reliability	Validity	Outcome methods	Outcome domain
				Trait scales for adults				
Mindful Attention Awareness Scale (MAAS; Brown & Ryan, 2003)	15	Theravādan Buddhist (scholarly, popular), clinical	Attention/ awareness	Undergraduate, community adult, experienced meditator, clinical	Internal consistency, test–retest, Parallel forms	Convergent, discriminant, concurrent, predictive, incremental	SR, EMA, Neuro, Physio, Task	CF, BR, ER, MH, PH
Philadelphia Mindfulness Scale (PHLMS; Cardaciotto et al., 2008)	20	Clinical	Awareness, Acceptance	Undergraduate, clinical	Internal consistency	Convergent, discriminant, concurrent, predictive	SR, Neuro	CF, MH
Trait Toronto Mindfulness Scale (TMS; Davis, Lau, & Cairns, 2009)	13	Clinical	Curiosity, Decentering	Undergraduate, experienced meditator, adult	Internal consistency	Convergent, discriminant, incremental	SR, Task	CF
Southampton Mindfulness Questionnaire (SMQ; Chadwick et al., 2008)	16	Clinical	Decentered awareness, Letting go of reacting, Accepting, Opening awareness to difficult experience	Meditator, adult, clinical	Internal consistency	Convergent, discriminant, Concurrent	SR	MH

158

State scales for adults

Scale	#	Basis	Facets	Populations	Reliability	Validity	Methods	Outcomes
State Mindful Attention Awareness Scale (State MAAS; Brown & Ryan, 2003)	5	See MAAS, above	Attention/ awareness	Undergraduate, community adult, experienced meditator, clinical	Internal consistency, test–retest, parallel forms	Convergent, discriminant, predictive, concurrent	SR, EMA, Task	CF, MH
State Toronto Mindfulness Scale (State TMS; Lau et al., 2006)	13	Clinical	Curiosity, Decentering	Undergraduate, experienced meditator, community adult	Internal consistency	Convergent, discriminant, incremental	SR, Task	ER, MH, PH

Trait scales for children/adolescents

Scale	#	Basis	Facets	Populations	Reliability	Validity	Methods	Outcomes
Child Acceptance and Mindfulness Measure (CAMM; Greco, Baer, & Smith, 2011)	10	Clinical (DBT)	Mindfulness	Community child, adolescent (grades 5–10)	Internal consistency	Convergent, discriminant	SR, 2nd-person	MH
Mindful Attention Awareness Scale— Adolescent (MAAS-A; Brown, West, Loverich, & Beigel, 2011)	14	See MAAS, above	Attention/ awareness	Community adolescent, clinical adolescent	Internal consistency, test–retest	Convergent, discriminant, concurrent	SR	MH

Note. DBT, dialectical behavior therapy; SR, self-report; Task, task performance behavioral measure; EMA, ecological momentary assessment; Neuro, neurophysiological measures (e.g., EEG, fMRI); Physio, peripheral physiological measures (e.g., cortisol); 2nd-person, second-person ratings of behavior; CF, cognitive functioning; BR, behavior regulation; ER, emotion regulation; MH, mental health; PH, physical health.

Complexity of the Construct

Mindfulness is a quality of mind that can both occur spontaneously and be developed or enhanced through practices such as meditation. Thus, expressions of mindfulness may be expected to show more subtleties among those with more training in mindfulness, just as our understanding of what it means to play a musical instrument, or perform any number of other skills, is subject to change according to level of experience.

Unquestionably, the current mindfulness scales primarily tap rudimentary expressions of mindfulness, and this is by design because all were developed with mindfulness naive or novice trainee respondents in mind. Yet just as the basic, brief training offered by current mindfulness interventions has shown remarkable effects on brain function, subjective experience, and behavior, so too have scaled measures of mindfulness predicted a range of subjective and objective outcomes consistent with mindfulness theory, as suggested by evidence we discuss later. Nonetheless, to date, subtly nuanced measurement of mindfulness has been neglected in efforts to establish the construct validity of the existing measures.

Scale Diversity

How should one best think about so many operationalizations of mindfulness? It has been argued that the diversity of scales, particularly the differing factor structures, reflects poor consensus about what mindfulness is, and without such consensus, these scales cannot be said to assess the phenomenon adequately (Grossman, 2011). We suggest, alternatively, that there are valid reasons for a diversity of measures, and researchers can make effective use of this diversity to address different research objectives. Mindfulness scale differences, particularly the differing factor structures, likely stem from at least two sources: (1) the explicit or implicit conceptual position driving the definition and operationalization, and (2) the intended uses of the scale.

Regarding the former, most extant scales were derived with one or more of three sources in mind: Buddhist scholarship, Buddhist popular writings, and clinical approaches (see Table 9.2). We regard a clinical source for definition and operationalization as one that applies mindfulness to clinical issues, but it is important to note that some clinical approaches (e.g., Kabat-Zinn, 1990; Linehan, 1993) have drawn on Buddhist and other contemplative sources. Calling a theoretical source *clinical* is in recognition that clinical applications, because they are oriented toward the goals of fostering adjustment and well-being, can involve particular, even unique, ways of conceptualizing mindfulness (also see Chiesa & Malinowski, 2011; Dreyfus, 2011). As examples of each source, the Kentucky Inventory of Mindfulness Skills (KIMS; Baer, Smith, & Allen, 2004) and its structurally similar descendant, the FFMQ, were developed from the dialectical behavior therapy (DBT) model of "mindfulness skills" (Linehan, 1993), cultivated through a variety of short exercises originally designed for individuals with borderline personality disorder. These exercises particularly focus on the elements of observing, describing, acting with awareness, nonjudgment of inner experience, and nonreactivity to emotional events, all of which are important tools in self-regulation specifically targeted within DBT, and thus have utility as outcomes measures. The Philadelphia Mindfulness Scale (PHLMS; Cardaciotto, Herbert, Forman, Moitra, & Farrow, 2008) was derived from Kabat-Zinn's model of mindfulness as nonjudgmental attention, which links this measurement approach with an emphasis on stress reduction, while the FMI and MAAS were developed primarily on the basis of canonical, and specifically Theravādin Buddhist, scholarship and popular writings, as well as clinical writings on mindfulness and its practice.

Despite the wide variance in sources and aims, all of the scales shown in Table 9.2 either focus on quality of attention and awareness as the central feature (e.g., MAAS) or include it among a set of factors (e.g., FFMQ Act with Awareness subscale). Beyond this factor, the scales differ widely in their inclusion of other factors (e.g., acceptance, nonjudgment). Thus, diversity of operationalizations primarily reflects conceptual divergences concerning what processes, aside from attention and awareness, are part of mindfulness and must therefore be part of its measurement. These conceptual differences have manifold implications for the ways in which mindfulness, its development, its antecedents, and its consequences are understood. For example, aside from the conceptual issue raised by the canonical perspective on mindfulness noted earlier, the acceptance or nonjudgment factor included in several scales is also considered a form of emotion regulation (e.g., Aldao, Nolen-Hoeksema, & Schweizer, 2010) and a coping strategy (Carver, Scheier, & Weintraub, 1989), making operational overlap between these constructs a key concern. Also, measures of mindfulness skills may be conflated with those outcomes of practicing mindfulness that reflect the development of introspective skills (e.g., the ability to describe internal events).

Differences between scales may also be attributed to their intended uses, particularly regarding the focal population. Some scales, such as the MAAS, which has state and trait versions, were developed for use in the general population to assess naturally occurring variations in mindfulness both between individuals and within persons as a function of current context or training. In contrast, the FMI and the state TMS were developed to measure mindfulness within mindfulness meditation training contexts. Similarly, the FFMQ was validated as a four-factor version for the general population and a five-factor version for practitioners (that includes the Observe factor), though the latter version is commonly used in both populations (but from a psychometric validation perspective, inappropriately so). Differences between scales according to target population are reasonable given that mindfulness may be understood differently by those with or without experience in it. Knowing the populations for which each scale has been designed and validated (see Table 9.2) better informs choices about which scale(s) to use for any given research situation.

In summary, understanding that different scales stem from differences in their conceptual starting points, intended applications, and target populations can inform choices about which to use in research. As we have reviewed, conceptions of mindfulness vary both between and within Buddhist and Western psychological traditions. Whereas all share a common focus on quality of attention to, or awareness of ongoing experience, they diverge in whether attitudinal and other features are part of the construct. Many of the measures were designed for particular populations and with particular aims in mind, such as assessing the lived, day-to-day experience of mindfulness, or measuring mindfulness practice skills. In the face of such differences in conception and intended use, researchers would do well to carefully consider scale choices and specify the guiding theory and intended use when describing the chosen measure in their research reports. Furthermore, empirical research is needed to show whether some mindfulness scale factors are better understood as representing other constructs, such as emotion regulation (e.g., Coffey, Hartman, & Fredrickson, 2010). Such research would not only clarify the nature of the selected measure but also foster clearer interpretation of research findings.

Dissociability from Other Attention Constructs

A second key issue in whether the extant self-report scales measure mindfulness concerns their discriminability from measures of other attention-related constructs. For example, attentional control measures, commonly understood as tapping the capacity to select deliberately and focus on a particular object over others have, like mindfulness, been associated with adaptive outcomes, such as lower attentional bias to threatening information among trait anxiety populations (Derryberry & Reed, 2002).

Attentional control and mindfulness appear to be overlapping constructs. Both capacities involve an increased stability, or continuity, of attention toward a focal object, and both may be trainable. Evidence also supports their relation (e.g., Brown, Goodman, & Inzlicht, 2013; Mrazek, Smallwood, & Schooler, 2012). Despite this similarity, there is theoretical divergence between the two constructs. In particular, mindfulness is distinct in its interrelation with meta-awareness and its receptivity to ongoing phenomena (see Goodman et al., 2014, for further discussion). If measures of mindfulness are dissociable from those of attentional control, the former should also predict theoretically relevant outcomes over and above the latter. Emerging evidence supports such incremental validity. For example, Brown and colleagues (2013) found that both the MAAS and FFMQ Act with Awareness subscale measures, but not a measure of attentional control, predicted reduced amplitudes of the *late positive potential* (LPP)—an electrocortical indicator of emotional reactivity—in response to unpleasant, high-arousal images. Quaglia, Goodman, and Brown (2014) also found that whereas the MAAS predicted electrocortical markers of top-down attention to socioemotional stimuli (the N100, N200, and No-Go P300), attentional control did not.

Grossman (2011) has argued that some mindfulness measures are merely capturing "experienced lapses of attention" (p. 1038). This charge has relied, to a considerable degree, on *face validity*—the superficial appearance, or face value—of scale items as reflections of a construct. Because it relies on subjective judgment, face validity is typically not a scientific criterion for judging the value of a measure (e.g., Gravetter & Forzano, 2009). Scale items may bear no obvious relation to the construct of interest (Walsh & Betz, 2001) and, as with some mindfulness scales (e.g., FFMQ, KIMS, MAAS), indirect assessment is sometimes necessary when self-knowledge or social desirability is a concern (Gravetter & Forzano, 2009; Walsh & Betz, 2001). Furthermore, the construct validity evidence reviewed here shows that measures of mindfulness and a key form of attention (attentional control) are dissociable, and only the former have predicted outcomes consistent with mindfulness theory. In summary, the meaning of a construct lies not in item content per se but in the entire body of theoretical and empirical relations with other constructs. Said differently, the meaning of the measure *is* its construct validity.

Yet during this still early stage of research on dispositional mindfulness, self-report measures of the construct should continue to be subjected to rigorous empirical scrutiny. Studies that use self-report measures of mindfulness should incorporate additional measures of attention that share variance with mindfulness to assess their relations and incremental validity. Aside from addressing validity concerns, such research will enhance our understanding of how mindfulness fits into the nomological network of other, established indices of attention (e.g., Posner & Rothbart, 2007).

Are Self-Report Measures Valid Predictors of Theoretically Meaningful Outcomes?

Whether mindfulness scales predict theoretically expected outcomes is a key issue concerning both their construct validity and their research and clinical value. As indicated in the rightmost columns of Table 9.2, research has examined whether trait and, to a lesser extent, state mindfulness are associated with, or predict a variety of outcomes, ranging from those in cognitive, affective, and mental/physical health domains. Whether individual differences in mindfulness show relations to such important outcomes can inform understanding of the value of more frequent mindful states. We have previously reviewed much of this literature (see Brown, Ryan, & Creswell, 2007; Goodman et al., in press), but in brief, several self-report measures of mindfulness are related to a broad range of objective behavioral and neurophysiological outcomes in theoretically expected directions. For example, in the cognitive domain, scores on the Cognitive and Affective Mindfulness Scale—Revised (CAMS-R) and MAAS were negatively correlated with target omissions on the Continuous Performance Test II, indicating fewer attention lapses during this focused task among more mindful individuals (Schmertz, Anderson, & Robins, 2009). Similarly, Mrazek and colleagues (2012) found that higher MAAS scores negatively related to the number of errors on the Sustained Attention to Response Task (SART), which is also used to index mind wandering. Finally, Moore and Malinowski (2009) found that global KIMS scores were positively correlated with sustained attention on the d2-Concentration and Endurance Test.

In the affective domain, multiple functional magnetic resonance imaging (fMRI) studies have demonstrated that mindfulness scale scores predict meaningful differences in neural activation soon after encountering emotionally salient stimuli. Amygdala activation appears to index emotional appraisal (Oschner & Gross, 2005; Damasio, 1994; Davidson, 2000), and MAAS scores have predicted greater activity in prefrontal cortical regions and decreased activity in the amygdala during emotion regulation tasks (Creswell, Way, Eisenberger, & Lieberman, 2007; Modinos, Ormel, & Aleman, 2010; cf. Frewen et al., 2010). Interestingly, Way, Creswell, Eisenberger, and Lieberman (2010) found that MAAS scores predicted lower bilateral amygdala activation at rest, suggesting lower susceptibility to threat-based appraisals. Consistent with these findings, Taren, Creswell, and Gianaros (2013) found a relation between MAAS-assessed trait mindfulness and decreased gray-matter amygdala volume in a large sample of community adults, providing evidence of a neurobiological pathway that may help explain how mindful attention alters stress and emotional responding. Mindfulness scale scores show a similar pattern of effects with ecological indicators of emotion regulation. Brown (2011) found that MAAS scores predicted less emotional lability on a day-to-day basis by using experience sampling, part of a family of ecological momentary assessment (EMA) methods that track participants' real-world subjective experience and behavior. Another EMA study revealed that the Nonreactivity subscale of the FFMQ predicted more subtle differentiation between types of positive and negative emotion, reflected in smaller correlations between ratings of similar emotions, as well as less emotional lability of both positive and negative emotion (Hill & Updegraff, 2012). Mindfulness scale associations have also been found in studies of adaptive behavior regulation in such domains as gambling (Lakey, Campbell, Brown, & Goodie, 2007), drinking (Garland, 2011), and smoking (Black, Sussman, Johnson, & Milam, 2011).

In the health domain, mindfulness scales have been associated with biological markers of stress and physical health. MAAS-measured mindfulness has in two studies been found to be associated with reduced psychological and biological (cortisol) stress reactivity to acute physical and social stressors (Arch & Craske, 2006, 2010; Brown, Weinstein, & Creswell, 2012). Mindfulness scales have also been associated with reduced physical symptoms and physician visits (Brown & Ryan, 2003).

This brief overview of some key findings, along with findings organized by domain in Table 9.2, indicate that several mindfulness measures, particularly the MAAS and KIMS/FFMQ Act with Awareness subscales, are related to, or predict cognitive, emotional, behavior regulatory, and physical health-relevant physiological outcomes in ways consistent with theoretical conceptions of mindfulness. The findings are also broadly consistent with those revealed by studies of mindfulness training (Goodman et al., in press), suggesting that the scale measures are tapping psychological phenomena fostered through such training.

How Can Mindfulness Assessment Be Improved?

Despite the variety of scale operationalizations, several extant self-report scales have shown strong construct validity, including the ability to predict outcomes consistent with both mindfulness theory and research based on experimental inductions of mindfulness and mindfulness training (also see Arch & Landy, Chapter 12, this volume). Further validation in both lay and trainee populations may extend the utility of these scales. Yet the question remains whether participants can accurately report their levels of mindfulness. Although we have described a number of theoretically consistent outcomes predicted by self-report scales, more objective measures of mindfulness may provide more precision. Initial steps have been taken to develop behavioral, second-person, and ecological/ambulatory measures of mindfulness, which we outline next.

Behavioral Measures of Mindfulness

The inherently subjective nature of mindfulness makes it unlikely that the construct could, even in principle, be reduced to behavioral assessment alone, but such measures could provide corroboration of mindful states or traits at a level of analysis not subject to the response biases that can creep into self-reports of behavior. Furthest along this line of investigation are behavioral measures of mind wandering, which have been conceptualized as occurrences of task-unrelated thoughts (Smallwood & Schooler, 2006). Mind wandering has been considered antithetical to mindfulness in some accounts (Christoff, Gordon, Smallwood, Smith, & Schooler, 2009; Davidson, 2000) and, as already noted, recent research shows a convergence of mind-wandering measures/tasks and self-reported mindfulness (Burg & Michalak, 2011; Mrazek et al., 2012). But definitions of mindfulness (see, e.g., Table 9.1) suggest that it is more than an absence of mind wandering; so assessing mindfulness behaviorally will require more than measures of mind wandering.

Naturally occurring, observable behaviors may also inform about level of state mindfulness. For example, though not yet tested for predictive validity, a measure of introspective accuracy of tactile sensitivity may help to index mindfulness. Fox and colleagues (2012) showed that expert meditators' subjective reports of tactile sensitivity during a body scan better matched objective measures than did the reports of novice meditators. These behavioral measures provide a promising avenue for further research.

Second-Person Structured Interviews

Mindfulness teachers and other experts on the subjective and objective markers of mindfulness may also provide assessments of individuals' level of mindfulness through targeted probing of subjective experience and observation of behavior. Qualitative interview techniques may be used to assess the training-related development of mindfulness (Garland & Gaylord, 2009), as well as to explore mechanisms of change in mindfulness interventions (Mackenzie, Carlson, Munoz, & Speca, 2007; Williams, McManus, Muse, & Williams, 2011). Investigators have recently begun to develop expert interview schedules to assess mindfulness in trainees (e.g., Stelter, 2010). Potential risks of this interview approach include self-presentation and other response biases, but the approach has a long history and holds promise for assessing trait and state mindfulness, as well as the developmental processes that may unfold through mindfulness training.

Ecological Momentary Assessment

EMA seeks to capture experience and behavior as it happens in day-to-day life, typically through the use of records made on mobile electronic devices (e.g., cell phones). The recording of cognitive processes during mindfulness practice sessions and normative daily activities may provide a useful index of mindful states (Garland & Gaylord, 2009) that, when examined over time, could inform about dispositions toward mindfulness (e.g., Brown & Ryan, 2003). Unlike single-occasion self-report measures, EMA does not require significant retrospection that may be tainted by memory biases, and it permits the study of how mindful states are related to behaviors of interest occurring in real-world contexts (Hill & Updegraff, 2012; Levesque & Brown, 2007). EMA recording is time-, labor-, and potentially cost-intensive, however, suggesting that its current utility as a measure of mindfulness will be to supplement more efficient means.

Conclusions

Research on the conceptualization and operationalization of mindfulness has been provocative, generating debates about the meaning, assessment, development, and training of this quality. In this chapter we have attempted to show that in the midst of these valuable debates, efforts to define and measure basic forms of mindfulness as a trait and state have contributed to a developing theory and to a growing, multi-faceted body of empirical findings on mindfulness. Such investigation of subjective states has also opened topics to inquiry not easily permissible by other means, and is increasingly being done in conjunction with neurophysiological and behavioral methods to better inform understanding of the underpinnings, processes, and outcomes of mindfulness.

Much work is needed to understand better the nature and expression of mindfulness, as suggested in our review. Research should further examine the close relations between mindfulness and well-researched cognitive functions, including neurally mediated systems of attention (Posner & Petersen, 1990) and working memory. Work is also clearly needed on mindfulness assessment. In the present review of mindfulness scales, few have been shown to predict objective outcomes. At this time, it is unclear whether the majority of scales lack predictive validity for such outcomes or simply have yet to be used in such research. More broadly, rigorous assessment research undertaken in intimate dialogue with scholarly conceptualization efforts will do much to enhance research using self-report, behavioral, or other means of tapping traits and states of mindfulness. These iterations among theory, measurement, and observation will help to expand and better integrate our scientific knowledge of mindfulness; more broadly, such research can also contribute to applying that science to its most beneficial ends.

REFERENCES

Aldao, A., Nolen-Hoeksema, S., & Schweizer, S. (2010). Emotion-regulation strategies across psychopathology: A meta-analytic review. *Clinical Psychology Review, 30*(2), 217–237.

Anālayo, B. (2013). *Mindfulness in early Buddhism.* Unpublished manuscript, University of Hamburg, Hamburg, Germany.

Anālayo, B. (2003). *Satipaṭṭhāna: The direct path to realization.* Birmingham, UK: Windhorse.

Arch, J. J., & Craske, M. G. (2006). Mechanisms of mindfulness: Emotion regulation following a focused breathing induction. *Behaviour Research and Therapy*, 44(12), 1849–1858.

Arch, J. J., & Craske, M. G. (2010). Laboratory stressors in clinically anxious and non-anxious individuals: The moderating role of mindfulness. *Behaviour Research and Therapy*, 48(6), 495–505.

Baer, R. A. (2003). Mindfulness training as a clinical intervention: A conceptual and empirical review. *Clinical Psychology Science and Practice*, 10(2), 125–143.

Baer, R. A., Smith, G. T., & Allen, K. B. (2004). Assessment of mindfulness by self-report: The Kentucky Inventory of Mindfulness Skills. *Assessment*, 11(3), 191–206.

Baer, R. A., Smith, G. T., Hopkins, J., Krietemeyer, J., & Toney, L. (2006). Using self-report assessment methods to explore facets of mindfulness. *Assessment*, 13, 27–45.

Bishop, S. R., Lau, M., Shapiro, S., Carlson, L., Anderson, N. D., Carmody, J., et al. (2004). Mindfulness: A proposed operational definition. *Clinical Psychology: Science and Practice*, 11(3), 230–241.

Black, D. S., Sussman, S., Johnson, C. A., & Milam, J. (2011). Testing the indirect effect of trait mindfulness on adolescent cigarette smoking through negative affect and perceived stress mediators. *Journal of Substance Use*, 17, 417–429.

Bhikkhu Bodhi. (2006). *The noble eightfold path: Way to the end of suffering*. Onalaska, WA: Pariyatti.

Bhikkhu Bodhi. (2011). What does mindfulness really mean?: A canonical perspective. *Contemporary Buddhism*, 12(1), 19–39.

Brown, K. W. (2011, July). *Mindfulness and emotional stability in day-to-day life: Findings from experience sampling research*. Paper presented at the 2nd World Congress on Positive Psychology, Philadelphia, PA.

Brown, K. W., Goodman, R. J., & Inzlicht, M. (2013). Dispositional mindfulness and the attenuation of neural responses to emotional stimuli. *Social Cognitive and Affective Neuroscience*, 8(1), 93–99.

Brown, K. W., & Ryan, R. M. (2003). The benefits of being present: Mindfulness and its role in psychological well-being. *Journal of Personality and Social Psychology*, 84(4), 822–848.

Brown, K. W., & Ryan, R. M. (2004). Perils and promise in defining and measuring mindfulness: Observations from experience. *Clinical Psychology: Science and Practice*, 11(3), 242–248.

Brown, K. W., Ryan, R. M., & Creswell, J. D. (2007). Mindfulness: Theoretical foundations and evidence for its salutary effects. *Psychological Inquiry*, 18(4), 211–237.

Brown, K. W., Ryan, R. M., Loverich, T. M., Biegel, G. M., & West, A. M. (2011). Out of the armchair and into the streets: Measuring mindfulness advances knowledge and improves interventions: Reply to Grossman (2011). *Psychological Assessment*, 23(4), 1041–1046.

Brown, K. W., Weinstein, N., & Creswell, J. D. (2012). Trait mindfulness modulates neuroendocrine and affective responses to social evaluative threat. *Psychoneuroendocrinology*, 37(12), 2037–2041.

Brown, K. W., West, A. M., Loverich, T. M., & Biegel, G. M. (2011). Assessing adolescent mindfulness: Validation of an adapted Mindful Attention Awareness Scale in adolescent normative and psychiatric populations. *Psychological Assessment*, 23, 1023–1033.

Burg, J. M., & Michalak, J. (2011). The healthy quality of mindful breathing: Associations with rumination and depression. *Cognitive Therapy and Research*, 35(2), 179–185.

Cardaciotto, L., Herbert, J. D., Forman, E. M., Moitra, E., & Farrow, V. (2008). The assessment of present-moment awareness and acceptance: The Philadelphia Mindfulness Scale. *Assessment*, 15, 204–223.

Carver, C. S., Scheier, M. F., & Weintraub, J. K. (1989). Assessing coping strategies: A theoretically based approach. *Journal of Personality and Social Psychology, 56*(2), 267–283.

Chadwick, P., Hember, M., Symes, J., Peters, E., Kuipers, E., & Dagnan, D. (2008). Responding mindfully to unpleasant thoughts and images: Reliability and validity of the Southampton Mindfulness Questionnaire (SMQ). *British Journal of Clinical Psychology, 47*(4), 451–455.

Chiesa, A., & Malinowski, P. (2011). Mindfulness based approaches: Are they all the same? *Journal of Clinical Psychology, 67,* 404–424.

Christoff, K., Gordon, A. M., Smallwood, J., Smith, R., & Schooler, J. W. (2009). Experience sampling during fMRI reveals default network and executive system contributions to mind wandering. *Proceedings of the National Academy of Sciences, 106*(21), 8719–8724.

Coffey, K. A., Hartman, M., & Fredrickson, B. L. (2010). Deconstructing mindfulness and constructing mental health: Understanding mindfulness and its mechanisms of action. *Mindfulness, 1,* 235–253.

Creswell, J. D., Way, B. M., Eisenberger, N. I., & Lieberman, M. D. (2007). Neural correlates of dispositional mindfulness during affect labeling. *Psychosomatic Medicine, 69,* 560–565.

Damasio, A. R. (1994). *Descartes' error.* New York: Putnam.

Davidson, R. J. (2000). Affective style, psychopathology, and resilience: Brain mechanisms and plasticity. *American Psychology, 55,* 1196–1214.

Davis, K. M., Lau, M. A., & Cairns, D. R. (2009). Development and preliminary validation of a trait version of the Toronto Mindfulness Scale. *Journal of Cognitive Psychotherapy, 23*(3), 185–197.

Derryberry, D., & Reed, M. A. (2002). Anxiety-related attentional biases and their regulation by attentional control. *Journal of Abnormal Psychology, 111*(2), 225–236.

Dreyfus, G. (2011). Is mindfulness present-centred and non-judgmental?: A discussion of the cognitive dimensions of mindfulness. *Contemporary Buddhism, 12*(1), 41–54.

Dunne, J. (2011). Toward an understanding of non-dual mindfulness. *Contemporary Buddhism, 12*(1), 71–88.

Feldman, G., Hayes, A., Kumar, S., Greeson, J., & Laurenceau, J. P. (2007). Mindfulness and emotion regulation: The development and initial validation of the Cognitive and Affective Mindfulness Scale—Revised (CAMS-R). *Journal of Psychopathology and Behavioral Assessment, 29*(3), 177–190.

Fox, K. C., Zakarauskas, P., Dixon, M., Ellamil, M., Thompson, E., & Christoff, K. (2012). Meditation experience predicts introspective accuracy. *PLoS ONE, 7*(9), e45370.

Frewen, P. A., Dozois, D. J., Neufeld, R. W., Lane, R. D., Densmore, M., Stevens, T. K., et al. (2010). Individual differences in trait mindfulness predict dorsomedial prefrontal and amygdala response during emotional imagery: An fMRI study. *Personality and Individual Differences, 49*(5), 479–484.

Garland, E., & Gaylord, S. (2009). Envisioning a future contemplative science of mindfulness: Fruitful methods and new content for the next wave of research. *Complementary Health Practice Review, 14*(1), 3–9.

Garland, E. L. (2011). Trait mindfulness predicts attentional and autonomic regulation of alcohol cue-reactivity. *Journal of Psychophysiology, 25*(4), 180–189.

Gethin, R. (2011). On some definitions of mindfulness. *Contemporary Buddhism, 12*(01), 263–279.

Goodman, R. J., Quaglia, J. T., & Brown, K. W. (in press). Burning issues in dispositional mindfulness research. In B. D. Ostafin, M. D. Robinson, & B. P. Meier (Eds.), *Mindfulness and self-regulation*. New York: Springer.

Gravetter, F. J., & Forzano, L.-A. B. (2009). *Research methods for the behavioral sciences* (3rd ed.). Belmont, CA: Wadsworth.

Greco, L. A., Baer, R. A., & Smith, G. T. (2011). Assessing mindfulness in children and adolescents: Development and validation of the Child and Adolescent Mindfulness Measure (CAMM). *Psychological Assessment, 23*(3), 606–614.

Grossman, P. (2011). Defining mindfulness by how poorly I think I pay attention during everyday awareness and other intractable problems for psychology's (re)invention of mindfulness: Comment on Brown et al. (2011). *Psychological Assessment, 23*(4), 1034–1040.

Hill, C. L. M., & Updegraff, J. A. (2012). Mindfulness and its relationship to emotional regulation. *Emotion, 12*(1), 81–90.

Kabat-Zinn, J. (1990). *Full catastrophe living: Using the wisdom of your body and mind to face stress, pain and illness*. New York: Delta.

Kabat-Zinn, J. (1994). *Wherever you go, there you are: Mindfulness meditation in everyday life*. New York: Hyperion.

Kabat-Zinn, J. (2011). Some reflections on the origins of MBSR, skillful means, and the trouble with maps. *Contemporary Buddhism, 12*(1), 281–306.

Koch, C., & Tsuchiya, N. (2012). Attention and consciousness: Related yet different. *Trends in Cognitive Sciences, 16*(2), 103–105.

Lakey, C. E., Campbell, W. K., Brown, K. W., & Goodie, A. S. (2007). Dispositional mindfulness as a predictor of the severity of gambling outcomes. *Personality and Individual Differences, 43*(7), 1698–1710.

Lamme, V. A. F. (2003). Why visual attention and awareness are different. *Trends in Cognitive Sciences, 7*(1), 12–18.

Lau, M., Bishop, S., & Segal, Z. (2006). The Toronto Mindfulness Scale: Development and validation. *Journal of Clinical Psychology, 62*(12), 1445–1467.

Levesque, C., & Brown, K. W. (2007). Mindfulness as a moderator of the effect of implicit motivational self-concept on day-to-day behavioral motivation. *Motivation and Emotion, 31*, 284–299.

Linehan, M. M. (1993). *Cognitive-behavioral treatment of borderline personality disorder*. New York: Guilford Press.

Mackenzie, M. J., Carlson, L. E., Munoz, M., & Speca, M. (2007). A qualitative study of self-perceived effects of mindfulness-based stress reduction (MBSR) in a psychosocial oncology setting. *Stress and Health, 23*(1), 59–69.

Merikle, P. M., & Joordens, S. (1997). Parallels between perception without attention and perception without awareness. *Consciousness and Cognition, 6*(2–3), 219–236.

Modinos, G., Ormel, J., & Aleman, A. (2010). Individual differences in dispositional mindfulness and brain activity involved in reappraisal of emotion. *Social Cognitive and Affective Neuroscience, 5*, 369–377.

Moore, A., & Malinowski, P. (2009). Meditation, mindfulness and cognitive flexibility. *Consciousness and Cognition, 18*(1), 176–186.

Mrazek, M. D., Smallwood, J., & Schooler, J. W. (2012). Mindfulness and mind-wandering: Finding convergence through opposing constructs. *Emotion, 12*(3), 442–448.

Ochsner, K. N., & Gross, J. J. (2005). The cognitive control of emotion. *Trends in Cognitive Sciences, 9*, 242–249.

Posner, M. I., & Petersen, S. E. (1990). The attention system of the human brain. *Annual Review of Neuroscience, 13*(1), 25–42.

Posner, M. I., & Rothbart, M. K. (2007). Research on attention networks as a model for the integration of psychological science. *Annual Review of Psychology, 58*, 1–23.

Quaglia, J. T., Goodman, R. J., & Brown, K. W. (2014). *Trait mindfulness predicts efficient top-down attention to and discrimination of facial expressions*. Manuscript in preparation.

Schmertz, S. K., Anderson, P. L., & Robins, D. L. (2009). The relation between self-report mindfulness and performance on tasks of sustained attention. *Journal of Psychopathology and Behavioral Assessment, 31*(1), 60–66.

Smallwood, J., & Schooler, J. W. (2006). The restless mind. *Psychological Bulletin, 132*(6), 946–958.

Stelter, R. (2010). Experience-based, body-anchored qualitative research interviewing. *Qualitative Health Research, 20*(6), 859–867.

Taren, A., Creswell, J. D., & Gianaros, P. (2013). Dispositional mindfulness co-varies with smaller amygdala and caudate volumes in community adults. *PloS ONE, 8*(5), e64574.

Walach, H., Buchheld, N., Buttenmuller, V., Kleinknecht, N., & Schmidt, S. (2006). Measuring mindfulness—the Freiburg Mindfulness Inventory (FMI). *Personality and Individual Differences, 40*(8), 1543–1555.

Wallace, B. A., & Bhikkhu Bodhi. (2006). *The nature of mindfulness and its role in Buddhist meditation: A correspondence between B. Alan Wallace and the Venerable Bhikkhu Bodhi*. Unpublished manuscript, Santa Barbara Institute for Consciousness Studies, Santa Barbara, CA.

Walsh, W. B., & Betz, N. E. (2001). *Tests and assessment* (4th ed.). Upper Saddle River, NJ: Prentice-Hall.

Watanabe, M., Cheng, K., Murayama, Y., Ueno, K., Asamizuya, T., Tanaka, K., et al. (2011). Attention but not awareness modulates the BOLD signal in the human V1 during binocular suppression. *Science, 334*, 829–831.

Way, B. M., Creswell, J. D., Eisenberger, N. I., & Lieberman, M. D. (2010). Dispositional mindfulness and depressive symptomatology: Correlations with limbic and self-referential neural activity during rest. *Emotion, 10*(1), 12–24.

Williams, M. J., McManus, F., Muse, K., & Williams, J. M. G. (2011). Mindfulness-based cognitive therapy for severe health anxiety (hypochondriasis): An interpretative phenomenological analysis of patients' experiences. *British Journal of Clinical Psychology, 50*(4), 379–397.

CHAPTER 10

The Neurobiology
of Mindfulness Meditation

Fadel Zeidan

For thousands of years, contemplatives have reported that enhancements in sensory awareness, cognition, and health can be accomplished through meditation practice. Before the development and utilization of neuroimaging and other scientific methodologies, the scientific world cast these descriptions as reflections of a relaxation response at best, and report biases associated with practitioner zeal at worst. The recent surge in number of mindfulness-based studies has supported the claim that mindfulness meditation can improve a range of mental and physical health outcomes, and neuroimaging studies are beginning to identify the brain mechanisms that mediate the relationships between mindfulness meditation and such outcomes. Although the neuroscientific investigation of mindfulness meditation is in its infancy, the premise of this chapter is that mindfulness meditation engages a unique, distributed network of brain regions.

Recent accounts of mindfulness meditation have delineated some of the psychoneurobiological mechanisms of action of this method of mental training (Austin, 1998; Cahn & Polich, 2006; Hölzel et al., 2011) and offered theoretical frameworks to describe and explain meditation-based changes in neurocognitive and self-related processes (Vago & Silbersweig, 2012). However, discrepancies between meditation traditions, and differing characteristics and durations of training highlight the importance of delineating the neurobiological mechanisms of mindfulness meditation from a longitudinal perspective. Therefore, a comprehensive description of the brain mechanisms supporting mindfulness meditation must consider commonalties and differences across training levels. This chapter builds on previous neuroscientific work by offering a complementary perspective that focuses on a temporal account of the neurobiology of mindfulness, which considers the neurobiological basis of *how* mindfulness engages the brain over time. In this chapter, I first provide a brief overview describing some key neuroimaging methodologies used in research. In the sections to follow, I provide a descriptive account of the neurobiological correlates of dispositional mindfulness, brief meditation training (1 week or less), the mindfulness-based stress reduction (MBSR) program (approximately 8 weeks), and finally expert meditators (more than 1,000 hours of practice). The subsequent section, concerning mindfulness and the default mode network, briefly describes how different levels of mindfulness-related experience affect task-independent neural processing. I then provide a longitudinal perspective of the brain structural correlates associated with different levels of mindfulness. Finally, I discuss considerations for future mindfulness-based and other contemplative practice research.

A Stage-Based Account of the Neurobiology of Mindfulness Meditation

In this chapter, I argue that the neurobiology of mindfulness varies across different levels of meditation training (Figure 10.1). The proposed neurobiological model of mindfulness meditation is quite consistent with and based on the underlying principles of mindfulness postulated to develop across varying levels of proficiency in different meditative practice traditions (Gunaratana, 2002; Lutz, Slagter, Dunne, & Davidson, 2008; Wallace, 2006). I propose that mindfulness meditation is associated with higher-order brain mechanisms such as the prefrontal cortex (PFC) and the anterior cingulate cortex (ACC) at early stages of this form of mental training. This pattern of neural activity is also evident in those who have never meditated, but whose reports indicate higher levels of trait mindfulness. Because some accounts of mindfulness meditation are based on attending to arising sensory events, sensory appraisal-based brain regions such as the anterior insula and the somatosensory cortices are activated across all meditation training levels. However, at early stages of mindfulness meditation training and development, practitioners engage brain mechanisms supporting an effortful top-down regulation of lower-level afferent processing, indicated by greater activation in the PFC and ACC and deactivation of the thalamus and the amygdala, brain regions involved in early stages of sensory and emotional processing, respectively. As the meditator becomes more skilled at attending to sensory and emotional experiences without interpretation or elaboration, a decoupling between brain mechanisms supporting appraisals of sensory processing develops, as indicated by decreases in higher-order brain activity (PFC) and increases in sensory-processing brain regions (anterior insula, somatosensory cortices). I also postulate that robust changes in brain structure are associated with extensive training in mindfulness meditation and higher levels of dispositional mindfulness. Some initial studies *suggest* that mindfulness meditation can offset and/or buffer against age-related cortical thinning (Grant, Courtemanche, Duerden, Duncan, & Rainville, 2010; Hölzel et al., 2008; Lazar et al., 2005). In fact, adept meditation practitioners exhibit significant reductions in neural structures associated with emotional processing (amygdala) and increased thickness in brain regions associated with sensory awareness (insula). These findings suggest that long-term training in mindfulness meditation

	Behavioral mechanisms	Brain mechanisms
Trait mindfulness	• Labeling emotions as they arise • Cognitive reappraisal • Reduced mind-wandering	• ↑ PFC → ↓ Amygdala • ↓ Default-mode network
Brief meditation training (<1 week)	• Cognitive reappraisal • Reduced mind-wandering • Interoceptive awareness • Reward processing	• ↑ OFC, rACC, pgACC, right anterior insula, S2, SI corresponding to breathing • ↓ Thalamus, default-mode network, amygdala
MBSR (8 weeks): State effects	• Interoceptive awareness • Sensory evaluation • Cognitive control	• ↑ PFC, right anterior insula, S2
MBSR (8 weeks): Trait effects	• Interoceptive awareness • Working memory • Cognitive control of emotion	• ↑ Gray matter in the hippocampus, PCC, TPJ • ↓ Gray matter in the amygdala
Expert meditators (>1,000 hours of meditation training)	• Interoceptive awareness • Cognitive control of emotion • Sensory evaluation • Reward processing • Reduced mind-wandering	• ↑ rACC, PFC, putamen, anterior insula • ↓ Default-mode network
Expert meditators (>1,000 hours of training): Trait effects	• Higher sensory processing • Reduced evaluation/appraisals • Reduced mind-wandering • Interoceptive awareness	• ↑ Thalamus, S2, posterior insula • ↑ Gray matter in S2, posterior insula, right anterior insula • ↓ PFC • ↓ Default-mode network

FIGURE 10.1. Current understanding of the neurobiology of mindfulness meditation. *First row:* Trait mindfulness has been associated with cognitive reappraisal processes and interoceptive awareness. The neural correlates of these behavioral outcomes are reflected in downregulation of the amygdala by the prefrontal cortex (PFC) as well as reduced default-mode network activation. *Second row:* Meditating after brief meditation training engages brain mechanisms supporting reduced mind wandering (default-mode network) and amygdala activation (emotional processing), and greater activation in brain regions involved in reward processing (orbitofrontal cortex [OFC]), cognitive control and emotion regulation (OFC, rostral anterior cingulate cortex [rACC], perigenual ACC [pgACC]), sensory evaluation (secondary somatosensory cortices [S2]), and interoceptive awareness (right anterior insula). *Third row:* After training in mindfulness-based stress reduction (MBSR) programs, meditation produces brain activation in the PFC (cognitive control), right anterior insula (interoceptive awareness), and S2 (sensory evaluation). Stabilized, trait-like effects associated with MBSR (*fourth row*) are associated with reducing structural gray-matter density in the amygdala (emotional processing), and increasing gray-matter density in the hippocampus (working memory), temporoparietal junction (TPJ), and posterior cingulate cortex (PCC), brain regions associated with self-referential processes. Adept meditators show activation in the rACC, right anterior insula, putamen, and PFC during meditation (*fifth row*) and deactivation in the default mode brain network. Long-term changes in expert meditators (*sixth row*) are reflected by increases in gray matter and regional blood signals in sensory processing brain regions (S2, thalamus, posterior insula), and reduced activation in higher-order evaluative neural regions (PFC) and the default mode network.

may produce stabilized, "plastic" changes that can potentially support mindfulness-related enhancements in cognition and health. Taken together, the proposed model (Figure 10.1) provides an initial neurobiological account for the ways in which mindfulness meditation differentially engages a unique set of brain regions across different stages of meditative training. Before turning to the evidence for this model, I first briefly describe the neuroscientific methods used in mindfulness meditation-related research (for more, see He, Yang, Wilke, & Yuan, 2011; Howseman & Bowtell, 1999; Tang & Posner, Chapter 5, this volume).

Overview of Neurophysiological Methodologies

Mindfulness-based neuroscience has used two primary neurophysiological methods to identify the brain mechanisms associated with meditation. First, electroencephalography (EEG) uses electrodes placed on the scalp to record activity of electrical currents produced by neural synaptic activity. The event-related potential (ERP) is a neural marker embedded within continuous EEG signals that corresponds to a singular (predetermined) external event (i.e., attending to an exogenously driven stimulus). Although the spatial resolution of EEG/ERP is not very high, it is suitable for capturing *when* a cognitive and/or sensory event occurs; that is, it has high temporal resolution, on the order of milliseconds.

The development of neuroimaging methods, such as functional magnetic resonance imaging (fMRI), positron emission tomography (PET), and arterial spin labeling (ASL) fMRI, has provided means to collect direct (perfusion-based fMRI; PET) and indirect (blood oxygen level–dependent [BOLD]; fMRI) measures of cerebral blood flow (CBF), which provide higher spatial resolution (i.e., indicating where neural activity may be occurring), although this comes at a tradeoff, with poorer temporal resolution (2–5 seconds) than EEG/ERP.

Neural Correlates of Dispositional Mindfulness

Although the focus of this chapter is on delineation of the neural mechanisms supporting the effects of mindfulness meditation across different mental training levels, it is important to recognize that self-reported dispositional mindfulness is also associated with engaging a unique set of brain mechanisms. In the research community, dispositional mindfulness is measured in a basic way and is typically considered an inherent ability to sustain nonevaluative attention and/or receptive awareness to ongoing events and experiences. Not surprisingly, there is considerable interindividual variability in this capacity, and such differences have been associated with mindfulness theory-consistent neurobiological and other outcomes. For example, individuals reporting higher levels of dispositional mindfulness exhibit reduced neuroendocrine stress reactivity (Brown, Weinstein, & Creswell, 2012; Ciesla, Reilly, Dickson, Emanuel, & Updegraff, 2012; Tamagawa et al., 2013), lower amygdala activity at rest (opposed to those reporting higher depressive symptoms) (Way, Creswell, Eisenberger, & Lieberman, 2010), fewer posttraumatic stress symptoms (Garland & Roberts-Lewis, 2013), better sleep quality and physical health (Murphy, Mermelstein, Edwards, & Gidycz, 2012), and report higher psychological well-being (Brown & Ryan, 2003).

A growing body of neuroscientific research on dispositional mindfulness also suggests that this quality of attention promotes emotion regulation, a key underpinning of the mental and physical health outcomes just noted. The PFC is involved in the metacognitive ability to identify and/or label ongoing subjective experiences (Cole & Schneider, 2007; Ochsner et al., 2004; Wager, Davidson, Hughes, Lindquist, & Ochsner, 2008). Top-down regulation of the amygdala, a brain region crucially involved in fear processing (LeDoux, 2013), anxiety, and affect (Bishop, 2007, 2009; Urry et al., 2006) by the PFC, has been implicated as a classical neural signature of cognitive reappraisal processes (i.e., reinterpreting the meaning of a sensory event) that are considered an important, adaptive form of emotion regulation (Banks, Eddy, Angstadt, Nathan, & Phan, 2007; Drabant, McRae, Manuck, Hariri, & Gross, 2009; Goldin, McRae, Ramel, & Gross, 2008). In a seminal study, Creswell, Way, Eisenberger, and Lieberman (2007) revealed that greater dispositional mindfulness was associated with greater top-down regulation of the right amygdala by the ventrolateral PFC (vlPFC) during an emotion regulation task (i.e., affect labeling). Moreover, some studies indicate that mindful individuals exhibit a unique form of cognitive reappraisal (Garland, Gaylord, & Park, 2009; Garland et al., 2010; Shapiro, Carlson, Astin, & Freedman, 2006; Vago & Silbersweig, 2012; Zeidan, Martucci, Kraft, McHaffie, & Coghill, 2014), namely, the cognitive ability to disengage from higher-order interpretations of sensory events while maintaining an objective cognitive stance. After instructing participants to reappraise negative emotion-inducing pictures (International Affective Picture System [IAPS; Lang, Bradley, & Cuthbert, 1997]), Modinos, Ormel, and Aleman (2010) found that participants higher in dispositional mindfulness were more successful at regulating affective responses to negative mood-inducing pictures. Modinos and colleagues, similar to Creswell and colleagues (2007), found that mindful subjects reappraising negative stimuli showed higher PFC activation (i.e., dorsomedial PFC [dmPFC]), which in turn was associated with less activity in the amygdala. Higher dispositional mindfulness appears to reflect top-down regulation of brain regions involved in early stages of emotional processing (Brown, Goodman, & Inzlicht, 2013), mechanisms also seen in later stages of mindfulness development (through meditation training; see Figure 10.1). Interestingly, we have found that self-reported mindfulness can be significantly increased (up to 16%) after only 3 or 4 days of mindfulness meditation training (Zeidan, Gordon, Merchant, & Goolkasian, 2010; Zeidan, Johnson, Diamond, David, & Goolkasian, 2010; Zeidan et al., 2011), suggesting that mindfulness-induced top-down regulation of affective processes can be enhanced even after brief mental training, an important consideration for the clinical utility of mindfulness.

Neural Correlates of Brief Training in Mindfulness Meditation

In this chapter, I propose (Figure 10.1 on page 173) that brief training in mindfulness meditation engages brain mechanisms that support unique cognitive reappraisal processes that are involved in higher-order cognitive and affective control, enhanced interoceptive and sensory evaluation, acceptance-based emotion regulation, and reductions in low-level afferent processes (Taylor et al., 2011, 2013; Zeidan et al., 2011, 2014). Brief mindfulness training (1 week or less of training) has also led to improvements across a wide spectrum of cognitive (Mirams, Poliakoff, Brown, & Lloyd, 2013; Tang et al., 2007, 2009; Zeidan, Johnson, Diamond, et al., 2010), pain, and stress reduction outcomes (Tang, Tang, & Posner, 2013; Zeidan, Johnson, Gordon, & Goolkasian, 2010; Zeidan et al., 2011, 2014). Using perfusion fMRI, we recently assessed the brain mechanisms supporting mindfulness meditation, the neural correlates of meditation-related pain attenuation, and anxiety relief after a brief mental training intervention (4 days, 20 minutes per day) that involved breath awareness and other Vipassanā-based meditation techniques (Zeidan et al., 2011). Across 4 days, healthy, pain-free subjects were taught to focus on the changing sensations of the breath and to "acknowledge" sensory events nonjudgmentally. Regarding the brain mechanisms supporting mindfulness meditation, our findings revealed that this training engaged multiple brain regions that process executive level cognitive control (PFC, ACC) and sensory evaluation (anterior insula; secondary somatosensory cortices). Meditation activated the bilateral orbitofrontal cortex (OFC), a brain region involved in reframing the interpretation of our sensory experiences (O'Doherty, Kringelbach, Rolls, Hornak, & Andrews, 2001; Peters & Buchel, 2010; Rolls & Grabenhorst, 2008; Schoenbaum, Takahashi, Liu, & McDannald, 2011). We also detected widespread activation of the ACC, specifically the rostral ACC (rACC) and perigenual ACC (pgACC), during meditation, replicating previous findings with other novice meditators (Manna et al., 2010). Regarding pain attenuation, greater meditation-related activation in aspects of the ACC was directly associated with reducing pain and state anxiety ratings (Zeidan et al., 2011, 2014). Regarding anxiety relief, regression analyses revealed that brain activation corresponding to meditation-related pain relief was different than that associated with meditation-induced anxiety reductions (Zeidan et al., 2014). Importantly, meditators uniquely activated brain regions associated with attending to ongoing sensory events. For instance, significant activation in the right anterior insula, a brain region associated with processing sensory experiences relating to the self (Critchley, 2004; Critchley, Wiens, Rotshtein, Ohman, & Dolan, 2004), and the primary somatosensory cortex (S1), corresponding to the somatotopographic representation of the nose and mouth (where subjects were taught to direct their attention), were significantly activated during meditation. Meditation also activated lower-level sensory processing regions such as the bilateral secondary somatosensory cortices (S2; Coghill, Gilron, & Iadarola, 2001). In summary, this research suggests that even brief and basic training in mindfulness meditation is associated with processing sensory information (S2, anterior insula) and the engagement of brain mechanisms (OFC, ACC) involved in the cognitive reappraisal of sensory information (O'Doherty et al., 2001; Rolls & Grabenhorst, 2008).

Considerable insight into the mechanisms involved in the neurobiology of mindfulness meditation can be gained by examining how meditation modulates nociceptive (painful, noxious) processing. Pain is constructed and modulated by a constellation of interactions among sensory, cognitive, and affective dimensions of our moment-to-moment subjective experience, the same factors that are modulated by mindfulness meditation. My colleagues and I found that mindfulness meditation, after 4 days of mental training, significantly attenuated S1 activation, corresponding to painful stimulation (right calf) (Zeidan et al., 2011). Furthermore, regression analyses revealed that meditation-related pain relief was associated with significant reductions in low-level nociceptive processing, evidenced by widespread thalamic deactivation. Within the same set of analyses, meditation-related pain relief was associated with increases in executive level brain regions, including the OFC and ACC. These findings illustrate that mindfulness meditation modulates ascending sensory information at thalamic levels before accessing cortical regions implicated in interpreting the meaning of afferent information (Crick, 1984).

Other studies assessing the effects of brief meditation training on neural processes in response to emotion-provoking experimental tasks reveal similar mechanisms corresponding to top-down regulation of lower-level afferent processing. For example, using BOLD fMRI, Taylor and colleagues (2011) examined behavioral and neural responses to emotion-inducing IAPS pictures (Lang et al., 1997) in a group of naive meditators after 7 days of self-facilitated mindfulness meditation training (i.e., listening to an audio recording of guided mindfulness meditation). When compared to attending to "neutral" pictures, "mindfully attending" to positive and negative emotion-inducing pictures produced significant activation in brain regions involved in cognitive control of emotion (e.g., medial PFC [mPFC], lateral PFC, rACC), interoceptive awareness (anterior insula), working memory (hippocampus), as well as deactivation of the amygdala. This network of brain activity was associated with reports of reduced emotional intensity when attending to negative and positive affect-inducing stimuli. Taken together, these findings reveal that brief training in meditation activates the ACC and the PFC to regulate lower-level, emotionally salient sensory processing. These findings also indicate that mechanistic distinctions between self-reported dispositional mindfulness and mindfulness meditation exist. For instance, while PFC activation during mindfulness meditation is similar to brain activity associated with dispositional mindfulness, activation in the ACC and sensory processing areas (anterior insula, somatosensory cortices) signify that the cognitive state of meditation engages brain regions associated with unique, effortful, and purposeful attention toward sensory and cognitive processes. However it bears noting that there are still comparatively few neuroscientific studies of both dispositional mindfulness and brief mindfulness training. As we will see, the neurobiological changes induced by mindfulness meditation after brief training are quite consistent with neural changes seen in mindfulness practitioners trained in the 8-week MBSR course.

Neural Correlates
of Mindfulness Meditation after 8-Week MBSR Training

The MBSR program is an 8-week, intensive meditation course (Kabat-Zinn, 1990) that involves weekly guided group meditation sessions, daily guided meditation exercises practiced at home with the aid of audio recordings (e.g., focusing on the breath and body sensations as the meditative object), and a daylong meditation retreat conducted largely in silence. MBSR has been shown to improve a variety of mental and physical health outcomes (Grossman, Niemann, Schmidt, & Walach, 2004). Similar to brief meditation training, MBSR has been shown to activate brain regions implicated in executive-level processes (Figure 10.1 on page 173). For example, evidence for neural processes involved in MBSR-related improvements has been found in clinical anxiety (patients with generalized anxiety disorder), with training-related reductions in amygdala activity (Goldin & Gross, 2010; Goldin, Manber-Ball, Werner, Heimberg, & Gross, 2009) and activation in brain regions supporting reappraisal (i.e., aspects of the PFC and rACC) (Goldin & Gross, 2010; Goldin, Ziv, Jazaieri, & Gross, 2012; Goldin et al., 2009; Goldin, Ziv, Jazaieri, Hahn, & Gross, 2013).

Studies assessing the efficacy and neural correlates of MBSR participation in healthy adults paint a similar picture. When instructed to mindfully attend to the sounds of the MRI scanner, Kilpatrick and colleagues (2011) revealed that meditation induced robust functional-neural connections between the bilateral anterior/posterior insula, the mPFC, and ACC. Attending to one's internal bodily sensations after MBSR produced significant activation in right-lateralized vlPFC, ventromedial PFC (vmPFC), anterior insula, and S2, brain areas previously associated with practicing mindfulness meditation (Farb et al., 2007). Comparing the effects of breath awareness in a group that completed an MBSR program with a wait-listed control group, Farb, Segal, and Anderson (2013) found through functional connectivity analyses a robust decoupling between the insula and mPFC. Whereas the right anterior insula processes interoceptive awareness (Critchley, 2004; Critchley et al., 2003, 2004), the mPFC is a central neural hub for integrating self-narrative thought processes. These findings suggest that participation in an 8-week MBSR course can produce conscious processing changes reflecting a shift from a self-focused mental stance to a more receptive, less evaluative engagement of ongoing sensory events (Farb et al., 2013), neural markers associated with adept meditators, which I discuss next.

Neural Correlates of Long-Term Mindfulness Meditation Training

The neuroscientific investigation of adept meditators (more than 1,000 hours of practice; Taylor et al., 2011) suggests that long-term mindfulness meditation training significantly changes the manner in which sensory and perceptual processing occurs in the brain. Whereas brief meditation training appears to produce activation in executive-level brain regions (e.g., PFC) and reductions in lower-level sensory processing, evidenced by deactivations in the thalamus and primary somatosensory cortices, here I propose (Figure 10.1) that long-term meditators exhibit neural activity associated with higher-order awareness reflecting a greater acceptance of sensory experiences without the contextual elaboration or interpretation of those respective events. Indeed, some initial studies suggest that this proposed *shift* in cognitive processing is positively correlated with cumulative time spent in meditation practice (Brefczynski-Lewis, Lutz, Schaefer, Levinson, & Davidson, 2007; Brown & Jones, 2010; Froeliger et al., 2012; Grant et al., 2010; Grant & Rainville, 2009; Hasenkamp & Barsalou,

2012; Lazar et al., 2000; Lutz, Greischar, Rawlings, Ricard, & Davidson, 2004; Saggar et al., 2013). The proposed *shift* in cognition between brief and extensive training can be first demonstrated during formal meditation practice. While beginning stages of mindfulness practice tend to reflect a more effortful, self-directed attentional and emotion-regulatory stance, long-term meditators are postulated to meditate with more efficiency and less effort (Brewer et al., 2011; Gard et al., 2011; Grant, Courtemanche, & Rainville, 2011; Lutz et al., 2008; Manna et al., 2010; Zeidan, Grant, Brown, McHaffie, & Coghill, 2012). Additionally, the neural changes corresponding to adept meditators are more stabilized, such that the cognitive *state* of mindfulness meditation has been transformed into a *trait* or temperament that continues outside of formal mindfulness meditation practice (Davidson et al., 2003; Dunne, 2011; Grant et al., 2011; Lutz, McFarlin, Perlman, Salomons, & Davidson, 2013).

During mindfulness meditation practice, long-term meditators exhibit *increased* activation in brain regions associated with (1) cognitive control, indexed by the rACC (Baerentsen et al., 2010; Brewer et al., 2011; Hölzel et al., 2007; Manna et al., 2010; Short et al., 2010) and aspects of the PFC (superior frontal gyrus, middle frontal gyrus, dlPFC—Baerentsen et al., 2010; Brefczynski-Lewis et al., 2007; Manna et al., 2010); (2) brain regions involved in reward processing (putamen—Baerentsen et al., 2010; Brefczynski-Lewis et al., 2007); and (3) sensory processing (anterior insula—Brewer et al., 2011; Hasenkamp & Barsalou, 2012; Manna et al., 2010). Findings from EEG studies reveal that long-term meditation practitioners process sensory information more quickly after stimulus presentation (Cahn & Polich, 2009), with reduced interference from distracting stimuli (Cahn, Delorme, & Polich, 2013; Cahn & Polich, 2009; Lutz, Slagter, et al., 2009; Slagter et al., 2007), reflecting an overall improvement in perceptual and attentional stability (Lutz et al., 2004; MacLean et al., 2010). These findings provide further evidence that extensive meditation practice can alter cognitive processing, indicated by brain activity corresponding to higher-level executive cognitive control, enhanced lower-level sensory processing, and reduced influences of distracting sensations.

One of the underlying principles of mindfulness-based mental training is the attenuation of affective interpretations (Gunaratana, 2002; Nhât Hanh, 1987; Shapiro et al., 2006). Neuroimaging research focused on elucidating the neural correlates of meditation-related pain relief revealed that long-term meditation practitioners exhibit a less evaluative cognitive stance, demonstrated by reductions in the dlPFC, in the presence of intrusive, painful stimulation (Gard et al., 2011; Grant et al., 2011; Lutz et al., 2013), while brain regions involved in lower-level sensory processing (S2, thalamus; posterior insula) were significantly activated. Interestingly, this decoupling between brain regions supporting appraisal-oriented and sensory processing was directly related to lower pain reports (Gard et al., 2011; Grant et al., 2011). Reductions in the interpretation of the subjective pain experience are associated with reduced anticipation of impending sensory stimuli (Brown & Jones, 2010; Gard et al., 2011; Lutz, Greischar, Perlman, & Davidson, 2009; Zeidan et al., 2012). While the neural correlates of meditation are quite similar between brief meditation training and long-term training, the transformative neural changes associated with long-term meditation practice have been most clearly exhibited when practitioners are instructed to attend to intrusive sensory events in a nonmeditative state or at rest. This is where we see a greater disengagement between higher-order and lower-level appraisal brain mechanisms, reflecting a temperamental change in higher-level sensory awareness that resembles the cognitive state of meditation but which, taking trait form, appears more stable and enduring.

Mindfulness and the Default Mode Network

The default mode network of the brain is characterized by a robust pattern of oscillating neural activity among the mPFC, posterior cingulate cortex (PCC)/precuneus, and medial parietal cortices, and is activated (and functionally connected) during passive resting states, such as passively viewing a fixation cross (Buckner, 2012; Fransson & Marrelec, 2008; Raichle et al., 2001; Scheeringa et al., 2008). The way in which meditation practitioners experience passive resting states (default mode, network-related cognitive processing) differs from that of nonmeditators, and suggests an enhanced capacity to engage moment-to-moment awareness in a nonjudgmental manner. The neural findings to date suggest that that meditators actively engage ongoing sensory events, with an accompanying significant reduction in mind wandering and self-referential evaluations that have been associated with negative mood states (Killingsworth & Gilbert, 2010; Smallwood, Fitzgerald, Miles, & Phillips, 2009). Some of the most common patterns of neural activity across meditative training levels are reflected within the default mode network (Figure 10.1 on page 173). Reductions in default mode network activation during meditation are reported in studies examining all three forms of training discussed here: brief meditation training (Taylor et al., 2013; Zeidan et al., 2011), 8 weeks of MBSR training (Farb et al., 2007, 2010), and long-term meditation practice (Brewer et al., 2011; Garrison et al., 2013; Grant et al., 2011; Pagnoni, 2012). While we found that greater meditation-related reductions in neural activation in aspects (PCC) of the default mode network were associated with lower anxiety reports after brief mental training (Zeidan et al., 2013), others have found that long-term meditators report significant reductions of mind wandering, with corresponding reductions in default-mode network brain activity, even during rest and when compared to novice meditators (Taylor et al., 2013). These findings support the notion that while all levels of mindfulness significantly reduce default mode related brain activity, only extensive mindfulness practice over years produces durable changes in moment-to-moment processing and corresponding neural activity.

Structural Correlates of Mindfulness: A Longitudinal Perspective

Mindful individuals and mindfulness meditation practitioners have recently been found to exhibit unique differences in brain structures when compared to controls, or to individuals reporting lower levels of mindfulness. In one of the largest known mindfulness and neuroimaging studies (155 participants), Taren, Creswell, and Gianaros (2013) revealed that higher trait mindfulness levels were associated with smaller gray-matter volumes in right-lateralized amygdala and left-sided caudate, brain regions associated with processing a wide spectrum of emotions. The structural density and gray-matter concentrations of the amygdala and other brain regions in dispositionally mindful individuals parallel the effects observed in meditation practitioners. Moreover, highly stressed individuals assessed before and after an 8-week MBSR course showed significant reductions in reported perceived stress, and these were associated with reductions in the right amygdala gray-matter density (Hölzel et al., 2010). Increases in gray-matter concentrations in the left hippocampus, PCC, temporopartietal junction, and cerebellum have also been exhibited after MBSR participation (Hölzel et al., 2008). These findings may mark the beginning stages of more stable neural and behavioral improvements exhibited by adept meditators. In fact, studies assessing structural changes in long-term meditators have found significant increases in cortical thickness in sensory processing regions such as the dorsal ACC, bilateral S2 (Grant et al., 2010), S1, and right anterior insula (reflecting greater self-awareness) (Lazar et al., 2005), when compared to controls (Hölzel et al., 2010, 2011).

Building Models of the Mindful Brain: Opportunities and Challenges

There are still significant gaps in our understanding of the neurobiology of mindfulness. For one, we have yet to determine the neurofunctional connections mediating the relationship between mindfulness meditation and improvements in mental health. There are aberrant functional connections corresponding to brain regions associated with self-referential processing and disorders such as depression (Anand et al., 2005; Sheline, Price, Yan, & Mintun, 2010; Zeng et al., 2012), chronic pain (Loggia et al., 2013), and addiction (Konova, Moeller, Tomasi, Volkow, & Goldstein, 2013; Sutherland, McHugh, Pariyadath, & Stein, 2012). Since mindfulness meditation has been found to improve several mental health outcomes significantly (Brewer, Elwafi, & Davis, 2013; Farb et al., 2010; Kabat-Zinn, Lipworth, & Burney, 1985; Westbrook et al., 2013), it would be fruitful to determine whether such meditation-related improvements are directly associated with changes in neurofunctional connectivity. We also have not determined the active neurotransmitters corresponding to mindfulness meditation-related improvements in mental health. Bridging these explanatory gaps may advance the field to understand how meditation improves health. Additionally, we still do not know how mindfulness meditation practice leads to more stabilized temperamental neural effects exhibited by long-term practitioners. In other words, how much training is needed before we see long-lasting changes in the brain? Must training be ongoing for such changes to endure?

Another important issue in neuroscientific investigations of meditation deals with the significant reduction in respiration rate during meditation and how this may affect neuroimaging measures of neural activity. In short, meditation alters respiration patterns (specifically, carbon dioxide output) (Farb et al., 2013; Grant & Rainville, 2009; Zeidan et al., 2011), which in turn are likely to affect CBF effects in the brain; might these changes bias our neuroimaging measures of brain activity? While employing perfusion fMRI may not correct the effects of respiration changes on CBF during meditation, it can identify whether CBF changes are exhibited. Another possibility for evaluating this issue is to measure markers of respiration rate and amplitude (via a respiration belt), which can then be included as covariates or outcomes in mindfulness meditation imaging study analyses.

New imaging technologies offer new opportunities to build models of the *mindful brain*, which can help in the development of mindfulness-based treatments that specifically target a spectrum of health outcomes. Imaging methodologies such as real-time fMRI have already begun to contribute novel mechanistic insights into how mindfulness affects self-referential processing, social interactions, and attention (Garrison et al., 2013). Real-time fMRI allows us to record moment-to-moment neural information in conjunction with first-person accounts. This technique can provide ample opportunities for individuals to learn, via real-time neurofeedback, how to modulate health-related outcomes such as pain (deCharms et al., 2005), affective disorders (Johnston et al., 2011), and craving (Brewer et al., 2013) through mindfulness-based treatment approaches. Studies assessing changes in gene expression through epigenetic methodologies are also making an impact in delineating the benefits of meditation-based cognitive practices (Black et al., 2013; Creswell et al., 2012; Qu, Olafsrud, Meza-Zepeda, & Saatcioglu, 2013). While MRI scanner technology is improving rapidly, and the use of imaging techniques are becoming more common, assessing and integrating neural, endocrine, physiological, and behavioral data will continue to provide novel and clinically relevant insights into mindfulness-based improvements in health outcomes such as cancer, chronic pain, posttraumatic stress disorder, and substance dependency outcomes.

This chapter has offered an initial account of the neurobiology of mindfulness meditation, and the coming years offer many opportunities to extend our understanding in this area. We will no doubt be better able to gauge how mindfulness meditation practice affects the neurobiological mechanisms that mediate mental and physical health outcomes. Furthermore, identifying the neural substrates of mindfulness-based interventions will help tailor interventions to specific mental and physical health outcomes and thereby perhaps reduce health care costs and medication dependency (Blumenthal et al., 2002; Herman, Craig, & Caspi, 2005; Teasdale et al., 2000). Understanding the nature and structure of the mindful brain is thus a worthy pursuit that may also help to bring more clarity to the still enigmatic world of human consciousness.

ACKNOWLEDGMENTS

This chapter benefited from the helpful input of Dr. David Vago, Eric Garland, and Judson Brewer.

REFERENCES

Anand, A., Li, Y., Wang, Y., Wu, J., Gao, S., Bukhari, L., et al. (2005). Activity and connectivity of brain mood regulating circuit in depression: A functional magnetic resonance study. *Biological Psychiatry, 57*(10), 1079–1088.

Austin, J. H. (1998). *Zen and the brain: Toward an understanding of meditation and consciousness.* Cambridge, MA: MIT Press.

Baerentsen, K. B., Stodkilde-Jorgensen, H., Sommerlund, B., Hartmann, T., Damsgaard-Madsen, J., Fosnaes, M., et al. (2010). An investigation of brain processes supporting meditation. *Cognitive Processing, 11*(1), 57–84.

Banks, S. J., Eddy, K. T., Angstadt, M., Nathan, P. J., & Phan, K. L. (2007). Amygdala-frontal connectivity during emotion regulation. *Social Cognitive and Affective Neuroscience, 2*(4), 303–312.

Bishop, S. J. (2007). Neurocognitive mechanisms of anxiety: An integrative account. *Trends in Cognitive Sciences, 11*(7), 307–316.

Bishop, S. J. (2009). Trait anxiety and impoverished prefrontal control of attention. *Nature Neuroscience, 12*(1), 92–98.

Black, D. S., Cole, S. W., Irwin, M. R., Breen, E., St Cyr, N. M., Nazarian, N., et al. (2013). Yogic meditation reverses NF-κB and IRF-related transcriptome dynamics in leukocytes of family dementia caregivers in a randomized controlled trial. *Psychoneuroendocrinology, 38*(3), 348–355.

Blumenthal, J. A., Babyak, M., Wei, J., O'Connor, C., Waugh, R., Eisenstein, E., et al. (2002). Usefulness of psychosocial treatment of mental stress-induced myocardial ischemia in men. *American Journal of Cardiology, 89*(2), 164–168.

Brefczynski-Lewis, J. A., Lutz, A., Schaefer, H. S., Levinson, D. B., & Davidson, R. J. (2007). Neural correlates of attentional expertise in long-term meditation practitioners. *Proceedings of the National Academy of Sciences USA, 104*(27), 11483–11488.

Brewer, J. A., Elwafi, H. M., & Davis, J. H. (2013). Craving to quit: psychological models and neurobiological mechanisms of mindfulness training as treatment for addictions. *Psychology of Addictive Behaviors, 27*(2), 366–379.

Brewer, J. A., Worhunsky, P. D., Gray, J. R., Tang, Y. Y., Weber, J., & Kober, H. (2011). Meditation experience is associated with differences in default mode network activity and connectivity. *Proceedings of the National Academy of Sciences USA, 108*(50), 20254–20259.

Brown, C. A., & Jones, A. K. (2010). Meditation experience predicts less negative appraisal of pain: Electrophysiological evidence for the involvement of anticipatory neural responses. *Pain, 150*(3), 428–438.

Brown, K. W., Goodman, R. J., & Inzlicht, M. (2013). Dispositional mindfulness and the attenuation of neural responses to emotional stimuli. *Social Cognitive and Affective Neuroscience, 8*(1), 93–99.

Brown, K. W., & Ryan, R. M. (2003). The benefits of being present: Mindfulness and its role in psychological well-being. *Journal of Personality and Social Psychology, 84*(4), 822–848.

Brown, K. W., Weinstein, N., & Creswell, J. D. (2012). Trait mindfulness modulates neuroendocrine and affective responses to social evaluative threat. *Psychoneuroendocrinology, 37*(12), 2037–2041.

Buckner, R. L. (2012). The serendipitous discovery of the brain's default network. *NeuroImage, 62*(2), 1137–1145.

Cahn, B. R., Delorme, A., & Polich, J. (2013). Event-related delta, theta, alpha and gamma correlates to auditory oddball processing during Vipassanā meditation. *Social Cognitive and Affective Neuroscience, 8*(1), 100–111.

Cahn, B. R., & Polich, J. (2006). Meditation states and traits: EEG, ERP, and neuroimaging studies. *Psychological Bulletin, 132*(2), 180–211.

Cahn, B. R., & Polich, J. (2009). Meditation (Vipassanā) and the P3a event-related brain potential. *International Journal of Psychophysiology, 72*(1), 51–60.

Ciesla, J. A., Reilly, L. C., Dickson, K. S., Emanuel, A. S., & Updegraff, J. A. (2012). Dispositional mindfulness moderates the effects of stress among adolescents: Rumination as a mediator. *Journal of Clinical Child and Adolescent Psychology, 41*(6), 760–770.

Coghill, R. C., Gilron, I., & Iadarola, M. J. (2001). Hemispheric lateralization of somatosensory processing. *Journal of Neurophysiology, 85*(6), 2602–2612.

Cole, M. W., & Schneider, W. (2007). The cognitive control network: Integrated cortical regions with dissociable functions. *NeuroImage, 37*(1), 343–360.

Creswell, J. D., Irwin, M. R., Burklund, L. J., Lieberman, M. D., Arevalo, J. M., Ma, J., et al. (2012). Mindfulness-based stress reduction training reduces loneliness and pro-inflammatory gene expression in older adults: A small randomized controlled trial. *Brain, Behavior, and Immunity, 26*(7), 1095–1101.

Creswell, J. D., Way, B. M., Eisenberger, N. I., & Lieberman, M. D. (2007). Neural correlates of dispositional mindfulness during affect labeling. *Psychosomatic Medicine, 69*(6), 560–565.

Crick, F. (1984). Function of the thalamic reticular complex: The searchlight hypothesis. *Proceedings of the National Academy of Sciences USA, 81*(14), 4586–4590.

Critchley, H. D. (2004). The human cortex responds to an interoceptive challenge. *Proceedings of the National Academy of Sciences USA, 101*(17), 6333–6334.

Critchley, H. D., Mathias, C. J., Josephs, O., O'Doherty, J., Zanini, S., Dewar, B. K., et al. (2003). Human cingulate cortex and autonomic control: Converging neuroimaging and clinical evidence. *Brain, 126*(10), 2139–2152.

Critchley, H. D., Wiens, S., Rotshtein, P., Ohman, A., & Dolan, R. J. (2004). Neural systems supporting interoceptive awareness. *Nature Neuroscience, 7*(2), 189–195.

Davidson, R. J., Kabat-Zinn, J., Schumacher, J., Rosenkranz, M., Muller, D., Santorelli, S. F., et al. (2003). Alterations in brain and immune function produced by mindfulness meditation. *Psychosomatic Medicine, 65*(4), 564–570.

deCharms, R. C., Maeda, F., Glover, G. H., Ludlow, D., Pauly, J. M., Soneji, D., et al. (2005). Control over brain activation and pain learned by using real-time functional MRI. *Proceedings of the National Academy of Sciences USA, 102*(51), 18626–18631.

Drabant, E. M., McRae, K., Manuck, S. B., Hariri, A. R., & Gross, J. J. (2009). Individual differences in typical reappraisal use predict amygdala and prefrontal responses. *Biological Psychiatry, 65*(5), 367–373.

Dunne, J. (2011). Toward an understanding of non-dual mindfulness. *Contemporary Buddhism, 12*(1), 69–86.

Farb, N. A., Anderson, A. K., Mayberg, H., Bean, J., McKeon, D., & Segal, Z. V. (2010). Minding one's emotions: Mindfulness training alters the neural expression of sadness. *Emotion, 10*(1), 25–33.

Farb, N. A., Segal, Z. V., & Anderson, A. K. (2013). Mindfulness meditation training alters cortical representations of interoceptive attention. *Social Cognitive and Affective Neuroscience, 8*(1), 15–26.

Farb, N. A., Segal, Z. V., Mayberg, H., Bean, J., McKeon, D., Fatima, Z., et al. (2007). Attending to the present: mindfulness meditation reveals distinct neural modes of self-reference. *Social Cognitive and Affective Neuroscience, 2*(4), 313–322.

Fransson, P., & Marrelec, G. (2008). The precuneus/posterior cingulate cortex plays a pivotal role in the default mode network: Evidence from a partial correlation network analysis. *NeuroImage, 42*(3), 1178–1184.

Froeliger, B., Garland, E. L., Kozink, R. V., Modlin, L. A., Chen, N. K., McClernon, F. J., et al. (2012). Meditation-state functional connectivity (msFC): Strengthening of the dorsal attention network and beyond. *Evidence-Based Complementary and Alternative Medicine, 2012*, Art. No. 680407.

Gard, T., Holzel, B. K., Sack, A. T., Hempel, H., Vaitl, D., & Ott, U. (2011). Pain attenuation through mindfulness is associated with decreased cognitive control and increased sensory processing in the brain. *Cerebral Cortex, 191*(1), 36–43.

Garland, E., Gaylord, S., & Park, J. (2009). The role of mindfulness in positive reappraisal. *Explore (NY), 5*(1), 37–44.

Garland, E. L., Fredrickson, B., Kring, A. M., Johnson, D. P., Meyer, P. S., & Penn, D. L. (2010). Upward spirals of positive emotions counter downward spirals of negativity: Insights from the broaden-and-build theory and affective neuroscience on the treatment of emotion dysfunctions and deficits in psychopathology. *Clinical Psychology Review, 30*, 849–864.

Garland, E. L., & Roberts-Lewis, A. (2013). Differential roles of thought suppression and dispositional mindfulness in posttraumatic stress symptoms and craving. *Addictive Behaviors, 38*(2), 1555–1562.

Garrison, K. A., Santoyo, J. F., Davis, J. H., Thornhill, T. A., IV, Kerr, C. E., & Brewer, J. A. (2013). Effortless awareness: Using real time neurofeedback to investigate correlates of posterior cingulate cortex activity in meditators' self-report. *Frontiers in Human Neuroscience, 7*, 440.

Goldin, P., Ziv, M., Jazaieri, H., & Gross, J. J. (2012). Randomized controlled trial of mindfulness-based stress reduction versus aerobic exercise: Effects on the self-referential brain network in social anxiety disorder. *Frontiers in Human Neuroscience, 6*, 295.

Goldin, P., Ziv, M., Jazaieri, H., Hahn, K., & Gross, J. J. (2013). MBSR vs aerobic exercise in social anxiety: fMRI of emotion regulation of negative self-beliefs. *Social Cognitive and Affective Neuroscience, 8*(1), 65–72.

Goldin, P. R., & Gross, J. J. (2010). Effects of mindfulness-based stress reduction (MBSR) on emotion regulation in social anxiety disorder. *Emotion, 10*(1), 83–91.

Goldin, P. R., Manber-Ball, T., Werner, K., Heimberg, R., & Gross, J. J. (2009). Neural mechanisms of cognitive reappraisal of negative self-beliefs in social anxiety disorder. *Biological Psychiatry, 66*(12), 1091–1099.

Goldin, P. R., McRae, K., Ramel, W., & Gross, J. J. (2008). The neural bases of emotion regulation: reappraisal and suppression of negative emotion. *Biological Psychiatry, 63*(6), 577–586.

Grant, J. A., Courtemanche, J., Duerden, E. G., Duncan, G. H., & Rainville, P. (2010). Cortical thickness and pain sensitivity in zen meditators. *Emotion, 10*(1), 43–53.

Grant, J. A., Courtemanche, J., & Rainville, P. (2011). A non-elaborative mental stance and decoupling of executive and pain-related cortices predicts low pain sensitivity in Zen meditators. *Pain, 152*(1), 150–156.

Grant, J. A., & Rainville, P. (2009). Pain sensitivity and analgesic effects of mindful states in Zen meditators: A cross-sectional study. *Psychosomatic Medicine, 71*(1), 106–114.

Grossman, P., Niemann, L., Schmidt, S., & Walach, H. (2004). Mindfulness-based stress reduction and health benefits: A meta-analysis. *Journal of Psychosomatic Research, 57*(1), 35–43.

Gunaratana, H. (2002). *Mindfulness in plain English.* Boston: Wisdom.

Hasenkamp, W., & Barsalou, L. W. (2012). Effects of meditation experience on functional connectivity of distributed brain networks. *Frontiers in Human Neuroscience, 6*, 38.

He, B., Yang, L., Wilke, C., & Yuan, H. (2011). Electrophysiological imaging of brain activity and connectivity-challenges and opportunities. *IEEE Transactions on Biomedical Engineering, 58*(7), 1918–1931.

Herman, P. M., Craig, B. M., & Caspi, O. (2005). Is complementary and alternative medicine (CAM) cost-effective?: A systematic review. *BMC Complementary and Alternative Medicine, 5*, 11.

Hölzel, B. K., Carmody, J., Evans, K. C., Hoge, E. A., Dusek, J. A., Morgan, L., et al. (2010). Stress reduction correlates with structural changes in the amygdala. *Social Cognitive and Affective Neuroscience, 5*(1), 11–17.

Hölzel, B. K., Lazar, S. W., Gard, T., Schuman-Olivier, Z., Vago, D. R., & Ott, U. (2011). How does mindfulness meditation work?: Proposing mechanisms of action from a conceptual and neural perspective. *Perspectives on Psychological Science, 6*, 537–559.

Hölzel, B. K., Ott, U., Gard, T., Hempel, H., Weygandt, M., Morgen, K., et al. (2008). Investigation of mindfulness meditation practitioners with voxel-based morphometry. *Social Cognitive and Affective Neuroscience, 3*(1), 55–61.

Hölzel, B. K., Ott, U., Hempel, H., Hackl, A., Wolf, K., Stark, R., et al. (2007). Differential engagement of anterior cingulate and adjacent medial frontal cortex in adept meditators and non-meditators. *Neuroscience Letters, 421*(1), 16–21.

Howseman, A. M., & Bowtell, R. W. (1999). Functional magnetic resonance imaging: imaging techniques and contrast mechanisms. *Philosophical Transactions of the Royal Society of London B: Biological Sciences, 354*, 1179–1194.

Johnston, S., Linden, D. E., Healy, D., Goebel, R., Habes, I., & Boehm, S. G. (2011). Upregulation of emotion areas through neurofeedback with a focus on positive mood. *Cognitive, Affective and Behavioral Neuroscience, 11*(1), 44–51.

Kabat-Zinn, J. (1990). *Full catastrophe living*. New York: Delta.

Kabat-Zinn, J., Lipworth, L., & Burney, R. (1985). The clinical use of mindfulness meditation for the self-regulation of chronic pain. *Journal of Behavioral Medicine, 8*(2), 163–190.

Killingsworth, M. A., & Gilbert, D. T. (2010). A wandering mind is an unhappy mind. *Science, 330*, 932.

Kilpatrick, L. A., Suyenobu, B. Y., Smith, S. R., Bueller, J. A., Goodman, T., Creswell, J. D., et al. (2011). Impact of mindfulness-based stress reduction training on intrinsic brain connectivity. *NeuroImage, 56*(1), 290–298.

Konova, A. B., Moeller, S. J., Tomasi, D., Volkow, N. D., & Goldstein, R. Z. (2013). Effects of methylphenidate on resting-state functional connectivity of the mesocorticolimbic dopamine pathways in cocaine addiction. *JAMA Psychiatry, 70*(8), 857–868.

Lang, P. J., Bradley, M. M., & Cuthbert, B. N. (1997). *International Affective Picture System (IAPS): Technical manual and affective ratings*. Gainsville: University of Florida.

Lazar, S. W., Bush, G., Gollub, R. L., Fricchione, G. L., Khalsa, G., & Benson, H. (2000). Functional brain mapping of the relaxation response and meditation. *NeuroReport, 11*(7), 1581–1585.

Lazar, S. W., Kerr, C. E., Wasserman, R. H., Gray, J. R., Greve, D. N., Treadway, M. T., et al. (2005). Meditation experience is associated with increased cortical thickness. *NeuroReport, 16*(17), 1893–1897.

LeDoux, J. E. (2013). The slippery slope of fear. *Trends in Cognitive Sciences, 17*(4), 155–156.

Loggia, M. L., Kim, J., Gollub, R. L., Vangel, M. G., Kirsch, I., Kong, J., et al. (2013). Default mode network connectivity encodes clinical pain: An arterial spin labeling study. *Pain, 154*(1), 24–33.

Lutz, A., Greischar, L. L., Perlman, D. M., & Davidson, R. J. (2009). BOLD signal in insula is differentially related to cardiac function during compassion meditation in experts vs. novices. *NeuroImage, 47*(3), 1038–1046.

Lutz, A., Greischar, L. L., Rawlings, N. B., Ricard, M., & Davidson, R. J. (2004). Long-term meditators self-induce high-amplitude gamma synchrony during mental practice. *Proceedings of the National Academy of Sciences USA, 101*(46), 16369–16373.

Lutz, A., McFarlin, D. R., Perlman, D. M., Salomons, T. V., & Davidson, R. J. (2013). Altered anterior insula activation during anticipation and experience of painful stimuli in expert meditators. *NeuroImage, 64,* 538–546.

Lutz, A., Slagter, H. A., Dunne, J. D., & Davidson, R. J. (2008). Attention regulation and monitoring in meditation. *Trends in Cognitive Sciences, 12*(4), 163–169.

Lutz, A., Slagter, H. A., Rawlings, N. B., Francis, A. D., Greischar, L. L., & Davidson, R. J. (2009). Mental training enhances attentional stability: neural and behavioral evidence. *Journal of Neuroscience, 29*(42), 13418–13427.

MacLean, K. A., Ferrer, E., Aichele, S. R., Bridwell, D. A., Zanesco, A. P., Jacobs, T. L., et al. (2010). Intensive meditation training improves perceptual discrimination and sustained attention. *Psychological Science, 21*(6), 829–839.

Manna, A., Raffone, A., Perrucci, M. G., Nardo, D., Ferretti, A., Tartaro, A., et al. (2010). Neural correlates of focused attention and cognitive monitoring in meditation. *Brain Research Bulletin, 82*(1–2), 46–56.

Mirams, L., Poliakoff, E., Brown, R. J., & Lloyd, D. M. (2013). Brief body-scan meditation practice improves somatosensory perceptual decision making. *Consciousness and Cognition, 22*(1), 348–359.

Modinos, G., Ormel, J., & Aleman, A. (2010). Individual differences in dispositional mindfulness and brain activity involved in reappraisal of emotion. *Social Cognitive and Affective Neuroscience, 5*(4), 369–377.

Murphy, M. J., Mermelstein, L. C., Edwards, K. M., & Gidycz, C. A. (2012). The benefits of dispositional mindfulness in physical health: A longitudinal study of female college students. *Journal of American College Health, 60*(5), 341–348.

Nhât Hanh, T. (1987). *The miracle of mindfulness: A manual on meditation* (rev. ed.). Boston: Beacon Press.

O'Doherty, J., Kringelbach, M. L., Rolls, E. T., Hornak, J., & Andrews, C. (2001). Abstract reward and punishment representations in the human orbitofrontal cortex. *Nature Neuroscience, 4*(1), 95–102.

Ochsner, K. N., Ray, R. D., Cooper, J. C., Robertson, E. R., Chopra, S., Gabrieli, J. D., et al. (2004). For better or for worse: Neural systems supporting the cognitive down- and up-regulation of negative emotion. *NeuroImage, 23*(2), 483–499.

Pagnoni, G. (2012). Dynamical properties of BOLD activity from the ventral posteromedial cortex associated with meditation and attentional skills. *Journal of Neuroscience, 32*(15), 5242–5249.

Peters, J., & Buchel, C. (2010). Neural representations of subjective reward value. *Behavioural Brain Research, 213*(2), 135–141.

Qu, S., Olafsrud, S. M., Meza-Zepeda, L. A., & Saatcioglu, F. (2013). Rapid gene expression changes in peripheral blood lymphocytes upon practice of a comprehensive yoga program. *PloS ONE, 8*(4), e61910.

Raichle, M. E., MacLeod, A. M., Snyder, A. Z., Powers, W. J., Gusnard, D. A., & Shulman, G. L. (2001). A default mode of brain function. *Proceedings of the National Academy of Sciences USA, 98*(2), 676–682.

Rolls, E. T., & Grabenhorst, F. (2008). The orbitofrontal cortex and beyond: From affect to decision-making. *Progress in Neurobiology, 86*(3), 216–244.

Saggar, M., King, B. G., Zanesco, A. P., Maclean, K. A., Aichele, S. R., Jacobs, T. L., et al. (2013). Intensive training induces longitudinal changes in meditation state-related EEG oscillatory activity. *Frontiers in Human Neuroscience, 6,* 256.

Scheeringa, R., Bastiaansen, M. C., Petersson, K. M., Oostenveld, R., Norris, D. G., & Hagoort, P. (2008). Frontal theta EEG activity correlates negatively with the default mode network in resting state. *International Journal of Psychophysiology, 67*(3), 242–251.

Schoenbaum, G., Takahashi, Y., Liu, T. L., & McDannald, M. A. (2011). Does the orbito-frontal cortex signal value? *Annals of the New York Academy of Sciences, 1239,* 87–99.

Shapiro, S. L., Carlson, L. E., Astin, J. A., & Freedman, B. (2006). Mechanisms of mindfulness. *Journal of Clinical Psychology, 62*(3), 373–386.

Sheline, Y. I., Price, J. L., Yan, Z., & Mintun, M. A. (2010). Resting-state functional MRI in depression unmasks increased connectivity between networks via the dorsal nexus. *Proceedings of the National Academy of Sciences USA, 107*(24), 11020–11025.

Short, B. E., Kose, S., Mu, Q., Borckardt, J., Newberg, A., George, M. S., et al. (2010). Regional brain activation during meditation shows time and practice effects: An exploratory FMRI study. *Evidence-Based Complementary and Alternative Medicine, 7*(1), 121–127.

Slagter, H. A., Lutz, A., Greischar, L. L., Francis, A. D., Nieuwenhuis, S., Davis, J. M., et al. (2007). Mental training affects distribution of limited brain resources. *PLoS Biology, 5*(6), e138.

Smallwood, J., Fitzgerald, A., Miles, L. K., & Phillips, L. H. (2009). Shifting moods, wandering minds: Negative moods lead the mind to wander. *Emotion, 9*(2), 271–276.

Sutherland, M. T., McHugh, M. J., Pariyadath, V., & Stein, E. A. (2012). Resting state functional connectivity in addiction: Lessons learned and a road ahead. *NeuroImage, 62*(4), 2281–2295.

Tamagawa, R., Giese-Davis, J., Speca, M., Doll, R., Stephen, J., & Carlson, L. E. (2013). Trait mindfulness, repression, suppression, and self-reported mood and stress symptoms among women with breast cancer. *Journal of Clinical Psychology, 69*(3), 264–277.

Tang, Y. Y., Ma, Y., Fan, Y., Feng, H., Wang, J., Feng, S., et al. (2009). Central and autonomic nervous system interaction is altered by short-term meditation. *Proceedings of the National Academy of Sciences USA, 106*(22), 8865–8870.

Tang, Y. Y., Ma, Y., Wang, J., Fan, Y., Feng, S., Lu, Q., et al. (2007). Short-term meditation training improves attention and self-regulation. *Proceedings of the National Academy of Sciences USA, 104*(43), 17152–17156.

Tang, Y. Y., Tang, R., & Posner, M. I. (2013). Brief meditation training induces smoking reduction. *Proceedings of the National Academy of Sciences USA, 110*(34), 13971–13975.

Taren, A. A., Creswell, J. D., & Gianaros, P. J. (2013). Dispositional mindfulness co-varies with smaller amygdala and caudate volumes in community adults. *PloS One, 8*(5), e64574.

Taylor, V. A., Daneault, V., Grant, J., Scavone, G., Breton, E., Roffe-Vidal, S., et al. (2013). Impact of meditation training on the default mode network during a restful state. *Social Cognitive and Affective Neuroscience, 8*(1), 4–14.

Taylor, V. A., Grant, J., Daneault, V., Scavone, G., Breton, E., Roffe-Vidal, S., et al. (2011). Impact of mindfulness on the neural responses to emotional pictures in experienced and beginner meditators. *NeuroImage, 57*(4), 1524–1533.

Teasdale, J. D., Segal, Z. V., Williams, J. M., Ridgeway, V. A., Soulsby, J. M., & Lau, M. A. (2000). Prevention of relapse/recurrence in major depression by mindfulness-based cognitive therapy. *Journal of Consulting and Clinical Psychology, 68*(4), 615–623.

Urry, H. L., van Reekum, C. M., Johnstone, T., Kalin, N. H., Thurow, M. E., Schaefer, H. S., et al. (2006). Amygdala and ventromedial prefrontal cortex are inversely coupled during regulation of negative affect and predict the diurnal pattern of cortisol secretion among older adults. *Journal of Neuroscience, 26*(16), 4415–4425.

Vago, D. R., & Silbersweig, D. A. (2012). Self-awareness, self-regulation, and self-transcendence (S-ART): A framework for understanding the neurobiological mechanisms of mindfulness. *Frontiers in Human Neuroscience, 6,* 296.

Wager, T. D., Davidson, M. L., Hughes, B. L., Lindquist, M. A., & Ochsner, K. N. (2008). Prefrontal-subcortical pathways mediating successful emotion regulation. *Neuron, 59*(6), 1037–1050.

Wallace, B. A. (2006). *The Attention Revolution: Unlocking the power of the focused mind.* Somerville, MA: Wisdom.

Way, B. M., Creswell, J. D., Eisenberger, N. I., & Lieberman, M. D. (2010). Dispositional mindfulness and depressive symptomatology: Correlations with limbic and self-referential neural activity during rest. *Emotion, 10*(1), 12–24.

Westbrook, C., Creswell, J. D., Tabibnia, G., Julson, E., Kober, H., & Tindle, H. A. (2013). Mindful attention reduces neural and self-reported cue-induced craving in smokers. *Social Cognitive and Affective Neuroscience, 8*(1), 73–84.

Zeidan, F., Gordon, N. S., Merchant, J., & Goolkasian, P. (2010). The effects of brief mindfulness meditation training on experimentally induced pain. *Journal of Pain, 11*(3), 199–209.

Zeidan, F., Grant, J. A., Brown, C. A., McHaffie, J. G., & Coghill, R. C. (2012). Mindfulness meditation-related pain relief: evidence for unique brain mechanisms in the regulation of pain. *Neuroscience Letters, 520*(2), 165–173.

Zeidan, F., Johnson, S. K., Diamond, B. J., David, Z., & Goolkasian, P. (2010). Mindfulness meditation improves cognition: evidence of brief mental training. *Consciousness and Cognition, 19*(2), 597–605.

Zeidan, F., Johnson, S. K., Gordon, N. S., & Goolkasian, P. (2010). Effects of brief and sham mindfulness meditation on mood and cardiovascular variables. *Journal of Alternative and Complementary Medicine, 16*(8), 867–873.

Zeidan, F., Martucci, K. T., Kraft, R. A., Gordon, N. S., McHaffie, J. G., & Coghill, R. C. (2011). Brain mechanisms supporting the modulation of pain by mindfulness meditation. *Journal of Neuroscience, 31*(14), 5540–5548.

Zeidan, F., Martucci, K. T., Kraft, R. A., McHaffie, J. G., & Coghill, R. C. (2014). Neural correlates of mindfulness meditation-related anxiety relief. *Social Cognitive and Affective Neuroscience, 9*(6), 751–759.

Zeng, L. L., Shen, H., Liu, L., Wang, L., Li, B., Fang, P., et al. (2012). Identifying major depression using whole-brain functional connectivity: A multivariate pattern analysis. *Brain, 135*(5), 1498–1507.

CHAPTER 11

Cognitive Benefits of Mindfulness Meditation

Marieke K. van Vugt

Given that mindfulness meditation is considered a method for training attention, and cognitive processes associated with it, including memory, can we observe the effects of such mental training with our cognitive science tools? To answer this question, it is important to separate two major styles of meditation practice: focused attention and open awareness. I use *focused attention* here to indicate the process of bringing attention to a particular object of focus and keeping it there, while with *open awareness* I mean the process of observing all salient stimuli as they occur without pursuing them in thought (or action) (Lutz, Slagter, Dunne, & Davidson, 2008). For example, when the thought "I want ice cream" arises, instead of immediately going after this thought of ice cream and creating many subsequent associated thoughts (e.g., about where to get the ice cream, how delicious it has been in the past, how it consoled me when I was little), I just watch the thought and allow it to pass (and get back to writing this chapter).

Different meditation types vary in the relative amounts of focused attention and open monitoring, and mindfulness practice can include both at, for example, different stages of practice. In this chapter I review the cognitive benefits of meditation while keeping this distinction in mind. Figure 11.1 outlines the effects of meditation on cognition that I discuss here. This chapter is not intended to be exhaustive, but I discuss a few representative studies in depth. Chiesa, Calati, and Serretti (2012) and Sedlmeier and colleagues (2012) provide extensive reviews of the effects of mindfulness training on cognition.

Figure 11.1 shows that meditative focused attention is theorized primarily to impact attention and, through that, memory and perception. Open awareness is theorized to impact cognitive monitoring and attention allocation, and through these, cognitive control and self-serving memory biases. Solid lines reflect links supported

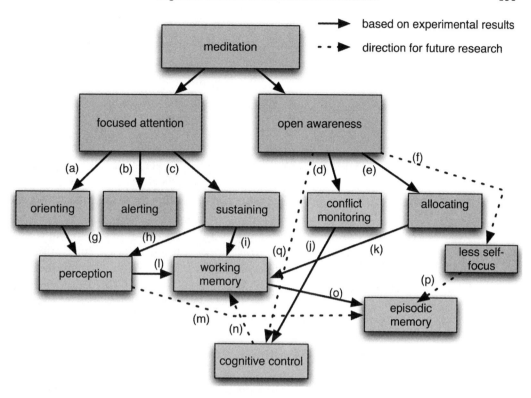

FIGURE 11.1. Conceptual overview of how the two main forms of meditative practice are associated with different parts of the cognitive system. Solid lines reflect links supported by evidence; dashed lines represent hypothesized links.

by data, whereas dashed lines represent hypothesized links to be tested in future experiments.

In this discussion, I pay special attention to an emerging approach to studying the effects of meditation on cognition that emphasizes computational modeling. Mathematical models, upon which this approach is built, can play an important role in clarifying mechanisms through which meditation practice affects cognition. Those models posit detailed mechanisms through which processes such as memory and decision making occur, then formalize those processes in equations or computer algorithms and make predictions about the behavior of people in certain (task) conditions. There is quite a lot of confusion in the literature about what processes compose meditation (e.g., Dunne, 2011), partly arising from the fact that the same words tend to be used for quite different processes by different authors, so using the less ambiguous mathematical models may be clarifying in this regard.

The study of the effects of meditation on cognition started with the idea that, at least in the beginning stages of the practice, the meditation instructions emphasize focused, or concentrated, attention (e.g., "Pay attention to your breath"; Austin, 2009; Wallace, 2008). For this reason, studying attention system processes in meditation seems a reasonable place to start. While the focused attention meditation style has a direct link to attention, the open awareness meditation style may be just as important in generating cognitive benefits of meditation, but it has been discussed much less in conceptualizations of meditation, especially in the context of cognitive science. In the latter, one practices nonattachment toward one's sensory and perceptual experiences, which results in an openness to the complete spectrum of one's conscious experience. It is easy to imagine that this changes not only the quality of attention but also how one remembers objects and events, and how one experiences one's life. In particular, being more open to the full spectrum of experience may make people more cognitively flexible and less susceptible to strong emotions. For example, in the earlier situation in which a thought of ice cream occurred in her or his mind, a practitioner of open monitoring would not completely focus his or her attention on ice-cream-related stimuli (i.e., a state of craving in which other thoughts are crowded out). Instead of being able to remember only things related to summer, eating, and ice cream, the practitioner would also be able to retrieve other memories, for example, about the next thing he or she was going to do, or about the person sitting next to him or her. Thus, these two meditation styles are thought to have differing implications for both attention and memory and, as we will see, other cognitive processes as well.

Benefits of Meditation for Attention

Given that the first instructions in mindfulness meditation and related forms are typically some variant of paying attention to the breath (or some other perceptual object), attention was the initial target for studies on the cognitive benefits of meditation. One of the first studies of the effects of meditation on attention came from Jha, Krompinger, and Baime (2007), who asked whether both short-term and long-term attentional training affected performance on a test assessing three key cognitively and neurally distinct aspects of attention, namely, the Attentional Network Test (ANT; Fan, McCandliss, Sommer, Raz, & Posner, 2002). The ANT indexes attentional orienting, alerting, and executive control. *Orienting* refers to voluntarily bringing attention to a particular object, as one does in locating one's luggage on an airport conveyer belt. *Alerting* refers to the ability to detect salient targets outside one's focus of attention, as one does in shifting focal attention to a prominent slippery floor warning sign. *Conflict monitoring* is the ability to prioritize among conflicting stimuli and responses, as one does in selectively attending to a stimulus from among multiple stimuli on a highway traffic sign. Jha and colleagues (2007) found that conflict monitoring was better for a group of experienced meditators compared to groups of controls and novice practitioners (path [d] in Figure 11.1; note that all future references to *path* refer to Figure 11.1). However, the novice practitioners showed improvements in orienting over the course of an 8-week mindfulness-based stress reduction (MBSR; Kabat-Zinn, 1990) training program (path [a]). In contrast, the experienced practitioners improved in alerting over the course of an intensive retreat (path [b]). The difference in conflict monitoring (path [d]) between experienced practitioners and controls was later replicated by van den Hurk, Giommi, Gielen, Speckens, and

Barendregt (2010), who further showed that the practitioners and controls also differed in orienting scores (path [a]).

The difference between these studies may be related to the different meditation practices in which the respective participants engaged. In the study by Jha and colleagues (2007), the practitioners came primarily from a Tibetan tradition, whereas those studied by van den Hurk and colleagues (2010) were primarily practitioners of Vipassanā meditation, which traditionally emphasizes long periods of formal practice in focused attention. Until recently, there has been little discussion in the literature about the differences between the cognitive capacities trained in different meditation traditions (but see Sedlmeier et al., 2012). However, meditation traditions, and various practices within those traditions, differ in the amount of emphasis placed on focused attention and open awareness meditation, which may therefore have different effects on cognition and emotion. Orienting and alerting may improve as the ability to focus on a single stimulus improves, whereas conflict monitoring (also called *executive function*) improvement may primarily be related to a reduction in stimulus attachment, which would make it easier to switch between competing responses.

In another early study in this vein, Slagter and colleagues (2007) examined the role of meditation training in ameliorating the temporal limits of attention using a rapid serial visual presentation task that can be used to measure the attentional blink (Raymond, Shapiro, & Arnell, 1992). In this task, participants try to detect two targets in a stream of very rapidly appearing stimuli (e.g., the targets might be two digits that appear in a stream of letters). The canonical observation is that people are unable to detect a second target when it follows the first target in close succession—that is, with only a few intervening stimuli. This has been termed the *attentional blink*, which is thought to result from an overinvestment of attentional resources in the first target (Shapiro, Arnell, & Raymond, 1997). If this is the case, and if meditation practice leads to an increase in attentional resources, then the attentional blink should decrease in meditators over the course of training. This is indeed what they found: The magnitude of the attentional blink decreased for meditators after a 3-month retreat, from a roughly 20% drop in performance for stimuli that occur close together in time to only a 10% drop in performance (path [e]). This improvement was not seen for nonmeditator controls.

They also showed that this reduction in attentional blink was accompanied by a decrease in the investment of mental effort, as indicated by the P3 event-related potential measured with scalp electroencephalography (EEG). In a second report on the same sample, Slagter, Lutz, Greischar, Nieuwenhuis, and Davidson (2008) showed that the meditators were more ready to process the second target, as indicated by a phase locking of brain oscillations in the 4–9 Hz theta frequency to this second target. Increased phase locking has been associated with better processing of a stimulus present at the time. This improved allocation of mental resources is likely to primarily result from the nonattachment aspect of meditation, in which the practitioner learned to see that perceptions, thoughts, and emotions are transient and fleeting, and is therefore less inclined to follow them. Nonattachment to perceptual stimuli should reduce the attentional blink, since it is essentially mental attachment to the first target stimulus (in an effort to remember this stimulus) that causes the attentional blink (see Taatgen, Juvina, Schipper, Borst, & Martens, 2009, for a detailed discussion and a computational model of the cognitive mechanisms behind the attentional blink). In fact, recently van Vugt and Slagter (2013) showed that the attentional blink was selectively reduced for open monitoring relative to focused-attention meditation.

Another facet of attention is the ability to sustain it over time. This aspect of attention is often measured by examining how attention declines over the course of a long and boring task. Typically, responses slow and errors increase in such tasks as time progresses. Better sustained attention is associated with less decline in performance. The ability to sustain attention for longer periods of time is likely to be the result of improvements in focused attention rather than open monitoring. In a study of the role of meditation on sustained attention (path 1 [c]), 30 people were randomized to a 3-month shamatha (a meditation practice which emphasizes focused attention) training retreat, whereas 30 others were wait-listed and completed the retreat 3 months later. MacLean and colleagues (2010) measured participants' sustained attention with a task in which they had to decide whether a vertical bar was long or short, and respond only to a short bar. The difference in length of the two bars was calibrated such that participants were only correct on 75% of the trials. This ensured that the task was sufficiently difficult to detect variability in responses. Vigilance was assessed by setting up the task such that participants only had to give a response (to long bars) on about 30% of the trials, while on 70% of the trials they did not (short bars). This meant they had to "do nothing" most of the time except to pay attention to appearing stimuli. While performance tends to deteriorate on this task over time, MacLean and colleagues found that attention could be sustained much longer at the end of the training retreat than at the beginning, and this effect persisted up to 5 months later (cf. Lutz et al., 2009).

In summary, it is clear that meditation impacts various components of attention, although the precise effects may depend on the meditation style practiced and the level of experience of the practitioner. Whereas initially mindfulness and other meditation trainings tend to train primarily focused attention, with less emphasis on developing awareness of the direction of attention (what is being attended to), later practices typically cultivate nonattachment, in which attention "broadens" to encompass more of the moment-to-moment perceptual field. Synthesizing the previous findings, it may be that initially the cultivation of focused attention results in improved ability to direct attention, measured by orienting scores in the ANT (path [a]; Jha et al., 2007). With greater experience in meditation practice, particularly through longer periods of meditation, one also trains sustained attention (path [c]; Lutz et al., 2009; MacLean et al., 2010; Pagnoni, 2012) and learns to allocate attention more effectively in space (path [e]) and time (path [b]). If one practices a meditation style emphasizing open monitoring, such as Tibetan Dzogchen and Mahamudra and Zen training, and perhaps also through the use of visualization, as in certain Tibetan practice traditions, one may develop nonattachment, and be better able to attend to and effectively respond when confronted with conflicting pieces of information (path [d]). Precisely mapping out how different types of meditation impact different aspects of attention is an important challenge for the coming years.

From Attention to Perception

Having established that meditation affects the attentional system, even though substantial variability may exist between different types of meditation and different levels of experience, a logical next step has been to examine whether meditation practice also affects perception (this section) and memory (following sections). *Perception* refers to the process by which we build representations of the external world through our sense organs. Perception is heavily influenced by what we pay attention to, and by what we expect to see (e.g., Summerfield & Egner, 2009). Interestingly, some of the most consistent reports from the meditative traditions themselves suggest that meditation practice can dramatically alter one's perception; it is said to become more vivid, more clear, and more intense (Wallace, 1999). In part, this may be a result of the improvements in attentional focus and quality (i.e., the amount of amplification of perceived stimuli due to directing attention to them). An obvious question is whether we can measure this clarity of perception objectively. The MacLean and colleagues (2010) study, discussed already in the context of sustained attention, can give some clues in this respect. They asked their participants to perceive very fine differences in length between two lines. And indeed, even halfway through their 3-month retreat, participants in this study showed an increased ability to perceive subtle differences in length of the lines. In addition, their discrimination ability covaried with the number of hours of practice completed by these participants (path [h]).

van Vugt and Jha (2011) also investigated perception, albeit indirectly, in the context of memory for face stimuli. Examining a sample of experienced practitioners beginning a 1-month meditation retreat in a Tibetan tradition, training primarily in focused attention, we asked them to perform a visual working memory task in which they had to remember sets of three very similar faces. They were then shown another face (the "probe") and asked whether it was identical to one of the face stimuli in the to-be-remembered list.

We then studied the clarity and quality of perception through fitting a mathematical model to the behavioral data that described performance in this task on the basis of stimulus similarities. This approach consisted of first fitting the behavioral data to a computational model that simulated the task with well-defined psychological mechanisms such as computing stimulus similarities, encoding items in memory, and so forth. During this fitting, various parameters of the model were adjusted to optimize the correspondence between the observed data and the model predictions. One could then see which parameters had to be adjusted to explain the differences in behavior between the practitioner and control groups, which would indicate something about the cognitive mechanisms involved (Forstmann, Wagenmakers, Eichele, Brown, & Serences, 2011).

The noisy exemplar model (Kahana & Sekuler, 2002; Figure 11.2[a]) explains recognition decisions (i.e., deciding "Have I seen this item before?") as follows. Participants implicitly compute a sum of the similarities between the probe and all study items, where similarity is a number that becomes higher as two items are more similar. As this "summed similarity" increases, participants are more likely to indicate they have seen the probe item before. This means that for list items that are identical

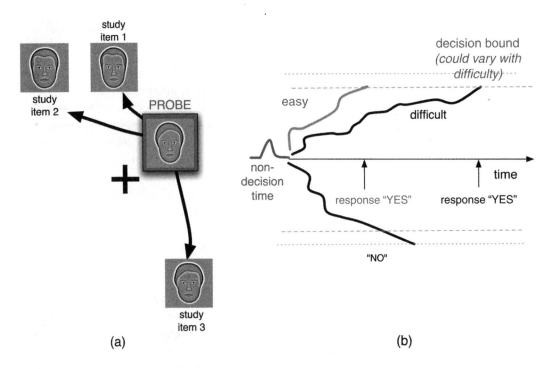

FIGURE 11.2. Models of cognition. (a) Noisy exemplar model of recognition memory. According to this model, the participant computes the probability endorsing a probe item (indicated by a square around the image) as a previously seen item (other faces) on the basis of the sum of the similarities between the probe and all study items (the other images). If this "summed similarity" is high enough (i.e., one of the study items is in the same location or very close to the probe), the participant will say, "Yes, this item was part of the studied list." (b) Drift diffusion model of decision making, which conceptualizes decisions between two alternatives as a noisy evidence accumulation that moves towards one of the decision thresholds corresponding to the response options (in this case, left and right). As soon as a decision threshold is reached, the participant makes the corresponding response.

to the probe, the similarity is very high, and the probability of saying "yes" (in that case the correct answer) also increases. However, if there are many list items that are similar, but not identical to the probe, this also increases the probability of saying "yes," which thereby causes a false alarm.

A strength of this model is that it exploits the similarity structure of the stimuli to make predictions about participants' behavior and can therefore offer insight into how people process stimuli that are highly similar visually. In this way, the model is an index of how clear the participants' mental representations of the stimuli are, and with how much detail they can encode and retrieve visual stimuli. Using the noisy exemplar model, van Vugt and Jha (2011) found that practitioners were able to discriminate between two very similar faces, which was captured by a parameter in the model that describes how sensitive behavioral judgments of similarity are to stimulus properties (see Figure 11.2[a] and Figure 11.1 path [g]).

This is one example of how mathematical models, which are abundant in psychophysics, and the study of perception can help to clarify exactly what components of the cognitive system are impacted by meditation practice.

From Attention to Working Memory

Another process that depends strongly on attention is memory. If one pays more attention, one can better remember the stimuli to which one attended (e.g., Chun & Turk-Browne, 2007). One form of memory, *working memory*, refers to the items in episodic memory that are in the current attentional spotlight (e.g., Oberauer, 2008). If this attentional spotlight is more flexible (as suggested by the just-discussed studies of Jha et al. [2007] and Slagter et al. [2007]), then it may be able to store more stimulus items. Moreover, being better able to sustain attention, through meditative practice, for example (Lutz et al., 2009; MacLean et al., 2010; Pagnoni, 2012), may make the representations in working memory more stable and less subject to interference or decay. How does meditation practice affect working memory?

In a seminal study, Jha, Stanley, Kiyonaga, Wong, and Gelfand (2010) examined the effects of mindfulness practice emphasizing open monitoring on working memory capacity in a cohort of predeployment military personnel (U.S. Marines). Over the course of the predeployment period, working memory capacity as assessed by the operation span task (OSPAN; Unsworth, Heitz, Schrock, & Engle, 2005) decreased in the control group that did not receive mindfulness training—perhaps due to the considerable stress that Marines experience during this period. Notably, mindfulness training seemed to prevent this working memory capacity decline. Moreover, working memory capacity at the end of the predeployment period was predicted by the amount of mindfulness practice in which participants engaged (path [k]). Focusing on a different type of working memory, Zeidan, Johnson, Diamond, and Goolkasian (2010) showed that for the "symbol digit modalities test," a complex visuospatial working memory task (Smith, 1982), participants showed performance increases immediately after a brief mindfulness intervention of 20 minutes' duration (relative to a control group that did not undergo such an intervention). In this task, participants have to decode a series of numbers on a piece of paper and match them to a set of geometrical figures. Their score is the number of correctly decoded symbols. The participants in the mindfulness intervention were thus able to manipulate these digits and geometrical figures in their minds more quickly, which is likely to be related to improvements in both focused attention and open awareness. If one can focus better, it is probably easier to keep items in memory, while allocating attention more flexibly can improve one's ability to manipulate information, which lies at the core of working memory.

Further evidence for the effect of meditation on working memory comes from Chambers, Lo, and Allen (2008), who showed that after a 10-day Vipassanā retreat, meditators improved more than a control group in a backward digit span task, wherein they were asked to remember sequences of digits and repeat them back in reverse order, suggesting that their practice of sustaining attention improved the representation of items in their working memory.

While Jha and colleagues (2010), Chambers and colleagues (2008), and Zeidan and colleagues (2010) studied working memory capacity, van Vugt and Jha (2011) instead focused on the entire sequence of cognitive operations underlying visual working memory, from encoding to response. In the previous tasks (OSPAN, backward digit span, symbol digit modalities), stimuli could be easily verbally encoded, while the stimuli in our study required perception and encoding of stimuli with substantial detail. Just like Lutz and colleagues (2009), we showed that after a retreat, meditation trainees showed a smaller and less variable response time, which may be another instance of the improvement in visuospatial working memory that Zeidan and colleagues observed.

Importantly, we used computational modeling to understand this decreased variability in response time. Since participants were making yes–no decisions, we could apply the drift diffusion model of decision making (see Figure 11.2(b); Ratcliff, 1978; Wagenmakers, van der Maas, & Grasman, 2007) to these data. While the noisy exemplar model explains how participants process stimulus similarity, the drift diffusion model explains how participants use evidence (either similarity-based or other) to make decisions. This model showed that the observed decrease in response time variability was associated with an increase in "drift rate" in the recognition decisions these participants made. In a drift diffusion model, participants accumulate evidence for each of their response options (in this case, "Yes, this face was in the list I had to remember" and "No, this face was not in the list I had to remember"). They make a response once they reach a decision threshold that corresponds to the response option. Drift rate is the model parameter that is thought to reflect the quality of evidence that participants accumulate in the decision process, which in our study was higher after a meditation retreat than before (Figure 11.1 path [l]). Since the quality of evidence in this case is based on the summed similarity that the noisy exemplar model describes, I posit that the improvement in working memory is at least partially mediated by improvements in perception.

The modeling approach that van Vugt and Jha (2011) took in these studies went beyond the directly observable behavioral data because it showed the mechanism by which behavior was changed rather than simply the behavior change by itself. Why is this useful? If we measure response time in a perceptual decision-making task, for example, it can not only increase because of increases in task difficulty, but also, for example, because of an increase in response caution by the participant. The drift diffusion model is able to disentangle these possibilities. If the task difficulty is the underlying cause, then the drift diffusion model fits would show a decrease in the drift rate parameter, while an increase in response caution would be associated with an increase in the decision threshold parameter (Figure 11.2 [b]).

We (van Vugt & Jha, 2011) then used another model to further probe this drift rate effect after meditation training. According to the noisy exemplar model of recognition memory (Figure 11.2[a]; Kahana & Sekuler, 2002; Nosofsky & Kantner, 2006), the drift rate increase should reflect a decrease in the "noise" with which stimuli are encoded. In the model, each item is encoded with noise to reflect the fact that our mental representations of stimuli are never completely veridical, but always some corrupted versions of the presented stimuli, particularly when those stimuli are relatively complex. The noise accounts for fluctuations in behavior in response to otherwise identical trials. Again, using a mathematical modeling approach, van Vugt and Jha (2011) found that meditators showed a decrease in a model parameter that reflects noise in the encoded mental representation of the stimuli. This suggests that meditators' memory becomes more accurate and vivid after intensive meditation practice (path [l]). Although I suggest here that this improvement is primarily related to improvements in focused attention, we do not yet know whether it depends on the type of practice in which participants engage.

In summary, we have shown that meditation not only trains attention but also affects working memory for both verbal (Jha et al., 2010) and nonverbal materials (Zeidan et al., 2010) even in novice practitioners. In more experienced practitioners, we showed that the quality of mental representations of the to-be-remembered stimuli increased after a meditation retreat (paths [i and l]; van Vugt & Jha, 2011). How this increased quality of representations relates to the working memory capacity results is an important question for future research. It may be the case that meditation improves the ability to encode stimuli, or it may increase the number of stimuli that can be held at the same time, or it may decrease degradation of the memories over time. Carefully designed studies with different types of practitioners and different tasks should address these questions. In particular, I expect that the strongest effects on visual working memory will come from forms of meditation that emphasize focused attention, while the capacity of working memory for more verbalizable materials may be more affected by practices that depend heavily on open monitoring and emphasize nonattachment, thereby promoting more flexibility in allocating attention (path [k]).

Episodic Memory: Changing Associative Patterns

If meditation affects attention and working memory, it may as a consequence also affect long-term episodic memory (path [o]). Episodic memories are those that are encoded with a particular temporal context associated with them. The relation between working memory and episodic memory is described in detail by computational memory models (e.g., Raaijmakers & Shiffrin, 1981), many of which posit that items sit in a working memory buffer in the process of being encoded into long-term episodic memory. As a result, if items are encoded with more fidelity into working memory (van Vugt & Jha, 2011), they can also be encoded into episodic memory with more detail. Can such improvements indeed be observed? And are there other effects of meditation on episodic memory? For example, does more clarity in perception lead to different encoding in episodic memory (path [m])?

One of the few studies reporting how meditation affects episodic memory was that of Lykins, Baer, and Gottlob (2012), who showed that meditators from a mixture of traditions recalled a larger number of words in a California Verbal Learning Test, in which participants are asked to learn and recall a list of words repeatedly over several trials. Nevertheless, this is only a very coarse index of episodic memory, and more research will be needed to probe whether meditation affects episodic memory, and if so, whether that effect depends on the type of meditation practiced. For example, does the content of episodic memory differ? If meditation reduces attachment, and especially attachment to the self (Sahdra, Shaver, & Brown, 2010), then meditators might tend to remember less self-related content and more other-related content (path [p]). In addition, the organization of memory recall may change. For example, it has been shown that free recall of word lists is more structured and organized for participants with higher working memory capacity (Spillers & Unsworth, 2011). Given that some types of meditation have been related to increased working memory capacity, this improvement in episodic memory organization may occur as well.

Another way of examining recall organization is on the basis of the valence of the remembered stimuli. For example, participants' recall of longer sequences of negative-valence stimuli may reflect a tendency toward depressive ruminations, which are trains of predominantly negative thoughts. We made use of this idea in a recent study (van Vugt, Hitchcock, Shahar, & Britton, 2012). While most studies of free recall focus on memory of the number of words of different types that participants remember, in that study we instead focused on the *mechanism by which* memory retrieval takes place, that is, how participants proceed from recalling one item of a particular valence to the next. Memory retrieval is driven by the patterns of association between memories: for example, "I should finish writing this chapter," which reminds me that "I should look up this new paper about meditation research." Considering that most of our thinking is driven by sequential patterns of associations, these determine to a large extent whether we are able to think of new things or we instead attend to habitual patterns of thought (which can lead to rumination; Lyubomirsky & Nolen-Hoeksema, 1993). They also determine whether we spend most of our time thinking happy thoughts (when we habitually keep recalling positive thoughts after recalling one positive thought) or alternatively, keep thinking unhappy thoughts (when we get "stuck" in recalling negative thoughts). Given that meditation is a practice in which one gets to know one's mind, including one's habitual patterns of mentation, it seems likely that episodic memory retrieval processes would change as a function of meditative practice. Instead of directly going with the dominant pattern of associations (e.g., Facebook—"I want to check whether my friend John has posted an update"), we can decide to instead focus on thoughts or actions that may be more productive (e.g., "I need to write this chapter"). Being aware of habitual patterns can therefore create a cognitive opening to pursue adaptive trains of associations.

In our study (van Vugt et al., 2012) of 52 depressed patients, we asked whether patterns of remembering positive-valence, negative-valence, and neutral words would change after participation in an 8-week mindfulness-based cognitive therapy (MBCT; Segal, Williams, & Teasdale, 2002) course. We measured how likely a person would continue recalling a word of a particular valence category given that he or she had just recalled a word from that category. Continuing to recall negative words could be the mechanism behind rumination, whereas continuing to recall positive words would reflect more healthy patterns of thoughts. We found that those patients who completed the MBCT course were more likely to repeatedly recall positive words once they were already recalling positive words, and they were less likely to "get stuck" in recalling negative words than were depressed patients in the control condition receiving treatment as usual. In addition, we found that MBCT may have protected them against the anxiety induced by the Trier Social Stress Test (TSST) that was administered to provoke rumination. We measured this by looking at the first recall a participant made. This gave us an idea of the mental context of the person at the start of recall because that context is what drives memory retrieval. In our study, this first recall occurred right after the TSST. While control patients increased in the probability of starting recall with a negative word, indicating that they were sensitized to the negative affect that is known to be induced by the TSST (Kirschbaum, Pirke, & Hellhammer, 1993), participants in the MBCT program did not do so (path [p]).

These findings indicate that free recall is a very useful tool to clarify how meditation practice affects the associations from one memory to another. Free recall can be used to track how our trains of thought may change as a function of meditation practice. For example, if meditation practice reduces attachment to the self, as it is claimed to do (e.g., Wallace, 2008), I would expect that presenting participants with stimuli related to the self would evoke shorter trains of self-related memories in meditators than in controls. Such a change in the dynamics of memory retrieval would particularly be associated with effects of meditative practice on (non)attachment. Importantly, these changes in the dynamics of memory associations may help prevent people from engaging in ruminative thinking and thereby enhance their mental health, potentially reducing the risk for depressive relapse (Mathew, Whitford, Kenny, & Denson, 2010).

Another reason for using free recall to study the cognitive benefits of meditation practice is that detailed computational models exist for this cognitive process (e.g., Howard & Kahana, 2002; Polyn, Norman, & Kahana, 2009). These models describe the cognitive processes involved in memory storage and retrieval, and can therefore provide insight into how these component processes may be modified by the practice of meditation. For example, according to these models, memories are associated with a temporal context that drifts over time. This temporal context includes the environment, mood, and other factors that were present at the time the memories were encoded. The temporal context is used as the main cue to retrieve the memories (Howard & Kahana, 2002). The speed of contextual drift is determined by the rate of incoming stimuli, with an increasing rate of stimuli leading to an increased rate of contextual drift. Would this context drift more slowly in meditators because they experience more cognitive control (i.e., are less distracted), and hence experience fewer incoming stimuli from mind wandering processes? The computational models also indicate how recall is organized by the temporal and semantic associations between stimuli. For example, items occurring in adjacent positions on the to-be-remembered list tend to be recalled together, just like semantically related items. Future studies should investigate whether and how the drift and recall organization change with meditative practice, and whether such change differs between types of meditation (e.g., path [n]).

Is Meditation an Exercise in Cognitive Control?

Anyone who has ever practiced meditation knows that a meditation session can be something like a battle for control of attention ("I want to go and eat that piece of pie"; "No, I should sit on this cushion"; "Where was I? I was supposed to pay attention to my breath."). Hence, an obvious hypothesis is that meditation teaches cognitive control: being aware of what one is thinking of and moving attention to a different focus if necessary. This also follows from the effects of meditation on conflict monitoring discussed in the section on attention. Since open awareness involves dealing with many different stimuli, I propose that improvements in cognitive control are primarily a result of the open awareness form of meditation practice. Cognitive control further involves monitoring and resisting temptations, such as the temptation to stop meditating and eat a piece of the pie about which one is thinking.

Cognitive control is operationalized in different ways, including the ability to deal with competing response options. For example, in the Stroop task (Stroop, 1935), participants see color names printed in different colors and must indicate the color of the ink. Sometimes the color of the ink and the word agree (no interference); at other times they conflict (interference). Moore and Malinowski (2009) found that mindfulness meditators (who practice predominantly open awareness) made fewer errors in trials where the color of the word and ink did not agree than in trials in which they agreed. In other words, meditators showed a reduced interference effect compared to nonmeditators (path [j]). It should be noted that in this study the observed effect may be confounded by demand characteristics because they were comparing a meditator group to a control group, with the former perhaps motivated to show there were beneficial effects of meditation. Nevertheless, Chan and Woollacott (2008) showed a similar effect in a different sample of meditators, in which the magnitude of the reduction in interference covaried with the amount of participants' meditation practice, and this held for both open awareness and focused attention meditation styles.

Another measure of cognitive control is the ability to inhibit responses. Sahdra and colleagues (2011) examined response inhibition in a sample of meditators on a 3-month retreat. In a task very similar to that of MacLean and colleagues (2010), participants were asked to judge the length of two similar lines. They had to respond to the majority of the stimuli (70%), which were long lines, and inhibit responses (i.e., withhold a button press) to short lines. The authors showed that after the 3-month retreat, people were better at inhibiting responses than before, and compared to a wait-list control group (path [j]). Interestingly, this improvement in performance was accompanied by self-reported increases in adaptive psychological functioning, an aggregate self-report measure that included anxious and avoidant attachment style, trait mindfulness, ego resilience, empathy, five broadband personality traits, emotion regulation capacities, depressive symptoms, anxiety, and psychological well-being. Yet these analyses cannot indicate whether adaptive functioning *caused* better cognitive control, or vice versa. As such, this study shows how intertwined the cognitive system and the emotional system are. In fact, the previously discussed effects of meditation practice on working memory could be related to improvements in cognitive control as well (path [n]).

Another very exciting avenue to study the effect of meditative practice on cognitive control is the use of decision-making paradigms from the field of neuroeconomics, which permit studies of the ability to control impulses and delay gratification (Glimcher, 2008). Just like perception, this field is based on well-developed cognitive theories, rich with computational models. Kirk, Downar, and Montague (2011) examined meditators' ability to decide rationally using the Ultimatum Game, a social decision-making paradigm. In this game, a sum of money is given and the proposer makes an offer to split up the money (e.g., $10 for you, $10 for me). Although it would be rational to accept any offer if one is the receiving party in this game, it has been found that receivers typically do not accept the offers when they receive less than 20% of the total sum available (Guth, Schmittenberger, & Schwarze, 1982). Kirk and colleagues (2011), however, found that meditators (whose meditation style was not reported) tended to accept larger inequalities in money (and therefore acted more rationally and were less swayed by their emotions) compared to a group of matched controls (path [f and j]). This finding suggests some important potential avenues for future investigations. For example, do meditators respond more optimally in a temporal discounting experiment, wherein participants have to choose between a smaller but earlier reward and a larger but later reward? Moreover, can these effects be explained by a reduction in meditators' attachment to positive outcomes and positive emotions (path [q])?

The Future: Modeling and Integrating Emotion and Cognition

This chapter has explored the emerging science describing how meditation affects cognition (see Figure 11.1 for an overview). Nevertheless, as I have noted, it is becoming clearer that cognition and emotion cannot be disentangled (e.g., Malinowski, 2013; Pessoa, Padmala, Kenzer, & Bauer, 2012), and that the meditation style (focused attention and open awareness) appears to affect both. While focused attention meditation primarily affects cognition, open awareness may also have important effects on cognition. But, notably, open awareness simultaneously affects emotion, suggesting that we should pay more attention to the cognition–emotion interaction in understanding the cognitive effects of meditation. This is even more so because as practice progresses, the focused attention and open awareness aspects of meditation become more and more entangled (or "non-dual"; Dunne, 2011), and therefore perhaps also the effects of the practice on emotion and cognition become more intertwined. These hypothesized distinctions between the open awareness and focused attention meditation styles should be studied more in the future by comparing groups of meditators who selectively focus on one of these meditation modes.

I believe that a real understanding of why meditation is so useful for many people (e.g., Grossman, Niemann, Schmidt, & Walach, 2004) depends on consideration of the effects of meditation on cognition and emotion simultaneously. For example, as discussed by Hölzel and colleagues (2011), changes in perspective on the self may underlie a large portion of the benefits of meditation practice. As one is less focused on oneself, one has more cognitive capacity (or mental resources) left to perform other cognitive tasks that require attention and working memory. At the same time, this shift away from an ego-involved perspective may reduce emotional biases in episodic memory (path [p]) and foster psychological adjustment.

Another important consideration for future studies is the need to distinguish the effects of different meditation styles and levels of experience in terms of effects on cognition (see also Sedlmeier et al., 2012). This volume focuses on mindfulness, the practice of which has been considered to involve both focused attention and open monitoring (Lutz et al., 2008). It is the latter that I predict mindfulness will affect most, with corresponding effects on conflict monitoring in attention tasks, the allocation of attention, cognitive control, and organization of episodic memory (paths [d, e, p]). For improvements in, for example, sustaining attention, I expect that the largest effects will come from shamatha and other meditation practices that emphasize focused attention (path [c]). The less-studied effects of meditation, including mindfulness practice, on the recollective processes that form our sense of self (path [f]) may require considerably more time to develop. For instance, as an individual gains experience with mindfulness and sees the transitory nature of thoughts and emotions more often, slowly the self-relevant associative structures and other habits of thoughts may start to change.

Studying the influence of meditation on the intertwined processes of cognition and emotion can benefit from computational or mathematical modeling to develop more detailed understandings of the *mechanisms* through which meditation exerts its effects. Because computational models describe the processes they model in great detail, they help to make fine-grained predictions about how the set of cognitive–emotional processes involved in meditation changes our habitual ways of processing.

Models can also point to the commonalities between seemingly different tasks. For example, in this chapter I have indicated that the drift diffusion model can be used to describe both response inhibition tasks and recognition memory decisions. And yet these models can also highlight subtle differences between behaviors that are not obvious from the verbal descriptions of the participants (cf. Marewski & Mehlhorn, 2011). By defining precisely what cognitive processes are involved in different tasks, including the task of meditation, this approach may lead to a more detailed understanding of how mindfulness impacts thought and emotion, and why mindfulness has the benefits that research has demonstrated.

REFERENCES

Austin, J. H. (2009). *Selfless Insight: Zen and the Meditative transformations of consciousness.* Cambridge, MA: MIT Press.

Chambers, R., Lo, B. C. Y., & Allen, N. B. (2008). The impact of intensive mindfulness training on attentional control, cognitive style, and affect. *Cognitive Therapy Research, 32,* 303–322.

Chan, D., & Woollacott, M. (2008). Effects of level of meditation experience on attentional focus: Is the efficiency of executive or orientation networks improved? *Journal of Alternative and Complementary Medicine, 13*(6), 651–657.

Chiesa, A., Calati, R., & Serretti, A. (2012). Does mindfulness training improve cognitive abilities?: A systematic review of neuropsychological findings. *Clinical Psychology Review, 31*, 449–464.

Chun, M., & Turk-Browne, N. (2007). Interactions between attention and memory. *Current Opinion in Neurobiology, 17*(2), 177–184.

Dunne, J. (2011). Toward an understanding of non-dual mindfulness. *Contemporary Buddhism, 12*(1), 69–86.

Fan, J., McCandliss, B. D., Sommer, R., Raz, A., & Posner, M. I. (2002). Testing the efficiency and independence of attentional networks. *Journal of Cognitive Neuroscience, 14*, 340–347.

Forstmann, B. U., Wagenmakers, E.-J., Eichele, T., Brown, S., & Serences, J. T. (2011) Reciprocal relations between cognitive neuroscience and formal cognitive models: Opposites attract? *Trends in Cognitive Sciences, 15*(6), 272–279.

Glimcher, P. W. (Ed.). (2008). *Neuroeconomics: Decision making and the brain*. London: Elsevier.

Grossman, P., Niemann, L., Schmidt, S., & Walach, H. (2004). Mindfulness-based stress reduction and health benefits: A meta-analysis. *Journal of Psychosomatic Research, 57*, 35–43.

Guth, W., Schmittenberger, R., & Schwarze, B. (1982). An experimental analysis of ultimatum bargaining. *Journal of Economic Behavior and Organisation, 3*(4), 367–388.

Hölzel, B. K., Lazar, S. W., Gard, T., Schuman-Olivier, Z., Vago, D. R., & Ott, U. (2011). How does mindfulness meditation work?: Proposing mechanisms of action from a conceptual and neural perspective. *Perspectives on Psychological Science, 6*, 537–559.

Howard, M. W., & Kahana, M. J. (2002). A distributed representation of temporal context. *Journal of Mathematical Psychology, 46*, 269–299.

Jha, A. P., Krompinger, J., & Baime, M. J. (2007). Mindfulness training modifies subsystems of attention. *Cognitive, Affective, and Behavioral Neuroscience, 7*(2), 109–119.

Jha, A. P., Stanley, E. A., Kiyonaga, A., Wong, L., & Gelfand, L. (2010). Examining the protective effects of mindfulness training on working memory capacity and affective experience. *Emotion, 10*(1), 54–64.

Kabat-Zinn, J. (1990). *Full catastrophe living: Using the wisdom of your body and mind to face stress, pain, and illness*. New York: Bantam Dell.

Kahana, M. J., & Sekuler, R. (2002). Recognizing spatial patterns: A noisy exemplar approach. *Vision Research, 42*, 2177–2192.

Kirk, U., Downar, J., & Montague, P. R. (2011). Interoception drives increased rational decision-making in meditators playing the ultimatum game. *Frontiers in Neuroscience, 5*, 49.

Kirschbaum, C., Pirke, K. M., & Hellhammer, D. H. (1993). The Trier Social Stress Test: A tool for investigating psychobiological stress response in a laboratory setting. *Neuropsychobiology, 28*, 76–81.

Lutz, A., Slagter, H. A., Dunne, J. D., & Davidson, R. J. (2008). Attention regulation and monitoring in meditation. *Trends in Cognitive Sciences, 12*(4), 163–169.

Lutz, A., Slagter, H. A., Rawlings, N. B., Francis, A. D., Greischar, L. L., & Davidson, R. J. (2009). Mental training enhances attentional stability: Neural and behavioral evidence. *Journal of Neuroscience, 29*(42), 13418–13427.

Lykins, E. L. B., Baer, R. A., & Gottlob, L. R. (2012). Performance-based tests of attention and memory in long-term mindfulness meditators and demographically matched non-meditators. *Cognitive Therapy and Research, 36*(1), 103–114.

Lyubomirsky, S., & Nolen-Hoeksema, S. (1993). Self-perpetuating properties of dysphoric rumination. *Journal of Personality and Social Psychology, 65*(2), 339–349.

MacLean, K. A., Ferrer, E., Aichele, S. R., Bridwell, D. A., Zanesco, A. P., Jacobs, T. L., et al. (2010). Intensive meditation training improves perceptual discrimination and sustained attention. *Psychological Science, 21*(6), 829–839.

Malinowski, P. (2013). Neural mechanisms of attentional control in mindfulness meditation. *Frontiers in Neuroscience, 7,* 8.

Marewski, J. N., & Mehlhorn, K. (2011). Using the ACT-R architecture to specify 39 quantitative process models of decision making. *Judgment and Decision Making, 6,* 439–519.

Mathew, K. L., Whitford, H. S., Kenny, M. A., & Denson, L. A. (2010). The long-term effects of mindfulness-based cognitive therapy as a relapse prevention treatment for major depressive disorder. *Behavioural and Cognitive Psychotherapy, 38*(5), 561–576.

Moore, A., & Malinowski, P. (2009). Meditation, mindfulness and cognitive flexibility. *Consciousness and Cognition, 18,* 176–186.

Nosofsky, R. M., & Kantner, J. (2006). Exemplar similarity, study list homogeneity, and short-term perceptual recognition. *Memory and Cognition, 34*(1), 112–124.

Oberauer, K. (2008). How to say no: Single- and dual-process theories of short-term recognition tested on negative probes. *Journal of Experimental Psychology: Learning, Memory, and Cognition, 34*(3), 439–459.

Pagnoni, G. (2012). Dynamical properties of bold activity from the ventral posteromedial cortex associated with meditation and attentional skills. *Journal of Neuroscience, 32*(15), 5242–5249.

Pessoa, L., Padmala, S., Kenzer, A., & Bauer, A. (2012). Interactions between cognition and emotion during response inhibition. *Emotion, 12*(1), 192–197.

Polyn, S. M., Norman, K. A., & Kahana, M. J. (2009). A context maintenance and retrieval model of organizational processes in free recall. *Psychological Review, 116,* 129–156.

Raaijmakers, J. G. W., & Shiffrin, R. M. (1981). Search of associative memory. *Psychological Review, 88,* 93–134.

Ratcliff, R. (1978). A theory of memory retrieval. *Psychological Review, 85,* 59–108.

Raymond, J. E., Shapiro, K. L., & Arnell, K. M. (1992). Temporary suppression of visual processing in an RSVP task: An attentional blink. *Journal of Experimental Psychology: Human Perception and Performance, 18,* 849–860.

Sahdra, B. K., MacLean, K. A., Ferrer, E., Shaver, P. R., Rosenberg, E. L., Jacobs, T. L., et al. (2011). Enhanced response inhibition during intensive meditation training predicts improvements in self-reported adaptive socioemotional functioning. *Emotion, 11*(2), 299–312.

Sahdra, B. K., Shaver, P. R., & Brown, K. W. (2010). A scale to measure non-attachment: A Buddhist complement to Western research on attachment and adaptive functioning. *Journal of Personality Assessment, 92*(2), 116–127.

Sedlmeier, P., Eberth, J., Schwarz, M., Zimmermann, D., Haarig, F., Jaeger, S., et al. (2012). The psychological effects of meditation: A meta-analysis. *Psychological Bulletin, 138*(6), 1139–1171.

Segal, Z. V., Williams, J. M. G., & Teasdale, J. D. (2002). *Mindfulness-based cognitive therapy for depression: A new approach to preventing relapse.* New York: Guilford Press.

Shapiro, K. L., Arnell, K. M., & Raymond, J. E. (1997). The attentional blink. *Trends in Cognitive Sciences, 1,* 291–296.

Slagter, H. A., Lutz, A., Greischar, L. L., Francis, A. D., Nieuwenhuis, S., Davis, J. M., et al. (2007). Mental training affects distribution of limited brain resources. *PLoS Biology, 5*(6), e138.

Slagter, H. A., Lutz, A., Greischar, L. L., Nieuwenhuis, S., & Davidson, R. J. (2008). Theta phase synchrony and conscious target perception: Impact of intensive mental training. *Journal of Cognitive Neuroscience, 21*(8), 1536–1549.

Smith, A. (1982). *Symbol-digit modalities test (SDMT) manual—revised.* Los Angeles: Western Psychological Services.

Spillers, G. J., & Unsworth, N. (2011). Variation in working memory capacity and temporal-contextual retrieval from episodic memory. *Journal of Experimental Psychology: Learning, Memory, and Cognition, 37*(6), 1532–1539.

Stroop, J. R. (1935). Studies of interference in serial verbal reactions. *Journal of Experimental Psychology, 18*, 643–662.

Summerfield, C., & Egner, T. (2009). Expectation (and attention) in visual cognition. *Trends in Cognitive Sciences, 13*(9), 403–409.

Taatgen, N. A., Juvina, I., Schipper, M., Borst, J. P., & Martens, S. (2009). Too much control can hurt: A threaded cognition model of the attentional blink. *Cognitive Psychology, 59*, 1–29.

Unsworth, N., Heitz, R. P., Schrock, J. C., & Engle, R. W. (2005). An automated version of the operation span task. *Behavior Research Methods, 37*, 498–505.

van den Hurk, P. A. M., Giommi, F., Gielen, S. C., Speckens, A. E. M., & Barendregt, H. P. (2010). Greater efficiency in attentional processing related to mindfulness meditation. *Quarterly Journal of Experimental Psychology, 63*(6), 1168–1180.

van den Hurk, P. A. M., Giommi, F., van Schie, H., & Barendregt, H. P. (2012). *Mindfulness meditation associated with changes in response bias: A study on the recognition of emotional facial expressions.* Manuscript submitted for publication.

van Vugt, M. K., Hitchcock, P., Shahar, B., & Britton, W. (2012). The effects of mindfulness-based cognitive therapy on affective memory recall dynamics in depression: A mechanistic model of rumination. *Frontiers in Human Neuroscience, 6*, 257.

van Vugt, M. K., & Jha, A. P. (2011). Investigating the impact of mindfulness meditation training on working memory: A mathematical modeling approach. *Cognitive, Affective, and Behavioral Neuroscience, 11*(3), 344–353.

van Vugt, M. K., & Slagter, H. A. (2013). Control over experience?: Magnitude of the attentional blink depends on meditative state. *Consciousness and Cognition, 23*, 32.

Wagenmakers, E., van der Maas, H. L. J., & Grasman, R. P. (2007). An EZ-diffusion model for response time and accuracy. *Psychonomic Bulletin and Review, 14*(1), 3–22.

Wallace, B. A. (1999). The Buddhist tradition of Samatha: Methods for refining and examining consciousness. *Journal of Consciousness Studies, 6*, 175–187.

Wallace, B. A. (2008). *The attention revolution.* Somerville, MA: Wisdom.

Zeidan, F., Johnson, S. K., Diamond, B. J., & Goolkasian, P. (2010). Mindfulness meditation improves cognition: Evidence of brief mental training. *Consciousness and Cognition, 19*, 597–605.

CHAPTER 12

Emotional Benefits of Mindfulness

Joanna J. Arch and Lauren N. Landy

Many Western theories of emotion (e.g., Ekman, 1992; Frijda, 1986), particularly those based on Darwinian evolutionary theory, argue that emotions—even negative ones—communicate important and adaptive information essential for survival. For example, emotions play a key role in making decisions, readying behavioral responses, and facilitating interpersonal interactions (Gross, 2007, 2014a). A large and growing body of evidence, however, demonstrates that emotions—particularly negative emotions—also can be maladaptive, dysregulated, or situationally inappropriate, fostering poor decisions, unhelpful behavioral responses, and interpersonal conflict (see Gross, 2007, 2014b, for a review). For example, ruminating on a minor annoyance in someone's behavior can lead to anger, which can then escalate into verbal or physical conflict. Thus, some emotions appear to be more intra- and interpersonally beneficial than others. Considerable research has addressed the emotional benefits of mindfulness and its cultivation, and this line of inquiry addresses the fundamental question of whether mindfulness helps us to lead happier lives. This focus also illuminates how mindfulness can contribute to our understanding of the potential to transform emotional experience.

The Study of Mindfulness in Emotion Contexts

Mindfulness has been studied in a variety of forms, including trait or dispositional mindfulness (e.g., Brown & Ryan, 2003), induced state mindfulness (e.g., Arch & Craske, 2006), and formally trained mindfulness (e.g., Kabat-Zinn, 1990). This chapter is structured in a way that treats evidence for the emotional benefits of mindfulness in a progression from trait to briefly induced state to trained forms of mindfulness. At a fundamental level, however, all forms of mindfulness represent variations on the theme of state mindfulness; that is, trait mindfulness represents the tendency to reside in mindful states over time, whereas trained mindfulness represents the trained capacity to cultivate and more frequently reside in mindful states. Despite this core link, inducing a brief mindful state on a onetime basis differs from the in-depth mindfulness training in interventions such as mindfulness-based stress reduction (MBSR; Kabat-Zinn, 1990) and still more so from the sustained training characteristic of lifelong commitment to mindfulness practices. One question we consider is whether different forms of mindfulness (trait, state, short and long-term trained) are associated with similar versus distinct emotional benefits—whether different forms of mindfulness represent distinct categorical entities with regard to emotional benefits or whether the evidence points to similar benefits across the three foci of mindfulness research (to varying degrees).

For this review, we selected studies that most strongly informed our understanding of the emotional benefits of mindfulness in normative, nonpatient samples. Due to space limitations and a desire to emphasize more rigorous studies, we omitted studies in which self-report questionnaires were correlated with one another at a single time point in the absence of experiential, longitudinal, or biobehavioral outcomes. Second, we selected studies in which affect, emotion, or reactivity in them (subjective, behavioral, or physiological) was measured as a primary dependent variable. Third, we excluded studies that focused primarily on clinical populations, including medical and psychiatric populations, because they represent the focus of other chapters (see Part V, this volume). Finally, we excluded studies that focused mainly on attentional, cognitive, social, or relational benefits of mindfulness; though linked to emotion, these topics represent the focus of other chapters in this volume.

In reviewing evidence for the emotional benefits of mindfulness, we remain within the long-standing Western tradition of distinguishing between emotions and other mental phenomenon (e.g., Ekman, 1992). Moreover, Western notions of positive and negative emotions (e.g., Watson, Clark, & Tellegen, 1988) frame the benefits of mindfulness discussed herein. To date, the vast majority of studies on this topic have focused on the benefits of mindfulness for negative emotional experience, and on the peripheral physiology and neural processing purported to instigate the manifestation of negative emotions, so it is to these emotions that we first turn our attention.

Benefits of Mindfulness for Negative Emotions

Negative emotions are a primary expression of human suffering, and reflected in rates of psychiatric disorders, human suffering is astounding: Over a lifetime, nearly half of the U.S. population will meet criteria for an anxiety, mood, substance use, or impulse control disorder (Kessler, Berglund, Demler, Jin, & Walters, 2005). Negative emotions are experienced normatively as well. We therefore investigate a question central to both normal and clinical psychology: the impact of mindfulness on reducing, regulating, and transforming the experience of negative emotion.

Trait Mindfulness Studies

The terms *trait* or *dispositional* mindfulness typically refer to the degree of day-to-day mindful attention that varies in quality and frequency between individuals (Brown & Ryan, 2003). Extant studies suggest that higher levels of trait mindfulness are associated with emotional benefits across self-report, behavioral, and neural outcomes. Such studies have assessed trait mindfulness using validated self-report questionnaires, most commonly the Mindful Attention Awareness Scale (MAAS; Brown & Ryan, 2003), or brief questions assessing present-moment focus in an experience-sampling context (e.g., Hill & Updegraff, 2012). We now review several of these studies in greater detail.

Laboratory studies have demonstrated benefits of trait mindfulness in coping with negative emotional provocation. For example, Arch and Craske (2010) demonstrated that higher trait mindfulness (as assessed by the MAAS; Brown & Ryan, 2003) predicted lower negative affect in response to a hyperventilation task (an interoceptive stressor). Barnes, Brown, Krusemark, Campbell, and Rogge (2007) found that higher trait mindfulness predicted lower anxiety and hostility in dating couples at baseline and following a relationship conflict discussion.

The notion that higher dispositional mindfulness provides a buffer or even inoculation to negative affectivity in interoceptive and relational contexts is consistent with neuroimaging findings. Creswell, Way, Eisenberger, and Lieberman (2007) used functional magnetic resonance imaging (fMRI) to show that dispositional mindfulness predicted greater prefrontal cortical activation, reduced bilateral amygdala activity, and stronger negative correlations between these two regions during affect labeling relative to a control task. High trait-mindful adults, therefore, more effectively down-regulated limbic brain regions. Using an event-related potential methodology, Brown, Goodman, and Inzlicht (2012) found that higher trait-mindful undergraduates showed reduced responses to both high arousal positive and negative images, even after accounting for trait attentional control. Trait differences emerged within the first *second* (500–900 ms) of image exposure in the late positive potential component of the EEG response, suggesting that trait mindfulness tempered the initial rise of emotions by reducing the appraisal of emotional stimuli.

Emerging evidence also indicates that mindfulness promotes increased voluntary exposure to aversive experiences. Arch and Craske (2010) found that higher trait-mindful adults showed a greater willingness to experience aversive physiological sensations, as evidenced by greater endurance in a voluntary hyperventilation task. In response to threatening information related to mortality, Niemiec and colleagues (2010) showed that higher trait mindfulness predicted less suppression of thoughts related to death, a greater willingness to engage in thoughts of death, and less defensiveness in response to self-relevant threats. Finally, Hill and Updegraff (2012) found that higher dispositional mindfulness, assessed by the Five Facet Mindfulness Questionnaire (full scale; Baer, Smith, Hopkins, Krietemeyer, & Toney, 2006), predicted lower emotional lability and dysregulation in daily life. Mediation analyses suggested that higher trait mindfulness enabled greater emotional clarity—the capacity to better differentiate between emotions and therefore more precisely and adaptively respond to them.

These sample findings suggest that trait mindfulness functions to promote more sustained contact with aversive experience (voluntary exposure), dampened appraisal of negative stimuli, less suppression and intensity of negative affect, greater emotional clarity, and more effective down-regulation of negative emotion. Perhaps higher trait mindfulness promotes nonjudgmental acceptance of stimuli and experiences as they occur, leading to more effective processing of initial or "primary" emotions and less need for secondary emotional responses such as rumination, suppression, and avoidance.

Many questions remain, however. For example, we know little about whether trait mindfulness has greater impact on some negative emotions than on others. That is, does trait mindfulness aid in recovering from anger to a greater extent than sadness, for instance, or does trait mindfulness impact the full range of negative emotions similarly? Relatedly, how does trait mindfulness impact the experience of healthy or normative negative emotions such as the sadness that accompanies the loss of a loved one? Given the correlational nature of these studies, it also remains unknown whether high levels of trait mindfulness promote emotional benefits, or whether it is easier for individuals who naturally experience less negative emotion to be mindful. Experimental studies that induce mindfulness or train individuals in cultivating mindfulness provide opportunities to test how mindful states causally impact emotional responding, which we consider next.

Brief Mindfulness Induction Studies

Brief, one-time mindfulness inductions, typically 3–15 minutes in length, aim to produce effects during the immediate laboratory experiment. Such studies have the advantage of isolating the effect of mindfulness instructions, in contrast to mindfulness interventions, which may include multiple active treatment components. Inductions typically make use of guided instructions delivered via audio recordings or spoken instructions. One-time mindfulness inductions are best conceptualized as the smallest "dose" of mindfulness that can be studied to assess the immediate impact of mindful states, representing one end of the mindfulness training continuum. These studies typically include naive participants without previous formal exposure to mindfulness exercises; thus, the quality of mindfulness induced during these brief manipulations is unlikely to approach the quality of mindfulness induced during long-term training. Nonetheless, this approach can be valuable for isolating and elucidating the immediate emotional effects of mindful states.

Studies to date have demonstrated the potential of brief mindfulness inductions to reduce negative affect and improve emotion regulation in response to varied stimuli, and to better tolerate and recover from negative provocation. For example, Broderick (2005) induced a sad mood in undergraduates, then randomized them to mindfulness (present-moment breath –focus), rumination, or distraction exercises. Brief mindfulness led to significantly faster recovery from dysphoric mood than the other conditions despite no difference in the number of positive or negative thoughts. Arch and Craske (2006) had university students view positive, negative, and neutral International Affective Picture Slides (IAPS; Lang, Bradley, & Cuthbert, 2008) before and after mindfulness, unfocused attention, or worry inductions. The mindfulness group reported more consistent positive affect in response to the neutral slides over time, whereas responses in the other two groups grew more negative over time. Furthermore, the mindfulness group reported lower negative affect and emotional volatility in response to the slides than the worry group and greater willingness to view a series of highly negative slides than the unfocused attention group. Similarly, Erisman and Roemer (2010) had high anxiety-sensitive undergraduates view positive, negative, and affectively mixed film clips before and after a mindfulness induction or neutral listening exercise. Medium to large group differences emerged following the affectively mixed clip, with the mindfulness group reporting less negative affect and more adaptive emotion regulation (assessed by the State Difficulties in Emotion Regulation Scale; McLaughlin, Mennin, & Farach, 2007). Regarding null findings after the negative clip, the authors propose that perhaps the mindfulness exercise was too brief to counter such a negative experience.

These latter two studies suggest that mindfulness may diminish "carryover" effects from affective to neutral stimuli. The mindfulness groups showed more stable, positive responses to neutral slides (embedded between positive and negative slides; Arch & Craske, 2006) and to affectively mixed visual stimuli (which included positive, neutral, and negative material; Erisman & Roemer, 2010). In a related study, sensory monitoring (similar to mindfulness of sensory experience) during pain resulted in less carryover effects to subsequent neutral vibration ratings (Cioffi & Holloway, 1993). In summary, there is initial evidence that brief mindfulness inductions facilitate recovery from high-arousal emotional states in a way that inhibits the "contamination" of responses to neutral or mixed material.

Several limitations of the experimental induction literature are worth noting. First, the extant studies involved university student samples using subjective outcomes. Broader community and clinical samples are now needed to establish generalizability of the immediate effects of mindful states. Future work would also benefit from adding more physiological and behavioral markers of emotion. Furthermore, future studies could consider examining affectively reactive populations (e.g., high anxiety, emotionally dysregulated) to determine whether mindful states foster adaptive emotion regulation in the "heat" of strong, difficult emotional reactions.

To determine the specificity of the effects of onetime mindfulness inductions, future studies also need to compare brief mindfulness to *adaptive* emotion regulation approaches that contrast with core components of mindfulness—for example, to cognitive reappraisal (vs. decentering from thought content in mindfulness). Similarly, to strengthen or lengthen mindfulness effects, induction studies could be expanded to brief mindfulness trainings that deliver multiple inductions over several days (see Zeidan, Gordon, Merchant, & Goolkasian, 2010).

Intervention Studies

In contrast to mindfulness induction studies, intervention studies examine benefits sustained beyond the immediate practice environment, allowing researchers to examine benefits that endure for weeks or months following the initial mindfulness training. Numerous clinical interventions offer mindfulness training as a core treatment component (e.g., Hayes, Strosahl, & Wilson, 2012; Linehan, 1993; Segal, Williams, & Teasdale, 2002), illustrating its growing popularity in treating psychiatric and physical health conditions. Mindfulness training also offers emotional benefits for healthy nonpatients—our current focus. We concentrate on studies in which mindfulness meditation and related practices comprise the major intervention component rather than an integrated or relatively minor component (e.g., Tang et al., 2007). In most reviewed studies, MBSR (Kabat-Zinn, 1990) or a variant or component thereof comprises the intervention.

Within our area of focus, at least 12 studies have examined negative affect and related outcomes following mindfulness training. A rigorous meta-analysis of mindfulness-based therapy, including MBSR, found medium effect size improvements in anxiety (Hedges's $g = 0.63$) and depression (Hedges's $g = 0.59$), helping to demonstrate the robustness of mindfulness training for negative affect related outcomes (Hofmann, Sawyer, Witt, & Oh, 2010). These findings, however, combined community and psychiatric sample studies.

Focusing specifically on a community sample, Robins, Keng, Ekblad, and Brantley (2012) found that relative to a wait-list control group, standard MBSR resulted in decreased reported fear of emotions, worry, rumination, and emotion regulation difficulties, with a group difference moderate to large in magnitude at postintervention and 2-month follow-up. Davidson and colleagues (2003) found that among healthy employees, MBSR led to significant reductions in trait anxiety and other negative emotions relative to wait-list control, as well as shifts in prefrontal alpha band electrocortical activity, consistent with greater approach motivation and emotions.

Shapiro and colleagues have conducted a considerable number of MBSR studies examining the beneficial effects of mindfulness training for negative emotions. For example, among premedical and medical students, a 7-week mindfulness training led to lower reported state and trait anxiety, distress, and depression relative to a wait-list control group (Shapiro, Schwartz, & Bonner, 1998). An MBSR study for psychotherapist trainees found decreases in stress, negative affect, rumination, and anxiety following MBSR versus an attention control group (Shapiro, Brown, & Biegel, 2007). In these studies, however, posttreatment measures were administered 15 to 20 minutes after the final group, complicating interpretation of whether results were due to feelings about the last group, a sense of accomplishment due to completing the course, or enduring effects of the mindfulness training. In a study with undergraduates, MBSR participation led to significant increases in MAAS-assessed trait mindfulness at 2-month follow up, which mediated reductions in rumination and perceived stress (Shapiro, Oman, Thoresen, Plante, & Flinders, 2008).

Several studies have examined briefer approaches to mindfulness training using interventions of 1 month or less. Jain and colleagues (2007) randomized health care profession students to a 12-hour mindfulness or somatic relaxation training delivered over 1 month. Both resulted in declines in distress at postintervention. Relative to relaxation, however, mindfulness led to larger decreases in distraction and rumination; reductions in rumination partially mediated declines in distress.

In a study assessing physiological and behavioral outcomes, Kingston, Chadwick, Meron, and Skinner (2007) randomized undergraduates to six twice-weekly mindfulness training sessions or two guided visual imagery sessions. Relative to the visual imagery group, the mindfulness group improved in pain tolerance but not in negative affect or blood pressure physiology, which suggests training that is a fraction of the length of MBSR produced more limited benefits.

Ortner, Kilner, and Zelazo (2007) compared the effects of a 7-week mindfulness meditation training, relaxation training, and wait-list control group. At posttraining, both training groups reported similar improvements on a variety of self-reported well-being measures and evidenced less intense affect and lower skin conductance responses in response to viewing negative slides. In the mindfulness group, however, these improvements further generalized to the positive slides and resulted in reduced emotional interference (defined by the speed of categorizing auditory tones as high- or low-pitched while viewing unpleasant compared to neutral pictures). Mindfulness group effects generalized to a broader range of slide types and were reliably distinguished from relaxation training, illustrating the broader benefits of sustained training in mindfulness over onetime mindfulness inductions.

Before and after MBSR training (vs. wait-list controls) in a community sample, Farb and colleagues (2010) induced sadness via film clips viewed in an fMRI scanner. Despite similar self-reported sadness in the two groups at baseline and posttraining, MBSR resulted in a different neural response to sadness, including greater activation of visceral and somatosensory areas linked with experiencing bodily sensations, relative to wait-listed controls. Greater activation of these regions correlated with lower depression scores, and negatively correlated with neural language centers. The authors argued that mindfulness training helped participants to direct more attention toward bodily sensations associated with emotion rather than remain dominated by conceptual, verbal, and elaborative processing of emotion, which may represent one pathway through which mindfulness training reduces vulnerability to sadness. Together with the Jain and colleagues (2007) study, these findings suggest that by directing attention toward present-moment, embodied experience, mindfulness training increases moment-by-moment contact with emotions and decreases verbal–conceptual elaboration in response to them (e.g., rumination) that can sustain or intensify the initial emotional response and lead to depression, anxiety, and other chronically negative states.

A few studies have examined the benefits of intensive mindfulness retreats. Though lacking randomized control groups (Chambers, Lo, & Allen, 2008; Orzech, Shapiro, Brown, & McKay, 2009), these studies demonstrated improvements in reported distress or anxiety following a 10-day (Chambers et al., 2008) or 1-month (Orzech et al., 2009) mindfulness meditation retreat. These studies promote an alternative format for delivering mindfulness-based training—an intensive mindfulness retreat—that appears to offer substantial benefits in exchange for short-term intensive practice. Future retreat studies should utilize random assignment and employ active intervention comparison conditions.

In summary, relatively short-term training in mindfulness meditation (2 months or less) can produce an array of benefits related to negative emotion relative to wait-list and active control conditions, including relaxation (Ditto, Eclache, & Goldman, 2006; Jain et al., 2007), a treatment sometimes confused with mindfulness practice. The length and intensity of mindfulness training appears to matter. Mindfulness training of 1 month or less has failed to yield the similar negative affect improvements as the full 8-week MBSR course except if conducted intensively (e.g., Jain et al., 2007). The number of months that negative affect benefits endure and the types of continued practice and booster training required to maintain emotional benefits over time remain important questions for future research. We now turn to studies on highly experienced meditators to address a different but related question: What are the emotional benefits of long-term training in mindfulness meditation?

Experienced Meditators

Within the contemplative traditions from which mindfulness practices arise, the cultivation of mindfulness is a process occurring over years rather than days, weeks, or months. Studying long-term practitioners provides a practical opportunity to investigate the benefits of engaging in mindfulness practice that is sustained over time. Given the considerable time, motivation, and commitment required, it is logistically challenging (and perhaps ethically so as well) to randomize participants to obtain such training or not. On the other hand, studying those already practicing mindfulness has inherent drawbacks. Individuals attracted to and successful at maintaining a long-term commitment to mindfulness training likely differ from others in important ways. Thus, cross-sectional comparisons between long-term practitioners and controls, even when findings correlate with mindfulness experience, fail to account for factors that drive certain individuals to commit more strongly to or succeed at this unusual path in the first place. Considering these qualifications, we review selected studies on highly experienced mindfulness practitioners.

Most studies with this population have compared experienced and novice meditators on neural structures and functions related to emotional processing and attention. For example, Perlman, Salomons, Davidson, and Lutz (2010) compared highly experienced meditators (HEMs; 10,000–54,000 hours of practice in the Tibetan Buddhist tradition) to novice meditators (1 week of meditation instructions) exposed to painful thermal (very hot temperature) skin stimulation during open-monitoring meditation (mindfulness cultivated broadly toward all present-moment experience). Relative to novices, HEMs reported lower unpleasantness but not lower intensity of painful stimuli, a finding consistent with superior regulation of negative emotional experiences without a change in sensory experience.

Ortner and colleagues (2007) assessed mindfulness meditators (with 1 month to 29 years' experience) on an IAPS picture rating and interference task. Participants with greater meditation experience showed less emotional interference (on the same task described in the previous section) but did not differ on picture intensity ratings, a finding that echoes the Perlman and colleagues (2010) thermal pain findings. A related fMRI study by Taylor and colleagues (2011) compared experienced (1000+ hours of Zen meditation) and novice (1 week of mindfulness meditation) meditators while instructed (vs. not instructed) to be mindfully attentive to IAPS photographic images. Viewing the pictures in a mindful (vs. nonmindful) state reduced emotional intensity ratings in both groups but activated a different set of brain regions in each. For novices, mindful viewing resulted in down-regulation of the left amygdala

through greater prefrontal cortical regulation and control. For experienced meditators, mindful viewing deactivated default mode network areas. The authors argued
that long-term meditation experience induced brain changes consistent with emotional acceptance, stability, and present-moment awareness, whereas novice meditators relied on emotional control. These findings are consistent with a recent review
by Chiesa, Serretti, and Jakobsen (2013) proposing that short-term mindfulness
practice is associated with "top-down" emotion regulation (e.g., prefrontal regulation of emotion-generative brain regions), whereas long-term mindfulness practice is
associated with "bottom-up" emotion regulation (e.g., directly reduced reactivity of
emotion-generative brain regions without active recruitment of prefrontal regions).

In comparing experienced meditators (averaging 3 years of practice) and non-
meditating controls, Teper and Inzlicht (2013) found that meditators had higher
self-rated emotional acceptance, which was significantly associated with years spent
meditating. Emotional acceptance mediated meditators' superior performance on the
color Stroop task (a measure of executive functioning), suggesting that "enhanced
acceptance of emotional states may be a key reason that meditation improves executive functioning" (p. 90). Perhaps emotional acceptance reflects the more "bottom-
up" approach associated with long-term meditators by Chiesa and colleagues (2013)
and prefrontal regions were therefore more available to focus on tasks of executive
functioning (e.g., the Stroop task).

In summary, findings suggest that experienced meditators respond with less
effort and with less distress to emotional provocation; one study also indicated less
emotional interference or "carryover" effects with experienced relative to less experienced meditators. Furthermore, when practicing mindfulness, different brain regions
appear to be activated in more versus less experienced meditators; that is, mindfulness may have a different quality and result in distinct emotion regulation approaches
(Chiesa et al., 2013) depending on degree of training and practice.

Benefits of Mindfulness for Positive Emotion

Our emphasis on the benefits of mindfulness for negative emotion-related neural processing, physiology, and experience reflects the fact that far more studies have examined those topics than the relation between mindfulness and positive emotion-related
outcomes. As discussed later, however, mindfulness as a form of attention deployment should influence the appraisal and response to *positive* as well as negative emotional experience (Gross, 1998, 2014b). In positive contexts, the mindful capacity to
more directly and receptively experience "what is" rather than process through layers
of conceptual thinking (see Brown & Ryan, 2003) may enhance pleasure, joy, contentment, and other positive emotions. In the simple experience of smelling a rose, for
example, mindfulness encourages one's full sensory engagement with this particular
rose, noticing its color, scent, and texture. A conceptually dominant experience of the
rose might lead to preoccupation with memories of receiving roses in the past, which
could trigger sadness, loss, longing, nostalgia, happy recalling, and a range of other
experiences disconnected from the immediate positivity of the current experience.

The relatively few mindfulness induction and intervention studies that assess positive emotion-related outcomes demonstrate increases in self-reported positive affect (e.g., Erisman & Roemer, 2010; Shapiro et al., 2007). This represents a promising start and, clearly, more research is needed to investigate further the benefits of mindfulness for positive emotion-related experiences. Research on mindfulness and positive emotion will inform our understanding of the breadth of the emotions influenced by mindfulness.

Toward a Theory of Mindful Emotion Regulation

From the perspective of the Gross's model of emotion regulation (1998, 2014b; see Figure 12.1), mindfulness appears to represent primarily an attention deployment approach to emotion regulation (see also Brown & Ryan, 2003; Wadlinger & Isaacowitz, 2011).According to Gross's model, attention deployment affects the downstream processes of appraisal and emotional response. We suggest that mindfulness can be conceptualized as a form of attention deployment that impacts emotion generation early, influencing downstream appraisals and emotional responses (Wadlinger & Isaacowitz, 2011). Specifically, mindfulness may reduce the threat value of aversive experiences (modify appraisal), alter the generation of emotional response to aversive experience (modify emotional response), or increase the capacity to tolerate, regulate, and recover from negative emotions triggered by aversive experience (e.g., enhance coping). Furthermore, Gross's model is not exclusive to negative emotional experiences. Appraisal and response to *positive* emotional experiences should also be influenced by mindfulness. For example, events may be appraised and responded to in ways that enhance a sense of gratitude or contentedness.

We now examine evidence for the hypothesis that mindfulness represents a form of attention deployment. The studies reviewed here indicate that mindfulness reduces negative appraisals of affective stimuli, as indicated by subjective ratings (e.g., Arch & Craske, 2006; Erisman & Roemer, 2010; Barnes et al., 2007; Cioffi & Holloway, 1993; Ortner et al., 2007), peripheral physiology (Ortner et al., 2007; Cioffi & Holloway, 1993), and neural responses associated with emotion processing (Brown et al., 2012; Creswell et al., 2007). Appraisals, however, unfold very rapidly after stimulus

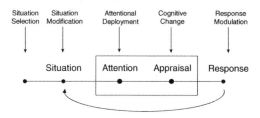

FIGURE 12.1. The modal model of emotion generation (lower portion) and associated model of emotion regulation strategies (upper portion). From Gross (2014b). Copyright 2014 by The Guilford Press. Reprinted by permission.

contact. Studies that have examined neural markers of appraisal over several seconds (with fMRI; e.g., Creswell et al., 2007; Perlman et al., 2010) or within a second (with EEG; e.g., Brown et al., 2013) provide some evidence that such rapid appraisals are altered among mindful individuals, but these studies were correlational or quasi-experimental in nature. Extant studies, therefore, provide consistent but still incomplete evidence for the impact of mindfulness on negative affective appraisal. Future research should examine the impact of mindfulness on very early stimulus responses within experimental designs using methodologies such as EEG that capture rapid appraisal-relevant responses.

More evidence supports the idea that mindfulness impacts emotional *responses*. Convergent findings from trait (e.g., Barnes et al., 2007; Brown & Ryan, 2003), briefly induced state (e.g., Broderick, 2005; Erisman & Roemer, 2010), daily state (Brown & Ryan, 2003), and intervention-based studies (e.g., Jain et al., 2007; Robins et al., 2012) indicate that mindfulness leads to dampened negative affect and, in several studies, greater positive affect in response to affective stimuli in the laboratory and in daily life.

Thus, mindful attention appears to impact downstream cognitive appraisals and particularly emotional responses. As an antecedent-focused strategy, mindful attention deployment represents an early and therefore highly efficient approach to regulating emotion. Furthermore, Sheppes and Gross (2011) note that regulation strategies that target an early stage of emotion processing are relatively uninfluenced by the intensity of the emotion that is being regulated. By contrast, strategies that target a late selection processing stage generally become less effective as the emotion that is being regulated becomes stronger. Training in mindfulness may therefore alter individual emotion regulatory profiles. Wadlinger and Isaacowitz (2011), in reviewing attention-based strategies for regulating emotion, conclude that "although [mindfulness] practices take the most cognitive effort to initially enact, they may create the most lasting regulatory outcomes of all training techniques" (p. 93). Thus, even among attention-based strategies (which also include distraction and others), mindfulness represents a particularly promising approach to regulating emotion.

Mindfulness may also offer advantages in regulating difficult emotions that have arisen, and such management is of clear importance in both normative and mental health populations. Regarding the latter, a growing number of mental health theories posit that *emotion dysregulation*—defined by Mennin (2005) as heightened intensity, poor understanding of emotions, negative reactivity, and maladaptive management of emotions—underlies many psychiatric disorders. Related theories of emotion in psychopathology (Hayes, Strosahl, & Wilson, 1999; Orsillo, Roemer, Lerner, & Tull, 2004) distinguish between "clean" and "clear" versus "dirty" and "muddied" emotions—the primary emotion response versus the secondary emotion response overlaid upon the initial response in attempts to avoid or rigidly control it (e.g., chronic worry, rumination, or avoidance). Growing evidence suggest that these secondary responses underlie much emotion dysregulation (Gratz & Roemer, 2004) and psychopathology (Gratz, Rosenthal, Tull, Lejuez, & Gunderson, 2006; Mennin, Heimberg, Turk, & Fresco, 2005). By promoting direct, early contact with primary emotions, mindfulness may represent a form of "emotional exposure" (see Brown, Ryan, & Creswell, 2007; Hölzel et al., 2011, for similar views)—deliberate, sustained, and repeated contact with the full range of present emotional experience, be it "good, bad, or ugly" (Kabat-Zinn, 1990). As such, mindfulness and training in it may offer a degree of protection from psychopathologies related to emotion dysregulation (e.g., unipolar mood and anxiety disorders).

Extant research supports the hypothesis that mindfulness fosters adaptive regulation of emotional responses that have arisen: Trait and induced mindfulness predict greater voluntary exposure to aversive stimuli (Arch & Craske, 2006, 2010) and self-threatening information (Niemiec et al., 2010), greater clarity about what emotions are felt (Hill & Updegraff, 2012), acceptance of emotions experienced (Teper & Inzlicht, 2013), and faster recovery from unpleasant emotions and aversive experiences (Broderick, 2005; Cioffi & Holloway, 1993).

Viewed through the lens of adaptive emotion regulation, this work also informs a working definition of the emotional benefits of mindfulness: greater attentiveness to and dampened appraisal of emotional stimuli; greater acceptance of emotions and clarity about what is felt; less intense, rigid, or enduring secondary emotional responses; faster recovery from negative emotions; and less interference of negative emotions with adaptive behavior. These benefits should promote flexible, contextually sensitive emotional responding. From the perspective of Gross's (1998, 2014b) emotion regulation model, these benefits stem from subsequently altered appraisal and response-related processes.

Conclusions and Future Research Directions

Findings from diverse studies demonstrate that trait, induced state, and trained forms of mindfulness yield emotional benefits. These three approaches address different questions regarding immediate (inductions), longer-term (training), and continual (trait) emotional benefits of mindfulness, but results from extant studies are quite consistent in their conclusions. However this area of investigation is still young, and we close by offering several suggestions that we believe will broaden and deepen our scientific understanding of this topic.

Methodological Improvements

To date, the majority of findings on mindfulness and emotion derive from self-reported outcomes. First-person accounts are important for capturing subjective experience, but future studies would benefit from integrating behavioral, neural, and psychophysiological markers of affect and emotion (Davidson, 2010). The integration of multiple forms of emotion measurement would address the issue that different dimensions of emotional experience—traditionally defined as subjective, behavioral, and physiological—do not always cohere (Mauss, Levenson, McCarter, Wilhelm, & Gross, 2005), a finding also observed in several mindfulness studies (e.g., Erisman

& Roemer, 2010; Farb et al., 2010). Examining only a single dimension of emotion, therefore, risks missing information about the impact of mindfulness on other dimensions, limiting our understanding of its effects.

Assessing the role of mindfulness within *personally relevant* emotion contexts represents another important avenue for research in this area. Specifically, in addition to what is observed in the laboratory, it is important to study whether mindfulness promotes the capacity to regulate emotions within daily life. Daily diary or ecological momentary assessment (EMA) studies have begun to examine this question (Brown & Ryan, 2003; Hill & Updegraff, 2012). However, these studies have examined a generic adaptive emotional profile (lower negative affect, higher positive affect, stable overall affect) across all days of people's lives rather than contextualizing people's affective experience through the lens of meaningful daily events. Future mindfulness research would benefit from using EMA methodologies to track meaningful emotional events and associated emotional responses with greater contextual sensitivity. For example, in examining daily emotions in response to a major loss (e.g., death of a loved one), we may find that mindfulness practice initially promotes *greater* engagement with loss and therefore more initially intense feelings of grief and sadness. Such a finding would contrast with the generic profile of desirable emotional responding that is often assumed, namely, that lower negative affect equates with more adaptive responding.

Greater Focus on Positive Emotional Experiences

Another area for future research lies in examining the influence of mindfulness on positive emotional experiences. Enhancing the experience, expression, and endurance of positive emotions represents an emotional benefit in many contexts. For example, experiencing greater positive emotions (e.g., joy, contentment, and gratitude) predicts "human flourishing," which includes resilience in the face of adversity (e.g., Fredrickson, 2001).

A few studies (e.g., Arch, Brown, Della Porta, Kiken, & Tillman, 2014; Erisman & Roemer, 2010) have indicated that mindfulness enhances the enjoyment of positive sensory stimuli (e.g., pleasant film clips, foods). In contrast, other studies suggest that mindfulness may *dampen* the strength of emotional response to positive sensory stimuli (Brown et al., 2012; Ortner et al., 2007). Thus, mindfulness does not appear simply to increase positive emotion. Assessing and differentiating between active and nonactive forms of positive affect (i.e., "excited" vs. "calm") may help to understand this mix of findings. Mindfulness-related positive emotional experience may take the profile of higher nonactive forms of positive affect (e.g., calm or contented) to a greater extent than active forms (e.g., excited)—and this is more consistent with Buddhist-informed notions of emotional well-being than Western notions (Ekman, Davidson, Ricard, & Wallace, 2005). It is also important to attend to the time frame in which emotions are studied. Mindfulness may, for example, be associated with lower state-positive affect but higher positive affect over time, a pattern perhaps attributable to lower emotional lability (cf. Hill & Updegraff, 2012). Directing greater research efforts toward investigating the positive emotional benefits of mindfulness will help to illuminate these complexities and further elucidate how mindfulness enhances human flourishing.

REFERENCES

Arch, J. J., Brown, K. W., Della Porta, M. D., Kiken, L. G., & Tillman, S. (2014). *Mindfulness enhances the positivity of sensory experience: Evidence from food tasting.* Manuscript in preparation.

Arch, J. J., & Craske, M. G. (2006). Mechanisms of mindfulness: Emotion regulation following a focused breathing induction. *Behaviour Research and Therapy, 44,* 1849–1858.

Arch, J. J., & Craske, M. G. (2010). Laboratory stressors in clinically anxious and non-anxious individuals: the moderating role of mindfulness. *Behaviour Research and Therapy, 48*(6), 495–505.

Baer, R. A., Smith, G. T., Hopkins, J., Krietemeyer, J., & Toney, L. (2006). Using self-report assessment methods to explore facets of mindfulness. *Assessment, 13*(1), 27–45.

Barnes, S., Brown, K. W., Krusemark, E., Campbell, W. K., & Rogge, R. D. (2007). The role of mindfulness in romantic relationship satisfaction and responses to relationship stress. *Journal of Marital and Family Therapy, 33*(4), 482–500.

Broderick, P. C. (2005). Mindfulness and coping with dysphoric mood: Contrasts with rumination and distraction. *Cognitive Therapy and Research, 29*(5), 501–510.

Brown, K. W., Goodman, R. J., & Inzlicht, M. (2013). Dispositional mindfulness and the attenuation of neural responses to emotional stimuli. *Social Cognitive and Affective Neuroscience, 8*(1), 93–99.

Brown, K. W., & Ryan, R. M. (2003). The benefits of being present: Mindfulness and its role in psychological well-being. *Journal of Personality and Social Psychology, 84*(4), 822–848.

Brown, K. W., Ryan, R. M., & Creswell, J. D. (2007). Mindfulness: Theoretical foundations and evidence for its salutary effects. *Psychological Inquiry, 18*(4), 211–237.

Chambers, R., Lo, B. C. Y., & Allen, N. B. (2008). The impact of intensive mindfulness training on attentional control, cognitive style, and affect. *Cognitive Therapy and Research, 32*(3), 303–322.

Chiesa, A., Serretti, A., & Jakobsen, J. C. (2013). Mindfulness: Top-down or bottom-up emotion regulation strategy? *Clinical Psychology Review, 33,* 82–96.

Cioffi, D., & Holloway, J. (1993). Delayed costs of suppressed pain. *Journal of Personality and Social Psychology, 64*(2), 274–282.

Creswell, J. D., Way, B. M., Eisenberger, N. I., & Lieberman, M. D. (2007). Neural correlates of dispositional mindfulness during affect labeling. *Psychosomatic Medicine, 69*(6), 560–565.

Davidson, R. J. (2010). Empirical explorations of mindfulness: Conceptual and methodological conundrums. *Emotion, 10*(1), 8–11.

Davidson, R. J., Kabat-Zinn, J., Schumacher, J., Rosenkranz, M., Muller, D., Santorelli, S. F., et al. (2003). Alterations in brain and immune function produced by mindfulness meditation. *Psychosomatic Medicine, 65*(4), 564–570.

Ditto, B., Eclache, M., & Goldman, N. (2006). Short-term autonomic and cardiovascular effects of mindfulness body scan meditation. *Annals of Behavioral Medicine, 32*(3), 227–234.

Ekman, P. (1992). An argument for basic emotions. *Cognition and Emotion, 6*(3–4), 169–200.

Ekman, P., Davidson, R. J., Ricard, M., & Wallace, B. A. (2005). Buddhist and psychological perspectives on emotions and well-being. *Current Directions in Psychological Science, 14*(2), 59–63.

Erisman, S. M., & Roemer, L. (2010). A preliminary investigation of the effects of experimentally induced mindfulness on emotional responding to film clips. *Emotion, 10*(1), 72–82.

Farb, N. A. S., Anderson, A. K., Mayberg, H., Bean, J., McKeon, D., & Segal, Z. V. (2010). Minding one's emotions: Mindfulness training alters the neural expression of sadness. *Emotion, 10*(1), 25–33.

Fredrickson, B. L. (2001). The role of positive emotions in positive psychology: The broaden-and-build theory of positive emotions. *American Psychologist, 56*(3), 218–226.

Frijda, N. H. (1986). *The emotions.* London: Cambridge University Press.

Gratz, K. L., & Roemer, L. (2004). Multidimensional assessment of emotion regulation and dysregulation: Development, factor structure, and initial validation of the Difficulties in Emotion Regulation Scale. *Journal of Psychopathology and Behavioral Assessment, 26*(1), 41–54.

Gratz, K. L., Rosenthal, M. Z., Tull, M. T., Lejuez, C. W., & Gunderson, J. G. (2006). An experimental investigation of emotion dysregulation in borderline personality disorder. *Journal of Abnormal Psychology, 115*(4), 850–855.

Gross, J. J. (1998). Antecedent- and response-focused emotion regulation: Divergent conseqeunces for experience, expression, and physiology. *Journal of Personality and Social Psychology, 74,* 224–237.

Gross, J. J. (Ed.). (2007). *Handbook of emotion regulation.* New York: Guilford Press.

Gross, J. J. (2014a). Emotion regulation: Conceptual and empirical foundations. In J. J. Gross (Ed.), *Handbook of emotion regulation* (2nd ed., pp. 3–20). New York: Guilford Press.

Gross, J. J. (Ed.). (2014b). *Handbook of emotion regulation* (2nd ed.). New York: Guilford Press.

Hayes, S. C., Strosahl, K. D., & Wilson, K. G. (1999). *Acceptance and commitment therapy: An experiential approach to behavior change.* New York: Guilford Press.

Hayes, S. C., Strosahl, K. D., & Wilson, K. G. (2012). *Acceptance and commitment therapy: The process and practice of mindful change* (2nd ed.). New York: Guilford Press.

Hill, C. L. M., & Updegraff, J. A. (2012). Mindfulness and its relationship to emotion regulation. *Emotion, 12*(1), 81–90.

Hofmann, S. G., Sawyer, A. T., Witt, A. A., & Oh, D. (2010). The effect of mindfulness-based therapy on anxiety and depression: A meta-analytic review. *Journal of Consulting and Clinical Psychology, 78*(2), 169–183.

Hölzer, B. K., Lazar, S. W., Gard, T., Schuman-Olivier, Z., Vago, D. R., & Ott, U. (2011). How does mindfulness meditation work?: Proposing mechanisms of action from a conceptual and neural perspective. *Perspectives on Psychological Science, 6*(6), 537–559.

Jain, S., Shapiro, S. L., Swanick, S., Roesch, S. C., Mills, P. J., Bell, I., et al. (2007). A randomized controlled trial of mindfulness meditation versus relaxation training: Effects on distress, positive states of mind, rumination, and distraction. *Annals of Behavioral Medicine, 33*(1), 11–21.

Kabat-Zinn, J. (1990). *Full catastrophe living: Using the wisdom of your body and mind to face stress, pain, and illness.* New York: Delta.

Kessler, R. C., Berglund, P., Demler, O., Jin, R., & Walters, E. E. (2005). Lifetime prevalence and age-of-onset distributions of DSM-IV disorders in the National Comorbidity Survey Replication. *Archives of General Psychiatry, 62*(6), 593–602.

Kingston, J., Chadwick, P., Meron, D., & Skinner, T. C. (2007). A pilot randomized control trial investigating the effect of mindfulness practice on pain tolerance, psychological well-being, and physiological activity. *Journal of Psychosomatic Research, 62*, 297–300.

Lang, P. J., Bradley, M. M., & Cuthbert, B. N. (2008). *International affective picture system (IAPS): Affective ratings of pictures and instruction manual* [Technical Report A-8]. Gainesville: University of Florida.

Linehan, M. M. (1993). *Cognitive-behavioral treatment of borderline personality disorder.* New York: Guilford Press.

Mauss, I. B., Levenson, R. W., McCarter, L., Wilhelm, F. H., & Gross, J. J. (2005). The tie that binds?: Coherence among emotion experience, behavior, and physiology. *Emotion, 5*(2), 175–190.

McLaughlin, K. A., Mennin, D. S., & Farach, F. J. (2007). The contributory role of worry in emotion generation and dysregulation in generalized anxiety disorder. *Behaviour Research and Therapy, 45*(8), 1735–1752.

Mennin, D. S. (2005). Emotion and the acceptance-based approaches to the anxiety disorders. In S. M. Orsillo & L. Roemer (Eds.), *Acceptance and mindfulness-based approaches to anxiety: Conceptualization and treatment* (pp. 37–70). New York: Springer.

Mennin, D. S., Heimberg, R. G., Turk, C. L., & Fresco, D. M. (2005). Preliminary evidence for an emotion dysregulation model of generalized anxiety disorder. *Behaviour Research and Therapy, 43*(10), 1281–1310.

Niemiec, C. P., Brown, K. W., Kashdan, T. B., Cozzolino, P. J., Breen, W. E., Levesque-Bristol, C., et al. (2010). Being present in the face of existential threat: The role of trait mindfulness in reducing defensive response to mortality salience. *Journal of Personality and Social Psychology, 99*(2), 344–365.

Orsillo, S. M., Roemer, L., Lerner, J. B., & Tull, M. T. (2004). Acceptance, mindfulness, and cognitive-behavioral therapy: Comparisons, contrasts, and application to anxiety. In S. C. Hayes, V. M. Follette, & M. M. Linehan (Eds.), *Mindfulness and acceptance: Expanding the cognitive-behavioral tradition* (pp. 66–95). New York: Guilford Press.

Ortner, C. N. M., Kilner, S. J., & Zelazo, P. D. (2007). Mindfulness meditation and reduced emotional interference on a cognitive task. *Motivation and Emotion, 31*(4), 271–283.

Orzech, K. M., Shapiro, S. L., Brown, K. W., & McKay, M. (2009). Intensive mindfulness training-related changes in cognitive and emotional experience. *Journal of Positive Psychology, 4*(3), 212–222.

Perlman, D. M., Salomons, T. V., Davidson, R. J., & Lutz, A. (2010). Different effects on pain intensity and unpleasantness of two meditation practices. *Emotion, 10*(1), 65–71.

Robins, C. J., Keng, S.-L., Ekblad, A. G., & Brantley, J. G. (2012). Effects of mindfulness-based stress reduction on emotional experience and expression: A randomized controlled trial. *Journal of Clinical Psychology, 68*(1), 117–131.

Segal, Z. V., Williams, J. M., & Teasdale, J. D. (2002). *Mindfulness-based cognitive therapy for depression: A new approach to preventing relapse.* New York: Guilford Press.

Shapiro, S. L., Brown, K. W., & Biegel, G. M. (2007). Teaching self-care to caregivers: Effects of mindfulness-based stress reduction on the mental health of therapists in training. *Training and Education in Professional Psychology, 1*(2), 105–115.

Shapiro, S. L., Oman, D., Thoresen, C. E., Plante, T. G., & Flinders, T. (2008). Cultivating mindfulness: Effects on well-being. *Journal of Clinical Psychology, 64*(7), 840–862.

Shapiro, S. L., Schwartz, S. A., & Bonner, G. (1998). Effects of mindfulness-based stress reduction on medical and premedical students. *Journal of Behavioral Medicine, 21*(6), 581–599.

Sheppes, G., & Gross, J. J. (2011). Is timing everything?: Temporal considerations in emotion regulation. *Personality and Social Psychology Review, 15*(4), 319–331.

Tang, Y.-Y., Ma, Y., Wang, J., Fan, Y., Feng, S., Lu, Q., et al. (2007). Short-term meditation training improves attention and self-regulation. *Proceedings of the National Academy of Science, 104*(43), 17152–17156.

Taylor, V. A., Grant, J., Daneault, V., Scavone, G., Breton, E., Roffe-Vidal, S., et al. (2011). Impact of mindfulness on the neural responses to emotional pictures in experienced and beginner meditators. *NeuroImage, 57*, 1524–1533.

Teper, R., & Inzlicht, M. (2013). Meditation, mindfulness and executive control: The importance of emotional acceptance and brain-based performance monitoring. *Social Cognitive and Affective Neuroscience, 8*(1), 85–92.

Wadlinger, H. A., & Isaacowitz, D. M. (2011). Fixing our focus: Training attention to regulate emotion. *Personality and Social Psychology Review, 15*(1), 75–102.

Watson, D., Clark, L. A., & Tellegen, A. (1988). Development and validation of brief measures of positive and negative affect: The PANAS scales. *Journal of Personality and Social Psychology, 54*(6), 1063–1070.

Zeidan, F., Gordon, N. S., Merchant, J., & Goolkasian, P. (2010). The effects of brief mindfulness training on experimentally induced pain. *Journal of Pain, 11*(3), 199–209.

CHAPTER 13

The Science of Presence

A Central Mediator of the Interpersonal Benefits of Mindfulness

Suzanne C. Parker, Benjamin W. Nelson, Elissa S. Epel, and Daniel J. Siegel

This chapter focuses on an intriguing question concerning mindfulness that is perhaps even paradoxical at first glance. How can mindfulness, often developed through a personal and solitary meditation practice, lead to interpersonal benefits off the meditation cushion? Put more briefly, how does the internal attunement and self-regulation of mindfulness foster interpersonal benefits when one interacts with other people? People high in dispositional mindfulness traits and experienced mindfulness meditators are often described as "warm" people, humans who are intimately in touch with the joys and sufferings of their fellow humans. Is this common perception true, and is there empirical evidence to support it? Herein we examine these and related questions in light of recent research from psychology, neuroscience, and biology.

We base this exploration within the framework of the interdisciplinary approach of *interpersonal neurobiology*, which examines the neural basis of relationships as the sharing of energy and information (Siegel, 2012a, 2012b). First, we pinpoint the quality and process of *presence* as an essential component of mindfulness that has a large role in mediating the relationship of mindfulness and *interpersonal attunement*, the ways in which we focus on the internal state of another individual with kindness and compassion (Siegel, 2012a). We explore the conceptual and scientific definitions of presence, as well as one of its opposites, *mind wandering*. We expand upon the neural bases of these two seemingly opposing processes, looking at the latest research on presence and mind wandering, and how the research provides a way to view their conceptual opposition in empirical terms. We then explore how presence, attunement, and resonance coalesce and lead to interpersonal benefits. Next, we explore the nature of relationships and how research findings on interpersonal experience intersect with those on mindful awareness. Here, we examine attachment and developmental neurobiology, and how emerging evidence from this area aligns with the benefits of mindfulness. Finally, we expand on the integration and self-organization of complex systems, focusing on how mindfulness ultimately creates the capacity for the self to be part of a "we" without losing the "me." Together, examination of these areas will shed light on how the presence at the base of mindfulness can nurture interpersonal benefits.

Presence: The Roles of Bare Attention and Mindful Awareness

In this discussion of the interpersonal benefits of mindfulness, we examine presence as a key element responsible for facilitating the resonance and attunement that mindfulness fosters. *Presence* is "the bare awareness of the receptive spaciousness of our mind," a "state of receptive awareness of our open minds to whatever arises as it arises" (Siegel, 2007a, p. 160–161). Presence combines a temporal quality of focusing on the immediate *now* with an intention to experience that *now* directly. To be present and experience directly means to minimize interpreting what occurs from within a framework of rigid mental constructs or ingrained emotional reactivity. Being present entails an intentional, receptive, and flexible state of attending to the moment of now.

Presence can be viewed as a state of open awareness to what emerges in the flow of conscious experience, moment by moment. We can identify multiple aspects of presence, using the qualifying term *bare attention* to refer to the quality of conscious experience that is filled with direct experience of here-and-now sensory information with little filtering by top-down processes acquired from prior events. We can also distinguish this bare attention from *mindful awareness*, in which we propose that there is the activation of an observing self that is "attuned" to an experiencing self: a witnessing circuit that is open and curious to what is happening in the sensory unfolding of the moment, along with the broader context of one's experience also within awareness. The *mindfulness* component adds to bare attention the quality of being aware without being swept up by judgments. This nonjudgmental awareness of being fully and intentionally present has emotional, physiological, and interpersonal impacts on experience.

Phelan (2010) describes *mindful practice* as "presence with the intention of becoming one with our activity, so that the gaps between body and mind, between our attention and our activity, close" (p. 131). Phelan illustrates the classic example of washing dishes with presence:

> You will not have to stop and ask yourself: "Are my hands in the water or out?" "Does the water feel hot or just lukewarm?" . . . When we wash dishes, we know directly and immediately the heat and sudsy quality of the water without needing to pull ourselves back from the situation to think about it. . . . *Once we step back*

to examine an experience, the original experience has ended and we begin a new experience, which is reflecting on the past. (pp. 132–133, emphasis added)

Phelan eloquently portrays the essence of presence: If you are not experiencing directly, then in your interpretation of what is happening you are already reflecting on the past, catapulted discreetly out of the present.

Such a process is similar to Csikszentmihalyi's (2008) sense of flow, of losing self-consciousness while becoming immersed in an experience. We propose that such flow is only one aspect of being present. This we might equate with what we are calling *bare attention*. As we'll see, mindful awareness, as opposed to bare attention, also involves in its essence an awareness of an observing self as it witnesses the direct experiencing self in the present moment—not as reflections on the past, interpretations of the present, or anticipations of the future—but with an attunement of the observing capacity of the perceptual system with the experiencing capacity of the self.

There are separate neurological circuits that underlie these different mental processes of awareness. Farb and colleagues (2007) have identified a midline observing–narrating–witnessing self-circuitry and a lateralized sensing–perceiving–experiencing self-circuitry. Our proposal is that mindfulness involves the integration of these two circuits in real time, honoring their differences, with the attunement of an observing self with what is happening in the here and now with the experiencing self (see Siegel, 2007a, 2007b). This is the *internal attunement* that arises with mindful awareness.

The contrast to reflecting on the past is anticipating the future, another mental process that illustrates what presence is by virtue of what it is not. "The brain is an anticipation machine, always readying itself for the next moment. It appears that this is a fundamental property of neural circuits—it is how as parallel distributed processors they learn from experience" (Siegel, 2007a, p. 187). Priming is an excellent example of the brain's continual preparation for the next moment. Priming is how the brain readies itself for the immediate horizon of the present, the "next event to follow now," based on what has happened in the past as embedded in implicit memory. Such priming can make us vigilant for danger based on what has happened before, shaping our perceptions of the present moment based on these implicit "top-down" filters that are shaped by the past, that mold how we experience the present, and that ready us—prime us—to respond in the future. However, it is important to distinguish the brain's automatic anticipation of the future from intentional future planning, which is driven by the prefrontal cortex. "This [intentional future planning] is anatomically, neurologically, and subjectively quite different from the priming sense of 'next'" (Siegel, 2007a, p. 187). *Being present* means gently reining in this natural tendency to be unintentionally preparing for the next thing in order to simply "be" with what is currently happening.

In this way, being present may initially require our effort to sense top-down influences on perception and "let them go" with intention. With practice, presence may become effortless as a trait, activated without conscious intention. To let vigilance be released, it may be necessary to achieve an inner state of safety, one that enables the brain to move from a reactive state of fight–flight–freeze in anticipation of danger to one of being open and receptive. This receptive state may involve activation of what

Porges (2011b) refers to as the ventral branch of the 10th cranial nerve, the vagus, as part of his *polyvagal theory*. Presence may therefore be fostered by a sense of safety. It is challenging, if not impossible, to dismiss an impending sense of "next" if one does not feel safe in this world, in an interpersonal context. In this way, presence as revealed in mindfulness traits may co-occur with secure attachment, as evidenced by a preliminary study of adults by DiNoble (2009).

Mind Wandering

Another way to understand the importance of presence is to examine what may be its most accurate opposite, mind wandering. Mind wandering is a universal experience, whether the mind is wandering away from one's reading, the breath, simple awareness, or any other present-moment focus. Mind wandering is an unintentional process, quite different from giving oneself permission to *free-associate*, which is letting the imagination explore spontaneous images and connections in a way that is at the heart of creativity and divergent thinking. Studies of creativity have in fact found that when people intentionally allow their minds to explore, there is an increased association with creative output, whereas when they are unaware that their minds are wandering there is no increase in creative productions (Sayette, Reichle, & Schooler, 2009). The key is intentionality: The choice to allow one's mind to roam may help inner understanding and facilitate creative insight. It is both possible and likely helpful to be present intentionally with spontaneous activations of the mind that are a part of exploring one's own imagination and creative thought. We refer to mind wandering as distinctly different from this more creative process that is characterized by more intention and self-reflection.

When looking at the capability to remain undistracted, mindfulness—especially the quality of presence—and (unintentional) mind wandering are seemingly at opposite ends of the spectrum (Mrazek, Smallwood, & Schooler, 2012). Though this spectrum might appear to be solely delineating the nature of attention, it becomes evident in light of mindfulness that this spectrum is a union of both attention and awareness. Studies suggest that mindfulness practice may even enhance the capacity to monitor when mind wandering has occurred, then to redirect attention toward appropriate mental processing (Hasenkamp, Wilson-Mendenhall, Duncan, & Barsalou, 2012). Brown and Cordon (2009) assert that presence itself is "the subjective experience of this refinement of the basic capacities of consciousness—*an immediacy of experience as it occurs*" (p. 65, emphasis added). Mind wandering would entail the opposite—not to be experiencing immediately as experience occurs, but rather to be in another mental timespace away from the sensory occurrence of the present moment.

In the framework of mindfulness theory, presence may be seen as the opposite of mind wandering in regard to one's activities. Phelan (2010) asserts that presence is the opposite of mind wandering because it is focusing on one thing at a time. In this sense, mind wandering represents a division of oneself, specifically, of one's attention and awareness, while presence might be seen as a unification of oneself. If, with mindfulness, we are aiming to bring a full mind to what we are doing, we would likely be focusing on many fewer things at a time than when mind wandering. Exercises such as mindful eating or mindful driving exemplify this goal in their focus on being solely present with the specific activity that is being carried out in the present moment.

Experimental Investigations of Mind Wandering

Mind wandering directly opposes a fundamental element of the definition of mindfulness, the component of sustained attention or nondistraction that is fundamental to presence. Mrazek and colleagues (2012) illustrate this relationship with eloquent brevity: "Where mindfulness ends, mind-wandering begins" (p. 443). Mrazek and colleagues conducted two studies examining the relationship between mindfulness and mind wandering. In the first study they looked at the correlation between dispositional mindfulness and indicators of mind wandering, while in the second study they administered a brief mindfulness exercise to determine whether the intervention affected subsequent mind wandering. The initial study, examining the correlation between dispositional mindfulness and mind wandering, indeed found that high levels of dispositional mindfulness were significantly negatively correlated with both trait mind wandering and task indications of mind wandering. Measurements used in this study to assess dispositional mindfulness included self-report questionnaires such as the Mindful Attention Awareness Scale (MAAS), while task-unrelated thought (TUT) and performance errors were used as a measure of mind wandering. The second study corroborated the oppositional relationship between mindfulness and mind wandering through a mindfulness induction exercise. A brief, 8-minute mindful breathing exercise lowered mind wandering in the postinduction phase, as measured by fewer task errors compared to those following a passive relaxation or reading induction. Thus, it is becoming well established that mindfulness and mind wandering are in direct contrast to each other.

Qualitative Assessments of Mind Wandering

Delving into mind wandering, especially as it relates to mindfulness, is crucial to this chapter because of how mind wandering is in direct opposition to presence and is therefore a hindrance rather than asset to promoting interpersonal connection. It is not possible simultaneously to be mind wandering and present. In addition to the contrast to presence, debate is long-standing about whether mind wandering can be distilled down to a label of "good" or "bad." In 2010, academic and journalistic article titles ranged from "A Wandering Mind Is an Unhappy Mind" (Killingsworth & Gilbert, 2010) to "Discovering the Virtues of a Wandering Mind" (Tierney, 2010). Studies that uncover associations between mind wandering and unhappiness or negative affect are quickly countered by people who assert that mind wandering is beneficial for processes such as creativity. As mentioned earlier, the difference that clarifies these contrary positions may rest in the intentionality of the way awareness is placed on the ongoing experience. Creativity is associated with intentionally letting into awareness spontaneously arising *s*ensations, *i*mages, *f*eelings, and *t*houghts (Siegel,

2010). This is how we can *SIFT* the mind to cultivate creativity. However, the bulk of the research has so far shown mind wandering—what we would clarify here as unintentional wanderings—generally to be associated with unhappiness and negative affect.

Many studies use "experience sampling" to probe participants throughout the day about their current mental state—on-task or mind wandering—and mood. Kane and colleagues (2007) found a correspondence between a higher degree of mind wandering and boredom, stress, and dislike of the current activity. Killingsworth and Gilbert (2010) went further with time-lag analyses to determine which was the cause of which: Does mind wandering lead to an unhappy mental state, or does unhappiness lead to mind wandering? Their results suggest that indeed mind wandering was what generally brought about unhappiness, not the other way around. Using a different approach to examine the interleaved factors of mind wandering, time frame, and unhappiness, Smallwood and O'Connor (2011) found that unhappy moods led to a past-related bias in mind wandering. In their study, inducing an unhappy mood qualitatively led subsequent mind wandering to be retrospective in nature, with a focus on events from the past instead of the present or future. The magnitude of the increase in past-related thoughts also led to higher scores on an evaluation of depressive symptoms, suggesting that the more one's mind wanders to the past, the more unhappy one becomes. Note that this does not counter Killingsworth and Gilbert's time-lag analysis finding that mind wandering is the cause of unhappiness; rather, it delineates how the time-bias of mind-wandering thoughts changes based on one's mood while mind wandering. Thus, mind wandering leads to unhappiness, and an unhappy mind tends to mind-wander specifically to thoughts of the past as opposed to those of the present or future. Together, these findings demonstrate the grounds to bring us back to the benefits of the opposite: presence.

The Biological Embedding of Presence

Can we empirically parse aspects of presence, such as bare attention and mindful awareness, to examine how they might be related to fundamental aspects of physiological health? A new measure of health status, one that can be examined at any age, is the length of one's *telomeres*, the protective caps at the ends of chromosomes. Telomeres serve as a measure of the rate of cellular aging, and they predict longevity (Epel, Daubenmier, Moskowitz, Folkman, & Blackburn, 2009). Telomerase is the enzyme that maintains and repairs telomeres. While normal chronological aging shortens telomere length slowly, stress has been found to accelerate the rate of this shortening (Epel et al., 2004).

Several recent studies have examined the correlations of meditation interventions or reports of attentional states on the rates of cell aging. In one study, participants who underwent a 3-month Shamatha meditation retreat—focused on cultivating both mindful awareness and benevolent states—had significantly greater telomerase activity at the end of the retreat when compared to controls, and this increase appeared to be mediated by increases in feelings of control and "purpose in life" (Jacobs et al.,

2010). This study also found that those who increased most in self-reported mindfulness (mainly aspects of mindful awareness) showed significant decreases in their daily cortisol levels (Jacobs et al., 2013).

In a new study that examined telomere length in relation to self-reported presence and mind wandering, utilizing a large sample of healthy, relatively low-stress women, Epel and colleagues (2012) found that *greater presence of mind, similar to flow or bare attention*, was related to longer telomere length. Conversely, more negative mind wandering—as assessed by thinking about other things or wanting to be somewhere else—was related to shorter telomere length. One limitation of this study is that it measured self-reported tendency to be present versus absent. The accuracy of self-reported measures of retrospective attentional behavior is limited, ironically, by how aware people have been of where their attention lies. Nevertheless, to the extent that self-reports truly isolated mind wandering versus presence (see Baer, Smith, Hopkins, Krietemeyer, & Toney, 2006), this finding suggests that presence has opposite effects on physiology than effects of mind wandering. No other studies thus far have examined whether a propensity for mind wandering as opposed to a proclivity for presence has a biological impact.

The salutary effects of presence on telomere length likely work through sending signals of safety and triggering reparative physiological housekeeping functions. Together, integrating findings across these studies, as well as studies on stress, it appears that mindfulness creates biological embedding over time through the combination of reduced negative emotionality and stress and increased positive states of mind, including development of a greater sense of personal control and purpose. In turn, the consequent decrease in stress-related catabolic activity (e.g., high cortisol) and enhancement of restorative physiology (increased vagal tone, anabolic activity) create a conducive environment to slow cellular aging (Epel et al., 2009). In summary, whereas mind wandering appears to be associated with greater levels of unhappiness and increased biological age, presence, a fundamental component of mindfulness, promotes well-being across biological, psychological, and, as described below, social domains.

Interpersonal Connections and the Biological Embedding of Presence

We know that people with close supportive relationships tend to have better health and longevity, and their related biological mechanisms, such as reduced inflammation, are starting to be elucidated (Fagundes, Bennett, Derry, & Kiecolt-Glaser, 2011). We speculate that these broad relationships may start early in life, based on processes of interpersonal attunement or lack of them. Early experience within supportive social relationships, as well as with social adversity, can shape neural systems and downstream biological functions such as cell aging. For example, emotional neglect and abuse early in life are related to shorter adult telomere length (Kiecolt-Glaser et al., 2011; O'Donovan et al., 2011; Tyrka et al., 2010), whereas social support is associated with longer telomere length (Carroll et al., 2012). Low maternal warmth can affect gene expression, shifting genes to create pro-aging proteins that lead to inflammation (Chen, Miller, Kobor, & Cole, 2011). It appears that early life shaping of the attachment system may influence rate of aging even late in life. The exact mechanisms are unknown but likely include early biological embedding, as well as shaping of stress-responsive systems and attentional states that tend to promote greater wear and tear on physiology throughout life.

Our proposal is that early experience may also shape mindfulness later in life. We speculate that secure attachment and a sense of safety and interpersonal trust may influence the propensity for the development of presence and mindful awareness. Fortunately, it appears that there is plasticity and the ability for even short-term training of mindful awareness to cultivate not only presence but also the enhancement of telomerase (Jacobs et al., 2010). In the next section we elaborate on these proposals as we describe how presence of mind may lead to presence with other people, and how these are fundamental components of healthy, fulfilling relationships.

Presence, Attunement, and Resonance

Presence is especially important in interpersonal attunement, whether within personal relationships or in a clinical setting. The importance of presence is largely in the ability to attend to the most authentic—the least automatic—experience possible. This authenticity of experience requires as much freedom as possible from previously established, "top-down" mental constructs that restrict our ability to be fully present. Top-down processing, in this perspective, is the perceptual, emotional, and cognitive mechanisms learned from the past that filter present experience and lead to restrictions, feelings, and categorizations that constrain how an individual experiences the present moment directly. Opening one's present experience to "bottom-up" processing means taking in present internal and external stimuli and sensing them as directly as possible, with a minimization of top-down filtering from past experience. Bottom-up processing permits us to be receptive to what is happening as it is happening. The receptivity of presence allows us to release these limiting structures that include ingrained emotional responses based on past experience, an inability to hear accurately what someone is saying based on anticipation of what is expected to come, and misinterpretation of emotional signals because of an ongoing internal narrative that distorts and confuses the ability to see clearly. Brown and Cordon (2009) eloquently describe how presence entails a suspension of the habitual, automatic mode of processing in favor of a receptive attentiveness that is focused on processing what occurs moment by moment. They assert that this flexibility of attention enables us to bring a sense of novelty and lucidity to our individual experience.

> In the presence mindful awareness reveals, top-down constraints that filter, distort, limit, and restrict sensation are minimized. . . . It seems that mindful awareness permits us to get as close as we can to clear vision, that there is some kind of "ground of being" or some grounded receptive state, some spaciousness of the mind, that is as free from top-down filter constraints as is humanly possible. (Siegel, 2007a, pp. 161–162)

The work on "grounded cognition" by Barsalou (2008) supports this notion of bottom-up processing.

Imagine an interpersonal interaction in which habit and ingrained emotional expectation could easily collide to leave parties hurt or misunderstood. Picture running into a good friend while walking, but your friend barely acknowledges you as she rushes by with a quick glance. You might understandably have a hurt and indignant reaction, attributing the blow-off to dispositional inferences that your friend must be mad at you, and your hurt continues to transform into anger directed at your friend that is based in rumination and expectation. However, imagine that same interaction, but upon feeling the first *reaction* of hurt you mindfully reflect, able to make a situational attribution to the interaction instead. You remember that your friend is under a great deal of stress due to a potential promotion at work and was likely unintentionally communicating that sense of being overwhelmed and distracted when she saw you, and that none of it is actually due to you. In this second situation, mindfulness enables the potential for a much more interpersonally attuned understanding that allows a more authentic, less automatic or reactive response. In a follow-up interaction with your friend, you gently question her about her current emotional state, as opposed to surprising her with an accusatory follow-up about how she intentionally ignored you.

Presence within interpersonal interactions can be delineated into two elements: what we are *doing* when we are present and what we are *experiencing*. Geller and Greenberg (2002) find that the core processes of *doing* while being present can be defined as engaging in receptivity before inwardly attending—fully aware of the resonance of being fully present with someone—then expressing that inner resonance to the other person. They further define this element of receptivity: "Receptivity demands a conscious intention and commitment to remain open, accepting, and allowing to all of the dimensions and experiences that arise. The allowing quality of receptivity is a distinct process of letting in experience and allowing it to flow through one's self, as opposed to observing experience from an emotional or clinical distance" (p. 78).

Here, the focus on being receptive includes welcoming the experience of the moment to actively "flow through oneself." In this way, being aware of one's inner response to being present with another person can even extend to processes such as interoception, the awareness of one's bodily response to the other person. Thus, one is fully present with the other person in both mind and body. This is how presence involves a connection of the interpersonal, the mental, and the somatic.

The receptivity scenario we have just described is the union of *intra*personal attunement and *inter*personal attunement. In other words, being present with another person while simultaneously being fully present with oneself and one's own experience is the synchrony of attunement and resonance, facilitated by mindful awareness. Internal attunement involves the "COAL" state of being *c*urious, *o*pen, *a*ccepting, and *l*oving in the focus of attention of an observing self on the experiencing self. This is how we can become mindfully aware of our interior world. The very circuitry of being aware of one's own inner life overlaps with that used in being aware of the internal life of another person. As such, the neural circuitry used for intrapersonal awareness when turned outwards has the possibility to facilitate interpersonal awareness. The mechanisms enabling this dual awareness may be seen as creating "maps of intention" that allow us to map the intentions of others, as well as our own intentional states (Siegel, 2007a). If mindfulness is indeed strengthening our ability to map our own intentional states, then we might also be able to do the reverse: to use these intrapersonal awareness circuits strengthened through mindfulness to map the intentional states of others, cultivating receptive forms of interpersonal awareness.

The Neural Circuitry of Intra- and Interpersonal Attunement

A demonstration of the integration or overlap of intrapersonal and interpersonal circuits in the context of presence is the neural contrast between two states of being: a present-focused, experiential state compared to a more elaborative, narrative-constructing state. As briefly noted earlier, Farb and colleagues (2007) distinguish a narrative self from an experiential self. The *narrative self* is the aspect of awareness that monitors enduring traits, often forming an autobiographical narrative around them and constructing the sense of self from the top down. In contrast, the experiential self is the aspect of awareness that is focused on moment-to-moment present experience. In regard to attention, narrative focus has been associated with increased ruminative self-related thoughts, whereas experiential focus "avoids rumination by disengaging attentional processes of self-referential elaboration" (Farb et al., 2007, p. 314). With respect to interpersonal attunement, being able to focus attention away from self-rumination is conducive to being able to devote attention to the experiential self and therefore to one's affective response to the person with whom one is interacting in the present moment. One intriguing idea this raises is the view that the self–other attunement in interpersonal mindfulness is parallel to the attunement of self-as-observing and self-as-experiencing. This is the proposal for how self-empathy and self-compassion are fundamental elements of internal attunement at the heart of mindful awareness. Internal attunement likely harnesses overlapping neural regions with the social circuits of the brain. In this way, the overlap between interpersonal and intrapersonal attunement circuits becomes apparent and we can see how mindful awareness—as a trait or a learned skill—would be associated with enhanced interpersonal skills.

A neural *resonance circuit* that facilitates these interpersonal benefits of mindfulness may be at the heart of the neural correlates of internal and interpersonal attunement (Siegel, 2007a). This resonance circuit enables us to attend to the intentions of ourselves and others and involves both mirror neurons and the superior temporal cortex. Such a circuit plays an important role in the ability to be emotionally resonant with others. Mirror neurons reveal a link between perception and action, and are present in various regions of the brain, including the frontal and parietal cortex (Uddin, Kaplan, Molnar-Szakacs, Zaidel, & Iacoboni, 2004). Activated both while perceiving an action and when preparing to produce that action, mirror neurons may also be involved in empathy and emotional resonance. The striking finding of Iacoboni, Kaplan, and Wilson (2007) is that these mirror neurons indeed engage our very emotional processes: "The observation of your smiling face triggers a cascade of neural activity in my brain, from inferior frontal (mirror) neurons controlling my facial musculature down to anterior insula neurons and to limbic neurons such that I suddenly and deeply feel your happiness. Your happiness is in my body" (p. 317). The process described here involves a series of associations among perceived physical motions, neural activity, and emotional activations.

Mirror neurons in the cortex drive information down to lower limbic levels more intimately associated with emotional processes by way of the insular cortex, or insula. The important communication with the insula then happens, as the brain responds to the information taken in and produces bodily effects, which are then experienced via activity in the insula. The "resonance" occurs as the body then feels the very information it is receiving from others, that is, the internal state of the other person. The resonance circuit is complete as information then travels back up through the insula to the prefrontal cortex and becomes interoceptive information that enables our perception of our internal bodily state. A range of studies has revealed that mindfulness practice is associated with increased insular activity and increased insular size in long-term meditators (Lazar et al., 2005; Luders, Toga, Lepore, & Gaser, 2009).

This resonance circuit—which includes the mirror neurons and the middle aspects of the prefrontal region including the insula—might be seen as the neural hub enabling the interpersonal benefits generated by mindfulness. The prefrontal functions that are part of this circuit, facilitating attunement, are associated with both mindful awareness practices and secure attachment (Siegel, 2007a, 2012a). If attunement were indeed a vital mechanism of both mindfulness and attachment, the prefrontal area's dual association might explain how this resonance circuit could be developed in these two very different ways. We now explore an interpersonal neurobiology view of the similar neural development that occurs through attachment, development, and mindful awareness practices, and how this commonality might be seen as a neural hub between presence and interpersonal attunement. We have seen how mindfulness enables us to have a deep sense of presence. The question now becomes, what is the role of presence in interpersonal relationships?

Defining Relationships

Interpersonal neurobiology provides a foundation upon which to view relationships as the sharing of energy and information (Siegel, 2009, 2012a, 2012b). This sharing of energy and information can arise through diverse modalities, including physical contact, verbal communication, nonverbal exchanges involving facial expression, tone of voice, gestures, postures, eye contact, timing of response between members of a dyad, and even the physical distance between two people. In one recent study, Hasson, Ghazanfar, Galantucci, Garrod, and Keysers (2012) termed this process *brain-to-brain coupling*, for example, "seeing or hearing the actions, sensations or emotions of an agent trigger cortical representations in the perceiver (so-called vicarious activations). If the agent has a similar brain and body, vicarious activations in the perceiver will approximate those of the agent, and the neural responses will become coupled" (p. 115). Hasson and colleagues explain that this happens during verbal, nonverbal, and gestural communication. Similarly, research studying affective information by Anders, Heinzle, Weiskopf, Ethofer, and Haynes (2011) furthers this claim. They state, "Distributed anterior temporal, insular and somato-motor brain regions that have been associated with 'embodied simulation' during affective communication not only show common activity during emotion observation and first-hand emotional experience, but indeed carry emotion-specific information in the sender and perceiver" (p. 444). This mechanism is the way in which the energy shared between a dyad has a direct impact on the neuronal circuits of the members' brains and corresponding states of mind, mental representations, and emotions. Thus, the brain is one of the mechanisms through which energy and information flow.

The human brain is an extremely complex system composed of parts in a hierarchical organization that are integrated into a larger whole, including neurons, groups of neurons connected by synapses, neural circuits, and hemispheres. The human brain comprises over 100 billion neurons, each with an average of 10,000 connections to other neurons, and is a living system that is open, dynamic, and nonlinear. It is *open* in that it is influenced by its environment, dynamic because it is in a constant state of change, and *nonlinear* in that small inputs can have a large effect on the system as a whole. As we have seen, interpersonal relationships have a major impact that can facilitate or inhibit this brain structure and its functioning. An example of one such relationship in which this sharing of energy and information takes place is that between infants and their attachment figures.

Developmental Neurobiology

Development occurs within a psychosocioemotional context because an individual develops in a relational setting, not in isolation. The emotional communication inherent to dyadic relationships at the heart of attachment experiences is the primary force "shapes, for better or worse, the experience-dependent maturation of the brain systems involved in attachment functions that are accessed throughout the life span" (Schore, 2011, p. 502). Emotional communication between infant and parent serves to organize the self not only in the physical sense (brain structure and function) but also in the subjective mental sense (memories, representations, and narratives), which coalesce to create who we are (Siegel, 2012a). In this way, the human brain matures within a context in which interpersonal relationships are vital for proper brain development.

The formative relationship of parent and child is particularly important because it takes place during a period of rapid brain development. Knickmeyer and colleagues (2008) posited the finding relative to early brain development that total brain volume is increased 101% in the first year, with another 15% increase in the second year. This critical time of brain development is directly impacted by the gene–environment interactions, which are controlled by epigenetic mechanisms that determine which genes are expressed or inhibited without changing the DNA sequence. Roth and Sweatt (2011) confirm the importance that caregivers have on epigenetics: "Epigenetic mechanisms, or the chemical markings of the DNA and the surrounding histone proteins that regulate gene activity in the CNS [central nervous system], are modified by experiences, particularly those occurring within the context of caregiving" (p. 398). While the brain is undergoing massive growth, the autonomic nervous system (ANS), which extends out from the brain into the body proper to regulate bodily arousal, is similarly being influenced by the communication patterns between parent and infant. This system comprises two branches with contrasting, yet balancing, functions: the sympathetic (excitatory) and parasympathetic (inhibitory) nervous systems. Early in life, the sympathetic nervous system is dominant, driving exploration, interest/excitement, and enjoyment/joy—in other words, states of arousal. Until the parasympathetic nervous system develops well enough to balance the arousing functions of the sympathetic nervous system, the parent serves as a stand-in parasympathetic nervous system to help regulate the infant (e.g., through soothing and calming). In this way, a parent's attunement to the infant's emotional states has an immense impact on neurodevelopment and self-regulation. Dyadic regulation during the early years is imprinted on the growing nervous system, enabling more autonomous forms of self-regulation (Dutra, Ilaria, Siegel, & Lyons-Ruth, 2009). The specific biological basis for this imprinting is apparent in part in the regulation of the vagus nerve, according to the polyvagal theory (Porges & Furman, 2011). Through positive social interactions, there is greater development of the myelinated ventral branch of the vagus nerve, which serves to promote positive social engagement and a receptive state of mind. In contrast, social neglect leads to an impaired ability of this aspect of the vagus nerve to function, leading to a poor vagal brake on the sympathetic nervous system and therefore exaggerated reactivity and less ability for social engagement. The myelinated vagus is also directly connected to motor neuron areas and indirectly to areas of the prefrontal cortex. The vagal system therefore appears to be a key player in facilitating interpersonal attunement, especially under states of challenge. It is the receptive ventral vagal state that activates the "social engagement system" that may be turned on within a state of mindful awareness, much like a "self-engagement system" that promotes receptivity to the inner life of the self, as well as openness to the internal life of others (Porges, 2011a; Siegel, 2007a).

Attachment Theory

Attachment is an inborn motivational system that influences infants to establish relationships with significant attachment figures. The attachment system shapes the organization of emotional and memory processes by the ways in which relational transactions between infant and parent influence the unfolding of neural circuits that regulate emotion, attention, and action. In this dyadic relationship, the parent serves to promote positive emotional experience, while minimizing negative states of arousal. These patterns of interaction form the attachment relationship that shapes how the infant's brain will be influenced by the functions of the parent's brain. Repeated patterns of communication become engrained in the infant, creating mental models or what Bowlby termed a "secure base" (Bowlby, 1969, 1988). Siegel (2012a) furthers this notion, stating, "Studies of attachment have revealed that the patterning or organization of attachment relationships during infancy is associated with characteristic processes of emotional regulation, social relatedness, access to autobiographical memory, and the development of self-reflection and narrative" (p. 91). Siegel continues: "Childhood patterns in the transfer of energy and information between minds can create organized strategies in relationships. These are revealed within characteristic behavioral responses in attachment-related situations" (p. 308). These patterns of relating are so pervasive that researchers have classified the communication patterns of infant-parent interaction into four categories with subsequent developmental outcomes. Sroufe and Siegel (2011) explain the long-term impact of attachment status throughout the lifetime: "In general, attachment predicted engagement in the preschool peer group, the capacity for close friendships in middle childhood, the ability to coordinate friendships and group functioning in adolescence, and the capacity to form trusting, non-hostile romantic relationships in adulthood" (p. 37). In this way, adaptations to early relationships affect our neurodevelopment, behavior, affective styles, susceptibility to psychopathology and health-related disorders, and the ways in which we respond in interpersonal relationships.

While attachment status confers a degree of resilience or risk, relationships continually impact development throughout the lifespan. For this reason, the attachment system is malleable, enabling the internal working model of attachment to change during childhood, adolescence, and adulthood. In fact, research has shown that in a subset of secure attachment called earned–secure, individuals alter their attachment status by creating a coherent narrative of their childhood experience (Siegel & Hartzell, 2003). With either continuous secure or earned–secure attachment status, one is better equipped to attune with others. In a previously mentioned preliminary study, DiNoble (2009) found that mindfulness traits in parents are associated with security in adult measures of attachment. Secure attachment is associated with attunement between parent and child, and with parents who have come to make sense of their own lives. Such a sense-making process may involve a form of self-attunement, possibly brought about through self-reflection, similar in nature to mindfulness practices.

Mindfulness, Secure Attachment, and the Middle Prefrontal Cortex

Earlier we explored the topic of how mindfulness and secure attachment can be seen to go hand in hand, along with the role that presence plays in this association. Secure attachment and mindfulness studies have a remarkable convergence in outcome measures (Kabat-Zinn, 2003; Stroufe, Egeland, Carlson, & Collins, 2005), and both are associated with functions of the middle aspects of the prefrontal cortex (Siegel, 2007a). This region of the brain remains plastic even into adulthood, corresponding with the notion in attachment theory and research that people can change their attachment classification across the lifespan, and the findings from mindfulness practice that training the mind can change the structure and function of the brain (Davidson & Begley, 2012). The prefrontal cortex is integrative, connecting widely distributed areas of the nervous system together as it links cortical, limbic, brainstem, and bodily neural signals with the neural input of the social world of other people. These are distinct, differentiated areas that are linked together into one functional whole, the essence of what we mean by "integration." Prefrontal cortex functionality includes bodily regulation, emotional balance, fear modulation, interpersonal attunement, response flexibility, insight, empathy, morality, and intuition. The first eight of these nine functions have been shown to be outcomes of secure parent–child attachment (intuition has not yet been explored); all nine of these functions are outcomes of mindfulness training (Siegel, 2007a). Our suggestion is that at the neural heart of both mindfulness and secure attachment are the integrative functions of the nervous system, especially these prefrontal regions central to self-regulation and interpersonal behavior.

Mindfulness, Positive Relationships, and Presence

While research on the effects of mindfulness within the context of relationships is relatively sparse, a few studies support the beneficial effects of mindfulness on relationships. Carson, Carson, Gil, and Baucom (2004) conducted a randomized waitlist controlled design of mindfulness-based relationship enhancement to investigate the potential beneficial effects of mindfulness within the context of happy couples. Participants reported a positive impact on satisfaction, relaxation, autonomy, spirituality, relationship, closeness, acceptance of their partner, and psychological and relationship distress. In addition, there were "significant improvements in day-to-day relationship happiness, relationship stress, stress coping efficacy, and overall stress" (p. 489). A dose–response relationship was also found between the amount of time participants spent on mindfulness exercises and the positive benefits that resulted from the practice. Interestingly, these positive effects were reported at 3-month follow-up, indicating a lasting positive effect.

Barnes, Brown, Krusemark, Cambell, and Rogge (2007) examined the connection between mindfulness traits and relationship satisfaction. They found that higher levels of trait mindfulness predicted higher relationship satisfaction, along with an increased ability to respond constructively and flexibly to friction in relationships. Mindfulness traits were correlated with lower stress in emotional responses, while mindfulness states were associated with improved quality of communication. In a similar study, Jones, Welton, Oliver, and Thoburn (2011) examined the relationships among mindfulness, spousal attachment, and marital satisfaction. They proposed that the status of spousal attachment might be the mediating mechanism of the relationship between trait mindfulness and marital satisfaction. There was a significant relationship between trait mindfulness and relationship satisfaction. They proposed that the practice of mindfulness might improve interpersonal attunement, which might increase satisfaction with one's relationship. According to these studies, mindfulness demonstrates a positive role in promoting relationship well-being and satisfaction.

Why would mindfulness and secure attachment seem to go hand in hand? Our proposal is that presence is the key mechanism at the heart of both the internal attunement of mindfulness and the interpersonal attunement of healthy, supportive relationships. Presence permits an individual to be receptive to what is emerging, moment by moment, both within and between attunement. In many ways, within- and between-attunement each reflect a form of integration that the field of interpersonal neurobiology views as a common mechanism underlying well-being. Integration is the linkage of differentiated parts of a system. For mindfulness, integration would entail honoring differences between the differentiated streams of the observing self and the experiencing self, and their linkage within mindful awareness; interpersonal attunement involves honoring differences between two individuals and the compassionate, caring communication that links them to one another. Secure attachment also provides a state of safety that down-regulates vigilance and a propensity to screen ongoing experience through the lens of top-down protective perceptual filters. This sense of safety, along with the activation of the social engagement system (Porges, 2011b), may enable the cultivation of presence. In these ways, presence may emerge with the internal and interpersonal state of safety and receptivity, supporting a decrease in stress and enhancing physiological well-being.

The Social Embedding of Presence

Energy and information flow can be seen as the fundamental essence of the system that comprises our self-experience. Within our inner somatic lives, we can view energy and information flow as riding along waves of neural firing patterns that are the embodied mechanism we can call the *embodied brain* or simply, *brain*. When we enable our observing circuits to honor the differentiated unfolding of our experiencing self without constraining this flow by prior expectations and judgments, we call this the presence at the heart of being mindful. This is an internal form of integration. How energy and information flow is shared between two people, or among one and several other people, is how we define a relationship. When this sharing is integrated, that is, when people are honored for their differences and compassionate communication links them, relationships thrive. In the brain itself, we can see that both internal and interpersonal forms of integration stimulate the neuronal activation and growth of integrative regions of the brain. Healthy relationships between child and parent are associated with integrative functioning (Teicher, 2002). Healthy relationships that one cultivates with oneself—for example, becoming one's own best friend within mindfulness practice—are associated with the growth of integrative fibers of the brain as well (Lazar et al., 2005; Luders et al., 2009).

The framework of interpersonal neurobiology offers the suggestion that beyond awareness and subjective experience, the mind can be seen as an emergent, self-organizing process that arises from energy and information flow patterns within both the nervous system distributed throughout the whole body (the "embodied brain") *and* our relationships with others. We are both embodied and embedded in a social network. As a self-organizing dimension of our lives, one aspect of the *mind* can be defined as "an embodied and relational process that regulates energy and information flow" (Siegel, 2010, 2012a, p. 2). The key is that *mind*—rarely defined in academic fields (Siegel, 2012b)—can be seen to both arise from and regulate energy and information flow that passes within the body and between ourselves and others within relationships. Two other foundational aspects of mind also related to presence, consciousness and subjective experience, may also be fundamentally influenced by both the embodied and relational nature of our mental life.

When we have presence in our lives, when we have the mental state of presence in our awareness, we invite a fundamental process of integration. From an interpersonal neurobiology point of view, integration is the heart of health. In this way, presence cultivates health internally and interpersonally. This state of mind—presence and mindful awareness—is therefore at the heart of resilience and healthy living.

Presence: The Hub of Integration from Me to We

Presence cultivates *integration*, the state of linking differentiated elements of a system that has the subjective feeling of harmony. When we are not present, when we are not moving toward integration, we may get stuck in states of chaos, rigidity, or both. Integration creates a relational experience of vitality and connection. *Mindsight* is a term (Siegel, 2012a) used to highlight this capacity to perceive the inner life of the mind of self and other, and move that energy and information flow toward integration. Mindsight skills cultivate the capacity for presence within an individual and between the individual and others. As the mechanism beneath emotional and social intelligence (Siegel, 2010), mindsight can be seen as the ways in which presence for oneself and presence for others in relationship with the self emerges in the moment-to-moment life experiences as they unfold. Cultivating integration, as with the origins of the mind itself, arises from both within us and between us, highlighting how presence is both an internal and an interpersonal process. Integration enables us to live life—internally and interpersonally—with flexibility, adaptability, coherence, energy, and stability. At the core of integration is presence. It is for this reason we can propose that one sees presence of mind associated with well-being in such widely distributed domains of life as telomeres and cellular health, and emotional closeness and resilient family functioning. Presence both emerges from and cultivates integration. This recursive quality of the system that is who we are as embodied and socially embedded beings reveals how mindfulness is naturally both an internal and interpersonal form of integration. Presence is fundamental to not only developing enhanced well-being but also promoting resiliency to stress. These ideas suggest that bringing more presence into people's lives may be a crucial goal for interventions at the individual, family, educational, and larger societal levels. There is now a broad empirical basis that demonstrates the damaging effects of stress, and in particular, the type of early life stress that impairs attachment and the development of presence, and cell health, described here. There is therefore a desperate need for "societal stress reduction" (Blackburn & Epel, 2012). Developing presence is both a critical path to and outcome of societal stress reduction. With these scientific foundations emerging from empirical research, the path is clear for a movement to bring presence into our larger culture as a means to create healthier individuals, healthier relationships, and a healthier world.

REFERENCES

Anders, S., Heinzle, J., Weiskopf, N., Ethofer, T., & Haynes, J. D. (2011). Flow of affective information between communicating brains. *NeuroImage, 54*(1), 439–446.

Baer, R., Smith, G., Hopkins, J., Krietemeyer, J., & Toney, L. (2006). Using self-report assessment methods to exploring facets of mindfulness. *Assessment, 13*(1), 27–45.

Barnes, S., Brown, K. W., Krusemark, E., Campbell, W. K., & Rogge, R. D. (2007). The role of mindfulness in romantic relationship satisfaction and responses to relationship stress. *Journal of Marital and Family Therapy, 33*(4), 482–500.

Barsalou, L. (2008). Grounded cognition. *Annual Review of Psychology, 59*, 617–645.

Blackburn E. H., & Epel, E. S. (2012). Telomeres and adversity: Too toxic to ignore. *Nature, 490*, 169–171.

Bowlby, J. (1969). *Attachment and loss: Vol. 1. Attachment.* New York: Basic Books.

Bowlby, J. (1988). *A secure base: Parent–child attachment and healthy human development.* New York: Basic Books.

Brown, K. W., & Cordon, S. L. (2009). Toward a phenomenology of mindfulness: Subjective experience and emotional correlates. In F. Didonna (Ed.), *Clinical handbook of mindfulness* (pp. 59–81). New York: Springer.

Carroll, J. E., Diez Roux, A. V., Fitzpatrick, A., & Seeman, T. (2012). *Emotional social support is positively associated with late life telomere length: The Multi-Ethnic Study of Atherosclerosis.* Paper presented at the 70th annual meeting of the American Psychosomatic Society, Athens, Greece.

Carson, J. W., Carson, K. M., Gil, K., & Baucom, D. H. (2004). Mindfulness-based relationship enhancement. *Behavior Therapy, 35*(3), 471–494.

Chen, E., Miller, G. E., Kobor, M. S., & Cole, S. W. (2011). Maternal warmth buffers the effects of low early-life socioeconomic status on pro-inflammatory signaling in adulthood. *Molecular Psychiatry, 16*(7), 729–737.

Csikszentmihalyi, M. (2008). *Flow: The psychology of optimal experience.* New York: HarperCollins.

Davidson, R. J., & Begley, S. (2012). *The emotional life of your brain: How its unique patterns affect the way you think, feel, and live—and how you can change them.* New York: Penguin Group/Hudson Street Press.

DiNoble, A. (2009). *Examining the relationship between adult attachment style and mindfulness traits.* Unpublished doctoral dissertation, California Graduate Institute of the Chicago School of Professional Psychology, Los Angeles.

Dutra, L., Ilaria, B., Siegel, D. J., & Lyons-Ruth, K. (2009). The relational context of dissociative phenomena. In P. F. Dell & J. A. O'Neil (Eds.), *Dissociation and the dissociative disorders, DSM-V and beyond* (pp. 83–92). New York: Routledge.

Epel, E., Daubenmier, J., Moskowitz, J. T., Folkman, S., & Blackburn, E. (2009). Can meditation slow rate of cellular aging?: Cognitive stress, mindfulness, and telomeres. *Annals of the New York Academy of Sciences, 1172*, 34–53.

Epel, E., Puterman, E., Lin, J., Blackburn, E., Lazaro, A., & Mendes, W. (2012). Wandering minds and aging cells. *Clinical Psychological Science, 1*(1), 75–83.

Epel, E. S., Blackburn, E. H., Lin, J., Dhabhar, F. S., Adler, N. E., Morrow, J. D., et al. (2004). Accelerated telomere shortening in response to life stress. *Proceedings of the National Academy of Sciences, 101*, 17312–17315.

Fagundes, C. P., Bennett, J. M., Derry, H. M., & Kiecolt-Glaser, J. K. (2011). Relationships and inflammation across the lifespan: Social developmental pathways to disease. *Social and Personality Psychology Compass, 5*(11), 891–903.

Farb, N. A. S., Segal, Z. V., Mayberg, H., Bean, J., McKeon, D., Fatima, Z., et al. (2007). Attending to the present: Mindfulness meditation reveals distinct neural modes of self-reference. *Social Cognitive and Affective Neuroscience, 2*(4), 313–322.

Geller, S. M., & Greenberg, L. S. (2002). Therapeutic presence: Therapists' experience of presence in the psychotherapy encounter. *Person-Centered and Experiential Psychotherapies, 1*(1–2), 71–86.

Hasenkamp, W., Wilson-Mendenhall, C., Duncan, E., & Barsalou, L. (2012). Mind wandering and attention during focused meditation: A fine-grained temporal analysis of fluctuating cognitive states. *NeuroImage, 59*, 750–760.

Hasson, U., Ghazanfar, A. A., Galantucci, B., Garrod, S., & Keysers, C. (2012). Brain-to-brain coupling: A mechanism for creating and sharing a social world. *Trends in Cognitive Sciences, 16*(2), 114–121.

Iacoboni, M., Kaplan, J., & Wilson, S. (2007). A neural architecture for imitation and intentional relations. In C. L. Nehaniv & K. Dautenhahn (Eds.), *Imitation and social learning in robots, humans and animals: Behavioural, social and communicative dimensions* (pp. 71–87). New York: Cambridge University Press.

Jacobs, T. L., Epel, E. S., Lin, J., Blackburn, E. H., Wolkowitz, O. M., Bridwell, D. A., et al. (2010). Intensive meditation training, immune cell telomerase activity, and psychological mediators. *Psychoneuroendocrinology, 36*(5), 664–681.

Jacobs, T. L., Shaver, P. R., Epel, E. S., Zanesco, A. P., Aichele, S. A., Bridwell, D. A., et al. (2013). Self-reported mindfulness and cortisol dynamics during a Shamatha meditation retreat. *Health Psychology, 32*(10), 1104–1109.

Jones, K. C., Welton, S. R., Oliver, T. C., & Thoburn, J. W. (2011). Mindfulness, spousal attachment, and marital satisfaction: A mediated model. *Family Journal, 19*(4), 357–361.

Kabat-Zinn, J. (2003). Mindfulness-based interventions in context: Past, present, and future. *Clinical Psychology: Science and Practice, 10*(2), 144–156.

Kane, M. J., Brown, L. H., McVay, J. C., Silvia, P. J., Myin-Germeys, I., & Kwapil, T. R. (2007). For whom the mind wanders, and when. *Psychological Science, 18*(7), 614–621.

Kiecolt-Glaser, J. K., Gouin, J. P., Weng, N. P., Malarkey, W. B., Beversdorf, D. Q., & Glaser, R. (2011). Childhood adversity heightens the impact of later-life caregiving stress on telomere length and inflammation. *Psychosomatic Medicine, 73*(1), 16–22.

Killingsworth, M. A., & Gilbert, D. T. (2010). A wandering mind is an unhappy mind. *Science, 330*, 932–932.

Knickmeyer, R. C., Gouttard, S., Kang, C., Evans, D., Wilber, K., Smith, J. K., et al. (2008). A structural MRI study of human brain development from birth to 2 years. *Journal of Neuroscience, 28*, 12176–12182.

Lazar, S. W., Kerr, C. E., Wasserman, R. H., Gray, J. R., Greve, D. N., Treadway, M. T., et al. (2005). Meditation experience is associated with increased cortical thickness. *NeuroReport, 16*, 1893–1897.

Luders, E., Toga, A. W., Lepore, N. & Gaser, C. (2009). The underlying anatomical correlates of long-term meditation: Larger hippocampal and frontal volumes of gray matter. *NeuroImage, 45*, 672–678.

Mrazek, M. D., Smallwood, J., & Schooler, J. W. (2012). Mindfulness and mind-wandering: Finding convergence through opposing constructs. *Emotion, 12*(3), 442–448.

O'Donovan, A., Epel, E., Lin, J., Wolkowitz, O., Cohen, B., Maquen, S., et al. (2011). Childhood trauma associated with short leukocyte telomere length in posttramatic stress disorder. *Biological Psychiatry, 70*(5), 465–471.

Phelan, J. P. (2010). Mindfulness as presence. *Mindfulness, 1*(2), 131–134.

Porges, S. W. (2011a, March). *Mindfulness and the polyvagal theory*. Paper presented at the Interpersonal Neurobiology Annual UCLA Conference, Los Angeles.

Porges, S. W. (2011b). *The polyvagal theory*. New York: Norton.

Porges, S. W., & Furman, S. A. (2011). The early development of the automatic nervous system provides a neural platform for social behavior: A polyvagal perspective. *Infant and Child Development, 20*(1), 106–118.

Roth, T. L., & Sweatt, J. D. (2011). Annual Research Review: Epigenetic mechanisms and environmental shaping of the brain during sensitive periods of development. *Journal of Child Psychology and Psychiatry and Allied Disciplines, 52*(4), 398–408.

Sayette, M., Reichle, E., & Schooler, J. (2009). Lost in the sauce: The effects of alcohol on mind wandering. *Psychological Science, 20,* 747–752.

Schore, A. (2011). Family law and the neuroscience of attachment, Part I. *Family Court Review, 49*(3), 501–512.

Siegel, D. J. (2007a). *The mindful brain: Reflection and attunement in the cultivation of well-being*. New York: Norton.

Siegel, D. J. (2007b). Mindfulness training and neural integration. *Journal of Social, Cognitive, and Affective Neuroscience, 2*(4), 259–263.

Siegel, D. J. (2009). Mindful awareness, mindsight, and neural integration. *Humanistic Psychologist, 37*(2), 137–158.

Siegel, D. J. (2010). *Mindsight: The new science of personal transformation*. New York: Bantam.

Siegel, D. J. (2012a). *The developing mind: How relationships and the brain interact to shape who we are* (2nd ed.). New York: Guilford Press.

Siegel, D. J. (2012b). *Pocket guide to interpersonal neurobiology: An integrative handbook of the mind*. New York: Norton.

Siegel, D. J., & Hartzell, M. (2003). *Parenting from the inside out: How a deeper self-understanding can help you raise children who thrive*. New York: Tarcher.

Smallwood, J., & O'Connor, R. C. (2011). Imprisoned by the past: Unhappy moods lead to a retrospective bias to mind wandering. *Cognition and Emotion, 25*(8), 1481–1490.

Sroufe, A., & Siegel, D. J. (2011, March–April). The verdict is in: The case for attachment theory. *Psychotherapy Networker*, pp. 34–39, 52–53.

Sroufe, L. A., Egeland, B., Carlson, E. A., & Collins, W. A. (2005). *The development of the person: The Minnesota study of risk and adaptation from birth to adulthood*. New York: Guilford Press.

Teicher, M. (2002). The neurobiology of child abuse. *Scientific American, 286*(3), 68–75.

Tierney, J. (2010, June 28). Discovering the virtues of a wandering mind. *New York Times*, p. D1.

Tyrka, A. R., Price, L. H., Kao, H.-T., Porton, B., Marsella, S. A., & Carpenter, L. L. (2010). Childhood maltreatment and telomere shortening: Preliminary support for an effect of early stress on cellular aging. *Biological Psychiatry, 67*(6), 531–534.

Uddin, L. Q., Kaplan, J. T., Molnar-Szakacs, I., Zaidel, E., & Iacoboni, M. (2004). Self-face recognition activates a frontoparietal "mirror" network in the right hemisphere: An event-related fMRI study. *NeuroImage, 25,* 926–935.

CHAPTER 14

Did the Buddha Have a Self?

No-Self, Self, and Mindfulness in Buddhist Thought and Western Psychologies

Richard M. Ryan and C. Scott Rigby

As the concept and practice of mindfulness has penetrated Western psychology and medicine, it has interfaced with conceptions and philosophies distinct from the Buddhist traditions from which it originally sprang. Among the most discussed and important topics at this interface is how mindfulness, both conceptually and in practice, relates to concepts and processes of *self*. The discussion is in part provoked by the contrast between Buddhist perspectives on mindfulness, which are famously founded on an idea of *no-self*, and Western psychological theories in which the self represents a central construct.

Most discussions of no-self versus self focus on their opposing implications. Yet the ways in which these perspectives on self connect with each other, and with mindfulness, is a complex issue concerning more than mere oppositions. The no-self doctrines of Buddhism clearly reject certain definitions of self but not others. Buddhist traditions also imply certain process views of integrated functioning that share similarities with some Western formulations of healthy self-regulation. For example, mindfulness practices have been empirically demonstrated to foster and support experiences of autonomy and other psychological attributes associated with more integrated self-functioning (Brown, Ryan, & Creswell, 2007).

In this chapter we examine this complex interface between mindfulness and varied conceptions of self, both Buddhist and Western. To do so we first recognize and define mindfulness not as a philosophy or a theory, but rather as a phenomenon. *Mindfulness* is the open and receptive awareness of what is occurring in the present moment (Bhikkhu Bodhi, 2011; Brown & Ryan, 2003). It is bare perception, in the sense that in being mindful, one attends to the bare facts of what is occurring, without habitual reacting, rebuking, or resolving (Nyaniponika Thera, 1972; see Gethin, Chapter 2, this volume). Within Buddhist frameworks, mindfulness is often described as observing without "grasping" or "clinging" to what unfolds—not burdening it with evaluation but simply being aware of what occurs.

As a fundamental human capacity, mindfulness does not inherently belong to or refer to any particular notion of self or philosophical perspective. That is, mindfulness has no ideological axes to grind, nor does it "belong" to any one school of philosophical thought. As such, mindfulness can be considered in its relations with both Buddhist conceptions of self and those prominent in Western psychology. Over many centuries, traditions within Buddhist thought have applied mindfulness in illuminating and refining a doctrine of *no-self*, which concerns the composite, impermanent, and illusory nature of the self (Collins, 1992; Hanh, 1998). Given this rich history, we turn first to Buddhist concepts of no-self (*anatta*) and *rigpa* (non–dual awareness), exploring both whether and how they might shed light on mindfulness, and its ameliorative effects on well-being.

Following this, we turn to the two major traditions of understanding self within Western psychological traditions. The first is the *me-self*, or *self-as-object* (e.g., James, 1890) that lies at the core of constructivist and social-cognitive views of development and personality (Harter, 2012; McAdams, 1990). The me-self concerns the conceptions, images, roles, statuses, and attributes associated with an identity. Western conceptions of the me-self parallel the depictions of self that are clearly rejected as delusional in Buddhist discourse, in which clinging to the me-self and identifying with self-conceptions leads to suffering (Sogyal, 2002). We therefore highlight some of the relations of no-self and me-self, and their implications for mindfulness and psychological wellness.

The second Western conception of self we consider is the *I-self*, or *self-as-process*, that is represented in a number of post-Kantian philosophies (Atkins, 2005; Organ, 1988) and prominently within organismic theories of personality development (e.g., Loevinger & Blasi, 1991; Ryan, 1995). Self-as-process concerns the inherent integrative tendencies of people to understand, grow, and create coherence in their experiences. Whereas regulation by the me-self is often associated with externally controlled behaviors, integrated "I" regulation is manifest in behaviors that are more fully self-endorsed and wholehearted, tending to be both higher quality and more positively experienced (Ryan, Legate, Niemiec, & Deci, 2012). Interestingly, there is considerable evidence that mindfulness facilitates more autonomous and integrated regulation, which are the hallmarks of healthy self-as-process functioning. Thus, an important question is how the sense of integrated, "true self" regulation as embodied in this concept of self-as-process can be reconciled with the "no-self" of Buddhist discourse, since both are seen to be promoted by mindfulness and positively related to well-being.

In what follows we review each of these three conceptions of self (i.e., no-self, self-as-object, and self-as-process) and how they relate to mindfulness. Although our task is primarily conceptual, an ever-growing body of empirical findings have a bearing on these matters. For instance, mindfulness has been measured in relation to many self-related attributes (e.g., Brown & Ryan, 2003). We use such findings to help clarify how concepts of self can have distinct relations with mindfulness.

On Mindfulness

Mindfulness is in one sense the simplest of human psychological phenomena, yet it is also nuanced, both as a concept and in practice. Mindfulness, first and foremost, concerns awareness (Bhikkhu Bodhi, 2011), but it is not just any awareness. As phenomenologists since Husserl (1931) have established, awareness of events and moments can occur in many different ways. Mindfulness is a quite specific way of being aware: It is an open and receptive awareness of what is occurring in the present (Brown & Ryan, 2003). When mindful, one is fully but impartially present for what is occurring; there is no judgment, investment, or antipathy for what appears. Stripped of the evaluations and judgments that often accompany other states of awareness, whatever arises is accepted without elaboration or reaction. Awareness is employed "equanimously" (Chambers, Lo, & Allen, 2008).

Because mindfulness is open and receptive, unburdened by filtering or censoring via judgments or social concerns, it is associated with a deeper awareness of the present moment and all that is occurring. Accordingly, people higher in mindfulness should be less "unconscious" or out of touch with internal feelings, attitudes, or prejudices. Brown and Ryan (2003) demonstrated that when people's explicit (self-report) and implicit (Implicit Association Test–measured) emotional states were assessed, overall, there was not a reliable association between them. Yet people high in mindfulness showed substantial congruence; their explicit reports of current feelings were positively associated with implicit measures of affect, providing evidence that mindfulness facilitates more integrated awareness of what is occurring (see also O'Loughlin & Zuckerman, 2008).

As a further conceptual nuance, mindfulness is both an individual difference (Baer, Walsh & Lykins, 2009; Brown & Ryan, 2003), and an internal state that varies. Using diary methods in which adults were paged multiple times a day, Brown and Ryan (2007) describe considerable variation in mindfulness at a within-person level, suggesting that people can be more or less present for, and nonavoidant of, what is occurring as a function of state-level factors. Clearly too, mindfulness can be cultivated as an individual attribute, which is why it is a promising point of leverage for efforts at both personal growth and clinical interventions (Brown et al., 2007; Segal, Williams, & Teasdale, 2002).

Rigpa ("Non-Dual Awareness") and *Anatta* ("No-Self")

Buddhism contains a rich and complex cannon of philosophical writings on the nature of the self and mindfulness. For instance, within the Nyingma school of Tibetan Buddhism, nine paths of various teachings are recognized, with the Dzogchen tradition focusing strongly on recognizing the true nature of mind and self. Discussions of concepts such as awareness, mindfulness, and self are common in the tradition (e.g., Gyatso, 2000).

A key aspect of these teachings is distinguishing between "reality" at both an absolute and a relative level. The *relative level* refers to what we experience through the senses—the warm breeze as it blows through the window, the hot cup of tea nearby, this page of this book. At the relative level, it would be inaccurate to deny that these experiences exist because, quite simply, they are here. You are reading this. In fact, they are often vivid and shared in common with other perceivers. The self we conceptualize and think about—our notion of "me"—can likewise fall into this category of perceptions, as we see ourselves engaging in particular roles and relations with others.

In Buddhism, the *absolute level* of reality is concerned with how things are in their true nature, and not simply how they appear at the relative level. Here, several qualities are emphasized. The first is the "empty essence" or impermanence of things. Everything that arises and exists at the relative level changes and recedes as other phenomena arise—like waves on the ocean (Sogyal, 2002). Fundamentally, things can be said to be simply like illusions or images in a dream—appearing, but not "real." It is in this spirit that Buddhism discusses concepts such as *anatta* or "no-self," because, as with all phenomena, there is no permanence to the self or the identities and self-conceptions one experiences. As with all phenomena, the self we conceptualize will not only one day cease to exist, but in fact is also constantly shifting moment to moment as thoughts, feelings, and sensations arise and pass away. We are happy one moment and disgruntled the next. We identify strongly today with one philosophy, only to find ourselves discarding it as "not me" a year later. In this way, although our experiences of both our own selves and the world around us may seem quite solid at the moment, much like a vivid dream that feels real as it is experienced, upon awakening, we realize that its solidity was in fact illusory. One quote from the *Bhadrahalpa Sutra* that integrates the ideas of relative and absolute states simply: "I manifested in a dreamlike way to dreamlike beings and gave a dreamlike Dharma, but in reality I never taught and never actually came." A second quality that is present at the absolute level is that of our *cognizant nature*, which is described as a knowing awareness that is spontaneously present and free from conceptualization and dualistic thinking (Gyatso, 2000). Thoughts and conceptualizations may be energized by cognizant nature, but they are not synonymous with it.

The term *rigpa* is used within the Dzogchen tradition of Buddhism to describe nondualistic awareness: being aware of experiences at the relative level, while simultaneously recognizing the absolute reality of phenomena (Gyatso, 2000). The Dzogchen tradition describes how the qualities of emptiness and cognizance create a "possibility space" for phenomena to arise, change, and recede. One Buddhist metaphor states that if our relative experiences are the images shown on a movie screen, our absolute nature is the bulb behind them: It shines forth and makes images possible, but it is fully impartial and uninvolved with those appearances (Sogyal, 2002).

In Dzogchen Buddhism, therefore, there is no inherent problem with fully experiencing the senses, thoughts, and emotions of relative reality, including self-reflections that naturally arise moment to moment. These transient events emerge within the relative level: We feel happy, frustrated, cold, anxious, or any number of things simultaneously. But in *rigpa*, one simultaneously recognizes that all of these "risings" are fundamentally impermanent: The "knowing" quality of our cognizant nature is merely expressing itself moment to moment, but by also seeing the empty essence of all phenomena at an absolute level, we are allowed the freedom simply to have these experiences without "grasping" or fixating on them as solid and unchanging. In this view, unhappiness begins only when we lose sight of this true nature and mistake the relative experience as being solid or permanent in some way. This understanding is similarly captured in this quote from the Zen tradition, depicting Chi-tsang's "two-fold truth at three levels" and the transcendence of duality (cf. Organ, 1988, p. 41):

- *Level 1:* Before I studied Zen for 30 years, I saw mountains as mountains, waters as waters.
- *Level 2:* When I arrived at more intimate knowledge, I came to the point where I saw that mountains are not mountains, and waters are not waters.
- *Level 3:* But now that I have got its very substance I am at rest. For it is just that I see mountains once again as mountains and waters once again as waters.

Here, Level 1 describes being "caught up" in the relative level alone, seeing phenomena as permanent. Level 2 represents a realization that the absolute nature of even the most "solid" of phenomena is impermanent, which in turn empowers a peaceful freedom (Level 3) simply to experience phenomena in the moment—to have the non–dual awareness of both the absolute and the relative that enables experience without the burden of grasping.

It is in this context of distinguishing between relative and absolute reality that we can understand the relationship between the Theravāda Buddhist concepts of self (*atta*) and no-self (*anatta*), and integrate these more fully with Western conceptualizations of the self and mindfulness. A core tenet of the Buddha's teachings is that although we experience a self at the relative level, no self actually exists at the absolute level. Subsequently, attachments to these concepts as being "real" are a cause of suffering. By contrast, the doctrine of *anatta*, often translated as "no-self," appears throughout Buddhist teachings (Collins, 1992; Hanh, 1998; Pfeil, 2000) and describes an understanding that, at an absolute level, there is no permanent or enduring self; like all phenomena, every aspect of who we "are" at a relative level is impermanent and ever-changing. Thus, even as we can reflect on our "self" at the relative level, at an absolute level, this concept of self refers to something ultimately nonexistent.

Understanding and remaining mindful of both the relative and absolute nature of self—as opposed to only maintaining awareness at a relative level—leads to a significantly different framing of experiences. When anger arises, holding an awareness of "no-self" (*anatta*) will lead to a recognition that "there is anger," but not grasping onto the emotion, as in "I am angry." Similarly, in mindfulness, "I am depressed" could become instead "I am aware of sadness and self-critical thoughts." The self-referent nature of the former statement presupposes a concrete thinker or self that is afflicted by the thoughts or experiences. This is so despite the fact that when we look for a thinker behind our thoughts, we find only another thought (Epstein, 2007).

In this respect, the Buddhist philosophy of no-self resonates with the work of Husserl, Heidegger, Merleau-Ponty and other Western phenomenologists who emphasized the fluidity of experience and the phenomenal absence of any concrete self. It is also echoed in the Gestalt approach (Perls, Hefferline & Goodman, 1958), in which the self is not perceived as a direct object of consciousness but as spontaneously arising at the *contact boundary*, an emergent, fluid, and changing point. For Perls and colleagues (1958), and later, cognitive theorists Varela, Thompson, and Rosch (1991), such contact arises in a "the middle mode," arising neither from the self nor the environment. This is only to highlight the rich convergences between Western phenomenological traditions and Buddhist observations regarding no-self and non-dual awareness (*rigpa*).

Buddhist philosophers point out that remaining aware of the absolute understanding of no-self is not nihilistic because relative reality is also respected (e.g., Lingpa, 1994). At the relative level, there is undeniably a functioning person, transacting with the world, having experiences through thought and the senses, and motivated to plan and to organize actions. Rather than negating this, the absolute understanding and awareness of the "dream-like" nature of the self creates an openness to experience and an equanimity even in the face of the constant change that occurs around us. Put differently, understanding that there is no self with which to be preoccupied frees us up to experience fully and relate to the world around us. Thus, paradoxically, Buddhist philosophy suggests that holding an awareness of no-self results in an increase in experiences of stability, peace, and confidence. Presumably, in fact, mindfulness fully practiced will lead one along the "middle way" (Hanh, 1998). Here an important distinction between mindfulness and self is apparent: Mindfulness is not synonymous with the "I-self"; rather, it describes a quality of awareness that potentiates or creates the fertile conditions for more integrated self-regulation. This occurs specifically because mindful states are free from the noise of the ego involvements and judgments that can lead to a walling off of emotions and experiences (through defensiveness and evaluations), thus suppressing an open, creative synthesis or integration of what is occurring.

Mindfulness Meditation and the No-Self

No-self is a doctrine, but it also relates directly to specific experiences in meditation and mindfulness practices. Images of self appear in mind, but because a typical meditative practice is to observe rather than grasp or engage these images, their relative nature becomes quite clear. Qualitatively, thoughts about the self are seen simply as arising—similar to a passing emotion or sensory observation. Views and concepts of both self and others arise, change, and disappear. In this way, mindfulness of the passing experiences teaches us about their variability, impermanence, and lack of essentialness. It also shows that one can simply observe such phenomena, positive or negative, and that attaching to them, processing them, or defending against them is not necessary to resolving them or experiencing them fully.

Mindfulness meditation practices also make salient the ongoing and transient upheavals of consciousness, and the lack of a continuous agent or entity standing behind them. Observing, one can see the spontaneous emergence of thoughts and urges not as "self"-initiated, but simply as arising from our true nature, which is the union of fundamental emptiness (the impermance of all phenomena that in turn creates a constant "possibility space") and cognizance (the energy behind the risings themselves). These "risings" of thought and emotion recede and exit naturally, without a self needing to exert any effort to close the door behind them. In this way, mindfulness practices highlight that the occupations of the mind can be spontaneous, variable, and impermanent.

Mindfulness practices therefore provide practical training in the idea that we need not attach to ideas of self as permanent. Buddhism describes such tendencies toward perceptions of permanence as habit and, like all habits, they can be softened and eliminated through practice of alternative behaviors. Yet for many, holding on to a permanent self is a strong habit, and the idea of disrupting this habit results in significant anxiety and defensiveness. For example, *terror management theory* (TMT; Solomon, Greenberg, & Pyszczynski, 2004) suggests that people's need to protect against awareness of impermanence and death drives much defensive behavior. A common technique in TMT research is to expose people to reminders of death, called *mortality salience* (MS) stimuli, then follow their reactions. Stimulated by thoughts of death, people often amplify their allegiance to their social worldviews and become more prone to derogate or exclude outgroup members, presumably to shore up self-esteem and feelings of significance. In other words, TMT research indicates that fear of impermanence leads to a defensive clinging to beliefs and identities to shore up (illusory) feelings of continuity and worth.

But, interestingly, mindfulness fully moderates this tendency to be reactive to MS manipulations, diminishing the defensive tendencies associated with terror management. Niemiec and colleagues (2010) did a series of experiments in which they presented persons with MS stimuli and measured their subsequent tendencies to derogate others from outgroups. They replicated the typical TMT effects (those exposed to MS conditions were more likely to derogate outgroup members), but this effect was carried entirely by participants with low trait mindfulness. People with higher trait mindfulness did not exhibit the defensive reactions predicted by TMT. Moreover, these experiments detailed some of the mechanisms underlying this effect. When first presented with death reminders, people higher in mindfulness were more open in processing them, whereas persons low in mindfulness showed less depth of processing of MS stimuli. Yet after the delay period that typifies TMT studies, findings revealed that the less mindful participants evidenced *higher* death accessibility, which means that death thoughts were still active (though not necessarily conscious) in their minds. By contrast, more mindful individuals, who had earlier more fully assimilated the experience, were no longer preoccupied, even implicitly, with death. They were not still holding on to, or resisting, awareness of impermanence by defending a self-identity.

Reconciling Buddhist Philosophy with Western Theories of Self

Turning now to Western psychology, it is clear that the term *self* carries quite different meanings in different psychological theories and traditions. We begin with the traditional social-cognitive view of the self as the *me-self*, or *self-as-object*. As Harter

(2012) summarized, historically, most of the empirical attention in psychology has been on the me-self, or self-as-object. This is most notably reflected in the extensive research on topics such as self-consciousness, identity, and self-esteem. But there is also a long-standing tradition in the West of viewing the self as an integrative or synthetic process, one that brings about both coherence and connectedness. We examine each of these conceptions of self in turn.

The "Me-Self" or Self-as-Object

Work on the me-self can be traced to the "looking glass" self of Cooley (1902) and Mead (1934), who both noted that we often employ the term *self* to represent ourselves as an *object* of perception. As an object of perception, the self is understood as a cognitive–affective construction, built largely from the internalization of other people's appraisals and perceptions of the individual (McAdams, 1990). In other words, individuals live in a social world where others respond and react to them, providing feedback and bases for evaluations and social comparisons. Based largely on this reflected feedback, individuals form identities and self-concepts that include various self-applied labels, roles, and attributes. In addition they internalize evaluations concerning how esteem-worthy they are in different domains (Harter, 2012; Wylie, 1989).

Identities and self-concepts often function to connect us with others and help us feel that we belong (Ryan & Deci, 2011; Sedikedies & Gaertner, 2001). The me-self thus functions to help us locate ourselves within social networks and groups. Here, identity statements take the basic form "I am . . ." filled in by roles, skills, abilities, interests and evaluations. "I am a retail clerk" is an identity, as is "I am poor at mechanical things." The value in this process is that identifying oneself as a "Girl Scout" or a "Republican" may help an individual feel connected with specific others. In fact, James (1890) argued that people create multiple "me selves," paralleling the different social roles and interactions in which they engage.

The me-self is thus an internalized and self-elaborated concept or representation, and comes with a collection of associated mechanisms, or self-schemas, for governing action (Oyserman, Elmore, & Smith, 2012; Sedikedies & Gaertner, 2001). Because we can take ourselves to be an object, we can form an objectifying and evaluative view of self that provides a reference point for who we are, and subsequently react to our ability to succeed in attaining the standards associated with that "me-self" role.

The notion of mindfulness is often loosely associated with conceptions of *self-awareness*, including awareness of self-as-object. Yet although Baer (2003) notes that "self-directed attention" is a central characteristic of mindfulness, it is clear that mindfulness is associated with only some types of self-directed attention and *not* others. In fact, consciousness of self-as-object can be negatively associated with mindfulness.

As an example, Fenigstein, Scheier, and Buss (1975) distinguished three types of self-awareness: *private self-consciousness*, or the tendency to reflect on inner feelings and thoughts; *public self-consciousness*, which is the tendency to view oneself from the perspective of others; and *social anxiety*, which assesses tendencies toward shyness and a focus on social fears. Brown and Ryan (2003) demonstrated that none of these is positively associated with mindfulness. Public self-consciousness and social anxiety, both of which involve objective self-awareness (Buss, 1980), were negatively associated with mindfulness; private self-consciousness was uncorrelated. Cramer (2000) suggested parsing private self-consciousness as two distinct components—*internal state awareness*, or the tendency to be aware of feelings and sensibilities; and *self-reflectiveness*—a tendency to direct attention to the self. Brown and Ryan found that only the former, internal state awareness, had positive relations with mindfulness. Self-reflectiveness, because it does not differentiate how one attends to self, was not a positive correlate. Still other measures that concern attention to self-as-object were not associated with mindfulness (Brown & Ryan, 2003). For example, *self-monitoring* (Snyder & Gangestad, 1986), the tendency to track and control behaviors and self-presentation, was not associated with mindfulness. Trapnell and Campbell (1999) distinguished two types of self-focus: *reflectiveness*, or the tendency to explore and contemplate the self, and *rumination*, the tendency to worry about events. Reflectiveness was weakly positively associated with mindfulness; rumination was negatively related.

What is clear here is that mindfulness is not about a focus on self. One can track, monitor, control, contemplate, worry about, narcissistically value, and in myriad other ways be attached to and engaged with the self as a concept or an object of perception. These do not all equate with being mindful. Indeed, many measures of self-awareness, being derived from the self-as-object tradition, require *objectifying* the self, making it concrete, and therefore creating a distinction between awareness and an "object" that is judged and evaluated. In contrast, mindfulness is not about creating such a judgmental duality; when mindful, one fully experiences the succession of feelings and self-thoughts that emerge spontaneously without judgment or prejudice.

Self-Esteem and Mindfulness

In me-self theories, people strive to meet the standards associated with internalized self-images, and they derive *self-esteem*, or feelings of worth and positive regard, when they succeed (Kernis, 2003). Indeed, people can put a lot of energy into maintaining or enhancing self-conceptions, and when this becomes a predominant goal it can bring with it a variety of anxieties, conflicts, and defensive reactions (Brown, Ryan, Creswell, & Niemiec, 2008; Weinstein, Przybylski, & Ryan, 2012). Ryan and Brown (2003) highlighted how being invested in particular identities fosters a need to defend against threats to them, as well as negative evaluations of self-worth that may arise when identity-related goals are not attained. For example, if I identify myself as a successful achiever, than setbacks in achievements are not just experiences; they represent a blow to my sense of "self" (Brown et al., 2008).

In self-determination theory (SDT; Deci & Ryan, 1985) this phenomenon is described as *ego-involvement* (Niemiec, Ryan, & Brown, 2008; Ryan, 1982). Such "self-esteem" is based on an internal pressure to meet constructed expectations, and is therefore seen as a form of introjected regulation (Rigby, Deci, Patrick, & Ryan, 1992). Within the SDT framework, because introjects and ego-involvements make worth contingent on specific outcomes, they are sources of instability and control rather than autonomy and liberation (see also Kernis, 2003). In parallel, Buddhism represents such investment in the me-self as a deluded state, being rooted in one's failure to recognize the true nature of experience and identity. This in turn results in mental suffering.

As it turns out, correlations between dispositional mindfulness and trait self-esteem are generally moderate to high (e.g., Brown & Ryan, 2003). This is because standard measures of self-esteem ask whether one generally regards oneself positively, and there is no reason to think that mindfulness would not be associated with positive regard. But esteeming oneself is a particularly interesting issue from a mindfulness perspective. As Ryan and Brown (2003) argued, if self-esteem is an ongoing concern or question, then whether it is low or high, it is a problem. When esteem is a concern, one is likely to be driven to act in accord with projections of others' views or opinions rather than on the basis of what is occurring, reflectively considered. Another consequence of these internalized self-concepts is that they become a source of bias in perception and a distorting filter through which other events and communications are processed. Events and interactions are appraised and processed not in a fully open way, but more in accord with how it affects the conception of "me" (Brown et al., 2008). In addition, such reactivity can frequently be nonconscious (Bargh & Chartrand, 1999).

Such nonconscious defenses of identity were recently highlighted in a series of studies by Weinstein, Ryan, and colleagues (2012). The investigators asked individuals explicitly to report their sexual identity on a scale from *very gay* (homosexual) to *very straight* (heterosexual). The researchers subsequently assessed same-sex attractions using implicit, reaction-time-based measures. They found in some individuals a significant discrepancy between explicit (conscious) reports of sexual orientations and nonconscious attractions. Moreover these participants were more likely than others to find gays and lesbians threatening, and they demonstrated higher signs of hostility and aggression toward homosexuals. This illustrates how attachments to specific identities (e.g., being straight) can lead to defense, and engender the kinds of negative emotions that Buddhism might predict in those who cling to self-concepts.

Indeed, within Buddhism the concept of ego itself is directly linked to a deluded sense of self-permanence (Sogyal, 2002); therefore, it follows that ego-involvement rises with one's experience of a permanent and reified "me-self." The result is attachment and being caught up in a cycle of suffering via the "eight winds" (Sogyal, 2002) designed to protect this dream-like self: the hope of gain and the fear of loss, the hope of fame and the fear of infamy, the hope of pleasure and the fear of pain, and the hope of praise and the fear of blame. All of these represent a form of preoccupied suffering that is rooted in one's protecting the concept of a me-self.

Insofar as mindfulness is associated with less attachment to identities and self-images, it should reduce the tendency to experience these "hopes and fears" and associated social threats (Hodgins, 2008). Evidence supporting this claim has come from a few recent studies. For example, Creswell, Eisenberger and Lieberman (2008) argued that social exclusion is an ego-threatening experience that often leads to reactivity and defense. Yet they found that people higher in trait mindfulness experienced significantly less distress upon being excluded. Moreover, functional magnetic resonance imaging (fMRI) data showed that this lowered reactivity was manifest in lower activation of the dorsal anterior cingulated cortex (dACC), an area of the brain associated with social pain. Thus, mindfulness predicted lower reactivity, both subjectively felt and as neurophysiologically observed.

Barnes, Brown, Krusemark, Campbell, and Rogge (2007) demonstrated in two studies how more mindful people are less threatened in relationships, and therefore less reactive when conflicts occur. Among couples engaged in a relationship conflict discussion, more mindful people showed lower distress (less hostility, less anxiety) entering the discussion. In turn, this baseline lower reactivity was associated with less anxiety and hostility postdiscussion (and mindfulness during the discussion predicted greater positive feelings toward the partner afterwards). Presumably, mindfulness allowed individuals to be more aware of the issues raised, without the distractions of a reactive threat response, thus facilitating more adaptive communication.

In short, mindfulness appears to moderate the defensive tendencies associated with the me-self, as evidenced by links between mindfulness and lower ego-involvement, defensive reactions, and stress appraisals (e.g., Kernis & Goldman, 2006; Weinstein, Brown, & Ryan, 2009). A central message from Buddhism is that the source of our suffering is our attachment to the self-as-object: a clinging to experience, permanence, or identity (Trungpa, 1976). Our litany of self-conceptualizations ("I am a researcher," "I am a father, " I am an athlete"), as well as our conscious and unconscious beliefs about the "enduring" qualities that define us, are attempts to construct an identity that provides solidity, even though ultimately this "self," however elaborately built, is fundamentally an illusion. To use the often-repeated Zen metaphor, believing these identities are "real" is no more accurate than believing one's clenched hand "is" fundamentally a fist. When the fingers stretch, where is the fist? Similarly, who we "are" is constantly changing. Each moment of self is merely a temporary experience that will naturally give way to the next. It is being able to experience the relative manifestations of "me" from moment to moment, while simultaneously being aware of the true dream-like nature of the self ("no-self") that is indispensible in working toward happiness.

Mindfulness Meditation and the Me-Self

In a sustained state of mindfulness, one remains aware of the transient nature of the cravings and desires, and observes them dispassionately. Thoughts, emotions, and concepts constantly arise and recede—and when simply observed are recognized as impermanent. In other words, mindfulness practices bear on the me-self by exposing its activity, revealing that however clamoring the objects of mind may be, nothing requires that we cling to—or identify with—the marchers in this parade.

As Brown and colleagues (2008) describe, mindfulness "entails a shift in the locus of personal subjectivity from conceptual representations of the self and others to awareness itself" (p. 82). As a consequence, it lessens the intra- and interpersonal pressures that the me-self entails, and liberates the individual from the often automatic cognitive distortions and defensive reactions that can disrupt the integrative process underlying self-regulation (Brown et al., 2008; Martin & Erber, 2005; Ryan & Brown, 2003). Stated differently, for highly mindful people, rejections or successes do not involve their self-worth and are thus less destabilizing. As a result, their egos are quieter, allowing them to behave volitionally and without the need to prove, maintain, or stay attached to conceptions of the me-self (Hodgins, 2008; Niemiec et al., 2008).

The "I"-Self, or Self-as-Process

Whereas the me-self, or self-as-object, has been the predominant tradition in the study of self (Harter, 2012), perhaps the second most salient tradition has been the "I"-self or "self-as-process" view (McAdams, 1990; Ryan, 1995). In this tradition, self is construed not as a concept or set of self-evaluations but rather as the synthetic and integrative process of the personality. The self-as-process view is represented in many theories, including in psychoanalysis with the *synthetic function of the ego* (Freud, 1961), in Jungian psychology by *individuation* (Jung, 1983), in person-centered psychology by *self-actualization* (Rogers, 1963), in cognitive-developmental theory with the concept of *organization* (e.g., Piaget, 1971), and within self-determination theory (Deci & Ryan, 2000) with the concept of *integration*. Self-as-process in all these frameworks concerns the assimilation of experiences to the self, and bringing unity and coherence to the regulation of experience and action.

Conceiving of the self not as a "thing," but, rather, as the process of synthesis and initiation, has deep roots within constructivist and phenomenological traditions of philosophy. For example, Kant (1990) emphasized that experience is produced by the synthetic activity of mind, and that consciousness of self is essentially awareness of this synthetic activity. He emphasized that apart from the experience of this synthetic activity, there is no direct apprehension of a *self* because, phenomenologically, the self can never directly appear as an object of consciousness. Put differently, the self cannot be experienced as a thing, but only as the means through which experience is ordered. This acknowledgment that the "I" that perceives the world cannot itself become a direct object of perception was further refined in the works of Husserl (1931), Heidegger (1962), Ricoeur (1966), and others, all of whom stressed that the self as an initiator or perceiver of events is not a phenomenal object in any direct way. Because the self-as-process is not a "thing" or object that can be directly apprehended, it is phenomenally accessed indirectly as the sense of activity in contacting, assimilating, and acting in the world.

Autonomy and the I-Self

To access this organizing activity of the self, particularly relevant is the issue of *autonomy*, which means "self-governing," or the regulation of behavior by the self. Autonomy's opposite is *heteronomy*, or being regulated by forces experienced as other than (or alien to) the self (*heteron* means "otherness"). People typically have a direct sense of whether they are willingly engaged in an activity, or being regulated and controlled. By understanding this phenomenal experience of autonomy versus heteronomy, it is possible to develop a fuller understanding of what it means for thoughts, feelings, and behaviors to be experienced as reflecting the I-self, or self-as-process, to varying degrees.

Pfander (1967), an early phenomenologist, distinguished self-determined acts from other forms of motivation. He observed that self-determined acts are experienced "precisely not as an occurrence caused by a different agent" but rather invariably involve the support of one's "ego-center" (p. 20). In Pfander's view, even if the actions one undertakes are initiated by strong external demands, they can be self-determined, so long as the actions are truly *endorsed* by the self. In contrast, non-self-determined acts are experienced as compelled by forces outside the self with which one does not concur. Ricoeur (1966) similarly underscored that people can willingly obey and yet be self-determined, such as when we follow a doctor's "orders" or a traffic officer's command. The issue of autonomy lies in one's *assent* to demands and the sense of their *legitimacy*. Self-determination describes willfully consenting to external obligations based on a sense of value, or following demands that are deemed legitimate.

Similarly, our inner workings can also make demands on us. From emotional urges and strong drives to compulsive pressures, there are many clamoring forces and mental orders we can witness that arise internally (Ryan, Deci, Grolnick, & La Guardia, 2006). Yet, as with external demands, the issue of autonomy lies in whether one reflectively endorses and willingly follows these inner demands versus feels controlled by them. So autonomy does not concern the source from which cues and demands arise (i.e., internally or externally), but rather one's volitional regulation with respect to them.

In summary, autonomy and self-determination pertain to acts that are experienced as freely done and holistically self-endorsed or valued. In addition, we highlight that the self-as-process, or I-self, is *phenomenologically* implicated in all actions, precisely as the experience of volition and/or inner endorsement and commitment as one acts. By contrast, *controlled* forms of motivation are heteronomous and lack self-endorsement, whether the controls stem from internal or external demands.

Analytical Perspectives

Modern analytical approaches to autonomy begin with Frankfurt (1971), who defined *autonomy* as an issue of authentic assent, or assent that is congruent with one's reflective considerations. To Frankfurt, autonomy is not defined by whether behavior is prompted by internal or outside influences, but whether one decisively supports the behaviors one does undertake. Building on Frankfurt, Dworkin (1988) and Freidman (2003) similarly argue that autonomy need not entail behaving without constraint; one can assent to particular constraints (e.g., laws or manners) and still experience autonomy.

An additional point is that for a behavior to be autonomous, it is not necessary that it always be consciously reflected upon in that moment. It does require, however, that the behavior be informed by one's sensibilities and values, and if reflected upon, be authentically endorsed (Ryan et al., 2012). We add further that a lack of autonomy is dynamically indicated when there is a resistance to openly processing what one is doing, and the motives and reasons for acting. Clearly, too, there are *degrees of autonomy*, and the extent of autonomy is often dependent on the extent to which the individual has mindfully and reflectively integrated a particular regulation or value (Schultz & Ryan, in press). Autonomy therefore entails awareness and evaluation based on a breadth of considerations. As we discuss later, mindfulness supplies the most appropriate breadth of considerations a person might employ.

Autonomy, Mindfulness, and No-Self

Buddhist concepts such as no-self (*anatta*) and *rigpa* (non–dual awareness)—concepts that are philosophically associated with greater awareness and happiness—can be related to autonomous versus heteronomous regulation. When there is an awareness of one's absolute nature and the impermanence of the self, there is less grasping and defensiveness, for there is no concrete "me" to defend rigorously, maintain, or enhance. Such concerns primarily lie in the domain of heteronomous regulation, notably through external or introjected regulation that is characterized by feelings of pressure, guilt, shame, and other emotional states that are fed by holding a strong me-self concept. More simply put, the emotional forces associated with controlled regulation require a me-self (and its attendant ego-involvement) to act as their object. By contrast, holding an awareness of no-self attenuates the power of these emotional dynamics by removing the self-as-object. If ego-involved feelings arise, in this case, they are like a thief entering an empty house: There is nothing to grasp onto. Instead, mindful of the impermanence of the self, one has greater openness of the self-as-process, facilitating autonomous functioning.

In fact, evidence is mounting that mindfulness is positively associated with more autonomous self-regulation. Brown and Ryan (2003) demonstrated that dispositional and state mindfulness are independently associated with increased autonomy on a day-to-day basis. Specifically, people were asked at various points in their day to rate their relative autonomy, current mindfulness, mood, and other state-related variables. Results revealed that the more mindful one is, both in general and in any given moment, the more one experiences his or her actions as autonomously undertaken and volitional (see also Levesque & Brown, 2007).

When mindful, decreases in defensiveness allow for a more open and engaged presence to circumstances, which is in turn expected to increase a sense of meaningful choice and volitional engagement—hallmark qualities of autonomy (Hodgins, 2008). Indeed, the Buddhist notions of our true nature being the combination of "empty essence" and "cognizant nature" suggest room for autonomous regulation. Impermanence implies the possibility for change and opportunity, and cognizance describes the innate capacity to engage this "limitless space" in meaningful ways.

Mindfulness therefore appears to promote the I-self and its integrative tendencies through open attention to the present moment, free of evaluative mental concepts and self-centered biases, allowing more clarity and deeper processing of experiences. In fact, even though organismic views of self-as-process vary across psychodynamic, humanistic, and modern personality traditions, they share a belief with each other and with Buddhism: that a healthy self-as-process is characterized by nondefensiveness, integrity, and authentic self-regulation. That is, the individual is volitionally and autonomously engaged, effectively regulating behavior, not occupied with internal conflict, and not defending against information or inputs that arise.

The receptive nature of mindful awareness yields immense value for self-functioning by being *informative*. In this way, Buddhist teachings align with the conditions traditionally associated with autonomous functioning, namely, seeing inputs and events as informational rather than controlling (Deci & Ryan, 2000). If we are nondefensively and nonjudgmentally interested in what is occurring, then we have the opportunity to experience more fully the multidimensional universe of events around us. Akin to a process of *relaxed interest* (Deci & Ryan, 1985) or *interest taking* (Weinstein, Przybylski, et al., 2012), mindful states are about allowing information to flow and letting what is salient arise, free of the controls that accompany more dualistic, defensive, or judgmental forms of experience.

Autonomous regulation is supported by mindfulness in multiple ways. When individuals are more open to what is occurring without distortion, subsequent behavior can be more informed, selective, and volitionally supported (Hodgins & Knee, 2002; Niemiec et al., 2008). Being mindful of the present, one can more reflectively follow important and currently interesting pursuits, making decisions with sensitivity to one's own and others' needs and desires. The characteristics of willingness, nonattachment, and more effective processing all bespeak the potentially central role of mindfulness in integrated self-functioning, in which individuals are more choiceful and openly attentive to the situations in which they find themselves, "all things considered" (Brown et al., 2007).

Weinstein and colleagues (2009) further proposed that people who are more mindful are more resilient to stress, in part because they make better choices and therefore incur less stress, and in part because they do not feel as negatively about potential stressors. They also hypothesized that mindfulness is associated with more effective coping when challenges occur. Weinstein and colleagues conducted four studies using varied methods, together showing that people higher in dispositional mindfulness both attributed less stress to events and used more active and nondefensive coping strategies in response to the stressors. These studies also indicated that these different attribution styles and coping mechanisms partially explained the greater vitality and positive mood associated with mindfulness.

In contrast, when mindfulness is low or impaired, capacities for autonomous regulation are diminished. For example, Ryan (2005) described how the developmental conditions endured by most individuals with borderline personality disorder (BPD) were such that they interfered with the capacity simply to be present for what is occurring (also see Fonagy & Target, 1997). Abuse and unpredictability precipitate both poor regulation of impulses and hypersensitivity to external threats, and a need for vigilance that interferes with open, receptive processing. It is exactly for these reasons that mindfulness practices have proven worthwhile in the treatment of BPD. For example, Linehan (1993) employs techniques such as "just notice the experience" and "stepping aside" to observe impulses and emotions nonjudgmentally. Mindfulness-based interventions are also becoming increasingly common in treatments of other personality and mood disorders (e.g., Segal et al., 2002).

Levesque and Brown (2007) suggested that one way in which mindfulness may contribute to autonomous functioning is by "undoing" the reflexive automation of some behaviors, particularly those that may be controlled or conditioned. Using multilevel modeling of diary (experience-sampled) data, their research indicated that more mindful people are more likely to act autonomously in daily life, regardless of their implicit (automatic) motivational orientations.

In summary, there are multiple positive connections between mindfulness and more autonomous forms of self-regulation. In these connections, we do not argue that mindfulness is equivalent to autonomy. Rather it appears that mindfulness *facilitates* autonomous functioning through its association with more open and less defensive processing, allowing more selective and informed regulation to occur, in which the person can more wholeheartedly stand behind his or her actions; that is, mindfulness is conducive to development of integrity.

Further Discussion

In this chapter, we have focused on the relations of mindfulness to conceptions of self. We have argued that mindfulness is not itself a theory or psychological perspective but rather an open and receptive form of awareness. Thus, its meaning and practice can be related to any and all theories of self and experience, Eastern or Western. Our focus has been on Buddhist conceptions of no-self, and the two major Western traditions of self, namely, the self-as-object (me-self) theories that predominate in social-cognitive approaches and the self-as-process (I-self) theories that predominate in organismic traditions.

As might be expected, mindfulness practices fit well with the rich Buddhist traditions of no-self. Mindfulness meditation experiences directly display how self-images arise and evaporate, and how all experiences appearing at a relative level are impermanent at an absolute level. Mindfulness also reveals another basis of no-self: When we mindfully observe events, we do not see the organizing self as a phenomenal object. This is a point on which both Western phenomenology and Buddhist thinkers concur (Varela et al., 1991).

Yet an important further consideration within Buddhism is the distinction between the absolute and relative levels of reality. At an absolute level, the impermanent nature of all things, including the self, is clear, even as we can construe at the relative level the impact and meaning of events, and our responsibilities in acting, in either open and authentic or defensive ways.

Regarding the me-self, or self-as-object, it seems clear that investing in it has many drawbacks associated with ego-involvement and its attendant pressures. Mindfulness practices can help to liberate one from the troubles of the me-self by allowing one to receptively observe events, including one's ever-passing self-related perceptions, without evaluative burden and anxiety, and without the distractions of self-objectification and ego-involvement. In doing so, suffering is decreased as people perceive less threat and stress in events (Weinstein et al., 2009).

The I-self is understood as a synthetic function, or as assimilation and integration (Ryan, 1995). The more self-as-process is active, the more the person experiences his or her behaviors as volitional and autonomous, and the more his or her actions are experienced as wholehearted and authentic. In a practical sense, there is greater ownership and responsibility for what he or she does. Interestingly, empirical research supports the view that mindfulness supports and enhances the self-as-process, and the healthier behavioral regulation associated with it (e.g., Brown & Ryan, 2003; Niemiec et al., 2010). Mindfulness facilitates autonomy or "true self" regulation by affording the individual fuller awareness that better informs choices and decisions regarding reactions and behaviors that might follow. In part, this is due to the lower defensiveness associated with mindfulness, and its nonselective, nonjudgmental mode. As expressed by Goldstein and Kornfield (1987, p. 57):

> When the mind ceases to want and judge and identify with whatever arises, we see the empty flow of experience as it is. We come to a ground of silence and inherent incompleteness. When we stop struggling and let be, the natural wisdom, joy, and freedom of our being emerges and expresses itself effortlessly.

It is the emergence of this natural wisdom that interests us most. Directing life from our hearts means acting from a quiescent confidence that allows us to be fully in the moment and to take actions that reflect our authentic and integrated understanding.

There is therefore an interplay between mindfulness and the functioning of a more healthy and autonomous self-as-process. Although mindfulness includes awareness that—on an absolute level—there is no-self, when mindful, one is also more open to experiences and more likely to endorse taking actions that represent the integration of these experiences through the self-as-process. Clearly, both the me-self and the I-self are readily available avenues for framing experience and action, and in fact, both operate continuously within each individual to varying degrees. Mindfulness constitutes a facilitator for I-self over me-self experience as people grapple within their relative realities; it is a resource for organizing behavior by supporting the synthetic tendencies of self-as-process. Centuries of Western and Eastern philosophy, as well as the empirical research reviewed here, support the idea that integrity and well-being are among the outcomes made more likely by mindfulness.

So, Did the Buddha Have a Self?

We began with this question in our title, and in the end we appear to have not one but several clear answers. First, the Buddha himself, in the Bhadrakalpa Sutra, stated that although manifest, in reality he "never came and never taught." On an absolute level, he was showing that he had no self to grab hold of, no identity to possess or defend, and no accomplishments to which he was attached. From what we know of his attitude and his words, he was, once enlightened, uninvolved with a me-self and unconcerned approval or self-esteem. Yet, clearly, he was fully functioning and vital, congruent, autonomous, and authentic (Armstrong, 2001; Hanh, 1998). His aware-ness of no-self on an absolute level enabled a self-as-process on the relative level that was in every respect healthy and beneficial, both to himself and to all those around him, then and since.

REFERENCES

Armstrong, K. (2001). *Buddha*. New York: Penguin Books.

Atkins, K. (2005). Introduction. In K. Atkins (Ed.), *Self and subjectivity* (pp. 1–4). Oxford, UK: Blackwell.

Baer, R. A. (2003). Mindfulness training as a clinical intervention: A conceptual and empiri-cal review. *Clinical Psychology: Science and Practice, 10*, 125–143.

Baer, R., Walsh, E., & Lykins, E. (2009) Assessment of mindfulness. In F. Didonna (Ed.), *Clinical handbook of mindfulness* (pp. 153–168). New York: Springer.

Bargh, J. A., & Chartrand, T. L. (1999). The unbearable automaticity of being. *American Psychologist, 54*, 462–479.

Barnes, S., Brown, K. W., Krusemark, E., Campbell, W. K., & Rogge, R. D. (2007). The role of mindfulness in romantic relationship satisfaction and responses to relationship stress. *Journal of Marital and Family Therapy, 33*, 482–500.

Bhikkhu Bodhi. (2011). What does mindfulness really mean?: A canonical perspective. *Con-temporary Buddhism, 12*, 19–39.

Brown, K. W., & Ryan, R. M. (2003). The benefits of being present: Mindfulness and its role in psychological well-being. *Journal of Personality and Social Psychology, 84*, 822–848.

Brown, K. W., & Ryan, R. M. (2007). Multilevel modeling of motivation: A self-determination theory analysis of basic psychological needs. In A. D. Ong & M. van Dulmen (Eds.), *Handbook of methods in positive psychology* (pp. 530–541). New York: Oxford Uni-versity Press.

Brown, K. W., Ryan, R. M., & Creswell, J. D. (2007). Mindfulness: Theoretical foundations and evidence for its salutary effects. *Psychological Inquiry, 18*, 211–237.

Brown, K. W., Ryan, R. M., Creswell, J. D., & Niemiec, C. P. (2008). Beyond me: Mind-ful responses to social threat. In H. A. Wayment & J. J. Bauer (Eds.), *Transcending self-interest: Psychological explorations of the quiet ego* (pp. 75–84). Washington, DC: American Psychological Association.

Buss, A. H. (1980). *Self-consciousness and social anxiety*. San Francisco: Freeman.

Chambers, R., Lo, B. C. Y., & Allen, N. B. (2008) The impact of intensive mindfulness train-ing on attentional control, cognitive style, and affect. *Cognitive Research and Therapy, 32*, 303–322.

Collins, S. (1992). *Selfless persons: Imagery and thought in Theravāda Buddhism*. Cam-bridge, UK: Cambridge University Press.

Cooley, C. H. (1902). *Human nature and the social order*. New York: Scribner's.

Cramer, K. M. (2000). Comparing the relative fit of various factor models of the self-consciousness scale in two independent samples. *Journal of Personality Assessment, 75*, 295–307.

Creswell, J. D., Eisenberger, N., & Lieberman, M. (2008). *Neural correlates of mindfulness during social exclusion*. Unpublished manuscript, University of California, Los Angeles.

Deci, E. L., & Ryan, R. M. (1985). *Intrinsic motivation and self-determination in human behavior*. New York: Plenum Press.

Deci, E. L., & Ryan, R. M. (2000). The "what" and "why" of goal pursuits: Human needs and the self-determination of behavior. *Psychological Inquiry, 11*, 227–268.

Dworkin, G. (1988). *The theory and practice of autonomy.* New York: Cambridge University Press.

Epstein, M. (2007). *Psychotherapy without a self.* New Haven, CT: Yale University Press.

Fenigstein, A., Scheier, M. F., & Buss, A. H. (1975). Public and private self-consciousness: Assessment and theory. *Journal of Consulting and Clinical Psychology, 43*, 522–527.

Frankfurt, H. (1971). Freedom of the will and the concept of person. *Journal of Philosophy, 68*, 5–20.

Friedman, M. (2003). *Autonomy, gender, politics.* New York: Oxford University Press.

Freud, S. (1961). The ego and the id. In J. Strachey (Ed. & Trans.), *The standard edition of the complete psychological works of Sigmund Freud* (Vol. 19, pp. 3–66). London: Hogarth.

Fonagy, P., & Target, M. (1997). Attachment and reflective function: Their role in self-organization. *Development and Psychopathology, 9*, 679–700.

Goldstein, J., & Kornfield, J. (1987). *Seeking the heart of wisdom: The path of insight meditation.* Boston: Shambala.

Gyatso, T. (2000), *Dzogchen: The Heart essence of the great perfection.* Ithaca, NY: Snow Lion.

Hanh, T. N. (1998). *The heart of Buddha's teaching: Transforming suffering into peace, joy, and liberation.* New York: Broadway Books.

Harter, S. (2012). *The construction of the self: Developmental and sociocultural foundations* (2nd ed.). New York: Guilford Press.

Heidegger, M. (1962). *Being and time.* New York: Harper & Row.

Hodgins, H. S. (2008). Motivation, threshold for threat, and quieting the ego. In H. A. Wayment & J. J. Bauer (Eds.), *Transcending self-interest: Psychological explorations of the quiet ego* (pp. 117–124). Washington, DC: American Psychological Association.

Hodgins, H. S., & Knee, C. R. (2002). The integrating self and conscious experience. In E. L. Deci & R. M. Ryan (Eds.), *Handbook of self-determination research* (pp. 87–100). Rochester, NY: University of Rochester Press.

Husserl, E. (1931). *Ideas: General introduction to pure phenomenology.* London: Allen & Unwin.

James, W. (1890). *The principles of psychology.* New York: Holt.

Jung, C. G. (1983). *The collected works of C. G. Jung* (H. Read, M. Fordham, & G. Adler, Eds.). New York: Pantheon.

Kant, I. (1990). *Critique of pure reason* (N. K. Smith, Trans.). London: Macmillan.

Kernis, M. H. (2003). Toward a conceptualization of optimal self-esteem. *Psychology Inquiry, 14*, 1–26.

Kernis, M. H., & Goldman, B. M. (2006). A multicomponent conceptualization of authenticity: Theory and research. In M. P. Zanna (Ed.), *Advances in experimental social psychology* (Vol. 38, pp. 284–357). San Diego, CA: Elsevier.

Levesque, C. S., & Brown, K. W. (2007). Mindfulness as a moderator of the effect of implicit motivational self-concept on day-to-day behavioral motivation. *Motivation and Emotion, 31*, 284–299.

Linehan, M. M. (1993). *Cognitive-behavioral treatment of borderline personality disorder.* New York: Guilford Press.

Lingpa, D. (1994). *Buddhahood without meditation.* Junction City, CA: Padma.

Loevinger, J., & Blasi, A. (1991). Development of the self as subject. In J. Stranss & G. Goethals (Eds.), *The self: Interdisciplinary approaches* (pp. 150–167). New York: Springer-Verlag.

Martin, L. L., & Erber, R. (2005). Commentary: The wisdom of social psychology: Five commonalities and one concern. *Psychological Inquiry, 16,* 194–202.

McAdams, D. P. (1990). *The person: An introduction to personality.* New York: Harcourt Brace Jovanovich.

Mead, G. H. (1934). *Mind, self, and society* (C. W. Morris, Ed.). Chicago: University of Chicago Press.

Niemiec, C. P., Brown, K. W., Kashdan, T. B., Cozzolino, P. J., Breen, W. E., Levesque-Bristol, C., et al. (2010). Being present in the face of existential threat: The role of trait mindfulness in reducing defensive responses to mortality salience. *Journal of Personality and Social Psychology, 99,* 344–365.

Niemiec, C. P., Ryan, R. M., & Brown, K. W. (2008). The role of awareness and autonomy in quieting the ego: A self-determination theory perspective. In H. A. Wayment & J. J. Bauer (Eds.), *Transcending self-interest: Psychological explorations of the quiet ego* (pp. 107–116). Washington, DC: American Psychological Association.

Nyanaponika Thera. (1972). *The power of mindfulness.* San Francisco: Unity Press.

O'Loughlin, R. E., & Zuckerman, M. (2008). Mindfulness as a moderator of the relationship between dehydroepiandrosterone and reported physical symptoms. *Personality and Individual Differences, 44,* 1193–1202.

Organ, T. W. (1988). *The self in its worlds: East and West.* London: Associated University Presses.

Oyserman, D., Elmore, K., & Smith, G. (2012). Self, self-concept, and identity. In M. R. Leary & J. P. Tangney (Eds.), *Handbook of self and identity* (2nd ed., pp. 69–104). New York: Guilford Press.

Perls, F., Hefferline, R. F., & Goodman, P. (1958). *Gestalt therapy.* New York: Julian Press.

Pfander, A. (1967). *Phenomenology of willing and motivation.* Chicago: Northwestern University Press.

Pfeil, F. (2000). Subjects without selves: Contemporary theory accounts for the "I." In G. Watson, S. Batchelor, & G. Claxton (Eds.), *The psychology of awakening.* York Beach, ME: Weiser.

Piaget, J. (1971). *Biology and knowledge.* Chicago: University of Chicago Press.

Ricoeur, P. (1966). *Freedom and nature: The voluntary and the involuntary* (E. V. Kohak, Trans.). Chicago: Northwestern University Press.

Rigby, C. S., Deci, E. L., Patrick, B. C., & Ryan, R. M. (1992). Beyond the intrinsic–extrinsic dichotomy: Self-determination in motivation and learning. *Motivation and Emotion, 16,* 165–185.

Rogers, C. (1963). The actualizing tendency in relation to "motives" and to consciousness. In M. R. Jones (Ed.), *Nebraska Symposium on Motivation* (Vol. 11, pp. 1–24). Lincoln: University of Nebraska Press.

Ryan, R. M. (1982). Control and information in the intrapersonal sphere: An extension of cognitive evaluation theory. *Journal of Personality and Social Psychology, 43,* 450–461.

Ryan, R. M. (1995). Psychological needs and the facilitation of integrative processes. *Journal of Personality, 63,* 397–427.

Ryan, R. M. (2005). The developmental line of autonomy in the etiology, dynamics and treatment of borderline personality disorders. *Development and Psychopathology, 17,* 987–1006.

Ryan, R. M., & Brown, K. W. (2003). Why we don't need self-esteem: Basic needs, mindfulness, and the authentic self. *Psychological Inquiry, 14,* 71–76.

Ryan, R. M., & Deci, E. L. (2011). Multiple identities within a single self: A self-determination theory perspective on internalization within contexts and cultures. In M. R. Leary &

J. P. Tangney (Eds.), *Handbook of self and identity* (2nd ed., pp. 253–274). New York: Guilford Press.

Ryan, R. M., Deci, E. L., Grolnick, W. S., & La Guardia, J. G. (2006). The significance of autonomy and autonomy support in psychological development and psychopathology. In D. Cicchetti & D. Cohen (Eds.), *Developmental psychopathology: Vol. 1. Theory and methods* (2nd ed., pp. 295–849). New York: Wiley.

Ryan, R. M., Legate, N., Niemiec, C. P., & Deci, E. L. (2012). Beyond illusions and defense: Exploring the possibilities and limits of human autonomy and responsibility through self-determination theory. In P. R. Shaver & M. Mikulincer (Eds.), *Meaning, mortality, and choice: The social psychology of existential concerns* (pp. 215–233). Washington, DC: American Psychological Association.

Schultz, P. P., & Ryan, R. M. (in press). The why, what, and how of healthy self-regulation: Mindfulness and eudaimonic living from a self-determination theory perspective. In B. Ostafin (Ed.), *Handbook of mindfulness and self-regulation*. New York: Springer.

Sedikedes, C., & Gaertner, L. (2001). A homecoming to the individual self: Emotional and motivational primacy. In C. Sedikides & M. B. Brewer (Eds.), *Individual self, relational self, collective self* (pp. 7–24). Philadelphia: Psychology Press.

Segal, Z., Williams, M., & Teasdale, J. (2002) *Mindfulness-based therapy for depression: A new approach to preventing relapse.* New York: Guilford Press.

Sogyal, R. (2002). *Tibetan book of living and dying.* New York: HarperCollins.

Solomon, S., Greenberg, J., & Pyszczynski, T. (2004). The cultural animal: Twenty years of terror management theory and research. In J. Greenberg, S. L. Koole, & T. Pyszcyzinski (Eds.), *Handbook of experimental existential psychology* (pp. 13–34). New York: Guilford Press.

Snyder, M., & Gangestad, S. (1986). On the nature of self-monitoring: Matters of assessment, matters of validity. *Journal of Personality and Social Psychology, 51,*125–139.

Trapnell, P. D., & Campbell, J. D. (1999). Private self-consciousness and the five-factor model of personality: Distinguishing rumination from reflection. *Journal of Personality and Social Psychology, 76,* 284–304.

Trungpa, C. (1976). *The myth of freedom and the way of meditation.* London: Shambhahla.

Varela, F., Thompson, E., & Rosch, E. (1991). *The embodied mind.* Cambridge, MA: MIT Press.

Weinstein, N., Brown, K. W., & Ryan, R. M. (2009). A multi-method examination of the effects of mindfulness on stress attribution, coping, and emotional well-being. *Journal of Research in Personality, 43,* 374–385.

Weinstein, N., Przybylski, A. K., & Ryan, R. M. (2012). The index of autonomous functioning: Development of a scale of human autonomy. *Journal of Research in Personality, 46*(4), 397–413.

Weinstein, N., Ryan, W. S., DeHaan, C. R., Przybylski, A. K., Legate, N. & Ryan, R. M. (2012). Parental autonomy support and discrepancies between implicit and explicit sexual identities: Dynamics of self-acceptance and defense. *Journal of Personality and Social Psychology, 102,* 815–832.

Wylie, R. C. (1989). *Measures of self-concept.* Lincoln, NE: Buros Institute.

PART IV

MINDFULNESS INTERVENTIONS FOR HEALTHY POPULATIONS

CHAPTER 15

Mindfulness-Based Stress Reduction for Healthy Stressed Adults

Shauna L. Shapiro and Hooria Jazaieri

To date, the vast majority of research on mindfulness training has focused on its effect on decreasing mental and physical pathology. But when we examine the historical record of the Buddha's teachings, it is clear that he did not set out to teach those obscured by significant states of mental or physical suffering. In the *Ayacana Sutra* (S. i. 136), the Buddha's teaching was aimed toward those "with little dust in their eyes," which refers to people without significant impediments to their capacity to understand and benefit from the teachings. Mindfulness training, therefore, was not simply a means to decrease pathology; the original intention was to help practitioners live lives of greater well-being and freedom. Thus, a contemporary focus of mindfulness training that includes its applications for healthy populations is congruent with the original intent.

This chapter examines the applications and benefits of mindfulness for healthy, community-dwelling adults who perceive themselves as stressed, which in contemporary societies includes many people. After first offering a broad definition of mindfulness training as it has been applied to healthy adults, we review the empirical literature, examining the value of mindfulness-based interventions for a variety of healthy adult populations, particularly community members, and recent research with health care professionals and trainees, romantic partners, expectant mothers, and parents are also noted. We follow this with a discussion of the research in this area and offer suggestions for future research directions.

Mindfulness Training for Healthy Adults Defined and Described

Mindfulness can be defined as both a state of mind (mindful awareness) and a practice. *Mindfulness training* can be understood as "awareness that arises through intentionally attending in an open, kind, and discerning way" (Shapiro & Carlson, 2009, p. 15). *Mindfulness practice* can be conceptualized as involving three synergistic processes: (1) intention, (2) attention, and (3) attitude. *Intention* refers to reflecting explicitly on why one is practicing; that is,,what the motivation, value, and aspiration is for the practice. This does not imply that mindfulness is a means to an end; in fact, this is the antithesis of mindfulness practice. Intention simply refers to setting a direction, not a destination (Kornfield, 2010, personal communication). *Attention* refers to the focus on present-moment experience. *Attitude* refers to the quality of attention, infusing it with openness, acceptance, and care. Mindfulness practice, therefore, involves intentionally attending to the present moment with openness, acceptance, and care (Shapiro & Carlson, 2009).

The training of mindfulness and its applications in daily life has been skillfully developed into mindfulness-based interventions offered in a group psychoeducational context. The majority of the research we describe in this chapter utilizes mindfulness-based stress reduction (MBSR), the original secular mindfulness-based program (Kabat-Zinn, 1990) and still the most commonly used in research with healthy stressed adults. Thus, we describe the intervention here briefly, and in the course of our review, will also briefly describe other mindfulness-based interventions derived from MBSR and applied to specific populations.

MBSR is an intensive training program using a variety of mindfulness practices, both formal and informal. In its standard form, MBSR is an 8-week group program with up to 35 participants who meet weekly for 2.5 to 3 hours, with a 6-hour silent retreat occurring on a weekend between Classes 6 and 7. Participants are required to practice mindfulness as "homework" for a total of 45 minutes, 6 days each week during the course of the program (guided CDs are provided to encourage practice). The primary mindfulness practices taught in MBSR include the body scan, sitting meditation, walking meditation, gentle yoga, and informal daily mindfulness practice. Some didactic teaching of mindfulness concepts occurs each week, with time for participant processing of their experience, feedback from facilitators, and group discussion around challenges to practice and insights that may have arisen from it. The course atmosphere is intended to be collaborative and encouraging, with the group facilitator both implicitly modeling and outwardly encouraging the application of mindfulness training-related attitudes of nonjudging, patience, acceptance, beginner's mind, non-striving, letting go, non-attachment, and trust (Shapiro & Carlson, 2009).

Evidence on Mindfulness Training for Healthy Adults

Space limitations preclude an exhaustive review of the now considerable body of research that has examined the effects of MBSR and other mindfulness-based interventions in healthy adult populations. Thus, herein we highlight research studies that have been rigorously designed (typically randomized trials) and/or that have recently opened new areas of investigation. Much of the research in this area has focused on intervention outcomes related to psychological well-being, cognition, and interpersonal relations in a variety of populations, particularly community adults, and more recently in health care professionals and trainees, romantic partners, pregnant women, and parents.

Community Adults

Psychological Distress and Well-Being

To date, much of the mindfulness training research with community adults has focused on reducing psychological distress and improving well-being. For example, in a community sample of distressed adults randomized to either MBSR ($n = 29$) or a wait-list control group ($n = 30$), Nyklíček and Kuijpers (2008) found that relative to controls, MBSR participants reported significant improvements in positive affect, quality of life, and trait mindfulness (Mindful Attention Awareness Scale [MAAS] and Kentucky Inventory of Mindfulness Skills [KIMS]), as well as reductions in perceived stress and vital exhaustion. Lastly, mediation analyses of the MBSR effects on perceived stress, quality of life, and vital exhaustion by improvements in general mindfulness (MAAS) provided evidence that changes in mindfulness were partially responsible for the benefits obtained.

There is also indication that mindfulness training benefits can be sustained for at least several months after training ends. Williams, Kolar, Reger, and Pearson (2001) found that following an MBSR intervention ($n = 59$), university student participants reported significant reductions in daily hassles, psychological distress, and medical symptoms compared to a randomized control group ($n = 44$). Not only were these improvements maintained at the 3-month follow-up, but 81% of the MBSR participants reported continuing to practice the sitting meditation, yoga, or informal practice skills learned during the course.

These studies, like numerous others that have been conducted over the past 15 years, indicate that 8 weeks of MBSR training can lead to improvements in well-being and reductions in stress and distress symptoms that can be sustained following training, although there is little evidence to date that mindfulness practice is responsible for these changes. Also, relatively few studies have tested mindfulness training effects against active control interventions. Such studies would help to determine whether observed benefits are unique to mindfulness training or are related to nonspecific factors such as relaxation, instructor attention, and social support.

One exemplar study conducted by Jain and colleagues (2007) compared a brief version of MBSR (6 hours total) to a somatic relaxation intervention. Medical students, graduate nursing students, and undergraduate students majoring in premedical or prehealth studies were randomized to an MBSR group ($n = 27$), a relaxation group ($n = 24$), or a wait-list control group ($n = 30$). Both intervention groups yielded significant decreases in subjective distress and increases in positive mood states when compared to the wait-list control condition. However, compared to the relaxation intervention, the brief version of MBSR led to reductions in rumination and distraction. Furthermore, reductions in distress were mediated by reductions in rumination. This study provides evidence that even a brief (or low-dose) mindfulness intervention may provide relief from negative mental states such as rumination. In a similar vein, Klatt, Buckworth, and Malarkey (2009) found reductions in perceived stress among university employees receiving a low dose MBSR intervention (n=24) relative to waitlist controls (n=24) (but there was no treatment group difference in sleep improvement).

There is some indication that mindfulness training improvements are not limited to subjective experiences, but extend the neurological and neurobiological outcomes associated with distress and well-being. For example, Davidson and colleagues (2003) conducted a randomized controlled trial of MBSR (vs. wait-list controls) in a work environment. The study examined MBSR's effects on subjective experience, hemispheric asymmetry in electrical activity in the brain associated with positive and negative affect, and immune functioning after vaccination with an influenza vaccine. Relative to control group employees ($n = 16$) those in the MBSR group ($n = 25$) showed significant reductions in trait anxiety and negative affect, and displayed a significant increase in resting alpha-band electrical activity in the left frontal region of the brain, which this and previous studies have associated with approach-oriented emotions. Blood draws obtained at 3–5 weeks and again at 8–9 weeks after the influenza vaccination indicated that the MBSR group exhibited significant increases in antibody titers compared to the control group.

Interestingly, the magnitude of increase in left-sided brain activation predicted the magnitude of antibody titer rise in response to the influenza vaccine, suggesting a neural link from positive affect to health-supportive changes in the immune system. This study also supported the feasibility and benefits of MBSR in a workplace setting. MBSR is brief in duration (8 weeks) and cost-effective (up to 35 individuals per course with one instructor), so mindfulness training might be creatively incorporated into work schedules.

The finding that mindfulness training can impact affect-related neural functioning has recently been extended to an examination of regions linked with emotional responses to distress provocation. Using functional magnetic resonance imaging (fMRI), Farb and colleagues (2010) examined the effects of a modified MBSR program on neural reactivity to a sadness provocation among healthy adult volunteers ($n = 20$) compared to wait-list control participants ($n = 16$). The provocation resulted in activation of neural regions associated with autobiographical memory retrieval and self-referential processing. But compared to wait-list controls, mindfulness trainees showed reduced neural reactivity in these midline cortical regions. They also showed greater activation of right lateralized brain regions associated with visceral and somatosensory areas, and these activations were associated with lower depressive symptoms scores. The authors argued that a balancing of affective and sensory neural networks, reflecting both conceptual and body-based representations of emotion, may support dysphoric emotion regulation, a key underpinning for mental health and well-being (Gross & Muñoz, 1995).

Cognitive Functioning

In addition to its impact on psychological well-being, there is some research indicating that MBSR may impact cognitive outcomes in healthy adult populations. Much of this work has focused on the value of mindfulness training for improving attention processes (see also Tang & Posner, Chapter 5, this volume; Chiesa, Calati, & Serretti, 2011). An early study in this area by Anderson, Lau, Segal, and Bishop (2007) examined the effects of a randomized controlled trial of MBSR on attentional control assessed with a series of computer tasks. Following the MBSR intervention (n = 39), there were no significant improvements in attentional control relative to a control condition (n = 33). Yet improvements in trait mindfulness (Toronto Mindfulness Scale; TMS) were related to improvements in object detection.

In a nonrandomized controlled trial, Jha, Krompinger, and Baime (2007) examined the impact of mindfulness training on attention using three conditions: an MBSR program (n = 17) for adults with no prior mindfulness experience, a retreat condition with experienced meditators (n = 17), and a no-attention control condition with adults without mindfulness experience (n = 17). Participants' attention was measured using the Attention Network Test (ANT; Fan, McCandliss, Sommer, Raz, & Posner, 2002). At Time 1, the experienced meditators in the retreat condition displayed better ANT Conflict Monitoring (ability to prioritize between conflicting tasks and responses) compared to those in the MBSR and control groups. At Time 2 (post 8-week MBSR course), MBSR participants showed significant improvements in their ability to endogenously or voluntarily orient attention compared to the control and retreat participants. The results from this study suggest that mindfulness meditation practice may improve attention-related behavioral responses by improving voluntary response-level and input-level selection processes (Jha et al., 2007). Even brief mindfulness training (4 days, 20 minutes/day) appears to enhance the ability to sustain attention (Zeidan, Johnson, Diamond, David, & Goolkasian, 2010).

Finally, there is evidence that mindfulness training can alter neural network functioning associated with attention. Using functional connectivity MRI (fcMRI), Kilpatrick and colleagues (2011) examined the effects of a standard, 8-week MBSR program on altering intrinsic connectivity networks (ICNs) related to focused attention. Relative to wait-list controls (n = 15), adult women randomly assigned to MBSR (n = 17) exhibited increased connectivity within auditory and visual networks associated with improved attentional focus, enhanced sensory processing, and reflective awareness of sensory experience. Together these studies suggest that even comparatively short-term mindfulness training can produce beneficial effects in attentional and perceptual processes.

Interim Summary

There is now substantial evidence that mindfulness training, particularly using the canonical MBSR program, can enhance mental health-related subjective experience, with some indication that gains are maintained up to several months following training. There is also evidence to suggest that this intervention can alter patterns of neurological functioning consistent with better mental health and attention capacities. There is a need for longer-term studies to address the sustainability of the self-reported and neurophysiological changes observed. Given the preponderance of MBSR studies relying on self-report-based outcomes, there is also a need for studies that can provide convergent, objective evidence to substantiate the reported subjective changes in psychological states given that self-report measures can be influenced by treatment expectancies, demand characteristics, and other response biases.

Evidence on Mindfulness Training for Specific Healthy Adult Populations

Recently, psychoeducational programs modeled after MBSR have begun to emerge in response to the needs of specific healthy adult populations. This research is still nascent and much of it has been based on suboptimal study designs. Yet the research reviewed in this section represents the initial application of mindfulness training to major, well-delineated segments of the adult population, including health care professionals, married couples, expectant mothers, and parents; therefore, the research with each deserves brief discussion.

Health Care Professionals and Trainees

There is considerable evidence that the stress inherent in health care can negatively impact health care professionals. Stress can lead to depression (Tyssen, Vaglum, Gronvold, & Ekeberg, 2001), decreased job satisfaction (Blegen, 1993; Flanagan & Flanagan, 2002), disrupted personal relationships (Gallegos, Bettinardi-Angres, & Talbott, 1990), psychological distress (Jain, Lall, McLaughlin, & Johnson, 1996), and even suicide (Richings, Khara, & McDowell, 1986). Stress also may harm professional effectiveness by disrupting attention (Smith, 1990), reducing concentration (Askenasy & Lewin, 1996), impinging on decision-making skills (Klein, 1996; Lehner, Seyed-Solorforough, O'Connor, Sak, & Mullin, 1997), and reducing providers' abilities to establish strong working relationships with patients (Pastore, Gambert, Plutchik, & Plutchik, 1995). Stress also may lead to increased *burnout* (Spickard, Gabbe, & Christensen, 2002), defined as a syndrome of depersonalization, emotional exhaustion, and a sense of low personal accomplishment. It is clear that health care professionals need support in addressing the numerous stressors inherent in their work.

A number of studies have examined the impact of mindfulness training on mental health and well-being in both physicians and medical students, as well as mental health professionals and trainees. An early randomized controlled trial examined the effects of MBSR on premedical and medical students' subjective experiences relative to wait-list controls (Shapiro, Schwartz, & Bonner, 1998). Increases in empathy and spirituality, and reductions in state and trait anxiety, depressive symptoms, and overall psychological distress, were found in MBSR graduates ($n = 37$). These results were replicated in the wait-list control group ($n = 36$), lending further support to the role of MBSR in distress reduction in these medical trainees.

A more recent randomized controlled trial tested the efficacy of MBSR with a variety of health care professionals—physicians, nurses, social workers, physical therapists, and psychologists (Shapiro, Astin, Bishop, & Cordova, 2005). Compared to the control participants ($n = 20$), those in the MBSR group ($n = 18$) reported increases in self-compassion, a stress resilience trait, and reductions in perceived stress. Because it involved an array of helping professionals, this study suggested that the benefits of MBSR for stress outcomes may generalize across helping professions. But because cohort differences were not tested, it is possible that only certain profession groups showed significant improvements.

Yet there is initial evidence that mindfulness training benefits not only medical personnel, but psychotherapists in training. In a cohort-controlled study with this population, Shapiro, Brown, and Biegel (2007) showed that following a standard MBSR course (n = 22), participants showed significant increases in MAAS mindfulness, positive affect, and self-compassion, and reductions in stress, negative affect, rumination, and both state and trait anxiety, relative to those in structurally equivalent control courses (Psychological Theory or Research Methods) (n = 32). Similar results were found in a recent, uncontrolled study with psychotherapist trainees (n = 25; Shapiro, Jazaieri, & Goldin, 2012), in which improvements in moral reasoning were also observed.

Romantic Partners

Despite their mental and physical health benefits (see Wilson & Oswald, 2005, for a review), romantic relationships at times, and in some couples, also represent a potent source of stress. In an effort to test the value of mindfulness for improving couple functioning, mindfulness-based relationship enhancement (MBRE; Carson, Carson, Gil, & Baucom, 2004; 2006) was developed and first tested in nondistressed couples seeking to enhance their relationships. The belief that healthy individual functioning is an important component to the success of couple functioning was the inspiration for the couple approach to MBSR. Modeled closely after MBSR in terms of format (8 weeks, 2.5-hour sessions, full-day retreat) and content, MBRE includes teaching in both formal (body scan, sitting meditation, walking meditation) and informal (mindfulness during routine activities) techniques, and home practice in them. However, many of the MBSR practices are modified in MBRE to include didactic exercises, and with a particular emphasis on loving-kindness. For example, yoga exercises are done in tandem, wherein one person in the couple supports or facilitates the other in the yoga postures. Other couple-focused adaptations include mindful communication and mindful touch exercises.

Carson and colleagues (2004) demonstrated that following an MBRE program, couples (n = 22) reported improvements in relationship satisfaction, autonomy, relatedness or closeness, acceptance of the other, optimism, spirituality, and relaxation relative to wait-list controls (n = 22). Reductions in relationship distress and psychological distress were also reported. These benefits were sustained at 3-month follow-up point. Also reported were positive associations between mindfulness practice on a given day, as assessed through experience sampling, and positive psychological and interpersonal outcomes up to 2 days following that practice.

Expectant Mothers

Stress during pregnancy can impact both the woman and the developing child (see Hobel, Goldstein, & Barrett, 2008, for a review). New adaptations of mindfulness training programs for pregnant women have been subject to preliminary investigation. In general, the intent of these programs is to improve pregnant women's mood and reduce stress through mindfulness of emotions, cognitions, and bodily sensations via the previously discussed practices used in other programs.

Duncan and Bardacke (2010) conducted a pilot study ($n = 27$) of a 9-week program for expectant couples. As with MBSR, participants were asked to practice formal mindfulness exercises (e.g., body scan, yoga) both during each class and at home. Participants were also encouraged to continue meeting after the course ended to support each other in their mindfulness practices. The study found significant increases in mindfulness practice skills (Five Factor Mindfulness Questionnaire [FFMQ] subscales of Nonjudging and Nonreactivity) and positive affect, and reductions in pregnancy anxiety, depression, and negative affect. While these results are promising, it is important to note that not all findings converge, particularly when examining the longitudinal effects. For example, in a small ($n = 31$) randomized trial of a "Mindful Motherhood" intervention (Vieten & Astin, 2008) with expectant mothers in their second or third trimester, results indicated that increases in positive affect and reductions in perceived stress, state anxiety, depression, and negative affect following the program did not differ from those in control-condition expectant women at the 3-month postnatal follow-up point (though significant and large effects were apparent immediately following the intervention).

Parents

Parenting is a demanding, challenging, and stressful job for many in contemporary societies. Due to associations between parental stress and effective parenting skills (e.g., Webster-Stratton, 1990), and romantic relationship satisfaction (e.g., Lavee, Sharlin, & Katz, 1996), an interest in mindful parenting appears a worthy endeavor. Mindful parenting calls for "a new awareness and intentionality, not only as if what we did mattered, but as if our conscious engagement in parenting were virtually the most important thing we could be doing, both for our children and for ourselves" (M. Kabat-Zinn & Kabat-Zinn, 1997, p. 22). Recently, MBSR and other mindfulness-based interventions have been adapted for stressed parents, including those with children with developmental disorders (e.g., Singh et al., 2007) and parents who are divorced or separated (e.g., Altmaier & Maloney, 2007; Bögels, Lehtonen, & Restifo, 2010). Conjoint parent–child mindfulness interventions have also appeared (e.g., Saltzman & Goldin, 2008).

As an illustration of this research, we briefly discuss findings from Bögels and colleagues' (2010) 12-week mindful parenting program, which was designed to sustain emotional and physical connectedness between parents and children during the parents' divorce. The intention behind this nonrandomized trial was to enhance parents' awareness of the impact of their behavior during interactions with their children, so that they could more skillfully respond in ways that enhanced positive emotional connection. Yet despite increases in TMS trait mindfulness, there were no program effects on parent–child connectedness or on parental stress. Similar null results were obtained by Altmaier and Maloney (2007) in a study of the effects of mindfulness training on parental stress and parent–child interaction among divorced or permanently separated adults.

Interim Summary

Studies of mindfulness training for a variety of specific stressed adult populations are less advanced than those targeting general community adults, and reports of mental health benefits for health care professionals and trainees are promising, as are those showing enhanced romantic relationship satisfaction and functioning; however, the latter findings are based on only one study. Finally, mindfulness-based interventions for parents and expectant parents have shown mixed or null findings. This research is very new, however, and much more is likely to appear in the coming years.

Suggestions for Future Research

In general, mindfulness-based interventions have demonstrated, or have begun to demonstrate, their value for improving cognitive functioning and mental health among nonclinical, community-dwelling adult populations. However, with some notable exceptions, previous research studies have been methodologically limited, and in this section we offer a number of suggestions to enhance the rigor of future research in this important area.

Importance of Randomized Trial Designs

The brevity of this review is testament to the relative paucity of randomized trials in this area of research. Even among those studies reviewed, relatively few used active control interventions, which at best are structurally equivalent to mindfulness interventions under study, and differ only on the purported active ingredients of explicit mindfulness instruction and practice. Active control interventions designed for use in mindfulness trials are now readily available (e.g., MacCoon et al., 2012). Randomized trial designs control for nonspecific factors such as participant expectancies, group support, and instructor attention, and are therefore essential in discerning to what extent the intervention itself contains the active ingredients responsible for change.

Choice of Dependent Variables

We also recommend expansion of the range of outcome data collected. The subtlety and depth of mindfulness training effects do not easily lend themselves to quantification, and qualitative data provide a means to access the subjective experience of trainees from a first-person perspective. By exploring the lived experience of trainees, a more in-depth understanding of the nature of mindfulness training and practices, and their effects, may be obtained than through a reliance on quantified subjective reports.

There is also a need for the collection of objective outcome data, very little of which has been used to demonstrate mindfulness intervention effects among healthy adults. Qualitative and self-report data are valuable in the investigation of subjective changes accruing from mindfulness interventions, which teach an inherently phenomenological quality. Yet behavioral measures of attention and other aspects of cognition, and neural and neurobiological markers of affect, stress, and other mental health and well-being outcomes, are essential both to corroborate subjective reports and to indicate how mindfulness training may impact the brain and body.

In addition, most mindfulness research to date, consistent with the traditional biomedical paradigm, has focused on symptom reduction. Future research with healthy adults might also examine the effects of mindfulness on symptom prevention and health enhancement, as well as on outcomes consistent with the classical goals of meditation, such as the development of exceptional maturity, love and compassion, and lifestyles of service and generosity (see Walsh & Shapiro, 2006). Such research may reveal the impact of mindfulness training on functioning that is both personally and interpersonally optimal.

Sustainability of Training Effects

Most research in this area has to date included only short-term follow-up assessments of the sustainability of intervention gains. We recommend the addition of longer-term follow-up assessments as well (e.g., Shapiro, Brown, Thoresen, & Plante, 2011). This is important not just to gauge the lasting value of intervention effects, but also because mindfulness is a skill that often develops over many months and years, and longer-term follow up is essential to determine the impact of mindfulness practice over time.

Deconstruction of Mindfulness Training Effects

Mindfulness-based interventions have multiple, potentially potent components. These range from nonspecific factors, such as expectancy of benefit and social support, to specific attentional and other factors. Research is needed to determine which components are active ingredients of intervention effects.

Explanation of Training Effects

It is still poorly understood why mindfulness training works, which calls for the study of mediating variables that may account for the changes observed. For example, *decentering* (Segal, Williams, & Teasdale, 2002) or *reperceiving* (Shapiro, Carlson, Astin, & Freedman, 2006), which concerns the capacity to shift perspective from a personal, egocentric viewpoint to a more objective perspective, may be one pathway through which mindfulness training produces salutary change (Shapiro & Carlson, 2009). Also, the frequency and duration of mindfulness practice is thought to be key to training effects, which calls for the careful recording of practice details to determine whether, for example, practice type or practice time can help to explain the effects observed.

Teaching Considerations

Little is known about the most effective methods of teaching mindfulness and for whom. Determining the most effective way to teach mindfulness can be done by comparing different lengths of mindfulness training, as well as different formats for the training, including in-person group versus individual versus Web-based training (e.g., Glück & Maercker, 2011).

Also, little is known about the importance of mindfulness instructors' personal practice of mindfulness for enhancing their ability to teach mindfulness and better understand the experiences of their trainees. There are no "gatekeepers" determining who is and is not qualified to teach mindfulness programs such as MBSR (certification as an MBSR instructor is available but not required to teach). Arguably, without direct experience, concepts remain devoid of experiential grounding, and instructors may lack the capacity to comprehend deeper grades of significance. As Huxley (1945, p. 1) noted, "Knowledge is a function of being." Novak (1989, p. 67) pointed out that in meditation, the "deepest insights are available to the intellect, and powerfully so, but it is only when those insights are discovered and absorbed by a psyche made especially keen and receptive by long coursing in meditative discipline, that they begin to find their fullest realization and effectiveness." Therefore, study of the role of the teacher in intervention effectiveness deserves research attention.

The Role of Instructional Context

A final direction for future research on mindfulness teaching is to examine the role of instructional context. Although Western scientists and therapists have attempted to "decontextualize" contemplative practices so they can be taught in a universally applicable way, there is always context, which, commonly today, is a Western scientific framework (Kabat-Zinn, 1990). It is important to examine the role that context plays in mindfulness and other contemplative practices (Dunne, 2011), including the goals, intentions, motivations, and explicit or implicit ethics embedded in mindfulness training. For example, does the goal of eliminating all suffering have an impact on mindfulness practice (Dunne, 2011) or the way in which it is taught? Are there dangers in stripping mindfulness training of an ethical context and of the traditional spiritual goals of mindfulness practice? And finally, does the specific context in which mindfulness is taught impact the effectiveness of the training?

Conclusions

During the past four decades, research in mindfulness-based interventions for healthy adults has demonstrated significant psychological, neurological, and neurophysiological benefits. We suggest that mindfulness training helps cultivate essential human capacities involving the regulation of intention and values, attention, and healthy attitudes, all of which serve as basic skills leading to greater health and well-being. Research into the applications of this form of mental training to healthy populations is still young, and there is clearly room for improvement in the choice of study designs, a broadening of the scope of outcomes addressed, and other considerations. The invitation to researchers in this area is to bring sensitivity, creativity, and the use of a range of methodological tools to help illuminate the richness, complexity, and possibilities of mindfulness to enhance human welfare.

REFERENCES

Altmaier, E., & Maloney, R. (2007). An initial evaluation of a mindful parenting program. *Journal of Clinical Psychology, 63,* 1231–1238.

Anderson, N. D., Lau, M. A., Segal, Z. V., & Bishop, S. R. (2007). Mindfulness-based stress reduction and attentional control. *Clinical Psychology and Psychotherapy, 14,* 449–463.

Askenasy, J., & Lewin, I. (1996). The impact of missile warfare on self-reported sleep quality. *Sleep, 19,* 47–51.

Blegen, M. A. (1993). Nurses' job satisfaction: A meta-analysis of related variables. *Nursing Research, 42,* 36–41.

Bögels, S. M., Lehtonen, A., & Restifo, K. (2010). Mindful parenting in mental health care. *Mindfulness, 1,* 107–120.

Carson, J. W., Carson, K. M., Gil, K. M., & Baucom, D. H. (2004). Mindfulness-based relationship enhancement. *Behavior Therapy, 35,* 471–494.

Carson, J. W., Carson, K. M., Gil, K. M., & Baucom, D. H. (2006). Mindfulness-based relationship enhancement in couples. In R. A. Baer (Ed.), *Mindfulness-based treatment approaches: Clinician's guide to evidence base and applications* (pp. 309–331). London: Academic Press.

Chiesa, A., Calati, R., & Serretti, A. (2011). Does mindfulness training improve cognitive abilities?: A systematic review of neuropsychological findings. *Clinical Psychology Review, 31,* 449–464.

Davidson, R. J., Kabat-Zinn, J., Schumacher, J., Rosenkranz, M., Muller, D., Santorelli, S. F., et al. (2003). Alterations in brain and immune function produced by mindfulness meditation. *Psychosomatic Medicine, 65*(4), 564–570.

Duncan, L. G., & Bardacke, N. (2010). Mindfulness-based childbirth and parenting education: Promoting family mindfulness during the perinatal period. *Journal of Child Family Studies, 19,* 190–202.

Dunne, J. (2011). Toward an understanding of non-dual mindfulness. *Contemporary Buddhism, 12,* 71–88.

Fan, J., McCandliss, B. D., Sommer, T., Raz, A., & Posner, M. I. (2002). Testing the efficiency and independence of attentional networks. *Journal of Cognitive Neuroscience, 14,* 340–347.

Farb, N. A., Anderson, A. K., Mayberg, H., Bean, J., McKeon, D., & Segal, Z. V. (2010). Minding one's emotions: Mindfulness training alters the neural expression of sadness. *Emotion, 10,* 25–33.

Flanagan, N. A., & Flanagan, T. J. (2002). An analysis of the relationship between job satisfaction and job stress in correctional nurses. *Research in Nursing and Health, 25,* 282–294.

Gallegos, K., Bettinardi-Angres, K., & Talbott, G. (1990). The effect of physician impairment on the family. *Maryland Medical Journal, 39,* 1001–1007.

Glück, T., & Maercker, A. (2011). A randomised controlled pilot study of a brief, web-based mindfulness training. *BMC Psychiatry, 11,* 1–12.

Gross, J. J., & Muñoz, R. F. (1995). Emotion regulation and mental health. *Clinical Psychology: Science and Practice, 2,* 151–164.

Hobel, C. J., Goldstein, A., & Barrett, E. S. (2008). Psychosocial stress and pregnancy outcome. *Clinical Obstetrics and Gynecology, 51,* 333–348.

Huxley, A. (1945). *The perennial philosophy.* London: Chatto & Windus.

Jain, S., Shapiro, S. L., Swanick, S., Roesch, S. C., Mills, P. J., Bell, I., et al. (2007). A randomized controlled trial of mindfulness meditation versus relaxation training: Effects on distress, positive states of mind, rumination, and distraction. *Annals of Behavioral Medicine, 33,* 11–21.

Jain, V., Lall, R., McLaughlin, D., & Johnson, W. (1996). Effects of locus of control, occupational stress, and psychological distress on job satisfaction among nurses. *Psychological Reports, 78,* 1256–1258.

Jha, A. P., Krompinger, J., & Baime, M. J. (2007). Mindfulness training modifies subsystems of attention. *Cognitive, Affective, and Behavioral Neuroscience, 7,* 109–119.

Kabat-Zinn, J. (1990). *Full catastrophe living: Using the wisdom of your body and mind to face stress, pain and illness.* New York: Delacorte.

Kabat-Zinn, M., & Kabat-Zinn, J. (1997). *Everyday blessings: The inner work of mindful parenting.* New York: Hyperion.

Kilpatrick, L. A., Suyenobu, B. Y., Smith, S. R., Bueller, J. A., Goodman, T., Creswell, J. D., et al. (2011). Impact of mindfulness-based stress reduction training on intrinsic brain connectivity. *NeuroImage, 56,* 290–298.

Klein, G. (1996). The effect of acute stressors on decision making. In J. Driskell & E. Salas (Eds.), *Stress and human performance* (pp. 48–88). Mahwah, NJ: Erlbaum.

Klatt, M. D., Buckworth, J., & Malarkey, W. B. (2009). Effects of low-dose mindfulness-based stress reduction (MBSR-ld) on working adults. *Health Education and Behavior, 36,* 601–614.

Lavee, Y., Sharlin, S., & Katz, R. (1996). The effect of parental stress on marital quality. *Journal of Family Studies, 17,* 114–135.

Lehner, P., Seyed-Solorforough, M., O'Connor, M., Sak, S., & Mullin, T. (1997). Cognitive biases and time stress in team decision making. *IEEE Transactions on Systems, Man, and Cybernetics, 27,* 698–703.

MacCoon, D. G., Imel, Z. E., Rosenkranz, M. A., Sheftel, J. G., Weng, H. Y., Sullivan, J. C., et al. (2012). The validation of an active control intervention for mindfulness based stress reduction (MBSR). *Behaviour Research and Therapy, 50,* 3–12.

Novak, P. (1989). Buddhist meditation and the great chain of being: Some misgivings. *Listening, 24,* 67–78.

Nyklíček, I., & Kuijpers, K. F. (2008). Effects of mindfulness-based stress reduction Intervention on psychological well-being and quality of life: Is increased mindfulness indeed the mechanism? *Annals of Behavior Medicine, 35,* 331–340.

Pastore, F. R., Gambert, S. R., Plutchik, A., & Plutchik, R. (1995). Empathy training for medical students. Unpublished manuscript, New York Medical College, Valhalla, NY.

Richings, J. C., Khara, G. S., & McDowell, M. (1986). Suicide in young doctors. *British Journal of Psychiatry, 149,* 475–478.

Roth, B. (2001). Mindfulness-based stress reduction at the Yale School of Nursing. *Yale Journal of Biology and Medicine, 74,* 249–258.

Saltzman, A., & Goldin, P. (2008). Mindfulness based stress reduction for school-age children. In S. C. Hayes & L. A. Greco (Eds.), *Acceptance and mindfulness interventions for children, adolescents and families* (pp. 139–161). Oakland, CA: New Harbinger.

Segal, Z. V., Williams, J. M. G., & Teasdale, J. (2002). *Mindfulness-based cognitive therapy for depression: A new approach to preventing relapse.* New York: Guilford Press.

Shapiro, S. L., Astin, J. A., Bishop, S. R., & Cordova, M. (2005). Mindfulness-based stress reduction for health care professionals: Results from a randomized trial. *International Journal of Stress Management, 12,* 164–176.

Shapiro, S. L., Brown, K. W., & Biegel, G. M. (2007). Teaching self-care to caregivers: Effects of mindfulness-based stress reduction on the mental health of therapists in training. *Training and Education in Professional Psychology, 1*(2), 105–115.

Shapiro, S. L., Brown, K. W., Thoresen, C., & Plante, T. G. (2011). The moderation of mindfulness-based stress reduction effects by trait mindfulness: Results from a randomized controlled trial. *Journal of Clinical Psychology, 67,* 267–277.

Shapiro, S. L., & Carlson, L. E. (2009). *The art and science of mindfulness: Integrating mindfulness into psychology and the helping professions.* Washington, DC: American Psychological Association Publications.

Shapiro, S. L., Carlson, L. E., Astin, J. A., & Freedman, B. (2006). Mechanisms of mindfulness. *Journal of Clinical Psychology, 62*(3), 373–386.

Shapiro, S. L., Jazaieri, H., & Goldin, P. R. (2012). Mindfulness-based stress reduction effects on moral reasoning and decision making. *Journal of Positive Psychology, 7*(6), 504–515.

Shapiro, S. L., Schwartz, G. E., & Bonner, G. (1998). Effects of mindfulness-based stress reduction on medical and premedical students. *Journal of Behavioral Medicine, 21*(6), 581–599.

Singh, N. N., Lancioni, G. E., Winton, A. S. W., Singh, J., Curtis, W. J., Wahler, R. G., et al. (2007). Mindful parenting decreases aggression and increases social behavior in children with developmental disabilities. *Behavior Modification, 31,* 749–771.

Smith, A. (1990). Stress and information processing. In M. Johnston & M. L. Wallace (Eds.), *Stress and medical procedures* (p. 184). Oxford, UK: Oxford University Press.

Spickard, A., Gabbe, S., & Christensen, J. (2002). Mid-career burnout in generalist and specialist physicians. *Journal of the American Medical Association, 288,* 1447–1450.

Tyssen, R., Vaglum, P., Gronvold, N. T., & Ekeberg, O. (2001). Suicidal ideation among medical students and young physicians: A nationwide and prospective study of prevalence and predictors. *Journal of Affective Disorders, 64,* 69–79.

Vieten, C., & Astin, J. (2008). Effects of a mindfulness-based intervention during pregnancy on prenatal stress and mood: results of a pilot study. *Archives of Women's Mental Health, 11,* 67–74.

Walsh, A. B., & Shapiro, S. L. (2006). The meeting of meditative disciplines and Western psychology. *American Psychologist, 61,* 1–13.

Webster-Stratton, C. (1990). Stress: A potential disruptor of parent perceptions and family interactions. *Journal of Clinical Child Psychology, 19,* 302–312.

Williams, K. A., Kolar, M. M., Reger, B. E., & Pearson, J. C. (2001). Evaluation of a wellness-based mindfulness stress reduction intervention: A controlled trial. *American Journal of Health Promotion, 15,* 422–432.

Wilson, C. M., & Oswald, A. J. (2005). How does marriage affect physical and psychological health?: A survey of the longitudinal evidence. *IZA Discussion Paper,* No. 1619.

Zeidan, F., Johnson, S. K., Diamond, B. J., David, Z., & Goolkasian, P. (2010). Mindfulness meditation improves cognition: Evidence of brief mental training. *Consciousness and Cognition, 19,* 597–605.

CHAPTER 16

Mindfulness Training for Children and Adolescents

A State-of-the-Science Review

David S. Black

Over 30 years of accumulated scientific research has shown that mindfulness training can benefit adults in numerous ways. Those who are healthy and those with psychiatric and physical health conditions often experience reductions in mental and physical health symptoms, as well as enhanced well-being (see Parts IV and V, this volume). Consequently, several versions of mindfulness training, including mindfulness-based stress reduction (MBSR; Kabat-Zinn, 1990) and mindfulness-based cognitive therapy (MBCT; Teasdale et al., 2000) have earned the designation of "probably efficacious" treatments (Baer, 2003) and have more recently received high (3+ out of 4) *quality of research* and *dissemination* scores as designated by the U.S. Department of Health and Human Services (USDHHS) National Registry of Evidence-Based Programs and Practices (Substance Abuse and Mental Health Services Administration, 2013).

Research on mindfulness training for children and youth has a much shorter history. As of 2013, less than 5% of the over 2,600 scholarly publications on mindfulness pertain to children and adolescents (Black, 2010, 2013). Yet a cursory Internet search indicates that organizations delivering mindfulness training to this population are growing in the United States and around the world. Given the paucity of empirical evidence to parallel this accelerating trajectory of program delivery, the prevailing rationale must be that what is good for adults must also be good for *youth*—a term I use in this chapter to refer collectively to children and adolescents.

However youth live in cognitive, emotional, social, and behavioral worlds that are qualitatively different from those of adults. Consequently, scientific evidence indicating that mindfulness training is beneficial for adults may not generalize to youth.

Additional evidence is needed to determine whether mindfulness training might benefit youth in the same or different ways than have been found to help adults in the various areas of enhanced human health and reduced psychological suffering.

My aim in this chapter is to (1) present a state-of-the-science review of the available empirical evidence on mindfulness training for youth, spanning kindergarten to late adolescent years; (2) provide a discussion on the aggregate evidence and note the most promising and replicated findings that suggest outcomes that yield "probably efficacious" treatment effects; and (3) note limitations in this compendium of literature, and highlight future directions needed to advance the field of research.

Review of Research on Mindfulness Training for Youth

Review Methodology

The terms *child, youth,* and *adolescent* were used to search the most comprehensive mindfulness database available (i.e., Mindfo) that warehouses over 3,000 empirically based mindfulness references, pulling from literature searches conducted every month from PubMed, Ovid, PsycINFO, Web of Science, and Google Scholar (Black, 2013). Mindfo searches the aforementioned databases with the following search terms: *mindfulness, mindfulness meditation, mindfulness-based,* and *mindfulness training,* as well as combinations of these terms. Additionally, citations are received from authors in the scientific community, and table of content searches are conducted for topic-specific journals (e.g., *Mindfulness*). Inclusion criteria for this review included samples under age 19 years (two studies with participants 19 years and older were included given that the vast majority of the sample was under age 19 years), and the study must have tested a mindfulness-based intervention. Excluded were etiological and conceptual studies, as well as articles not written in English.

The current search scanned articles published between January 1966 and March 2013. The year 1966 was selected as a start date because this was when the first empirical paper on mindfulness training appeared. In addition to the computer-assisted searches, bibliographies of previous review papers on the topic (Black, Milam, & Sussman, 2009; Burke, 2010) were scanned to crosscheck for comprehensiveness.

Results of the Review

Table 16.1 presents the sample characteristics, intervention type, study design, treatment modality, and findings for all studies included in the review. The 41 included studies comprised 13 experimental trials (i.e., randomized controlled trials) and 28 quasi-experimental trials (i.e., seven nonrandomized controlled trials, 15 cohort studies, and six case studies). The first-ever study on the topic was published in 2002, indicating a relatively short (11 year) publication history. Training was administered as early as the kindergarten years, and delivery occurred most often in schools (*n* = 18), followed by clinics (*n* = 15), homes (*n* = 4), correctional facilities (*n* = 2), and community locales (*n* = 1). The majority of studies (*n* = 32; 78%) administered training to youth at risk for a prespecified health condition (e.g., heightened blood pressure, psychiatric disorder, conduct problems, drug use), while nine studies intervened with "healthy" youth, indicating that the majority of research is based on *secondary* rather than *primary* prevention of health risk outcomes.

The majority of mindfulness training programs were adapted from the MBSR and MBCT interventions, originally developed for the adult population. Other studies administered select components of these programs or provided mindfulness training in tandem with other psychotherapeutic modalities not part of the original MBSR family of interventions. Where indicated, most all studies reported that adaptations to the adult program were needed for the intervention to be suitable for youth. Examples of adaptations included shortening both the program and the individual training sessions, making didactic instruction relevant for the developmental needs of children, modifying intervention activities (e.g., focusing attention on a stuffed animal rising and falling on the belly), and reducing or omitting home mindfulness practice time.

Study Design Characteristics

Of the 13 randomized controlled trials (RCTs), almost half ($n = 6$) included an active control condition, while the remaining trials implemented a wait-list, treatment-as-usual, or presumed inert (e.g., silent reading) condition as a comparison group. Active control conditions included health education only ($n = 3$), health education or Botvin Lifeskills Training ($n = 1$; two control groups included within this study; Botvin, Eng, & Williams, 1980), arts and crafts ($n = 1$), and problem solving ($n = 1$). Of the seven nonrandomized controlled trials (NCTs), two (29%) used an active control condition, namely, health education ($n = 1$) and arts and crafts ($n = 1$). NCTs with inactive control conditions included wait-list ($n = 4$) and unspecified ($n = 1$) conditions. The 20 remaining quasi-experimental studies comprised small-cohort and single-case study designs, which indicates that almost half of the available literature is limited by lack of appropriate controls to account for artifactual effects on observed outcomes.

Neurocognitive Outcomes

Mindfulness training includes the practice of sustained and nonjudgmental attention to present moment experience—a type of attention that is not bound to habitual, discursive thinking, as is common in daily life. Repeated practice of directing attention in this manner is thought to "strengthen" associated neurocognitive capacities much in the same way that exercise strengthens muscle fibers associated with the specific physical targets of strength training. Therefore, the practice of intentionally directing this form of attention should strengthen the development of executive networks that oversee higher-order control of attention and awareness.

Executive function refers to the "higher order, self-regulatory, cognitive processes that aid in the monitoring and control of thought and action [including] inhibitory control, planning, attentional flexibility, error correction and detection, and resistance to interference" (Carlson, 2005, p. 595). In brief, it is an umbrella term for the system that coordinates attention, planning, decision-making, self-regulation, and goal-directed behaviors (Suchy, 2009), and is associated with brain activity in the posterior medial frontal cortex and the lateral prefrontal cortex (Ridderinkhof, Ullsperger, Crone, & Nieuwenhuis, 2004).

TABLE 16.1. Description of Studies Examining Mindfulness Training among Youth

Study	Age (M ± SD), age range, or grade	N	Program origin/ sample	Study design/ location	Control group	Data points	Treatment duration	Observed changes
Barnert et al. (2014)	14–18 y	29	MM/ incarcerated males	Cohort/ corrections	None	Pre Post	60 min, 1 time/w for 10 w + 7 h retreat	MT group showed improvement in self-regulation at posttest; mindfulness, impulsivity, and perceived stress scores improved but did not reach significance.
Barnes et al. (2004)	12.3 ± 0.6 y	73	MBSR/ healthy, majority AA	RCT/ school	HE	Pre Post	10 min, 2 times/ day for 12 w	MT group showed lowered resting systolic blood pressure, afterschool ambulatory systolic and diastolic blood pressure, afterschool heart rate, and nighttime heart rate compared to controls.
Barnes et al. (2008)	15.0 ± 0.7 y	66	MBSR/AA with eBP	RCT/ school	HE	Pre Post	10 min, 2 times/ day for 12 w	MT group showed lower systolic blood pressure and heart rate during school, and nighttime urinary sodium excretion rate and sodium content compared to controls.

Study	Age	N	Intervention/population	Design	Control	Assessment	Dosage	Outcomes
Beauchemin et al. (2008)	13–18 y	34	MBSR/ learning disabled	Cohort/ school	None	Pre Post	5–10 min, 5 d/w for 5 w	MT associated with reduced trait and state anxiety scores at posttest, and teacher ratings of decreased problem behavior.
Bei et al. (2012)	13–15 y	10	MBCT/poor sleepers	Cohort/ school	None	Pre Post	90 min, 1 time/w for 6 w	MT associated with objective and subjective improvements in sleep quality with effect sizes ranging from small (e.g., total sleep time) to large (e.g., sleep onset latency and sleep quality); small effect size for improvement in anxiety symptoms.
Biegel et al. (2009)	15.4 ± 1.2 y	102	MBSR/ outpatient psychiatry	RCT/clinic	TAU	Pre Post 3-m FU	120 min, 1 time/w for 8 w	MT group showed self-reported improvements in anxiety, depressive symptoms, somatization, self-esteem, mental health, and sleep quality relative to controls; clinicians rated higher DSM Global Assessment of Functioning and diagnosis change for MT group compared to controls at posttest and 3-m FU.

(continued)

TABLE 16.1. *(continued)*

Study	Age (M ± SD), age range, or grade	N	Program origin/ sample	Study design/ location	Control group	Data points	Treatment duration	Observed changes
Black & Fernando (2014)	K–grade 6	409	MM/low SES ethnic minority	Cohort	None	Pre Post 7-w FU	15 min, 3 times/w for 5 w	MT associated with teacher-reported improvements in classroom behavior of their students (i.e., paying attention, self-control, participation in activities, and caring/ respect for others) that lasted up to 7-w FU.
Bögels et al. (2008)	11–17 y	14	MBCT/ external disorder	NCT/clinic	WLC	Pre Post 2-m FU	90 min, 1 time/w for 8 w	MT associated with improvements in personal goal attainment, social and attention problems, self-control, sustained attention, and mindfulness relative to controls at posttest and FU.
Britton et al. (2010)	16.4 ± 1.3 y	55	MBSR/drug abuse	Cohort/ clinic	None	Pre Post 3-m FU 12 m	10 min, 6 times/w for 6 w	Female MT completers showed reduced substance use and substance-related problems at 20-week FU; frequency of MT practice correlated with improved sleep quality and substance use resistance self-efficacy.

288

Study	Age	N	Intervention/population	Design/setting	Control	Assessment	Dose	Outcomes
Broderick & Metz (2009)	16–19 y	137	MBSR/ healthy females	NCT/ school	HE	Pre Post	32–43 min, 2 times/w for 5 w	MT group reported improvements in tiredness, aches/pains, negative affect, sense of calmness, relaxation, and self-acceptance relative to controls.
Coholic et al. (2012)	8–14 y	21	MM/ behavior concern	NCT/ school	Arts and crafts	Pre Post	120 min, 1 time/w for 12 w	MT youth self-reported improved emotional reactivity (i.e., improved ability to regulate the speed and intensity of negative emotional response) relative to controls.
Dellbridge & Lubbe (2009)	17 y	1	MBSR/ healthy females	Case/home	None	Qual	? min, 5 times over 10 w	MT associated with qualitative reports of increased task orientation, personal growth, and self-regulation of attention.
Flook et al. (2010)	7–9 y	64	MBSR/ healthy	RCT/ school	Silent reading	Pre Post	30 min, 2 times/w for 8 w	MT group showed increased behavioral regulation, metacognition, and executive function relative to controls; The largest improvements found for those with low executive function at baseline.

(continued)

TABLE 16.1. *(continued)*

Study	Age (M ± SD), age range, or grade	N	Program origin/ sample	Study design/ location	Control group	Data points	Treatment duration	Observed changes
Gregoski et al. (2011, 2012)	15.1 ± 0.7 y	166	MBSR/AA with eBP	RCT/ school	LifeSkills training and HE	Pre Post	10 min, 7 times/w for 12 w	MT group showed improved hemodynamic function (i.e., systolic blood pressure, diastolic blood pressure, and heart rate) and a trend for sodium handling compared to controls; Only MT reduced blood pressure in those who reported high social stress from exposure to discrimination.
Haydicky et al. (2012)	12–18 y	60	MM/ learning disabled	NCT/clinic	WLC	Pre Post	90 min, 1 time/w for 20 w	MT group improved on parent-rated externalizing behavior, oppositional defiant problems, and conduct problems compared to controls.
Hilt & Pollak (2012)	9–14 y	102	MM/healthy	RCT/ community	Problem solving	Pre Post	One-time 8-min audio	MT and distraction training both reduced state rumination after negative mood induction compared to the problem-solving group.

Study	Age	N	Intervention/population	Design/setting	Control		Duration	Outcomes
Himelstein et al. (2012)	14–18 y	32	MBSR/incarcerated; ethnic minority	Cohort/corrections	None	Pre Post	60 min, 1 time/w for 10 w	MT associated with improvements in self-reported perceived stress and self-regulation.
Joyce et al. (2010)	10–12 y	141	MBSR/healthy	Cohort/school	None	Pre Post	Ten 45-min lessons	MT associated with reduced emotional and behavioral problems and depressive symptoms.
Kerrigan et al. (2011)	13–19 y	10	MBSR/AA high risk	Cohort/clinic	None	Qual	"Standard MBSR" for 8 w	MT associated with qualitative reports of greater awareness and acceptance of thoughts and feelings, reduced stress and hostility, and increased relaxation.
Lau & Hue (2011)	14–16 y	48	MBSR/low achieving	NCT/school	Unspecified	Pre Post	120 min, 1 time/w for 6 w + retreat	MT group self-reported reduced depression and stress combined score, increased mindful presence and personal growth compared to controls.
Lee et al. (2008)	9–13 y	25	MBCT/learning delayed	RCT/clinic	WLC	Pre Post	90 min, 3 times/w for 12 w	MT group showed lower Child Behavior Checklist total score and externalizing problems compared to controls.

(continued)

TABLE 16.1. *(continued)*

Study	Age ($M \pm SD$), age range, or grade	N	Program origin/ sample	Study design/ location	Control group	Data points	Treatment duration	Observed changes
Liehr et al. (2010)	9.5 ± 1.6 y	18	MBSR/ ethnic minority	RCT/ school	HE	Pre Post	15 min, 5 times/w for 10 w	MT group self-reported reduced depressive and anxiety symptoms compared to controls.
Mendelson et al. (2010)	Grades 4–5	98	MM/ethnic minority	RCT/ school	WLC	Pre Post	45 min, 4 times/w for 12 w	MT group reduced problematic involuntary responses to social stress and subcales of rumination, intrusive thoughts, and emotional arousal ($p < .01$) compared to controls.
Napoli et al. (2005)	Grades 1–3	194	MBSR/ healthy	RCT/ school	TAU	Pre Post	45 min, bimonthly for 24 w	MT group self-reported decreased test anxiety scores and increased selected visual attention, and had fewer teacher-rated problems in attention and social skills compared to controls.
Ott (2002)	9 y	1	MBSR/ GERD, nausea	Case/clinic	None	Qual	10 min, twice daily for ? w	MT associated with self-reported improvements in GERD symptoms, medication use, and sleep disturbances.

Study	Age	N	Intervention/Population	Design/Setting	Control	Assessment	Dose	Findings
Pace et al. (2013)	13–17 y	71	MM/foster care, most AA	RCT/clinic	WLC	Pre Post	60 min, 2 times/w for 6 w	MT group showed number of meditation practice sessions inversely correlated with changes in C-reactive protein levels.
Schonert-Reichl & Lawlor (2010)	9–13 y	246	MM/healthy	NCT/school	WLC	Pre Post	45 min, 1 time/w for 9 w	MT group showed self-reported improvements in optimism, teacher-reported domains of socioemotional and attention/concentration competence compared to controls.
Semple et al. (2005)	7–8 y	5	MBCT/anxiety	Cohort/school	None	Pre Post	45 min, 1 time/w for 6 w	MT associated with teacher-rated improvements in adaptive functioning and total internalizing and externalizing problems.
Semple et al. (2010)	9–13 y	25	MBCT/academic problems	RCT/clinic	WLC	Pre Post 3-m FU	90 min, 1 time/w for 12 w	MT group showed fewer attentional problems up to 3-m FU compared to controls; In children with elevated levels of anxiety or behavior problems at baseline, the MT group showed decreased anxiety and behavior problems.
Sibinga et al. (2008)	13–21 y	5	MBSR/AA HIV+	Cohort/clinic	None	Qual	120 min, 1 time/w for 8 w + 3-h retreat	MT associated with self-reported qualitative improvements in positive attitude, behavior regulation, and self-care.

(continued)

TABLE 16.1. (continued)

Study	Age ($M \pm SD$), age range, or grade	N	Program origin/ sample	Study design/ location	Control group	Data points	Treatment duration	Observed changes
Sibinga et al. (2011)	$16.8 \pm ?$ y	33	MBSR/HIV+ at risk	Cohort/ clinic	None	Pre Post	? min, 1 time/w for 9 w	MT associated with reduced hostility, general discomfort, and emotional discomfort; qualitative improvements observed in relationships, schoolwork, physical health, and stress.
Singh et al. (2007)	13.3 ± 0.6 y	3	MM/ conduct disorder	Case/ school	None	Pre Post 6-m FU	15 min, 3 times/w for 4 w	MT associated with decreased aggressive behavior/ bullying at posttest and FU.
Singh et al. (2010)	10–12 y	2	MM/ADHD	Case/home	None	Pre Post 6-m FU	? min, 1 time/w for 12 w	MT associated with maternal report of improved child compliance to parent requests.
Singh, Lancioni, Manikam, et al. (2011)	14–17 y	3	MM/male, autism	Case/home	None	Pre Post 3-y FU	30 min daily for 5 d	MT associated with decreases in sibling- and parent-reported aggressive behavior at posttest and FU.

Study	Age	N	Type/Population	Design/Setting	Control	Measures	Dose	Results
Singh, Lancioni, Singh, et al. (2011)	13–18 y	3	MM/male, Aspergers	Case/home	None	Pre Post 4-y FU	15 min twice daily for 5 d	MT associated with decreases in sibling- and parent-reported aggressive behavior at posttest and FU.
Tan & Martin (2013)	14–17 y	10	MBSR/psychiatric outpatient	Cohort/clinic	None	Pre Post 3-m FU	60 min, 1 time/w for 5 w	MT completers showed improvement in psychological distress, self-esteem, mindfulness, psychological flexibility, and parent-rated child behavior at posttest. At FU, psychological distress decreased from posttest, and all other outcomes maintained their improved posttest levels.
van der Oord et al. (2012)	8–12 y	22	MBSR/ADHD	NCT/clinic	WLC	Pre Post 2-m FU	90 min, 1 time/w for 8 w	MT group showed parent- and teacher-rated improvements in ADHD symptoms of inattention and hyperactivity/impulsivity; Parent-rated improvements were maintained at FU. Self-reported levels of child mindfulness increased at posttest.

(continued)

TABLE 16.1. *(continued)*

Study	Age ($M \pm SD$), age range, or grade	N	Program origin/ sample	Study design/ location	Control group	Data points	Treatment duration	Observed changes
Waltman et al. (2012)	14–17 y	7	MM/ disruptive behavior disorder	Cohort/ clinic	None	Pre Post 1-m FU	60 min, 2 times/w for 7 sessions	MT program completers showed improvement in residential treatment compliance scores at posttest; 50% of completers showed continued improvement at FU.
van de Weijer-Bergsma et al. (2012)	11–15 y	10	MBSR/ ADHD	Cohort/ school	None	Pre Post 2-m FU 4-m FU	90 min, 1 time/w for 8 w	MT associated with improvement in externalizing problems (by father report at posttest), attention problems (by self-report and father-report at 2-m FU), metacognition and behavioral regulation (by father-report at 2-m FU), and computerized attention test speed and false alarms (at posttest).

Study	Age	N	Program/Population	Design/Setting	Control	Assessment	Session	Results
van de Weijer-Bergsma et al. (2014)	8–12 y	199	MBSR/healthy, ethnically diverse	RCT/school	WLC	Base, Pre, Post, 7-w FU	30 min, 2 times/w for 6 w	MT group showed child-reported improvements in analysis of emotions, rumination, and parent-reported excessive somnolence compared to controls; poorest scoring children at baseline showed the most improvement.
Zylowska et al. (2008)	15.6 ± 1.1 y	8	MBSR/ADHD	Cohort/clinic	None	Pre, Post	150 min, 1 time/w for 8 w	MT associated with improvements in ADHD inattention and hyperactivity, attention conflict test, Stroop color–word test, and digit span test; however, youth results could not be independently extracted from those of adults.

Note. $N = 40$ studies. Light gray indicates randomized controlled trial (RCT); dark gray indicates nonrandomized controlled trial (NCT); WLC, wait-list control; TAU, treatment as usual; HE, health education; MBSR, mindfulness-based stress reduction; MBCT, mindfulness-based cognitive therapy; MM, mindfulness meditation (program used mindfulness components drawn from MBSR and related programs); eBP, elevated blood pressure; y, year(s); m, month(s); w, week(s); h, hour(s); Base, baseline; Pre, pretest assessment; Post, posttest assessment; FU, follow-up assessment; Qual, qualitative interview assessment. Copyright 2014 by David S. Black.

Executive function positively correlates with school readiness, prosocial behavior, and enhanced academic achievement (Brock, Rimm-Kaufman, Nathanson, & Grimm, 2009; Bull, Espy, & Wiebe, 2008). Conversely, impairments in childhood executive function are typically identified by poor impulse control, lagged working memory, failure to complete tasks, and disruptive behavior (Anderson, 2002). Therefore, mental training that bolsters executive function may support positive neurocognitive changes in the developing brains of youth. A recent review indicated that attention training methods, including mindfulness training, can improve executive function in children from preschool up to age 7, especially among those with the poorest scores on executive function (Diamond & Lee, 2011).

Evidence for Mindfulness Training

In the current review, three RCTs assessed outcomes that served as proxies for neurocognitive function (see Table 16.1). The aggregated evidence from these experimental studies indicates that among youth ages 6–13, mindfulness training (i.e., mindfulness-based cognitive therapy for children [MBCT-C], Mindful Awareness Practices [MAPs] program, and the Attention Academy Program [AAP]) can produce immediate improvements in measures of executive function, with one study indicating effects lasting up to 3 months in youth with academic problems.

Administering a randomized cross-lagged design with a wait-list control group, Semple, Lee, Rosa, and Miller (2010) tested the effect of MBCT-C among inner-city ethnic/minority youth (ages 9–13 years) with academic problems and elevated levels of anxiety. Parents rated their child's attention using the Attention Problems subscale from the Child Behavior Checklist (Achenbach, 1991). Youth who completed eight or more treatment sessions had fewer parent-rated attention problems than controls, and the improvement persisted at 3-month postintervention follow-up. The clinical significance of this treatment effect was moderate in size (Cohen's $d = 0.42$).

Flook and colleagues (2010) randomized 64 ethnically diverse schoolchildren to the MAPs program or to a silent reading control group. Parents and teachers completed the Behavior Rating Inventory of Executive Function (BRIEF; Gioia, Isquith, Guy, & Kenworthy, 2000) to assess the executive function of the children. Results showed that children with poorer initial executive function showed improved parent- and teacher-reported scores on overall executive function, metacognition, and behavioral regulation after MAPS training compared to controls, with a small effect size (partial $\eta^2 = 0.20$).

Napoli, Krech, and Holley (2005) randomized 194 schoolchildren in grades 1 through 3 to AAP or to class time as usual. Teachers rated children with the Attention Deficit Disorder with Hyperactivity (ADD-H) Comprehensive Teacher's Rating Scale (ACTeRS; Ullmann, Sleator, & Sprague, 1988), and children completed the Test of Everyday Attention for Children (TEA–Ch; Manly, Robertson, Anderson, & Nimmo-Smith, 1998). At posttest, results showed child improvement on the Attention subscale of the ACTeRS ($d = 0.49$) and increased Selective Attention scores on the TEA–Ch ($d = 0.60$) compared to controls.

Given this experimental RCT evidence examining the impact of mindfulness training on neurocognitive outcomes, such training may be considered "probably efficacious" for improving certain executive function measures, especially those of attention in younger youth. This determination is based on that fact that at least two RCTs have shown that mindfulness training outperforms an active or wait-list control group on outcome measures of attention (criteria based on Division 12 Task Force on Promotion and Dissemination of Psychological Procedures [TFPDPP], 1995). However, the outcomes used to date have been self-or second-person reports, and more objective measures of executive function are needed. Aside from assessing executive functioning more directly, such measures sidestep the potential biasing effect that knowledge of group allocation may create in self-, parent-, and teacher reports.

Aggregate findings from quasi-experimental studies generally support findings from the three RCTs outlined earlier, in that mindfulness training was found to be associated with various improvements in self-, parent, and teacher reports, as well as objective measures of attention, with improvements commonly of medium-to-large effect size, maintained in some cases up to 2 months postintervention. There is indication from at least one study that the lowest performing youth on neurocognitive performance measures may benefit most from mindfulness training (e.g., Flook et al., 2010). Child self-reported changes in dispositional mindfulness scores on the Mindful Attention Awareness Scale for Adolescents (MAAS-A; Brown, West, Loverich, & Biegel, 2011) have improved simultaneously with postintervention improvement on parent- and child-rated self-control, as well as attention task performance (Bögels, Hoogstad, van Dun, de Schutter, & Restifo, 2008; van der Oord, Bögels, & Peijnenburg, 2012), suggesting that changes in the active ingredient of training, mindful attention, may partially drive improvements in executive function.

Psychosocial Outcomes

Positive emotions such as joy, hope, and pride are positively associated with academic interest and achievement (Pekrun, Goetz, Titz, & Perry, 2002), whereas negative emotions such as anger, sadness, and anxiety are associated with poorer academic performance, including lower high school completion rates (Pekrun et al., 2002; Roeser, Eccles, & Freedman-Doan, 1999). Greater emotion regulation skills predict children's academic success and productivity in the classroom and on standardized tests, even after researchers control for IQ (Graziano, Reavis, Keane, & Calkins, 2007). To address the importance of socioemotional factors on child development and academic success, the field of study that has emerged—social and emotional learning (SEL)—theorizes that children require socioemotional skills for optimal learning, academic achievement, interpersonal relationships, and health.

SEL skills include recognition and management of emotions, empathy, and maintenance of positive interpersonal relationships (Durlak, Weissberg, Dymnicki, Taylor, & Schellinger, 2011). Developing these skills can provide a foundation for prosocial behaviors, academic achievement, emotional health, and adaptive conduct (Greenberg et al., 2003; Steinberg, 2009). A recent meta-analysis of 213 school-based

SEL interventions targeting youth from kindergarten through high school (Durlak et al., 2011) showed that SEL programs significantly improved prosocial attitudes and behavior, as well as academic test scores and course grades.

Mindfulness training is relevant to this discussion of SEL because the former also aims to develop competence in certain social and emotional faculties. For example, mindfulness training fosters self-awareness of cognitions and emotions, regulation of them, and the cultivation of kindness toward the self and empathy for others. Research findings among adults offer support for the proposal that mindfulness practice can impact psychosocial variables, including socioemotional outcomes. Experimental and correlational studies collectively show that mindfulness training is associated with improvements in emotion regulation, emotional well-being, interpersonal relationships, and stress reduction (in this volume, see Arch & Landy, Chapter 12; Parker, Nelson, Epel, & Siegel, Chapter 13; Shapiro & Jazaieri, Chapter 15; Lynch, Lazarus, & Cheavens, Chapter 18; see also Black, 2014; Black, Sussman, Johnson, & Milam, 2012; Galla, O'Reilly, Kitil, Smalley, & Black, 2014; Greeson, Garland, & Black, 2014). There is also indication of increases in neural activity and gray-matter volume in regions implicated in socioemotional functioning, including the frontoinsular, prefrontal, and limbic regions (see Hölzel et al., 2011, for a review).

Evidence for Mindfulness Training

In this review, nine RCTs assessed psychosocial outcomes of mindfulness training (see Table 16.1). The aggregate evidence from these experimental studies indicates that in youth ages approximately 6 to 18, mindfulness training can produce immediate improvements in depressive symptoms, anxiety symptoms, rumination, externalizing problems, and prosocial skills, with one study indicating some effects lasting up to 3 months postintervention among youth in an outpatient psychiatry clinic. Several of these studies are highlighted below.

Biegel, Brown, Shapiro, and Schubert (2009) randomized 102 children to MBSR + treatment at usual (TAU) or TAU only in an outpatient psychiatric clinic. Participants completed a self-report survey at preintervention, postintervention, and 3-month postintervention follow-up. Results indicated that the MBSR group showed significant improvements in anxiety symptoms ($d = 0.70$), perceived stress ($d = 0.89$), self-esteem ($d = 0.59$), depressive symptoms ($d = 0.95$), and interpersonal sensitivity ($d = 0.82$) at postintervention compared to controls. These medium-to-large effect sizes persisted at the follow-up assessment. MBSR participants were also more likely to show diagnostic improvements in mental health (as rated by treatment allocation-blinded clinicians) over the course of the study, as compared to controls (54 vs. 2%, respectively), especially among those with mood disorders at preintervention assessment. Dosage of sitting mindfulness practice was significantly associated with postintervention and follow-up improvements in depressive and anxiety symptoms, as well as diagnostic change.

In another RCT (Liehr & Diaz, 2010), 18 minority youth in the Mindful Schools program reported significantly reduced depressive symptoms and a trend toward a decrease in anxiety symptoms at postintervention compared to those in a health education condition. Semple and colleagues (2010) reported RCT results indicating that among youth with clinically elevated levels of anxiety at preintervention, mindfulness training produced significant reductions in anxiety symptoms at postintervention. Perhaps this is because a separate RCT showed that even a brief, single-session of mindfulness training can get youth out of a ruminative state after a negative mood induction compared to problem-solving techniques (Hilt & Pollak, 2012); also in youth, rumination has been found to have a strong positive association with anxiety (Muris, Roelofs, Meesters, & Boomsma, 2004).

Given the experimental RCT evidence to date that has examined the impact of mindfulness training on psychosocial outcomes, it may be concluded that such training is "probably efficacious" for reducing anxiety and depressive symptoms among normative youth (i.e., ages approximately 9 to 18) given that at least two RCTs have shown that mindfulness training outperformed an active or wait-list control group on self-report measures of anxiety and depressive symptoms (TFPDPP, 1995). Aggregate findings from quasi-experimental studies mainly support findings from the previously noted RCTs, in that mindfulness training has been associated with improvements in self- and parent-reported measures of youth anxiety, negative affect, hostility, prosocial skills, and externalizing behavior in clinical and healthy samples of youth (e.g., Black & Fernando, 2014; Sibinga et al., 2011; Tan & Martin, 2013). There is initial evidence that some of these psychosocial improvements are associated with increases in dispositional mindfulness (Brown et al., 2011; see, e.g., Tan & Martin, 2013).

Psychobiological Outcomes

A psychobiological perspective on stress can guide our understanding of how mindfulness training may get "under the skin" to modulate biological markers implicated in health and disease states. When the brain receives signals that a stressor exists, it activates a cascade of biological responses in an attempt to meet the demand. The sequence is elaborate and only briefly discussed here (for a review, see Glaser & Kiecolt-Glaser, 2005). First, the hypothalamic–pituitary–adrenal (HPA) axis is activated, and adrenocorticotropic hormone is secreted by the brain's pituitary gland. This hormone circulates in the peripheral blood and triggers the adrenal gland to release additional hormones into circulation—cortisol, adrenaline, and noradrenaline—in order to modulate cardiovascular output, energy, cognition, and behavior. HPA by-products help regulate the sympathetic–adrenal–medullary (SAM) axis inflammatory response to stress, coordinated by the immune system.

This biological cascade initiated by an acute stressor provides energy needed to combat or escape a stressor and promotes immunity against infection and injury (Chrousos & Gold, 1992). Acute stress responses are adaptive to survival; however, chronic stressors represent evolutionarily recent challenges that drive a prolonged and repetitive biological response cascade that can disrupt the ongoing health of the organism. Research has linked chronic stress exposure to cardiovascular disease (e.g., Black & Garbutt, 2002; Everson-Rose & Lewis, 2005) and reduced immunocompetence in adults (Kiecolt-Glaser, Dura, Speicher, Trask, & Glaser, 1991; Kiecolt-Glaser, Glaser, Gravenstein, Malarkey, & Sheridan, 1996; Uddin et al., 2010).

The developing nervous and immune system is sensitive to the psychobiological artifacts of early life stressors (Andersen & Teicher, 2008). Research shows that early childhood exposure to psychosocial stressors, such as physical or sexual abuse or parental loss, predicts changes in the expression of genes for glucocorticoid receptors that are involved in the regulation of the stress hormone cortisol (McGowan et al., 2009). Such exposure alters brain regions critical to stress reactivity and emotion regulation (Hanson et al., 2010). Childhood stressors also predict long-term dysregulation of the HPA axis and neuropeptide function that are important to development of later-life psychopathology such as anxiety and mood disorders (Bremner et al., 2003; Heim & Nemeroff, 2001; Tyrka et al., 2008).

Training in mindfulness appears to encourage stress reduction by curtailing stress-inducing mental "time travel" (e.g., rumination on the past, fear-laden thoughts about the future), which may foster relaxation and promote approach and acceptance stress-coping strategies rather than avoidance strategies. Mindfulness training may also alter brain structure and function in a manner that helps to buffer against dysregulated stress reactivity. For example, evidence indicates that mindfulness training and meditation can (1) activate neural structures that regulate the autonomic nervous system in a manner that increases opportunities for relaxation (Hölzel et al., 2010; Lazar et al., 2000), (2) reduces perceptions of psychological stress (de Vibe, Bjørndal, Tipton, Hammerstrøm, & Kowalski, 2012), (3) boosts immune function parameters (Davidson et al., 2003; SeyedAlinaghi et al., 2012), and (4) attenuates biomarkers of inflammation (Black et al., 2012, 2014; Creswell et al., 2012)—all possibly indicative of a healthy psychobiological profile.

Most studies linking mindfulness training to psychobiological outcomes have focused on adults. However, such training may show similar effects in youth. Children experiencing traumatic stress or low socioeconomic status show elevations in cortisol and other markers of a dysregulated HPA axis (Cicchetti & Rogosch, 2001; Lupien et al., 2005; Tarullo & Gunnar, 2006) that can persist into adulthood (Bremner et al., 2003; Tyrka et al., 2008). Thus, equipping children to manage stress early in life through mindfulness training may help them to regulate psychobiological stress reactivity.

Evidence for Mindfulness Training

In this review, four RCTs assessed psychobiological outcomes (see Table 16.1). Three of these studies examined the effects of a breathing awareness meditation (BAM; Session 1 from MBSR) against active health education control conditions on cardiovascular outcomes in mainly African American youth, with mean ages ranging from 12.3 to 15.1 years (range = 12 to 18 years; Barnes, Davis, Murzynowski, & Treiber, 2004; Barnes, Pendergrast, Harshfield, & Treiber, 2008; Gregoski, Barnes, Tingen, Harshfield, & Treiber, 2011). All three studies had adequately sized samples (range = 66 to 166 participants) with training administered approximately 10 minutes daily for 12 weeks. The aggregate evidence from the three studies indicates that in the mainly African American youth with normotensive or elevated blood pressure, mindfulness training produced immediate postintervention improvements in systolic blood pressure (SBP; daytime SBP d = 0.57–0.81), diastolic blood pressure (DBP; daytime DBP d = 0.41–1.03), and heart rate (HR; daytime HR d = 0.18–0.51). No studies have yet to provide follow-up data, so longer-term effects of such training are unknown.

A separate RCT allocated 71 foster care youth ages 13–17 to either a 6-week program including aspects of mindfulness practice (cognitive-based compassion training; CBCT) or to a wait-list control (Pace et al., 2013). Between-group effects were not significant for C-reactive protein levels (an inflammatory biomarker); however, youth in the CBCT group showed pre- to postintervention reductions in morning salivary C-reactive protein, and this reduction was significantly moderately correlated with the number of homework practice sessions, indicating a health-relevant dosage effect of practice time.

Given the experimental RCT evidence to date that has examined the impact of mindfulness training on physiological outcomes, it may be safe to say that such training is "probably efficacious" for improving systolic blood pressure, diastolic blood pressure, and heart rate in normotensive and high-normotensive African American youth (approximately 12 to 18 years of age) given that mindfulness training outperformed active control conditions in at least two RCTs (criteria based on Division 12 TFPDPP; 1995). Aggregate findings from quasi-experimental studies (see Table 16.1) indicate that mindfulness training was also associated with improvements in self-perceived stress, involuntary reactions to stress, calmness, and relaxation.

Next Steps in Mindfulness Research with Youth

The first review of mindfulness training for youth, published in 2009, documented 10 intervention studies (Black et al., 2009). This review yields four times that number of studies now published, indicating a growing interest in mindfulness training for youth and scientific evaluation of such programs. The currently available studies support the conclusion that mindfulness training is efficacious for some neurocognitive, psychosocial, and psychobiological outcomes, and that this training approach is feasible and acceptable for diverse groups of youth, with no published reports of treatment contraindications. Anecdotes from psychiatric clinical practice suggests that sensory exposure activities used in mindfulness training might aggravate symptoms in youth with a history of bodily trauma (e.g., sexual abuse), but published evidence is needed to address this claim. This is an exciting time for research exploration in this area, yet limitations of the extant research should be considered in order to strengthen the evidence base underlying mindfulness training for youth. Based on the current state of the research, I offer several recommendations for future research.

First, 68% of studies reviewed are quasi-experimental, cohort, and case studies, making much of the available evidence vulnerable to numerous validity threats. More studies are needed that use stringent study designs with active and structurally equivalent control conditions. Second, the majority of studies had sample sizes with less than 40 participants, and assessed multiple outcomes. Future studies will benefit from larger sample sizes, both to power statistical analyses adequately and to aid in generalizability of the obtained findings. Third, more research is needed to test training effects on objective outcomes. Many outcomes reviewed here were based on self- or second-person reports of a subjective nature, which, although informative, are limited by possible response biases and retrospective memory biases, and do not inform about neural and other biological markers of mental and physical health states.

Fourth, mechanisms of action linking mindfulness training to health outcomes are not well understood. More studies are needed to measure training-related change mechanisms. For example, a small number of the studies reviewed here (e.g., Barnert et al., 2014; Bögels et al., 2008) assessed changes in trait mindfulness with scales such as the validated MAAS-A (Brown et al., 2011). Moreover, mindfulness practice time is important to capture because this measure can inform the dosage needed for bringing about significant intervention effects.

Fifth, mindfulness training is highly variable across studies. Research is needed to determine the specific mindfulness practices (e.g., sitting meditation, body scan, movement meditations) and program delivery aspects (e.g., duration of training, level of teacher training) that best fit the needs of youth and induce the largest intervention effects. Also, careful session-by-session descriptions of mindfulness training programs in publications will aid in replication, as will publicly available manualized curricula.

In conclusion, interest in mindfulness training for youth continues to grow, and a stronger evidence base is needed if this training is to demonstrate value in engendering health and preventing disease in youth. High-quality evidence on mindfulness training for youth is relatively sparse, based on an array of training programs, and many studies are plagued by methodological weaknesses. However, evidence is strengthening in specific areas, especially in executive function, depressive and anxiety symptoms, and cardiovascular physiology. Carefully conducted research in the years ahead will offer a more definitive answer as to whether mindfulness training for youth significantly improves neurocognitive, psychosocial, and psychobiological functioning, and beneficially alters developmental trajectories within these important domains.

ACKNOWLEDGMENTS

This project was supported by a research fellowship (No. 5T32MH019925-13 to David S. Black). I would like to thank Kirk Warren Brown for insightful comments on earlier versions of this chapter.

REFERENCES

Studies included in the review are indicated by asterisks (*).

Achenbach, T. M. (1991). *Manual for the Child Behavior Checklist: Ages 4–18, and 1991 profile.* Burlington: University of Vermont, Department of Psychiatry.

Andersen, S. L., & Teicher, M. H. (2008). Stress, sensitive periods and maturational events in adolescent depression. *Trends in Neurosciences, 31*(4), 183–191.

Anderson, P. (2002). Assessment and development of executive function (EF) during childhood. *Child Neuropsychology, 8*(2), 71–82.

Baer, R. A. (2003). Mindfulness training as a clinical intervention: A conceptual and empirical review. *Clinical Psychology: Science and Practice, 10*(2), 125–143.

Barnert, E. S., Himelstein, S., Herbert, S., Garcia-Romeu, A., & Chamberlain, L. J. (2014). Innovations in practice: Exploring an intensive meditation intervention for incarcerated youth. *Child and Adolescent Mental Health, 19*(1), 69–73. (*)

Barnes, V. A., Davis, H. C., Murzynowski, J. B., & Treiber, F. A. (2004). Impact of meditation on resting and ambulatory blood pressure and heart rate in youth. *Psychosomatic Medicine, 66*(6), 909–914. (*)

Barnes, V. A., Pendergrast, R. A., Harshfield, G. A., & Treiber, F. A. (2008). Impact of breathing awareness meditation on ambulatory blood pressure and sodium handling in prehypertensive African American adolescents. *Ethnicity and Disease, 18*(1), 1–5. (*)

Beauchemin, J., Hutchins, T. L., & Patterson, F. (2008). Mindfulness meditation may lessen anxiety, promote social skills, and improve academic performance among adolescents with learning disabilities. *Complementary Health Practice Review, 13*(1), 34–45. (*)

Bei, B., Byrne, M. L., Ivens, C., Waloszek, J., Woods, M. J., Dudgeon, P., et al. (2012). Pilot study of a mindfulness-based, multi-component, in-school group sleep intervention in adolescent girls. *Early Intervention in Psychiatry, 7*(2), 213–220. (*)

Biegel, G. M., Brown, K. W., Shapiro, S. L., & Schubert, C. M. (2009). Mindfulness-based stress reduction for the treatment of adolescent psychiatric outpatients: A randomized clinical trial. *Journal of Consulting and Clinical Psychology, 77*(5), 855–866. (*)

Black, D. S. (2010). Mindfulness research guide: A new paradigm for managing empirical health information. *Mindfulness, 1*(3), 174–176.

Black, D. S. (2013). *Mindfo database.* Los Angeles: Mindfulness Research Guide. Retrieved February 10, 2013, from *www.mindfulexperience.org/mindfo.php.*

Black, D. S. (2014). Mindfulness-based interventions: An antidote to suffering in the context of substance use, misuse, and addiction. *Substance Use and Misuse, 49*(5), 487–491.

Black, D. S., Cole, S. W., Irwin, M. R., Breen, E., St Cyr, N. M., Nazarian, N., et al. (2012). Yogic meditation reverses NF-κB and IRF-related transcriptome dynamics in leukocytes of family dementia caregivers in a randomized controlled trial. *Psychoneuroendocrinology, 38*(3), 348–355.

Black, D. S., & Fernando, R. (2014). Mindfulness training and classroom behavior among lower-income and ethnic minority elementary school children. *Journal of Child and Family Studies, 23*(7), 1242–1246.

Black, D. S., Irwin, M., Olmstead, R., Ji, E., Crabb Breen, E. & Motivala, S. (2014). Tai chi effects on nuclear factor-κB signaling in lonely older adults: A randomized controlled trial. *Psychotherapy and Psychosomatics, 83*(5), 315–317.

Black, D. S., Milam, J., & Sussman, S. (2009). Sitting-meditation interventions among youth: A review of treatment efficacy. *Pediatrics, 124*(3), 532–541.

Black, D. S., Sussman, S., Johnson, C. A., & Milam, J. (2012). Testing the indirect effect of trait mindfulness on adolescent cigarette smoking through negative affect and perceived stress mediators. *Journal of Substance Use, 17*(5–6), 417–429.

Black, P. H., & Garbutt, L. D. (2002). Stress, inflammation and cardiovascular disease. *Journal of Psychosomatic Research, 52*(1), 1–23.

Bögels, S., Hoogstad, B., van Dun, L., de Schutter, S., & Restifo, K. (2008). Mindfulness training for adolescents with externalizing disorders and their parents. *Behavioural and Cognitive Psychotherapy, 36*(02), 193–209. (*)

Botvin, G. J., Eng, A., & Williams, C. L. (1980). Preventing the onset of cigarette smoking through life skills training. *Preventive Medicine, 9*(1), 135–143.

Bremner, J. D., Vythilingam, M., Anderson, G., Vermetten, E., McGlashan, T., Heninger, G., et al. (2003). Assessment of the hypothalamic–pituitary–adrenal axis over a 24-hour diurnal period and in response to neurophysiological challenges in women with and without childhood sexual abuse and posttraumatic stress disorder. *Biological Psychiatry, 54*(7), 710–718.

Britton, W. B., Bootzin, R. R., Cousins, J. C., Hasler, B. P., Peck, T., & Shapiro, S. L. (2010). The contribution of mindfulness practice to a multicomponent behavioral sleep intervention following substance abuse treatment in adolescents: A treatment-development study. *Substance Abuse, 31*(2), 86–97.(*)

Brock, L. L., Rimm-Kaufman, S. E., Nathanson, L., & Grimm, K. J. (2009). The contributions of "hot" and "cool" executive function to children's academic achievement, learning-related behaviors, and engagement in kindergarten. *Early Childhood Research Quarterly, 24*(3), 337–349.

Broderick, P. C., & Metz, S. (2009). Learning to BREATHE: A pilot trial of a mindfulness curriculum for adolescents. *Advances in School Mental Health Promotion, 2*(1), 35–46. (*)

Brown, K. W., West, A. M., Loverich, T. M., & Biegel, G. M. (2011). Assessing adolescent mindfulness: Validation of an adapted mindful attention awareness scale in adolescent normative and psychiatric populations. *Psychological Assessment, 23*(4), 1023–1033. (*)

Bull, R., Espy, K. A., & Wiebe, S. A. (2008). Short-term memory, working memory, and executive functioning in preschoolers: Longitudinal predictors of mathematical achievement at age 7 years. *Developmental Neuropsychology, 33*(3), 205–228.

Burke, C. A. (2010). Mindfulness-based approaches with children and adolescents: A preliminary review of current research in an emergent field. *Journal of Child and Family Studies, 19*(2), 133–144.

Carlson, S. M. (2005). Developmentally sensitive measures of executive function in preschool children. *Developmental Neuropsychology, 28*(2), 595–616.

Chrousos, G. P., & Gold, P. W. (1992). The concepts of stress and stress system disorders. *Journal of the American Medical Association, 267*(9), 1244–1252.

Cicchetti, D., & Rogosch, F. A. (2001). Diverse patterns of neurophysiological activity in maltreated children. *Development and Psychopathology, 13*(3), 677–693.

Coholic, D., Eys, M., & Lougheed, S. (2012). Investigating the effectiveness of an arts-based and mindfulness-based group program for the improvement of resilience in children in need. *Journal of Child and Family Studies, 21*(5), 833–844. (*)

Creswell, J. D., Irwin, M. R., Burklund, L. J., Lieberman, M. D., Arevalo, J. M., Ma, J., et al. (2012). Mindfulness-based stress reduction training reduces loneliness and pro-inflammatory gene expression in older adults: A small randomized controlled trial. *Brain, Behavior, and Immunity, 26*(7), 1095–1101.

Davidson, R. J., Kabat-Zinn, J., Schumacher, J., Rosenkranz, M., Muller, D., Santorelli, S. F., et al. (2003). Alterations in brain and immune function produced by mindfulness meditation. *Psychosomatic Medicine, 65*(4), 564–570.

Dellbridge, C. A., & Lubbe, C. (2009). An adolescent's subjective experiences of mindfulness. *Journal of Child and Adolescent Mental Health, 21*(2), 167–180. (*)

de Vibe, M., Bjørndal, A., Tipton, E., Hammerstrøm, K. T., & Kowalski, K. (2012). Mindfulness based stress reduction (MBSR) for improving health, quality of life, and social functioning in adults. *Campbell Systematic Reviews, 3*, 1–127.

Diamond, A., & Lee, K. (2011). Interventions shown to aid executive function development in children 4 to 12 years old. *Science, 333*, 959–964.

Durlak, J. A., Weissberg, R. P., Dymnicki, A. B., Taylor, R. D., & Schellinger, K. B. (2011). The impact of enhancing students' social and emotional learning: A meta-analysis of school-based universal interventions. *Child Development, 82*(1), 405–432.

Everson-Rose, S. A., & Lewis, T. T. (2005). Psychosocial factors and cardiovascular diseases. *Annual Review of Public Health, 26*, 469–500.

Flook, L., Smalley, S. L., Kitil, M. J., Galla, B. M., Kaiser-Greenland, S., Locke, J., et al. (2010). Effects of mindful awareness practices on executive functions in elementary school children. *Journal of Applied School Psychology, 26*(1), 70–95. (*)

Galla, B., O'Reilly, G., Kitil, J., Smalley, S. L., & Black, D. S. (2014). Community-based mindfulness program for disease prevention and health promotion: Targeting stress reduction. *American Journal of Health Promotion, 29*(2).

Gioia, G. A., Isquith, P. K., Guy, S. C., & Kenworthy, L. (2000). *Behavior Rating Inventory of Executive Function*. Lutz, FL: Psychological Assessment Resources.

Glaser, R., & Kiecolt-Glaser, J. K. (2005). Stress-induced immune dysfunction: Implications for health. *Nature Reviews Immunology, 5*(3), 243–251.

Graziano, P. A., Reavis, R. D., Keane, S. P., & Calkins, S. D. (2007). The role of emotion regulation and children's early academic success. *Journal of School Psychology, 45*(1), 3–19.

Greenberg, M. T., Weissberg, R. P., O'Brien, M. U., Zins, J. E., Fredericks, L., Resnik, H., et al. (2003). Enhancing school-based prevention and youth development through coordinated social, emotional, and academic learning. *American Psychologist, 58*(6–7), 466–474.

Greeson, J., Garland, E., & Black, D. S. (2014). Mindfulness: A transtherapeutic approach for transdiagnostic mental processes. In A. Ie, C. Ngnoumen, & E. Langer (Eds.), *The Wiley Blackwell handbook of mindfulness* (Vol. II, pp. 533–562). Oxford, UK: Wiley Blackwell.

Gregoski, M. J., Barnes, V. A., Tingen, M. S., Dong, Y., Zhu, H., & Treiber, F. A. (2012). Differential impact of stress reduction programs upon ambulatory blood pressure among African American adolescents: Influences of endothelin-1 gene and chronic stress exposure. *International Journal of Hypertension, 2012*, Article No. 510291. (*)

Gregoski, M. J., Barnes, V. A., Tingen, M. S., Harshfield, G. A., & Treiber, F. A. (2011). Breathing awareness meditation and lifeskills training programs influence upon ambulatory blood pressure and sodium excretion among African American adolescents. *Journal of Adolescent Health, 48*(1), 59–64. (*)

Hanson, J. L., Chung, M. K., Avants, B. B., Shirtcliff, E. A., Gee, J. C., Davidson, R. J., et al. (2010). Early stress is associated with alterations in the orbitofrontal cortex: A tensor-based morphometry investigation of brain structure and behavioral risk. *Journal of Neuroscience, 30*(22), 7466–7472.

Haydicky, J., Wiener, J., Badali, P., Milligan, K., & Ducharme, J. M. (2012). Evaluation of a mindfulness-based intervention for adolescents with learning disabilities and co-occurring ADHD and anxiety. *Mindfulness, 3*(2), 151–164. (*)

Heim, C., & Nemeroff, C. B. (2001). The role of childhood trauma in the neurobiology of mood and anxiety disorders: Preclinical and clinical studies. *Biological Psychiatry, 49*(12), 1023–1039.

Hilt, L. M., & Pollak, S. D. (2012). Getting out of rumination: Comparison of three brief interventions in a sample of youth. *Journal of Abnormal Child Psychology, 40*(7), 1157–1165. (*)

Himelstein, S., Hastings, A., Shapiro, S., & Heery, M. (2012). Mindfulness training for self-regulation and stress with incarcerated youth: A pilot study. *Probation Journal,* *59*(2), 151–165. (*)

Hölzel, B. K., Carmody, J., Evans, K. C., Hoge, E. A., Dusek, J. A., Morgan, L., et al. (2010). Stress reduction correlates with structural changes in the amygdala. *Social Cognitive and Affective Neuroscience, 5*(1), 11–17.

Hölzel, B. K., Lazar, S. W., Gard, T., Schuman-Olivier, Z., Vago, D. R., & Ott, U. (2011). How does mindfulness meditation work?: Proposing mechanisms of action from a conceptual and neural perspective. *Perspectives on Psychological Science, 6*(6), 537–559.

Joyce, A., Etty-Leal, J., Zazryn, T., & Hamilton, A. (2010). Exploring a mindfulness meditation program on the mental health of upper primary children: A pilot study. *Advances in School Mental Health Promotion, 3*(2), 17–25. (*)

Kabat-Zinn, J. (1990). *Full catastrophe living: Using the wisdom of your body and mind to face stress, pain, and illness.* New York: Dell.

Kerrigan, D., Johnson, K., Stewart, M., Magyari, T., Hutton, N., Ellen, J. M., et al. (2011). Perceptions, experiences, and shifts in perspective occurring among urban youth participating in a mindfulness-based stress reduction program. *Complementary Therapies in Clinical Practice, 17*(2), 96–101. (*)

Kiecolt-Glaser, J. K., Dura, J. R., Speicher, C. E., Trask, O. J., & Glaser, R. (1991). Spousal caregivers of dementia victims: Longitudinal changes in immunity and health. *Psychosomatic Medicine, 53*(4), 345–362.

Kiecolt-Glaser, J. K., Glaser, R., Gravenstein, S., Malarkey, W. B., & Sheridan, J. (1996). Chronic stress alters the immune response to influenza virus vaccine in older adults. *Proceedings of the National Academy of Sciences, 93*(7), 3043–3047.

Lau, N. & Hue, M. (2011). Preliminary outcomes of a mindfulness-based programme for Hong Kong adolescents in schools: Well-being, stress and depressive symptoms. *International Journal of Children's Spirituality, 16*(4), 315–330. (*)

Lazar, S. W., Bush, G., Gollub, R. L., Fricchione, G. L., Khalsa, G., & Benson, H. (2000). Functional brain mapping of the relaxation response and meditation. *NeuroReport, 11*(7), 1581–1585.

Lee, J., Semple, R. J., Rosa, D., & Miller, L. (2008). Mindfulness-based cognitive therapy for children: Results of a pilot study. *Journal of Cognitive Psychotherapy, 22*(1), 15–28. (*)

Liehr, P., & Diaz, N. (2010). A pilot study examining the effect of mindfulness on depression and anxiety for minority children. *Archives of Psychiatric Nursing, 24*(1), 69–71. (*)

Lupien, S. J., Fiocco, A., Wan, N., Maheu, F., Lord, C., Schramek, T., et al. (2005). Stress hormones and human memory function across the lifespan. *Psychoneuroendocrinology, 30*(3), 225–242.

Manly, T., Robertson, I. H., Anderson, V., & Nimmo-Smith, I. (1998). *Test of Everyday Attention for Children, The (TEA–Ch).* San Antonio, TX: Pearson.

McGowan, P. O., Sasaki, A., D'Alessio, A. C., Dymov, S., Labonté, B., Szyf, M., et al. (2009). Epigenetic regulation of the glucocorticoid receptor in human brain associates with childhood abuse. *Nature Neuroscience, 12*(3), 342–348.

Mendelson, T., Greenberg, M. T., Dariotis, J. K., Gould, L. F., Rhoades, B. L., & Leaf, P. J. (2010). Feasibility and preliminary outcomes of a school-based mindfulness intervention for urban youth. *Journal of Abnormal Child Psychology, 38*(7), 985–994. (*)

Muris, P., Roelofs, J., Meesters, C., & Boomsma, P. (2004). Rumination and worry in non-clinical adolescents. *Cognitive Therapy and Research, 28*(4), 539–554.

Napoli, M., Krech, P. R., & Holley, L. C. (2005). Mindfulness training for elementary school students: The Attention Academy. *Journal of Applied School Psychology, 21*(1), 99–123. (*)

Ott, M. J. (2002). Mindfulness meditation in pediatric clinical practice. *Pediatric Nursing, 28*(5), 487–490. (*)

Pace, T. W. W., Negi, L. T., Dodson-Lavelle, B., Ozawa-de Silva, B., Reddy, S. D., Cole, S. P., et al. (2013). Engagement with cognitively-based compassion training is associated with reduced salivary C-reactive protein from before to after training in foster care program adolescents. *Psychoneuroendocrinology, 38*(2), 294–299. (*)

Pekrun, R., Goetz, T., Titz, W., & Perry, R. P. (2002). Academic emotions in students' self-regulated learning and achievement: A program of qualitative and quantitative research. *Educational Psychologist, 37*(2), 91–105.

Ridderinkhof, K. R., Ullsperger, M., Crone, E. A., & Nieuwenhuis, S. (2004). The role of the medial frontal cortex in cognitive control. *Science, 306*, 443–447.

Roeser, R. W., Eccles, J. S., & Freedman-Doan, C. (1999). Academic functioning and mental health in adolescence patterns, progressions, and routes from childhood. *Journal of Adolescent Research, 14*(2), 135–174.

Schonert-Reichl, K. A., & Lawlor, M. S. (2010). The effects of a mindfulness-based education program on pre-and early adolescents' well-being and social and emotional competence. *Mindfulness, 1*(3), 137–151. (*)

Semple, R. J., Lee, J., Rosa, D., & Miller, L. F. (2010). A randomized trial of mindfulness-based cognitive therapy for children: Promoting mindful attention to enhance social-emotional resiliency in children. *Journal of Child and Family Studies, 19*(2), 218–229. (*)

Semple, R. J., Reid, E. F. G., & Miller, L. (2005). Treating anxiety with mindfulness: An open trial of mindfulness training for anxious children. *Journal of Cognitive Psychotherapy, 19*(4), 379–392. (*)

SeyedAlinaghi, S., Jam, S., Foroughi, M., Imani, A., Mohraz, M., Djavid, G. E., et al. (2012). Randomized controlled trial of mindfulness-based stress reduction delivered to human immunodeficiency virus-positive patients in Iran: Effects on CD4+ T lymphocyte count and medical and psychological symptoms. *Psychosomatic Medicine, 74*(6), 620–627.

Sibinga, E. M. S., Kerrigan, D., Stewart, M., Johnson, K., Magyari, T., & Ellen, J. M. (2011). Mindfulness-based stress reduction for urban youth. *Journal of Alternative and Complementary Medicine, 17*(3), 213–218. (*)

Sibinga, E. M., Stewart, M., Magyari, T., Welsh, C. K., Hutton, N., & Ellen, J. M. (2008). Mindfulness-based stress reduction for HIV-infected youth: A pilot study. *Explore, 4*(1), 36–37. (*)

Singh, N. N., Lancioni, G. E., Manikam, R., Winton, A. S. W., Singh, A. N. A., Singh, J., et al. (2011). A mindfulness-based strategy for self-management of aggressive behavior in adolescents with autism. *Research in Autism Spectrum Disorders, 5*(3), 1153–1158. (*)

Singh, N. N., Lancioni, G. E., Singh, A. D. A., Winton, A. S. W., Singh, A. N., & Singh, J. (2011). Adolescents with Asperger syndrome can use a mindfulness-based strategy to control their aggressive behavior. *Research in Autism Spectrum Disorders, 5*(3), 1103–1109. (*)

Singh, N. N., Lancioni, G. E., Singh Joy, S. D., Winton, A. S. W., Sabaawi, M., Wahler, R. G., et al. (2007). Adolescents with conduct disorder can be mindful of their aggressive behavior. *Journal of Emotional and Behavioral Disorders, 15*(1), 56–63. (*)

Singh, N. N., Singh, A. N., Lancioni, G. E., Singh, J., Winton, A. S. W., & Adkins, A. D. (2010). Mindfulness training for parents and their children with ADHD increases the children's compliance. *Journal of Child and Family Studies, 19*(2), 157–166. (*)

Steinberg, L. (2009). Adolescent development and juvenile justice. *Annual Review of Clinical Psychology, 5*, 459–485.

Substance Abuse and Mental Health Services Administration. (2013). National Registry of Evidence-Based Programs and Practices (NREPP). Retrieved May 28, 2013, from *www.nrepp.samhsa.gov*.

Suchy, Y. (2009). Executive functioning: Overview, assessment, and research issues for non-neuropsychologists. *Annals of Behavioral Medicine, 37*(2), 106–116.

Tan, L., & Martin, G. (2013). Taming the adolescent mind: Preliminary report of a mindfulness-based psychological intervention for adolescents with clinical heterogeneous mental health diagnoses. *Clinical Child Psychology and Psychiatry, 18*(2), 300–312. (*)

Tarullo, A. R., & Gunnar, M. R. (2006). Child maltreatment and the developing HPA axis. *Hormones and Behavior, 50*(4), 632–639.

Task Force on Promotion and Dissemination of Psychological Procedures. (1995). Training in and dissemination of empirically validated psychological treatments: Report and recommendations. *Clinical Psychologist, 48*, 3–23.

Teasdale, J. D., Segal, Z. V., Williams, J. M., Ridgeway, V. A., Soulsby, J. M., & Lau, M. A. (2000). Prevention of relapse/recurrence in major depression by mindfulness-based cognitive therapy. *Journal of Consulting and Clinical Psychology, 68*(4), 615–623.

Tyrka, A. R., Wier, L., Price, L. H., Ross, N., Anderson, G. M., Wilkinson, C. W., et al. (2008). Childhood parental loss and adult hypothalamic–pituitary–adrenal function. *Biological Psychiatry, 63*(12), 1147–1154.

Uddin, M., Aiello, A. E., Wildman, D. E., Koenen, K. C., Pawelec, G., de Los Santos, R., et al. (2010). Epigenetic and immune function profiles associated with posttraumatic stress disorder. *Proceedings of the National Academy of Sciences, 107*(20), 9470–9475.

Ullmann, R. K., Sleator, E. K., & Sprague, R. L. (1988). *ADD-H Comprehensive Teache's Rating Scale (ACTeRS)*. Torrance, CA: Western Psychological Services.

van der Oord, S., Bögels, S. M., & Peijnenburg, D. (2012). The effectiveness of mindfulness training for children with ADHD and mindful parenting for their parents. *Journal of Child and Family Studies, 21*(1), 139–147. (*)

van de Weijer-Bergsma, E., Formsma, A. R., de Bruin, E. I., & Bögels, S. M. (2012). The effectiveness of mindfulness training on behavioral problems and attentional functioning in 1 adolescents with ADHD. *Journal of Child and Family Studies, 21*(5), 775–787. (*)

van de Weijer-Bergsma, E., Langenberg, G., Brandsma, R., Oort, F. J., & Bögels, S. M. (2014). The effectiveness of a school-based mindfulness training as a program to prevent stress in elementary school children. *Mindfulness, 5*, 238–248. (*)

Waltman, S. H., Hetrick, H., & Tasker, T. E. (2012). Designing, implementing, and evaluating a group therapy for underserved populations. *Residential Treatment for Children and Youth, 29*(4), 305–323. (*)

Zylowska, L., Ackerman, D. L., Yang, M. H., Futrell, J. L., Horton, N. L., Hale, T. S., et al. (2008). Mindfulness meditation training in adults and adolescents with ADHD: A feasibility study. *Journal of Attention Disorders, 11*(6), 737–746. (*)

CHAPTER 17

Mindfulness Training to Enhance Positive Functioning

Kirk Warren Brown

Research exploring the benefits of mindfulness training began in clinical settings wherein the predominant focus was the reduction of suffering, both physical and psychological (e.g., Kabat-Zinn, Lipworth, & Burney, 1985). Over the past 40-plus years, the focus of mindfulness training (MT) research on symptom remission and reduction has remained, and indeed has expanded to a broad range of clinical syndromes, including chronic depression, anxiety, personality disorder, chronic pain, psoriasis, and many other conditions. This befits not only the primary mandate of both Western psychology and psychiatry but also that of the historical Buddha, among whose key teachings was concern about the reduction of human suffering in all its forms.

In recent years, another goal shared by psychology and Buddhism has gained attention in mindfulness research, namely, the capacity of MT to optimize psychological functioning. The Buddha's teaching did not stop with suffering reduction; it also emphasized the capacities of mindfulness-based and other forms of contemplative training for the development of wisdom, compassion, and other embodied qualities carrying both personal and interpersonal benefits. The surge of scholarly and empirical research interest in "positive psychology" over the past decade has emphasized a complementary goal, and perhaps because of this convergence, research examining the effect of MT to optimize psychological and behavioral functioning has gained momentum. My goal in this chapter is to show how this research has developed over the past decade and to offer possible directions for the future of this nascent line of inquiry. Along the way, I hope to show that this research can help to support the potential of mindfulness to optimize psychological well-being, not merely as an absence of disease (World Health Organization, 1948) but as a fulfillment of human potentials.

Positive psychology seeks to shift the standard of mental health from what is normative to what represents full or optimal functioning. Sheldon (2011, p. 423) defines the field of study as follows:

> Positive psychology is a positive science . . . with an eye to improving human life and functioning; its practitioners . . . take an appreciative view of the positive aspects of human nature, even if they do not go so far as to assume that human nature is "basically good"; they tend to study topics that are framed in positive terms rather than in polar negative terms; . . . even as they try . . . not to fall prey to wishful thinking and overly rosy visions and so as not to ignore important "negative" aspects of human nature that impact upon their topics.

Scholarly interest in positive psychological functioning is not new; it dates back at least to Aristotle (*eudaimonia*; 1992) and more recently, William James (*healthy mindedness*; 1902). In the 1950s and 1960s, humanistic and existential psychology's emphasis on full functioning (Rogers, 1959), self-actualization (Maslow, 1954), and other hypothesized features of mental health became a self-proclaimed "third force" in psychology (joining psychodynamics and behaviorism). Empirical and particularly quantitative research in positive mental health has gained considerable traction within the past 15 years (e.g., Seligman & Csikszentmihalyi, 2000), and is examining a broad range of qualities, including gratitude, forgiveness, stress resilience, and character expressions of long-standing interest to Buddhism, such as wisdom and compassion. Investigations of the effects of MT on positive functioning have largely followed the pluralistic lead of positive psychology as a whole, examining a range of features that have been ascribed to positive mental health and adaptive functioning.

Evidence for Mindfulness Intervention Effects on Positive Functioning

Mindfulness concerns a fundamental aspect of human functioning—attention—so it may be expected to have impact across numerous psychological domains. And indeed, the effects of MT have been investigated in several major domains wherein positive functioning (as defined already) can occur, specifically, cognition, motivation, emotion, and interpersonal relations. I review evidence for each of these domains in turn, particularly highlighting experimental studies in which random assignment to MT and control conditions occurred because these provide the most compelling evidence that MT, rather than other, perhaps related factors, was responsible for the observed effects. In this review I define MT broadly to include short-term mindfulness trainings (brief laboratory inductions and trainings over several days) and longer-term trainings as exemplified by 8-week mindfulness-based programs such as mindfulness-based stress reduction (MBSR; Kabat-Zinn, 1990), and intensive mindfulness trainings that occur over days or weeks, typically conducted in residential retreat contexts.

Attention

A number of recent studies support the utility of MT for enhancing attentional capacities and attention-related behavioral responses. Much of this work has examined three functionally and neuroanatomically distinct but overlapping attentional subsystems: alerting, orienting, and conflict monitoring. *Alerting* involves achieving and maintaining a state of preparedness; *orienting* directs and limits attention to a subset of possible stimulus inputs; and *conflict monitoring* (or executive control) prioritizes among competing tasks and responses (Fan & Posner, 2004). Also examined in some research is attention switching, the ability to alter the focus of attention in a "flexible and adaptive manner" (Mirsky, Anthony, Duncan, Ahearn, & Kellam, 1991, p. 112). A recent meta-analysis of meditation (including MT) research (Sedlmeier et al., 2012) indicated that MT has a medium effect on attention improvement, broadly construed (average $r = .32$).

A recent review of controlled MT trial effects specifically on cognitive functions (Chiesa, Calati, & Serretti, 2011) indicated that training in focused attention, as is commonly trained in the early stages of mindfulness-based interventions and in intensive mindfulness retreats, was associated with significant enhancements in selective attention (alerting) and executive control. Training in open monitoring, wherein attention is broadened to all salient internal and external stimuli, is sometimes introduced into later stages of some mindfulness interventions and intensive trainings. Several case-controlled studied reviewed by Chiesa and colleagues (2011) indicated that this form of MT enhanced sustained, distributed (unfocused) attention.

Qualifying these findings is the fact that studies are still relatively few, and they examine quite heterogeneous types of MT in terms of the form (e.g., intensive vs. spaced practice), total training duration, and other mindfulness training-specific and nonspecific factors. As Chiesa and colleagues (2011) noted, several methodological limits to extant studies are also apparent, including nonrandomized designs, which leave open the possibility that condition differences on outcomes may be due to pre-existing individual differences and problematic control group conditions (e.g., wait-list controls).

Research conducted since the Chiesa and colleagues (2011) review has lent further support to the claim that MT may improve attention capacities. For example, in an attempt to deconfound attention capacity from task effort on neuropsychological tests of attention, Jensen, Vangkilde, Frokjaer, and Hasselbalch (2012) found that a monetary incentive improved attention task performance across participants randomly assigned to MBSR, nonmindfulness stress reduction, and inactive control groups. Yet from pre- to postintervention, selective attention (alerting) in the MBSR participants improved significantly more than that among participants in the other groups. This finding suggests that mindfulness training itself is associated with attention enhancement, rather than task effort by trainees who may be motivated to perform well, or through indirect stress reduction effects on attention task performance. Further indication that the enhancement of mindfulness is producing improvements in attention comes from research examining the association of dispositional mindfulness with attention capacities. Cheyne, Carriere, and Smilek (2006) found that higher scores on the Mindful Attention Awareness Scale (MAAS; Brown & Ryan, 2003) were related to better regulation of attention, as indicated by fewer attention task-based errors and quicker reaction time. Results from such correlational research are limited by the fact that other factors associated with trait mindfulness may be responsible for better attention performance, but their convergence with the MT research reported already lends support to the conclusion that enhancements in mindful attention can produce improvements in certain types of attentional processing.

Researchers have also begun to investigate neural processes associated with attention enhancements among mindfulness trainees. For example, in an encephalographic (EEG) study of trainees with short-term, intermediate-term, and long-term mindfulness practice experience, Berkovich-Ohana, Glicksohn, and Goldstein (2012) found increases in electrocortical activity in the gamma power range in posterior scalp sites, suggesting increased attention and sensory awareness (for reviews see Lutz, Slagter, Dunne, & Davidson, 2008; Tang & Posner, Chapter 5, this volume).

As stated earlier, attention is a fundamental capacity whose enhancement may have benefits for a wide range of adaptive behaviors. For example, attention is critically important to the mental processing that is central to learning (LaBerge, 1995). Research indicating that MT may enhance alerting (selective attention) points to the possibility that MT may improve children's capacity to learn. In a recent study of multitasking (Foerde, Knowlton, & Poldrack, 2006), attention to a single task produced not just rote learning but an additional ability to generalize the learned information to new situations. There is preliminary evidence that MT may improve attentional capacities in even young children. Biegel and Brown (2011) found that following 5 weeks of MT, children in grades 2 and 3 showed significant improvements in executive attention on the Attention Network Task (ANT), compared to baseline (but not in alerting or orienting). This improvement was sustained at a 3-month follow-up point. This raises the possibility, to be explored in future research, that MT for children may foster not only learning but also the attention-related development of cognitive, emotional, self-regulatory, and social skills associated with positive functioning.

Psychological Well-Being

Over four decades of research with adult student, community, and clinical populations has provided evidence that meditation may reduce negative mental health symptoms and enhance psychological well-being (e.g., Baer, 2003; Brown, Ryan, & Creswell, 2007; Hofmann, Sawyer, Witt, & Oh, 2010). Much of this research has examined the potential benefits of mindfulness-based meditation using the MBSR intervention model (for review, see Shapiro & Jazaieri, Chapter 15, this volume), while several studies have examined intensive retreat experience. For example, in a recent study of individuals engaged in daily mindfulness practice during a 1-month retreat, Orzech, Shapiro, Brown, and McKay (2009) found that relative to wait-list control participants, the retreatants showed significant preretreat to 1-month postretreat follow-up increases in subjective well-being and self-compassion, as well as declines in anxiety.

Importantly, the effects of mindfulness meditation on mental health in students appear to extend beyond those of relaxation, a form of psychophysical self-regulation with which meditation is frequently conjoined and even confused. Common to various relaxation practices is a self-directed intent to relax through imagery techniques or through guided mental, emotional, or somatic exercises. With relaxation comes a release of physical tension that acts to oppose the stress response and creates a calm state of mind and body. In contrast, mindfulness meditation involves a simple noticing of what is taking place in the mind and body without attempts to alter experience.

Recent research provides evidence for unique patterns of psychological response in mindfulness- versus relaxation-based practices. In a randomized controlled trial with 83 medical students, graduate nursing students, and undergraduate students majoring in premedical or prehealth studies, all of whom reported distress, Jain and colleagues (2007) found that monthlong programs in mindfulness meditation and somatic relaxation produced similar salutary effects on distress reduction, while mindfulness was associated with a stronger enhancement of positive mood relative to the relaxation control students (see also Tang et al., 2007). Differences between these practices also appear to translate into psychophysiological effects (e.g., Ditto, Eclache, & Goldman, 2006; Tang et al., 2007).

Such results are potentially important not only for enhancing well-being but also, potentially, for reducing vulnerability to mental health problems (Joseph & Wood, 2010; Ryan, 2005). In addition, positive emotional states in particular have value in enhancing abilities to process and retain new information, and to create patterns of thought that are flexible and creative (Fredrickson, 1998). Furthermore, individuals who report more positive emotions show more constructive and flexible coping, more abstract and long-term thinking, and more successful emotion regulation following stressful events (Fredrickson, 1998).

Many MT studies rely solely on self-reported outcomes, which are vulnerable to response biases, particularly in the short-term interval following training, when responses may be influenced by a positive emotional afterglow of the intervention, or by demand characteristics and other artifacts. Such concerns are ameliorated to an extent by the fact that a number of studies indicate that self-reported gains are maintained months after training ends (e.g., Shapiro, Brown, Thoresen, & Plante, 2011), but the use of more objective measures, including neurological, other psychophysiological, and ecological momentary assessment outcomes, are effective in reducing or eliminating response biases and thereby provide valuable evidence for the mental health effects of MT.

Several studies have examined the impact of MT on neural functioning associated with positive mental states. For example, evidence from electroencephalography (EEG) indicates that at rest, higher alpha-band power in the left prefrontal cortex (PFC), relative to the right PFC, denotes approach motivation and positive affect (Davidson, 1998). In an initial study of the impact of MT on this prefrontal alpha asymmetry, Davidson and colleagues (2003) found that relative to wait-list controls, participant employees in a biotechnology firm receiving MBSR showed more left-sided alpha asymmetry immediately following and 4 months after training, both while at rest and in response to positive and negative autobiographical recall. The magnitude of asymmetry was in turn related to stronger antibody titer response to an influenza vaccine, suggesting a neural correlate of immunological robustness.

There is also an indication that the alpha asymmetrical pattern associated with positive, approach-oriented emotion can occur after only brief MT. College participants trained by Moyer and colleagues (2011) practiced a focused attention form of meditation for 5 to 16 minutes/day for 5 weeks. They exhibited a significant pre- to posttraining shifts toward left-sided alpha asymmetry compared to a wait-list group, though the conditions did not differ in reported positive affect after the training period (perhaps due to low statistical power associated with the small sample). A number of well-conducted, short-term meditation training studies have been reported (see also Tang et al., 2007, 2009) but it remains unknown whether such brief training can produce sustained changes in neural functioning.

Positive Interpersonal Relating

A variety of contemplative traditions emphasize the value of meditation for the cultivation of empathy, compassion, and other positive interpersonal qualities (Walsh & Shapiro, 2006). Mindfulness practice is believed to lead to a felt sense of trust and closeness with others, as well as an enhanced ability to approach stressful interpersonal events as challenges rather than threats (Kabat-Zinn, 1993), perhaps by promoting a capacity to witness thought and emotion so as to inhibit impulsive or destructive actions. Thus, meditation may foster not only healthy day-to-day interpersonal functioning but also adaptive responses to social conflict.

Research examining the effects of meditation on positive interpersonal functioning is still nascent, but is worth noting, given the importance of quality relationships for psychological and even physical well-being (Baumeister & Leary, 1995; Gable & Gosnell, 2011; Ryan & Deci, 2000). In an early report, Tloczynski and Tantriella (1998) examined the effects of focused attention practice via Zen meditation, which bears hallmarks of MT, on college adjustment. Seventy-five undergraduates reporting heightened anxiety were randomized into meditation, relaxation, and control groups. Only the meditation group demonstrated significant improvements in self-reported interpersonal relationship quality. Using an adaptation of the MBSR program for married couples, Carson, Carson, Gil, and Baucom (2004) found that relative to wait-list controls, participants in the mindfulness-based relationship enhancement (MBRE) program reported higher relationship satisfaction, closeness, and acceptance of one another, and lower relationship distress, both at postintervention and 3 months later. Interestingly, more time spent in mindfulness practice on a given day predicted several consecutive days of higher relationship happiness and stress coping efficacy, and lower relationship stress.

Recently, Kemeny and colleagues (2012) trained schoolteachers in mindfulness and other regulatory skills. Compared to wait-list controls in this randomized trial, intervention participants reported increased trait positive affect and showed increased recognition of emotions in others on a behavioral task. They also appeared to activate cognitive networks associated with compassion, and showed reduced hostile behavior in a marital interaction task. These positive interpersonal changes were maintained at 5 months following the intervention.

Empathy is a key social skill that concerns a capacity to understand and identify with the emotional states of others (Deutsch & Madle, 1975). Several recent studies suggest that MT may foster this beneficial quality. For example, Shapiro, Schwartz, and Bonner (1998) found that MBSR increased self-reported empathy in premedical and medical students relative to wait-list controls. Interestingly, these results obtained during a stressful examination period. Similar findings were reported by Shapiro, Brown, and Biegel (2007) among graduate counseling students, and by Birnie, Speca, and Carlson (2010) among community adults.

Group training programs such as MBSR and its adaptations are typically multimodal, and other ingredients besides an increase in mindfulness, such as didactic instruction and social support, may carry responsibility for any MT effects observed. But dispositional mindfulness has also predicted a felt sense of relatedness and interpersonal closeness, as well as more adaptive responses to romantic partner conflict (Barnes, Brown, Krusemark, Campbell, & Rogge, 2007). Since MT has been linked with increased dispositional mindfulness (e.g., Shapiro et al., 2007), Barnes and colleagues' (2007) findings lend support to the claim that MT may help to enhance interpersonal relationship quality.

The research reviewed here suggests that MT may foster capacities for positive interpersonal behavior and healthy social relationships. However, studies are still few in number, and similar to the research on mental health reported earlier, much of the extant evidence is self-reported, which makes it unclear whether MT facilitates changes in observable behavior, and particularly in naturalistic (normal day-to-day) contexts. There is a clear need for behavior-based research in this area, where observable actions are what matter most. Studies could, for example, address the effect of MT on positive interpersonal responses in parent–child, occupational, and other contexts wherein conflicts frequently arise and healthy relationships are key to well-being and adaptive behavior regulation.

Why Should MT Enhance Positive Functioning?

The range of positive outcomes with which MT has been linked suggests a variety of cognitive and emotional processes through which it operates. Efforts to understand these processes are valuable for refining MT programs and interventions to better hone in on and highlight their active ingredients. This may also facilitate the expansion of outcomes under study, and even lead to the development of new training models that highlight the most effective change processes.

Attention

Most fundamentally, as a form of training in attention, MT is thought to foster one or more networks in the attention system, including alerting, orienting, and/or executive control (e.g., Fan & Posner, 2004). The implications of enhanced attentional capacities are broad, as James (1890) recognized, and not just for educational, occupational, and other task-related outcomes, but potentially for many psychological functions and behaviors for which the voluntary control of thought, emotion, and action provide a key support, including emotion regulation, behavior regulation, and mental and physical health. Indeed, there may be few aspects of human behavior for which attention training would not have a positive impact.

Interest and Enjoyment

One way in which attention training may contribute to well-being and happiness is via higher-quality moment-to-moment experiences. Through the direction of attention to present-moment occurrences, mindfulness is thought to add clarity and vividness to experience (Brown & Ryan, 2003), and research indicates that intrinsically motivated and "flow" activities marked by engagement with and attention to what is occurring, yield a sense of enjoyment and vitality (Csikszentmihalyi, 1990; Deci & Ryan, 1985). MT programs such as MBSR emphasize the simple pleasures to be found in the most mundane of activities, and research suggests that mindful attention to quotidian activities such as eating can enhance the enjoyment to be taken in them (e.g., Arch, Brown, Della Porta, & Kiken, 2014).

Self-Regulation

Several psychological theories, including control theory (Carver & Scheier, 1981), processing mode theory (Watkins, 2004; see Chapter 6, this volume), and self-determination theory (Deci & Ryan, 1985; Deci, Ryan, Schultz, & Niemiec, Chapter 7, this volume) propose that attention is fundamental to the regulation of many forms of behavior, and mindful attention may be especially valuable in facilitating the choice of behaviors that are consistent with one's needs, values, and interests (Deci & Ryan, 1980). Enhanced attention may also offer benefit in the automatic, often nonconscious realm of thought, emotion, and behavior, some of which can be maladaptive if unregulated (e.g., depressed mood, unhealthy eating patterns, stereotyping; Langer, 2002). MT may help to disengage individuals from such automaticity, and thereby foster informed and self-endorsed behavioral regulation, as Levesque and Brown (2007) showed in a study of individuals varying in trait mindfulness. Effective self-regulation is a key determinant of psychological well-being, creativity, and other valued outcomes (Ryan & Deci, 2000), so MT may facilitate positive functioning through its effect on self-regulated activity. Research by Tang and colleagues (e.g., 2007, 2009) suggests that mindfulness-integrated training may enhance self-regulation, but it is unclear whether this leads to the kinds of positive outcomes noted previously. Evidence pointing in this direction comes from a series of four studies (Weinstein, Brown, & Ryan, 2009) that examined the role of mindfulness in supporting self-regulation in people under stress. These authors found that dispositionally mindful college students facing various academic stressors made more benign stress appraisals and used more adaptive coping strategies. In turn these more adaptive appraisal and coping responses partially or fully explained the relation between mindfulness and subjective well-being.

Disidentification

Most contemporary forms of MT involve the direction of attention inward to thoughts, emotions, and kinesthetic sensations. Perhaps fundamental to the effects of MT on positive functioning is the disidentification from these phenomena that an individual normally takes to be "me." In what has been called *cognitive defusion* (Hayes, Strosahl, & Wilson, 2012), *decentering* (Fresco et al., 2007), *deautomatization* (Diekman, 1983), *metacognitive awareness* (Bishop et al., 2004), and related terms, the mindfulness trainee can sooner or later learn to recognize and disidentify not just from maladaptive thoughts, emotions, and sensations, which psychotherapy also promotes, but from *all* such experiences; with a capacity for sustained observation of internal experience is theorized to come a deep sense of calm and equanimity (Walsh & Shapiro, 2006).

Learning to bring mindful attention to personal preferences, biases, and emotional tendencies can foster the recognition that awareness of these particular perspectives and tendencies opens possibilities for response that are not caught in or limited by those overlearned, often habitual patterns of thought and emotion (Segal, Williams, & Teasdale, 2002). Indication of this possibility comes from research with both dispositionally mindful individuals and mindfulness-based cognitive therapy (MBCT; Segal et al., 2002) graduates. For example, Brown, Weinstein, and Creswell (2012) found that in a social-evaluative threat context, dispositionally mindful individuals showed lower neuroendocrine (cortisol) activation and lower negative affect in response to stress, and even at baseline, before the stressor began. Brown, Goodman, and Inzlicht (2013) found that more mindful individuals showed lower electrocortical responses to highly arousing emotional images within a second after stimulus presentation, suggesting that early processing of emotionally provocative stimuli may dampen the arising of negative emotional responses. In these studies, mindfulness helped to inoculate against the rising of psychobiological stress and distress rather than simply enhancing better coping with cognitive and emotional responses that had already arisen. A follow-up study of MBCT graduates found lower susceptibility to depressive relapse/recurrence up to a year after mindfulness training among those scoring higher in dispositional mindfulness at the end of training (Michalak, Heidenreich, Meibert, & Schulte, 2008).

Disidentification from personal views and emotional response tendencies may also aid the development of critical thinking skills, including the ability to examine assumptions, discern hidden values, evaluate evidence, and assess conclusions in an objective manner. Such skills may also foster interpersonal harmony and more creative collective thought and action.

Nonattachment

Related to the capacity to disidentify, mindfulness is also thought to promote *nonattachment*, an absence of fixation on rigid ideas about how things ought, should, or need to be, and initial evidence supports this relation (Sahdra, Shaver, & Brown, 2010). The nonattached person is less likely to grasp onto and seek to maintain pleasant events and experiences or to resist unpleasant ones, and this acceptance of the flow of events and circumstances has been shown to promote a variety of forms of subjective well-being and mental health (Sahdra et al., 2010). The practice of mindfulness entails an objective stance on what is occurring—for example, to witness the flow of thought, emotion, and sensation—and this likely fosters a lessening of attachment to what is inherently subject to change in daily life and, consequently, a greater capacity to abide or enjoy what is. Research on nonattachment is still preliminary but may represent an important means through which MT leads to a variety of personal and interpersonal benefits.

Insight

Several of the processes described here, including disidentification and nonattachment, likely encourage insight into psychological and behavioral sources of suffering, which may leverage well-being enhancement or actions taken to facilitate it (Brown et al., 2007). Greater insight into self, others, and human nature promoted by mindfulness is also thought to encourage greater compassion for oneself and for others (Davidson & Harrington, 2002), but research has yet to be conducted to test these relations.

Hypoegoic Functioning

Perhaps underlying many of these processes is a disengagement from *self-concern—* the perceptions, thoughts, beliefs, evaluations, and related feelings people have about themselves that tend to channel and filter contact with reality in self-serving ways (Brown, Ryan, Creswell, & Niemiec, 2008; Leary, 2004; Ryan & Brown, 2003). Mindfulness involves a capacity to "step outside" the cognitive operations that fuel such egoic functioning and its vulnerability to suffering. Without the implicit or explicitly recognized need that reality match or conform to one's desires and expectations can come a greater capacity to meet life on its own terms, and a corresponding sense of ease with oneself and with others. When well-being is no longer contingent on obtaining what is "good" and avoiding what is "bad"—that is, for "me," as viewed through the eyes of the egoic self—the struggle to manage events and experiences lessens considerably, and a capacity to relax into life takes its place.

Future Directions for Mindfulness Interventions to Enhance Positive Functioning

Along with research on positive psychology interventions as a whole, investigation of the value of MT in fostering positive functioning is still in an early stage, but it has enormous potential for informing us about human flourishing. By way of encouragement, I offer two suggestions for future research in this area. First, there is a clear need for inclusion of objective outcomes to complement the study of subjective indices of positive psychological states and behavior. As valuable as self-report measures can be for tapping subjective states, their limits are also well known, especially when solely relied upon to infer ongoing behavior. Measures of brain activation, function, and dynamics, including EEG and functional magnetic resonance imaging (fMRI), provide a window into attention and other cognitive processes, emotional states and traits, and their downstream effects on somatic functioning (e.g., stress responses).

Aside from informing about neural correlates and substrates of these psychological phenomena, neural measures provide key convergent evidence on subjective experiences (see Zeidan, Chapter 10, this volume).

A number of behavioral indices of positive functioning—of an interpersonal nature, for example—are objectively observable and, ultimately, what most matter when evaluating any training program or intervention. For example, altruism is expressed by helping, supporting, and giving, and can be easily observed, as demonstrated in a recent study of compassion training (Davidson, 2012). Even subjective experiences can be tapped more directly (i.e., without memory and other response biases) through ecological momentary assessment methods that capture internal experiences and behaviors as they occur in individuals' day-to-day lives (e.g., Brown & Ryan, 2003; Carson et al., 2004; Hill & Updegraff, 2012).

Second, there is also room to expand the range of outcomes to the study of behaviors, including sustainable happiness (Ekman, Davidson, Ricard, & Wallace, 2005), equanimity, moral maturity, and compassion, that are associated with full human functioning and of increasing interest to mental health professionals (Germer & Siegel, 2012), educators (Shapiro, Brown, & Astin, 2011), and political leaders (Ryan, 2012). Perhaps a key challenge for mindfulness researchers who are interested in optimal functioning will be to focus efforts on the study of highly valued outcomes, not simply familiar ones (Walsh & Shapiro, 2006).

Conclusions

There are enormous benefits to making optimal functioning the standard of mental and physical health, and a perusal of bookstore shelves and best-seller lists suggests that contemporary Western culture is hungry for methods and means that promise a more fulfilling life. Centuries of mindfulness practitioners have attested to the value of this state of mind (and indeed, way of life) for fostering full functioning. Many positive psychological interventions focus on specific behaviors, such as gratitude, forgiveness, and positive emotional states. With its focus on the cultivation of attention, MT trains a fundamental aspect of human functioning and therefore suggests a broad spectrum of benefits, including the enhancements in attention, psychological well-being, and interpersonal relations discussed herein. The science of MT, which early in its fifth decade is still young, is just beginning to disclose those benefits.

REFERENCES

Arch, J., Brown, K. W., Della Porta, M., & Kiken, L. G. (2014). *Mindfulness enhances the positivity of sensory experience: Evidence from food tasting.* Manuscript in preparation.
Aristotle. (1992). *Eudemian ethics, books I, II, and VIII* (Michael Woods, Ed. & Trans.). Oxford, UK: Clarendon Press.
Baer, R. A. (2003). Mindfulness training as a clinical intervention: A conceptual and empirical review. *Clinical Psychology: Science and Practice, 10,* 125–143.
Barnes, S., Brown, K. W., Krusemark, E., Campbell, W. K., & Rogge, R. D. (2007). The role

of mindfulness in romantic relationship satisfaction and responses to relationship stress. *Journal of Marital and Family Therapy, 33,* 482–500.

Baumeister, R. F., & Leary, M. R. (1995). The need to belong: Desire for interpersonal attachments as a fundamental human motivation. *Psychological Bulletin, 117,* 497–529.

Berkovich-Ohana, A., Glicksohn, J., & Goldstein, A. (2012). Mindfulness-induced changes in gamma band activity—implications for the default mode network, self-reference and attention. *Clinical Neurophysiology, 123,* 700–710.

Biegel, G., & Brown, K. W. (2011, April). *Assessing the efficacy of an adapted in-class mindfulness-based training program for school-age children: A pilot study.* Paper presented at the 9th annual conference on Integrating Mindfulness-Based Interventions into Medicine, Health Care, and Society, University of Massachusetts Medical School, Worcester, MA.

Birnie, K., Speca, M., & Carlson, L. E. (2010). Exploring self-compassion and empathy in the context of mindfulness-based stress reduction (MBSR). *Stress and Health: Journal of the International Society for the Investigation of Stress, 26,* 359–371.

Bishop, S. R., Lau, M., Shapiro, S., Carlson, L., Anderson, N. D., Carmody, J., et al. (2004). Mindfulness: A proposed operational definition. *Clinical Psychology: Science and Practice, 11,* 230–241.

Brown, K. W., Goodman, R., & Inzlicht, M. (2013). Dispositional mindfulness and the attenuation of neural responses to emotional stimuli. *Social Cognitive and Affective Neuroscience, 8*(1), 93–99.

Brown, K. W., & Ryan, R. M. (2003). The benefits of being present: Mindfulness and its role in psychological well-being. *Journal of Personality and Social Psychology, 84,* 822–848.

Brown, K. W., Ryan, R. M., & Creswell, J. D. (2007). Mindfulness: Theoretical foundations and evidence for its salutary effects. *Psychological Inquiry, 18,* 211–237.

Brown, K. W., Ryan, R. M., Creswell, J. D., & Niemiec, C. P. (2008). Beyond me: Mindful responses to social threat. In H. A. Wayment & J. J. Bauer (Eds.), *Transcending self-interest: Psychological explorations of the quiet ego* (pp. 75–84). Washington, DC: American Psychological Association.

Brown, K. W., Weinstein, N., & Creswell, J. D. (2012). Trait mindfulness modulates neuroendocrine and affective responses to social evaluative threat. *Psychoneuroendocrinology, 37*(12), 2037–2041.

Carson, J. W., Carson, K. M., Gil, K. M., & Baucom, D. H. (2004). Mindfulness-based relationship enhancement. *Behavior Therapy, 35,* 471–494.

Carver, C. S., & Scheier, M. F. (1981). *Attention and self-regulation: A control-theory approach to human behavior.* New York: Springer-Verlag.

Cheyne, J. A., Carriere, J. S. A., & Smilek, D. (2006). Absent-mindedness: Lapses of conscious awareness and everyday cognitive failures. *Consciousness and Cognition, 15,* 578–592.

Chiesa, A., Calati, R., & Serretti, A. (2011). Does mindfulness training improve cognitive abilities?: A systematic review of neuropsychological findings. *Clinical Psychology Review, 31,* 449–464.

Csikszentmihalyi, M. (1990). *Flow: The psychology of optimal experience.* New York: HarperCollins.

Davidson, R. J. (1998). Affective style and affective disorders: Perspectives from affective neuroscience. *Cognition and Emotion, 12,* 307–330.

Davidson, R. J. (2012). The neurobiology of compassion. In C. K. Germer & R. D. Siegel (Eds.), *Wisdom and compassion in psychotherapy* (pp. 111–118). New York: Guilford Press.

Davidson, R. J., & Harrington A. (Eds.). (2002). *Visions of compassion: Western scientists and Tibetan Buddhists examine human nature.* New York: Oxford University Press.

Davidson, R. J., Kabat-Zinn, J., Schumacher, J., Rosenkranz, M., Muller, D., Santorelli, S. F., et al. (2003). Alterations in brain and immune function produced by mindfulness meditation. *Psychosomatic Medicine, 65*, 564–570.

Deci, E. L., & Ryan, R. M. (1980). Self-determination theory: When mind mediates behavior. *Journal of Mind and Behavior, 1*, 33–43.

Deci, E. L., & Ryan, R. M. (1985). *Intrinsic motivation and self-determination in human behavior.* New York: Plenum Press.

Deutsch, F., & Madle, R. A. (1975). Empathy: historic and current conceptualizations, measurement, and a cognitive theoretical perspective. *Human Development, 18*, 267–287.

Diekman, A. (1983). *The observing self.* Boston: Beacon Press.

Ditto, B., Eclache, M., & Goldman, N. (2006). Short-term autonomic and cardiovascular effects of mindfulness body scan meditation. *Annals of Behavioral Medicine, 32*, 227–234.

Ekman, P., Davidson, R. J., Ricard, M., & Wallace, B. A. (2005). Buddhist and psychological perspectives on emotions and well-being. *Current Directions in Psychological Science, 14*, 59–63.

Fan, J., & Posner, M. I. (2004). Human attentional networks. *Psychiatrische Praxis, 31*, S210–S214.

Foerde, K., Knowlton, B. J., & Poldrack, R. A. (2006). Modulation of competing memory systems by distraction. *Proceedings of the National Academy of Sciences USA, 103*, 11778–11783.

Fredrickson, B. L. (1998). What good are positive emotions? *Review of General Psychology, 2*, 300–319.

Fresco, D. M., Moore, M. T., van Dulmen, M. H., Segal, Z. V., Ma, S. H., Teasdale, J. D., et al. (2007). Initial psychometric properties of the experiences questionnaire: Validation of a self-report measure of decentering. *Behavior Therapy, 38*, 234–246.

Gable, S. L., & Gosnell, C. L. (2011). The positive side of close relationships. In K. M. Sheldon, T. B. Kashdan, & M. F. Steger (Eds.), *Designing the future of positive psychology: Taking stock and moving forward* (pp. 265–279). New York: Oxford University Press.

Germer, C. K., & Siegel, R. D. (Eds.). (2012). *Wisdom and compassion in psychotherapy: Deepening mindfulness in clinical practice.* New York: Guilford Press.

Hayes, S. C., Strosahl, K. D., & Wilson, K. G. (2012). *Acceptance and commitment therapy: The process and practice of mindful change* (2nd ed.). New York: Guilford Press.

Hill, C. L. M., & Updegraff, J. A. (2012). Mindfulness and its relationship to emotional regulation. *Emotion, 12*, 81–90.

Hofmann, S. G., Sawyer, A. T., Witt, A. A., & Oh, D. (2010). The effect of mindfulness-based therapy on anxiety and depression: A meta-analytic review. *Journal of Consulting and Clinical Psychology, 78*, 169–183.

Jain, S., Shapiro, S. L., Swanick, S., Roesch, S. C., Mills, P. J., Bell, I., et al. (2007). A randomized controlled trial of mindfulness meditation versus relaxation training: Effects on distress, positive states of mind, rumination, and distraction. *Annals of Behavioral Medicine, 33*, 11–21.

James, W. (1890). *The principles of psychology, Vols. I and II.* London: Macmillan.

James, W. (1902). *The varieties of religious experience: A study in human nature.* New York: Longman, Green.

Jensen, C. G., Vangkilde, S., Frokjaer, V., & Hasselbalch, S. G. (2012). Mindfulness training affects attention—or is it attentional effort? *Journal of Experimental Psychology: General, 141*, 106–123.

Joseph, S., & Wood, A. (2010). Assessment of positive functioning in clinical psychology: Theoretical and practical issues. *Clinical Psychology Review, 30*, 830–838.

Kabat-Zinn, J. (1990). *Full catastrophe living: Using the wisdom of your body and mind to face stress, pain and illness.* New York: Delacourt.

Kabat-Zinn, J. (1993). Mindfulness meditation: Health benefits of an ancient Buddhist practice. In D. Goleman & J. Garin (Eds.), *Mind/body medicine.* Yonkers, NY: Consumer Reports.

Kabat-Zinn, J., Lipworth, L., & Burney, R. (1985). The clinical use of mindfulness meditation for the self-regulation of chronic pain. *Journal of Behavioral Medicine, 8,* 163–190.

Kemeny, M. E., Foltz, C., Cavanagh, J. F., Cullen, M., Giese-Davis, J., Jennings, P., et al. (2012). Contemplative/emotion training reduces negative emotional behavior and promotes prosocial responses. *Emotion, 12,* 338–350.

LaBerge, D. (1995). *Attentional processing: The brain's art of mindfulness.* Cambridge, MA: Harvard University Press.

Langer, E. (2002). Well-being: Mindfulness versus positive evaluation. In C. R. Snyder & S. J. Lopez (Eds.), *Handbook of positive psychology* (pp. 214–230). New York: Oxford University Press.

Leary, M. R. (2004). *The curse of the self: Self-awareness, egotism, and the quality of human life.* New York: Oxford University Press.

Levesque, C., & Brown, K. W. (2007). Mindfulness as a moderator of the effect of implicit motivational self-concept on day-to-day behavioral motivation. *Motivation and Emotion, 31,* 284–299.

Lutz, A., Slagter, H. A., Dunne, J. D., & Davidson, R. J. (2008). Attention regulation and monitoring in meditation. *Trends in Cognitive Sciences, 12,* 163–169.

Maslow, A. H. (1954). *Motivation and personality.* New York: Harper.

Michalak, J., Heidenreich, T., Meibert, P., & Schulte, D. (2008). Mindfulness predicts relapse/recurrence in major depressive disorder after mindfulness-based cognitive therapy. *Journal of Nervous and Mental Disease, 196,* 630–633.

Mirsky, A. F., Anthony, B. J., Duncan, C. C., Ahearn, M. B., & Kellam, S. G. (1991). Analysis of the elements of attention: A neuropsychological approach. *Neuropsychology Review, 2,* 109–145.

Moyer, C. A., Donnelly, M. P. W., Anderson, J. C., Valek, K. C., Huckaby, S. J., Wiederholt, D. A., et al. (2011). Frontal electroencephalographic asymmetry associated with positive emotion is produced by very brief meditation training. *Psychological Science, 22,* 1277–1279.

Orzech, K. M., Shapiro, S. L., Brown, K. W., & McKay, M. (2009). Intensive mindfulness training-related changes in cognitive and emotional experience. *Journal of Positive Psychology, 4,* 212–222.

Rogers, C. R. (1959). A theory of therapy, personality, and interpersonal relationships as developed in the client-centred framework. In S. Koch (Ed.), *Psychology: A study of a science: Vol. 3. Formulations of the person and the social context* (pp. 184–256). New York: McGraw-Hill.

Ryan, R. M. (2005). The developmental line of autonomy in the etiology, dynamics and treatment of borderline personality disorders. *Development and Psychopathology, 17,* 987–1006.

Ryan, R. M., & Brown, K. W. (2003). Why we don't need self-esteem: On fundamental needs, contingent love, and mindfulness: Comment. *Psychological Inquiry, 14,* 71–76.

Ryan, R. M., & Deci, E. L. (2000). Self-determination theory and the facilitation of intrinsic motivation, social development, and well-being. *American Psychologist, 55,* 68–78.

Ryan, T. (2012). *A mindful nation: How a simple practice can help us reduce stress, improve performance, and recapture the American spirit.* New York: Hay House.

Sahdra, B. K., Shaver, P. R., & Brown, K. W. (2010). A scale to measure nonattachment: A Buddhist complement to Western research on attachment and adaptive functioning. *Journal of Personality Assessment, 92*, 116–127.

Sedlmeier, P., Eberth, J., Schwarz, M., Zimmermann, D., Haarig, F., Jaeger, S., et al. (2012). The psychological effects of meditation: A meta-analysis. *Psychological Bulletin, 138*(6), 1139–1171.

Segal, Z. V., Williams, J. M., & Teasdale, J. D. (2002). *Mindfulness-based cognitive therapy for depression: A new approach to preventing relapse.* New York: Guilford Press.

Seligman, M. E. P., & Csikszentmihalyi, M. (2000). Positive psychology: An introduction. *American Psychologist, 55*, 5–14.

Shapiro, S. L., Brown, K. W., & Astin, J. (2011). Toward the integration of meditation into higher education: A review of research evidence. *Teachers College Record, 113*, 493–528.

Shapiro, S. L., Brown, K. W., & Biegel, G. M. (2007). Teaching self-care to caregivers: Effects of mindfulness-based stress reduction on the mental health of therapists in training. *Training and Education in Professional Psychology, 1*, 105–115.

Shapiro, S. L., Brown, K. W., Thoresen, C., & Plante, T. G. (2011). The moderation of mindfulness-based stress reduction effects by trait mindfulness: Results from a randomized controlled trial. *Journal of Clinical Psychology, 67*, 267–277.

Shapiro, S. L., Schwartz, G. E., & Bonner, G. (1998). Effects of mindfulness-based stress reduction on medical and premedical students. *Journal of Behavioral Medicine, 21*, 581–599.

Sheldon, K. M. (2011). What's positive about positive psychology?: Reducing value-bias and enhancing integration within the field. In K. M. Sheldon, T. B. Kashdan, & M. F. Steger (Eds.), *Designing the future of positive psychology: Taking stock and moving forward* (pp. 421–429). New York: Oxford University Press.

Tang, Y., Ma, Y., Fan, Y., Feng, H., Wang, J., Feng, S., et al. (2009). Central and autonomic nervous system interaction is altered by short-term meditation. *Proceedings of the National Academy of Sciences USA, 106*, 8865–8870.

Tang, Y., Ma, Y., Wang, J., Fan, Y., Feng, S., Lu, Q., et al. (2007). Short-term meditation training improves attention and self-regulation. *Proceedings of the National Academy of Sciences USA, 104*, 17152–17156.

Tloczynski, J., & Tantriella, M. (1998). A comparison of the effects of Zen breath meditation or relaxation on college adjustment. *Psychologia: An International Journal of Psychology in the Orient, 41*, 32–43.

Walsh, R., & Shapiro, S. L. (2006). The meeting of meditative disciplines and Western psychology: A mutually enriching dialogue. *American Psychologist, 61*, 227–239.

Watkins, E. (2004). Adaptive and maladaptive ruminative self-focus during emotional processing. *Behaviour Research and Therapy, 42*, 1037–1052.

Weinstein, N., Brown, K. W., & Ryan, R. M. (2009). A multimethod examination of the effects of mindfulness on stress attribution, coping, and emotional well-being. *Journal of Research in Personality, 43*, 374–385.

World Health Organization. (1948). Preamble to the Constitution of the World Health Organization as adopted by the International Health Conference, New York, 19–22 June, 1946. Retrieved from *www.who.int/about/definition/en/print.html*.

PART V

MINDFULNESS INTERVENTIONS FOR CLINICAL POPULATIONS

CHAPTER 18

Mindfulness Interventions for Undercontrolled and Overcontrolled Disorders

From Self-Control to Self-Regulation

Thomas R. Lynch, Sophie A. Lazarus,
and Jennifer S. Cheavens

Many theoretical accounts of emotion describe emotions as being linked with behavioral *response tendencies* (e.g., Gross, 1998) that have evolved over millennia to serve humans in their quest for survival (LeDoux, 2003). However, success and happiness are often equated with the *ability to inhibit emotion-based response* tendencies—a form of self-control that is often equated with the ability to postpone or suspend acting upon desires, urges, or impulses for immediate gratification in "exchange" for greater future benefits. Indeed, the capacity for self-control is highly valued by most societies, and failures in self-control or 'undercontrol' characterize many of the personal and social problems afflicting modern civilization—including substance abuse, many criminal activities, domestic violence, financial difficulties, teen pregnancy, smoking, and obesity (Baumeister, Heatherton, & Tice, 1994; Moffitt et al., 2011). Yet, too much self-control also can be problematic. Excessive self-control or 'overcontrol' has been linked to social isolation, poor interpersonal functioning, hyperperfectionism, rigidity, lack of emotional expression, and the development of severe and difficult-to-treat mental health problems, such as chronic depression (Asendorpf, Denissen, & van Aken, 2008; Asendorpf & van Aken, 1999; Chapman & Goldberg, 2011; Eisenberg, Fabes, Guthrie, & Reiser, 2000; Lynch & Cheavens, 2008; Meeus, Van de Schoot, Klimstra, & Branje, 2011; Newton & Contrada, 1994; Riso et al., 2003; Zucker et al., 2007). Thus, both ends of the self-regulation spectrum (i.e., undercontrol or overcontrol) are associated with poor social and emotional functioning.

Our purpose in this chapter is to provide an overview of mindfulness-based approaches that target emotion dysregulation—and introduce a theoretical perspective that links mindfulness to the development of optimal self-regulation. We begin our chapter by proposing the utility of accounting for habitual self-control tendencies and introducing a novel neuroregulatory model of socioemotional functioning that outlines a basis for understanding optimal well-being. We also account for individual differences in self-control tendencies that are posited to mediate treatment responses. We then move to a discussion of how mindfulness may be incorporated into the treatment of overcontrolled and undercontrolled personality disorders and related treatment-resistant or chronic problems. We restrict our focus in this chapter to mindfulness-based skills used within dialectical behavior therapy (DBT; Linehan, 1993), a treatment developed for borderline personality disorder (BPD) and related undercontrolled problems that is hypothesized to be effective largely via *the reduction of ineffective action tendencies associated with dysregulated emotion* (Lynch, Chapman, Rosenthal, Kuo, & Linehan, 2006), and radically open dialectical behavior therapy (RODBT; Lynch, in press), a treatment developed for overcontrolled disorders and hypothesized effective largely via *reductions in social-signaling deficits linked to emotional loneliness* (Lynch, Hempel, & Dunkley, in press). Mindfulness training is considered *the core skill* in standard DBT (Linehan, 1993) and is *a crucial skill* in RODBT (Lynch et al., 2013; Lynch, Hempel, & Dunkley, in press). The efficacy of DBT for the treatment of BPD has been demonstrated in several randomized controlled trials (Koons et al., 2001; Linehan, Armstrong, Suarez, Allmon, & Heard, 1991; Linehan et al., 1999, 2006; Turner, 2000; Verheul et al., 2003; see Lynch, Trost, Salsman, & Linehan, 2007, for review). The efficacy of RODBT for overcontrol (OC) has been established in two randomized controlled trials (Lynch, Cheavens, et al., 2007; Lynch, Morse, Mendelson, & Robins, 2003), and two open trials targeting adult anorexia nervosa (Chen et al., 2014; Lynch et al., 2013), and is being further evaluated in an ongoing multicenter randomized controlled study for individuals with OC treatment-refractory depression (Project REFRAMED [REFRActory depression—Mechanisms and Efficacy of radically open Dialectical behavior therapy]). Here we present an overview of mindfulness approaches used both in standard DBT (Linehan, 1993) and in RODBT (Lynch, in press; Lynch et al., 2013; Lynch, Hempel, & Dunkley, in press) and review empirical support or associated relevant literature when it exists. We also briefly review the theoretical and empirical conceptualizations of the mechanisms of mindfulness in DBT treatment—and account for possible differences between strategies targeting BPD and OC. We conclude the chapter by challenging some general assumptions that we believe permeate a majority of mindfulness-based approaches—and outline an alternative means of addressing these limitations.

The Underdeveloped Dialectic

One problem in studying disorders of emotion dysregulation is that researchers have operationalized the construct of dysregulation in differing ways and/or collapsed emotion-eliciting factors and emotion regulatory factors into one construct, which makes comparisons across studies difficult. Moreover, a great deal of theory and research into this area has focused on disorders such as BPD, which is characterized by low inhibitory control, mood dependency, and low distress tolerance (Rosenthal et al., 2008). For this chapter, we define *emotion dysregulation* as broadly referring to deficits in understanding, responding to, and managing emotional responses (see Mennin, Holaway, Fresco, Moore, & Heimberg, 2007). Our definition of dysregulation purposefully separates regulatory factors (e.g., emotion dysregulation) from perceptual or reactive factors (e.g., threat or reward sensitivity or vulnerability factors). This approach allows the model to account for a wider range of disorders that may exhibit differing vulnerability, perceptual, or regulatory styles (see Lynch et al., 2013). Importantly, in contrast to standard DBT, which posits *emotion dysregulation* as the core problem for BPD (Linehan, 1993) and similar undercontrolled problems (Lynch et al., 2006), RO-DBT contends that *emotional loneliness* secondary to *social-signaling deficits* represent the core problem for disorders of overcontrol (Lynch, Hempel, & Dunkley, in press; Lynch et al., 2013).

The three core features most often linked to BPD manifest as extreme emotion dysregulation and labile mood, impulsive responding, and chaotic/disturbed interpersonal relationships (Clarkin, Hull, & Hurt, 1993; Sanislow, Grilo, & McGlashan, 2000; Skodol, Gunderson, et al., 2002; Skodol, Siever, et al., 2002) and involve *failures in being able to apply inhibitory control*. The biosocial theory in standard DBT (Linehan, 1993) was formulated to explain the development and maintenance of BPD. The biosocial theory accounts for the criterion behaviors associated with BPD by proposing a biological–genetic predisposition for heightened emotional vulnerability and impulsivity that transacts with a pervasive invalidating environment to produce the emotion dysregulation, risky behavior, and chaotic interpersonal relationships characteristic of BPD (Crowell, Beauchaine, & Linehan, 2009; Linehan, 1993). In many ways, BPD represents the quintessential undercontrolled (UC) disorder. Yet for individuals characterized by OC, we speculate that there are fundamental genetic–biological and sociobiographical differences that set them apart from UC individuals, and these differences function to create the unique patterns of responding associated with OC (Lynch & Cheavens, 2008; Lynch et al., 2013; Lynch, Hempel, & Dunkley, in press). For example, one fairly obvious theoretical difference between UC and OC is that is that individuals with BPD, and other UC presentations, are hypothesized to be intermittently reinforced for dramatic displays of emotion and/or impulsive behavior (Crowell et al., 2009; Linehan, 1993), whereas persons with OC are hypothesized to be reinforced for appearing to be in control, following rules, being correct, and acting calm or controlled. This has clear implications for incorporating mindfulness into treatments for these disorders; UC problems require interventions designed to enhance constraint or inhibitory control; whereas people with OC problems require interventions designed to relax inhibition and constraint (Lynch, in press; Lynch et al., 2013).

Our approaches in applying mindfulness-based interventions for individuals who represent extreme ends of OC or UC emotional responding are based on a transdiagnostic neuroregulatory model of personality and socioemotional functioning (Lynch et al., 2013). In this model, we posit three basic neuroregulatory components to be important: (1) *neuroceptive tendencies*: the degree to which incoming stimuli are perceived as safe, novel, threatening, rewarding, or overwhelming; these are influenced by individuals' basic temperament interacting with their sociobiographical history; (2) *response tendencies*: the degree to which the evolutionarily disposed autonomic nervous system (ANS) is activated and corresponding behaviors are potentiated by neuroceptive tendencies; and (3) *self-control tendencies*: the degree to which individuals yield to versus inhibit these response tendencies; this tendency also is influenced by both basic temperament and sociobiographical history.

The model addresses prior limitations in the literature regarding the development and maintenance of two broad classes of psychopathology, UC and OC disorders, which largely parallel the well-established division between internalizing and externalizing disorders, first introduced by Achenbach and colleagues (Crijnen, Achenbach, & Verhulst, 1997). Self-control tendencies are hypothesized to exhibit quadratic (inverted-U) relations with psychological well-being with either extreme of chronic OC or UC predicted as most treatment-resistant. UC individuals are hypothesized to be low in constraint, disinhibited, to act impulsively in response to current stimuli, to be high on impulsive risk taking, to lack planning, and to tolerate disorganization. OC individuals are hypothesized to be high in constraint, inhibited, to base actions on consequences, to be risk averse and nonimpulsive, and to prefer structure and order. Importantly, *undercontrol* and *overcontrol* are *not* one-dimensional constructs—that is, overcontrol and undercontrol are not simply opposite ends of a self-control continuum. Instead, they are "labels" used to describe a complex set of biopsychosocial behaviors that can guide treatment decisions. The three core components are embedded into a cyclical process/structure, in which an individual's perceptions of the environment and the accompanying response tendencies are updated continuously (Figure 18.1).

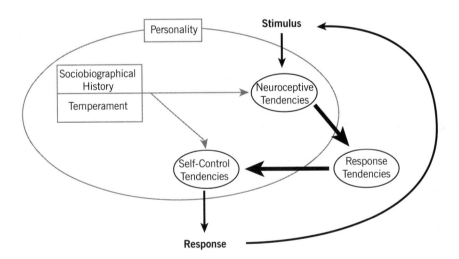

FIGURE 18.1. Neuroregulatory model for personality and socioemotional functioning.

In addition, self-control tendencies are hypothesized to be *key mediators* of subsequent behavioral outputs.[1] Temperamental factors such as positive or negative affectivity, or sociobiographical influences such as trauma or attachment history, are considered important moderators rather than mediators of socioemotional functioning. Thus, from this perspective, what matters most in psychological well-being is the habitual means by which a person regulates or controls internal (e.g., thoughts, sensations, emotions) and external responses/expressions (e.g., facial expressions, verbal expressions, displays of emotion or vulnerability) rather than the absolute degree of emotional experience or severity of traumatic experience. It follows from this that two individuals may share the same traumatic background, but how this negative life event impacts them will vary as a function of self-control or regulatory style. In addition, whereas it is impossible or difficult to change genetic–biological predispositions and/or one's past experiences, it is possible to improve how one controls or regulates one's emotions and interpersonal patterns of relating with others.[2] Thus, targeting self-control tendencies provides an avenue for introducing therapeutic change—and mindfulness is considered an essential means for achieving this.

An Overview of Mindfulness Approaches in DBT Approaches

Mindfulness is an essential component of DBT, and this is evident in several ways. For example, the mindfulness module is repeated formally during the overall sequence of skills training. Additionally, clients receive informal exposure to mindfulness skills and practices via short practices that typically start each DBT skills training class. At the therapist level, mindfulness is singled out as the only component of DBT that is explicitly required to be practiced by the therapist in order to be considered for DBT credentialing (see *depts.washington.edu/brtc/dbtca/wp-content/uploads/2012/01/prerequisites-for-credentialing.pdf*). Additionally, each consultation team meeting commences with a group mindfulness practice, enabling therapists to engage in a practice of mindfulness at least once a week. In some ways, mindfulness, and the larger construct of acceptance, is the component that most distinguishes DBT and other third-wave behavioral treatments from the change-focused behavioral interventions associated with the cognitive revolution.

The mindfulness component of DBT was derived from Christian contemplative practices and Zen practice, and has as its goal "keeping one's consciousness alive to the present reality" (Hahn, 1976, p. 11). RODBT replaces core Zen principles found in standard DBT with principles derived from Malmati-Sufism (Toussulis, 2010; Lynch, Hempel, & Dunkley, in press). The Malamatis are not interested so much in the acceptance of reality or seeing "what is" without illusion (central Zen principles); rather, they look to find fault within themselves and question their self-centered desires for power, recognition, or self-aggrandizement. Mindfulness, within the context of DBT, also stresses letting go of attachments and reducing judgment in the service of acting in a skillful, balanced way. Attachments can be responses to an emotion, material objects, environmental contexts, and/or relationships, among other things. Judgments involve labeling experiences as "good" or "bad" or "should" or "shouldn't" in a way that loses contact with "what is" in a given moment. For example, if something is indeed occurring in the present moment, labeling that very circumstance as something that "should not" happen removes an individual from reality for an instance. Cultivating a mindful stance therefore allows one to experience thoughts, feelings, sensations, and environments as they arise, moment by moment, without harsh judgment or insistence that an experience either change or remain.

Mindfulness as incorporated in DBT differs from other mindfulness approaches such as Mindfulness-Based Stress Reduction (Kabat-Zinn, 1990) and mindfulness-based cognitive therapy (Segal, Williams, & Teasdale, 2002) in several ways. First, given the foundation of behaviorist principles in DBT, mindfulness is viewed as a set of component parts, or behaviors, that is subject to the same principles of reinforcement and punishment as other behaviors. In this vein, the meditation process is distilled down to component parts that are then taught as psychological and behavioral skills to be used in various circumstances (Linehan & Dimidjian, 2003). The consequence of this view of mindfulness is that most DBT mindfulness exercises are shorter and less formal than typical meditation practices—the idea being that one does not need to remove oneself from one's life to practice mindfulness, nor is this considered the goal of practice (Lynch et al., 2006).

Practice Reminders: DBT and RODBT States of Mind

An essential component of mindfulness training in DBT involves the use of disorder-specific "states of mind" that metaphorically represent experiential state(s) linked to both maladaptive and optimal/effective coping. Mindful awareness of these "experiential states" allows an individual to predict response tendencies that may exacerbate difficulties—and remind the client of prior commitments made in therapy to practice skillful means. In her seminal work, Linehan developed states of mind specific for BPD (Linehan, 1993), then later added differing states of mind for substance dependence and suicidal adolescent populations (Linehan et al., 1999; Miller, Rathus, & Linehan, 2007). The state of mind identified by Linehan (1993) as most problematic for individuals with BPD, referred to as *emotion mind*, has clear links to BPD-relevant maladaptive behavioral responses, including intentional self-injury, dysregulated/extreme expressions of emotion, chaotic relationships, and risky or impulsive responding. The dialectical opposite of emotion mind is a nonemotional or rationale experiential state called *reasonable mind*—a state, that, for the most part, is not linked with BPD-relevant maladaptive responding. *Emotion mind*, as conceptualized in the context of BPD, represents primarily bottom-up processes that are influenced by neuroceptive tendencies (e.g., whether a particular stimulus is perceived as safe or threatening) that influence subsequent behavioral responses, which, when maladaptive, primarily reflect problems associated with poor inhibitory control (Lynch, in press). When reasonable mind and emotion mind are integrated, with representations of the truth of both states present, a basis for wisdom or effective responding emerges, a state that in standard DBT is called *wise mind*. Decisions made from wise mind often serve an individual's life values and/or balance long-term goals with short-term abilities for tolerating distress. Moreover, though wise mind requires inhibitory control—in order to block ineffective emotion mind response tendencies—it simultaneously encourages flexible control. Thus, wise mind allows the individual with BPD to take into account both emotional and rational ways of coping and to be more receptive to new ways of responding.

Genotypic and phenotypic differences between undercontrolled and overcontrolled disorders have necessitated the development of new disorder-specific states of mind for OC—experiential states linked to core maladaptive OC behaviors, including avoidance of novelty/risk, masking inner feelings, lack of openness, denial/minimization, and aloof/distant interpersonal relationships. Problematic OC states of mind typically arise secondary to disconfirming social–environmental feedback suggesting that change is needed and/or involve a novel situation requiring exhibition of unplanned or spontaneous behavior. Perhaps the most common OC response when challenged or stressed is to search immediately for a means to minimize, dismiss, or disconfirm feedback in order to reduce anxiety—without pausing to consider that there may be something to be learned from the situation. This experiential state in RODBT is referred to as *fixed-mind*. Fixed mind is generally painful because it frequently involves rejecting reality and is associated with anger, tension, or a feeling of being "pressured." Fixed mind is like the captain of the *Titanic*, who, despite repeated warnings, insists "full speed ahead and icebergs be damned." Essentially, a person with fixed mind says, "Change is unnecessary because I already know the answer." The opposite of compulsive fixedness or resistance to change is referred to as *fatalistic mind*. Whereas *fixed mind* involves vigorous resistance and energetic opposition to disconfirming feedback, fatalistic mind involves action tendencies and behaviors associated with appeasing, abandoning, and surrendering. Fatalistic mind may often appear to be submissive or nonaggressive, yet this state of mind functions as disguised resistance—an operant behavioral response oftentimes expressed via pouty silences, stonewalling, refusals to participate, and/or sudden acquiescence. In addition, when attempts to fight or flee disconfirming feedback (i.e., fixed mind) are perceived to be futile, fatalistic mind can involve the literal suspension of goal-directed behavior; resulting in numbness, anhedonia, immobilization, or complete shutdown. Fatalistic mind is like the Captain of the Titanic who, after hitting the fatal iceberg, retreats to his cabin, locks the door, and refuses to help passengers safely abandon ship. Essentially, someone with fatalistic mind eliminates personal responsibility by saying, "Change is unnecessary because there is no viable answer." Importantly, fixed mind and fatalistic mind are not necessarily always problematic—indeed, sometimes a rigid or fixed way of responding can be essential (e.g., a soldier in combat may need to rigidly obey orders in order to survive) or wild abandonment of self-control is needed (e.g., yelling to stop a mugger). Difficulties emerge when closed-minded, rule-governed, and/or passive responses are mindlessly enacted and negative consequences are ignored. *Flexible mind* is a synthesis of fixed mind and fatalistic mind: It involves purposeful self-inquiry, exploration, and openness to new experience, while honoring one's past and accepting responsibility for prior actions. Importantly, the goal of flexible mind is not equanimity; instead, flexible mind acknowledges the value of both disinhibition (e.g., dancing with abandon, yelling wildly to stop a mugger) and inhibition (e.g., not sharing a silly joke during a serious faculty meeting).

In summary, emotion mind represents primarily bottom-up processing and emotional response tendencies that, if mindlessly acted upon, can result in the maladaptive dysregulated behavior characterizing BPD. Consequently, wise mind often involves top-down inhibitory control processes that curb inappropriate emotion-based actions—and increase the prospect of effective responding. In contrast, fixed mind and fatalistic mind represent the inappropriate use of top-down inhibitory control processes that, if mindlessly and repetitively employed, can result in the maladaptive constricted behavior characterizing OC. Similar to wise mind, flexible mind requires activation of adaptive context-appropriate top-down control processes. Although the function of the two states of mind is similar, the behavioral manifestations of wise mind and flexible mind may frequently be disorder-specific; thus, flexible mind responses for OC often promote relaxation of rigid, rule-governed control efforts and an increase in context-appropriate disinhibition and/or emotional expression, whereas wise mind responses for BPD may tend to focus on reducing mood-dependent impulsive responding and increasing abilities to delay immediate gratification in order to pursue distal goals.

"What" Skills in DBT Mindfulness

Mindfulness skills in DBT are divided into "what" and "how" skills. As the names imply, the "what" skills are verbs that alert an individual as to the action or skill required, whereas the "how" skills are adverbs that instruct an individual as to the most effective way to use the "what" skills. The three "what" skills (i.e., observing, describing, and participating) tend to be necessary only when a new behavior is being learned, a difficulty has arisen, or change is required (Linehan, 1993). Because these skills require dedicated attention, clients are instructed to use and practice the "what" skills one at a time, without trying to use other skill use simultaneously. The first of the three skills, *observing*, is the practice of attending to, noticing, and sensing what is occurring in the present moment, without trying to change or label it. This includes observing bodily sensations, thoughts, and urges, as well as qualities of the external environment (e.g.,the quality of sights, sounds, textures, and smells). In addition, the act of observing one's thinking is differentiated from the act of thinking itself, giving clients some distance from their immediate experiences. Clients may practice observing through a variety of exercises, such as noticing the texture of some surface, the urge to scratch or move during a practice, or sensations related to the chair or floor upon which one is sitting. Another practice involves viewing one's mind as a conveyer belt and simply observing thoughts, sensations, feelings, and any wandering of the mind. Instead of interpreting their experience, group participants are simply noticing the flow of these events from moment to moment.

Once a thought, feeling, sensation, or urge has been noticed and experienced, an individual is able to move to communicating, with self or others, about this experience. *Describing* is the mindfulness "what" skill that involves putting a label or words to one's experience. The act of labeling one's experience can be especially use-ful when it comes to thoughts, feelings, and urges. In this case, the process of labeling a thought as a thought, no more and no less, can help group participants appreciate that just because a thought is internally generated does not inherently mean that it is or is not true. For example, having the thought "I am stupid" is different than actually being stupid, and group participants are encouraged to view their thoughts as thoughts rather than as truths. Simply recognizing the presence of such thoughts, feelings, and urges may reduce the likelihood of acting on them in problematic ways. In addition, it may help group participants to see that they have a choice in whether or not they act on the thoughts and feelings they have, and this may open them up to new, potentially more effective, behaviors in which to engage, even in the presence of painful thoughts or emotions. Mindfulness exercises used to practice describing skills include the conveyer belt example described earlier, with the addition of put-ting words to the observations, such as "I notice a thought about a to-do list" and "I observe an itch on my leg." In fact, any observe activity can be used to practice the describing skill.

Participating is the "what" skill that allows an individual to enter completely into the moment in a holistic way. Thus, an individual is involved in the activity and envi-ronment in a way that does not require a more removed observation or description; instead, the individual is at one with the activities of the current moment. Fully par-ticipating means to act with spontaneity and precludes the presence of self-evaluative thoughts. Group members can practice this by engaging in activities such as singing songs, dancing, or playing a short game. During these activities, group participants are asked to practice throwing themselves into the activity, even in the presence of feelings of self-consciousness or embarrassment. Outside of group, clients can prac-tice participating in conversations with others or physical activities, such as dancing, exercising, cooking, and showering. Participating reflects an important goal of mind-fulness skills, which is to combat patterns of acting mindlessly without awareness, which can result in impulsive or mood-dependent behavior. Instead, the goal is to act with awareness and engage fully in one's daily life. Because OC individuals spend a great deal of time "thinking about" rather than "experiencing life," they are likely to prefer practices associated with dispassionate awareness and may find participation practices difficult or stressful. Spontaneity may be considered foolish or a recipe for disaster—and expressions of trust or vulnerability, naive or possibly dangerous. As such, *graded* participation practices are considered an essential component of DBT for OC (Lynch, in press).

"How" Skills in DBT and RODBT Mindfulness

While the core mindfulness "what" skills are designed to be used one at a time, the "how" skills can (and are encouraged to be) used simultaneously and in concert with each "what" skill. Thus, although a client would be discouraged from attempting to use observing and describing skills at the same time, he or she would be encour-aged to observe nonjudgmentally, one-mindfully, and effectively. RODBT uses all three standard DBT "how" skills and adds a fourth, named *"with self-inquiry."* In DBT and RODBT, to be *nonjudgmental* means generally to take a nonevaluative stance toward one's experience (including both internal and external experience) and try to refrain from categorizing experiences as either negative (i.e., bad) or positive (i.e., good). Thus, all experiences are accepted as they are. Group participants are encouraged to note the desirable or aversive consequences of an experience or situation, as well as their feelings toward the experience, without judging it. This is to emphasize that being nonjudgmental does not mean that one does not or cannot have likes and dislikes or negative–positive emotional reactions to experiences. Clients are encouraged to change experiences that have aversive consequences or bump up against important values; this change can occur without judgment. In order to practice being nonjudgmental, clients are encouraged to observe and describe various objects, sensations, and experiences, providing "just the facts," without associated evaluation. Being nonjudgmental is practiced throughout skills group whenever any judgmental thoughts arise, and group participants are encouraged to use their "what" skills to observe and describe the situation using nonjudgmental language. Harsh self-judgmental thinking is common among both among BPD and OC individuals; with BPD it often reflects admonishments regarding failures at self-control, whereas, for OC, judgmental thinking often reflects annoyance at not being able to predict or control situations or shameful reactions following undesired emotional leakage.

Doing things *one-mindfully*, the second of the "how" skills, is to focus on one thing, and just one thing, in the moment. As opposed to acting without awareness, which is typical of many people's daily experience, group participants are encouraged to focus their full attention on only one activity or thing at a time. Although it is acknowledged that we are often required to do many things at once (i.e., the ever-encouraged multitasking), a DBT mindfulness perspective suggests that group participants would benefit from remaining one-mindful by devoting their full attention to each task and switching back and forth quickly between tasks. This might have the appearance of multitasking given that several activities might be worked on within a short time frame, but from the experience of the individual, each task is the sole focus of attention during the time in which it is engaged. In a group setting, this can be practiced by devoting full attention to eating, listening to a piece of music, or watching a video clip. It can be applied outside of group to almost any activity in which group participants engage, such as cooking, washing dishes, or driving.

The third standard DBT "how" skill, *acting effectively*, is behaving in a way that highlights what is needed in a given instance as opposed to becoming overly focused on what is "right" or "should" happen. By doing "what works" in a particular situation, clients are more likely to reach their valued goals rather than when their actions are based on their perceptions of what is fair or ideal. This involves identifying the contingencies of the situations, as well as one's goals, then doing what is needed to achieve those goals given the limitations of the environment. This requires letting go of ideas about how the situation should be and acting based on how it is. Acting effectively sometimes includes being political or savvy about people and may at time requires relaxing one's principles on some matter to achieve a larger goal. In skills class, acting effectively can be practiced when a group participant feels that a homework assignment is unfair or someone else in group is not engaging in group appropriately. This component of mindfulness is particularly salient for OC individuals because core issues revolve around following rules, doing what is "right," and behaving properly or consistently in all situations. Whereas, doing what is necessary to achieve one's objectives sometimes means not following "the rules" and often requires behaving politically (i.e., looking for compromise or synthesis).

RODBT adds a fourth "how" skill; namely, *"with self-inquiry."* Self-inquiry *challenges our perceptions of reality* by assuming that *we are unable to see things as "they are"; rather, we see things as "we are"* (Lynch, in press; Lynch, Hempel, & Dunkley, in press). From an RODBT perspective, our "observations" and "intuitions" are often misleading because "we don't know what we don't know," things are constantly changing, and there is a great deal of experience occurring outside of our conscious awareness. Self-inquiry requires a willingness to doubt or question our inner convictions without falling apart or mindlessly giving in. This contrasts with the concept of wise mind in standard DBT that emphasizes the value of intuitive knowledge, the possibility of fundamentally knowing something as true or valid, and posits inner knowing as "almost always quiet" and to involve a sense of "peace" (Linehan, 1993). In contrast, self-inquiry is "almost always painful" because it involves directing attention toward areas of our life that we may want to avoid (known as "finding one's edge"; Lynch, in press). Rather than seeking equanimity, wisdom, or a sense of peace, self-inquiry helps us learn because it doesn't assume we already know the answer. Self-inquiry practices in RODBT can be traced to similar Malamati-Sufi practices encouraging sustained self-observation and healthy self-criticism in order to understand one's true motivations (Toussulis, 2010). Malamatis believe that one cannot achieve heightened self-awareness in isolation and as a consequence emphasize spiritual dialogue and companionship. Thus, mindfulness practice in RODBT not only emphasizes self-inquiry but also a willingness to reveal what is discovered to a fellow practitioner—a process known as "outing oneself" (see Lynch, in press, for practice examples). Outing one's inner experience to another person goes opposite to OC tendencies to mask inner feelings and when generalized to other areas of life can become a powerful means for OC clients to rejoin the tribe. More globally, self-inquiry is particularly useful whenever we find ourselves strongly rejecting, defending against, or agreeing with feedback that we find challenging or unexpected—it begins by asking, "Is there something to learn here?"

Empirical Research and Proposed Mechanisms of Change

As articulated by Lynch and colleagues (2006), there are at least four routes through which mindfulness skills are hypothesized to function to influence emotional responding and increase effective responding. First, mindfulness is proposed to function as *exposure to emotions* that heretofore have been avoided, or partially experienced. Styles of coping associated with undercontrolled disorders (BPD), as postulated by Linehan (1993), are related to OC and are related to attempts to avoid unwanted emotional and cognitive experiences (e.g., Cheavens et al., 2005; Cukrow-icz, Franzese, Thorp, Cheavens, & Lynch, 2008; Lynch, Robins, Morse, & Krause, 2001); mindfulness skills, in contrast, call for the observation and acceptance of one's thoughts and emotions. Clients are taught to control the focus of attention rather than attempting to control the environment or their experiences that arise from an interaction with the environment. Some propose that observing and describing experiences, as opposed to attempting to avoid or control these experiences, functions as interoceptive exposure and, over time, leads to reduced intensity of emotions (e.g., Craske, Barlow, & Meadows, 2000; Lynch et al., 2006). Through nonjudgmental observation of emotions, thoughts, and sensations, clients come in contact with their internal experience. With repeated exposure or practice, clients can learn new associations between emotionally evocative stimuli or rule-governed behavior and mindful behavior, instead of automatic avoidance or problematic coping.

Second, mindfulness can function as an *emotional regulation* strategy. As new emotional and behavioral responses are acquired in response to stressful stimuli through mindfulness, clients may have a change in their experience of emotions. Specifically, mindfulness may change the automatic response tendencies associated with certain thoughts and emotions. For example, imagine a case in which the feeling of guilt has typically been associated with myriad escape behaviors as a means to avoid aversive arousal associated with this emotion. Through the use of mindfulness, this person may acquire new associations to stimuli that previously triggered unjustified guilt. Mindfulness may change automatic response tendencies when the client observes, describes, and participates in feelings of guilt—without acting on urges to inappropriately repair or fix the situation. This suggests that mindfulness may influence not only the behavioral response to emotions but also the associated thoughts, images, and/or memories linked to a maladaptive response. By observing rather than immediately avoiding or acting upon a response tendency, mindfulness automatically changes what was previously experienced to be a crisis to an experience in this moment that, although perhaps painful, does not necessarily require action or steps to be taken to reduce the pain. Indeed, mindfulness would not necessarily be considered a means to reduce the overall intensity of the primary emotional response; but with practice; rather, with repeated practice, associations between emotionally evocative stimuli and maladaptive responses can become increasingly less salient and more adaptive responses become increasingly dominant (Lynch et al., 2006). Although few studies have examined the influence of mindfulness on emotional responding, there is some thought that mindfulness may influence emotional experience at the level of neural responding (Davidson, 2003).

Third, mindfulness is hypothesized to reduce rule-governed behavior with respect to private experiences—a component that is particularly useful for OC clients. Specifically, *rule-governed behaviors* occur in response to some verbal rule about the relationship between a behavior (i.e., asking for help) and the consequence (i.e., being rejected). Some research suggests that rule-governed behavior reduces contact with the real contingencies of the environment (Hayes, Kohlenberg, & Melancon, 1989). For example, someone who is socially anxious may think, "If I ask for something, I will be rejected," and never learn that asking for help is not a dangerous situation in which they are invariably going to be rejected. Instead of trying to change or control these types of thoughts, mindfulness encourages clients to see them as mental events instead of literal statements or "truths." Therefore, mindfulness would not be expected to reduce the frequency of one's distressing thoughts but instead cause one to consider them as "just a thought"—not literal truth. For many OC individuals, rule-governance may become a "way of being" that is intermittently reinforced, despite evidence suggesting that the "rule" may not apply in a particular situation. As such, a major component of mindfulness practices with OC individuals involves nonjudgmental acknowledgment of desires for compliance and rule adherence—while cultivating a compassionate, nonjudgmental stance that appreciates *both* rules and spontaneity. Doing so is thought to maximize possibilities for full participation in the current moment and greater awareness of the natural contingencies operating in the environment.

Fourth, mindfulness would also be expected to increase the ability of clients to disengage from emotional stimuli (Lynch et al., 2006). Linehan (1993) posited that difficulties in being able to disengage from intense emotional experiences is particularly relevant for individuals with BPD. Indeed, mindfulness is hypothesized to increase one's ability to turn attention away from aversive emotional experiences, such as rumination and worry, toward experiences in the present moment that are consistent with one's goals. Consistent with this, one recent study showed that focusing on the nonemotional contextual details of an emotional memory can decrease the emotional intensity of the memory (Philippot, Schaefer, & Herbette, 2003). Thus, teaching clients to observe, describe, and decrease attachment with emotional stimuli may decrease the distress associated with aversive emotional reactions.

From Self-Control to Self-Regulation

Importantly, our neuroregulatory model (Lynch, in press) challenges linear assumptions regarding the nature of self-control (i.e., that one can never have too much self-control) by offering a developmental trajectory that accounts for both quadratic and linear relationships. We contend that optimal self-control is an emergent capacity requiring receptivity or openness and the capacity to flexibly adapt to changing environmental contingencies. Thus, whereas one can have "too much self-control" (quadratic model), by definition, it is impossible to have "too much self-regulation" (linear model) because a well-regulated person adjusts in whatever way is needed for optimal performance. For example, a person with highly flexible self-control tendencies or high self-regulation (1) strives for perfection but stops when it becomes clear that striving is counterproductive, (2) is rule-governed except when it is better to break the rules (e.g., to prevent a serious accident), (3) is polite and cooperative except when it is better not to be (e.g., when quality or safety concerns are overriding), and so on.

From this perspective, mental health and well-being are less about achieving happiness or success—as these are transitory—and more about being able to respond flexibly to changing environmental contingencies. Radical openness is the core philosophical principle and core skill in RODBT, a term representing the confluence of three capacities involved in emotional well-being: openness, flexibility, and social connectedness (Lynch, in press). Radical openness involves developing a passion for going opposite to where you are—it represents an intention to explore more deeply areas in our lives that are difficult, painful, or disturbing. It requires courage and is the opposite of complacency, passivity, or resignation (see "with self-inquiry," above). Though both openness and mindfulness require willingness, radical openness is more than awareness or simply engaging in new behavior; at its most extreme it involves actively seeking the things one wants to avoid or may find uncomfortable, in order to learn. Radical openness differs from *radical acceptance* skills taught as part of standard DBT (Linehan, 1993). Radical acceptance involves acknowledgment, in the present moment, of those things that cannot be changed, whereas, radical openness involves purposefully turning one's mind to the possibility of change and being willing to do something different. As a change strategy, radical openness requires one to be open to corrective feedback, to identify needed changes, and to fully participate in trying out the new behavior with compassionate awareness. An important outcome for the practitioner of radical openness is an improved capacity to respond flexibly to changing circumstances. However, as reviewed earlier, differing biotemperamental and sociobiographical influences can severely handicap capacities or opportunities to learn flexible control, resulting in the development and maintenance of maladaptive patterns of self-control—represented by extreme OC and UC behavioral responses.

Challenging Assumptions

Our clinical experience in applying RODBT to overcontrolled problems prompted us to reconsider some of our basic concepts and formulations about emotional well-being and therapy more broadly. Overcontrolled individuals tend to be perfectionists—that is, they don't need to learn how to be more serious, try harder, or be more composed. Thus, RODBT does not believe "one size fits all"—an intervention found to work with one disorder or several disorders does not necessarily mean it will work with all others. Mindfulness training exemplifies this. For example, the cultivation of equanimity or dispassionate awareness (i.e., calmness, poise, composure, self-control, and levelheadedness) common to many mindfulness-based interventions, may be iatrogenic for some OC individuals. OC individuals are "masters of self-control" (or at least they strive to appear so) and even unintended communication emphasizing the importance of composure or equanimity to an OC individual is like teaching a compulsive hand-washer the importance of being germ-free—their maladaptive coping style may only strengthened. Thus, to be effective, mindfulness training when working with OC ideally values both equanimity and disinhibition.

Moreover, a core focus of treatment involves welcoming the OC individual "back to the tribe" by encouraging participation in community and rediscovery of the value of intimate relationships. Thus, mindfulness training in RODBT involves practices designed to facilitate connection with others combined with practices designed to promote detached observation. Mindfulness training with OC also emphasizes the cultivation of a perspective that appreciates the importance of context-appropriate and mindful expression of extreme distress or excitement—for example, in order to validate another person's experience, to alert others of serious danger or to prevent serious injury, or to have peak experiences or passionately immerse oneself in activities, such as dancing, lovemaking, or creating. Consequently, mindfulness training for OC balances *dispassionate awareness* with *passionate participation*. Dispassionate awareness involves nonjudgmental awareness of thoughts, emotions, images, and sensations in a manner that implies they are not "literal truth," whereas passionate participation involves an active nonjudgmental engagement with one's community and a willingness to courageously immerse oneself in the current context in order to experience the moment fully.

Conclusion

The essence of mindfulness practices from a DBT perspective is the cultivation of a state of being in which one is fully awake to the present moment, without preconception or harsh judgment. The practice of mindfulness in DBT subtly differs from that of other approaches (e.g., Kabat-Zinn, 1990; Segal et al., 2002) in that the ultimate goal is not to achieve an objective distance from one's experience but rather to enter into, participate in, and become "one with" experience (Lynch et al., 2006). In addition, RODBT posits that we bring perceptual and regulatory biases with us no matter where we go or what we do—including our practice of mindfulness—thereby adding a fourth "how" skill *"with self-inquiry."* Though mindfulness is an acceptance technology, mindful awareness itself may function to change what is observed by the mere process of conscious awareness or observation itself (e.g., anger observed mindfully is qualitatively different from anger experienced mindlessly; Lynch & Bronner, 2006; Lynch et al., 2006). In addition, for OC individuals, the DBT mindfulness skill known as "participation" may be essential as a means to increase social connectedness.

Finally, we contend that core genotypic/phenotypic differences between groups of disorders (e.g., undercontrol and overcontrol) necessitate oftentimes vastly different treatment approaches—including in how mindfulness-based interventions are applied (Lynch, in press). For example, OC mindfulness states of mind and practices target rigid adherence to rules, extreme need for structure, and excessive desire to avoid making mistakes rather than the dysregulated emotions or impulsive responding that are core targets for BPD. Indeed, mindfulness training in standard DBT may work with BPD because it encourages inhibitory control and dispassionate awareness (e.g., mindful observing rather than impulsively acting on an automatic, emotion-based action tendency). However, for overcontrolled disorders, mindfulness training emphasizing equanimity and the importance of appearing calm, composed, or in control may be iatrogenic. For many OC individuals, a single-minded pursuit of composure is precisely what prevents them from fully experiencing emotions and/or participating in the community. Moreover, we posit that optimal self-regulation is an emergent capacity that requires receptivity or openness, self-inquiry, and a capacity to flexibly inhibit or disinhibit responses depending on what might be most effective in the moment. As such, we contend that mindfulness-based approaches may benefit from strategies that purposefully promote an appreciation for self-inquiry, a stance that requires openness to painful disconfirming feedback as a means for personal growth. This way of behaving has been reflected throughout human history in stories and myths involving heroism and courage. It involves advancing courageously to the source of the unknown with proper humility and a willingness to sacrifice in order to learn more from what the world has to offer.

NOTES

1. A "response" or behavioral output in Figure 18.1, the neuroregulatory model of personality and socioemotional functioning, refers to *private* (e.g., thoughts, sensations, emotions, memories, images) and *public* (e.g., actions, verbal speech, facial expression) responses. Responses in this model are both consequences and antecedents; that is, "responses" are both consequences of self-control (inhibited or disinhibited response tendencies) and an antecedent for neuroception via their impact on the environment and/or internal experience. Thus, responses are one component of a feedback loop—with each element influencing subsequent elements.

2. It is important to note that "self-control tendencies" can be effortless, quick (in milliseconds), and occur without conscious awareness *or* involve higher-order processes that are effortful and involve conscious intention.

REFERENCES

Asendorpf, J. B., Denissen, J. J. A., & van Aken, M. A. G. (2008). Inhibited and aggressive preschool children at 23 years of age: Personality and social transitions into adulthood. *Developmental Psychology, 44*(4), 997–1011.

Asendorpf, J. B., & van Aken, M. A. (1999). Resilient, overcontrolled, and undercontroleed personality prototypes in childhood: Replicability, predictive power, and the trait-type issue. *Journal of Personality and Social Psychology, 77*(4), 815–832.

Baumeister, R. F., Heatherton, T. F., & Tice, D. M. (1994). *Losing control: How and why people fail at self-regulation.* San Diego, CA: Academic Press.

Chapman, B. P., & Goldberg, L. R. (2011). Replicability and 40-year predictive power of childhood ARC types. *Journal of Personality and Social Psychology, 101*(3), 593–606.

Chen, E., Segal, K., Weissman, J. A., Zeffiro, T., Linehan, M. M., Bohus, M., et al. (2014). Radically open dialectical behavior therapy: A case series study examining adults with anorexia nervosa. In K. S. LaBar (Chair), *Novel treatments for difficult-to-treat anorexia nervosa.* Symposium conducted at the 48th annual convention of the Association for Behavioral and Cognitive Therapies, Philadelphia, PA.

Cheavens, J. S., Rosenthal, M. Z., Daughters, S. B., Nowak, J., Kosson, D., Lynch, T. R., et al. (2005). An analogue investigation of the relationships among perceived parental criticism, negative affect, and borderline personality disorder features: The role of thought suppression. *Behaviour Research and Therapy, 43,* 257–268.

Clarkin, J. F., Hull, J. W., & Hurt, S. W. (1993). Factor structure of borderline personality-disorder criteria. *Journal of Personality Disorders, 7*(2), 137–143.

Craske, M. G., Barlow, D. H., & Meadows, E. (2000). *Mastery of Your Anxiety and Panic*

(MAP-3): Therapist guide for anxiety, panic, and agoraphobia (3rd ed.). San Antonio, TX: Graywind/Psychological Corporation.

Crijnen, A. A., Achenbach, T. M., & Verhulst, F. C. (1997). Comparisons of problems reported by parents of children in 12 cultures: total problems, externalizing, and internalizing [Comparative Study Meta-Analysis Research Support, U.S. Gov't, P.H.S.]. *Journal of the American Academy of Child and Adolescent Psychiatry, 36*(9), 1269–1277.

Crowell, S. E., Beauchaine, T. P., & Linehan, M. M. (2009). A biosocial developmental model of borderline personality: Elaborating and extending Linehan's theory. *Psychological Bulletin, 135*(3), 495–510.

Cukrowicz, K. C., Franzese, A. T., Thorp, S. R., Cheavens, J. S., & Lynch, T. R. (2008). Personality traits and perceived social support among depressed older adults. *Aging and Mental Health, 12*(5), 662–669.

Davidson, R. J. (2003). *Darwin and the neural bases of emotion and affective style.* New York: New York University Press.

Eisenberg, N., Fabes, R. A., Guthrie, I. K., & Reiser, M. (2000). Dispositional emotionality and regulation: Their role in predicting quality of social functioning. *Journal of Personality and Social Psychology, 78*(1), 136–157.

Gross, J. J. (1998). Antecedent- and response-focused emotion regulation: Divergent consequences for experience, expression, and physiology. *Journal of Personality and Social Psychology, 74*(1), 224–237.

Gross, L. (2006). How the human brain detects unexpected events. *PLoS Biology, 4*(12), e443.

Hahn, T. N. (1976). *The miracle of mindfulness: A manual on meditation.* Boston: Beacon Press.

Hayes, S. C., Kohlenberg, B. S., & Melancon, S. M. (1989). *Avoiding and altering rule-control as a strategy of clinical intervention.* New York: Plenum Press.

Kabat-Zinn, J. (1990). *Full catastrophe living: Using the wisdom of your body and mind to face stress, pain, and illness.* New York: Delacourt.

Koons, C. R., Robins, C. J., Tweed, J. L., Lynch, T. R., Gonzalez, A. M., Morse, J. Q., et al. (2001). Efficacy of dialectical behavior therapy in women veterans with borderline personality disorder. *Behavior Therapy, 32*, 371–390.

LeDoux, J. (1996). *The emotional brain.* New York: Simon & Schuster.

LeDoux, J. (2003). *Synaptic self: How our brains become who we are.* New York: Penguin.

Linehan, M. M. (1993). *Cognitive-behavioral treatment of borderline personality disorder.* New York: Guilford Press.

Linehan, M. M., Armstrong, H. E., Suarez, A., Allmon, D., & Heard, H. L. (1991). Cognitive-behavioral treatment of chronically parasuicidal borderline clients. *Archives of General Psychiatry, 48*, 1060–1064.

Linehan, M. M., Comtois, K. A., Murray, A. M., Brown, M. Z., Gallop, R. J., Heard, H. L., et al. (2006). Suicidal and behavioral outcomes from a one year randomized trial and one year follow-up of dialectical behavior therapy for borderline personality disorder. *Archives of General Psychiatry, 63*, 757–766.

Linehan, M. M., Dimeff, L. A., Reynolds, S. K., Comtois, K. A., Welch, S. S., Heagerty, P., et al. (2002). Dialectical behavior therapy versus comprehensive validation therapy plus 12-step for the treatment of opioid dependent women meeting criteria for borderline personality disorder. *Drug and Alcohol Abuse, 67*, 13–26.

Linehan, M. M., & Dimidjian, S. (2003). Mindfulness practice. In W. O'Donohue, J. E. Fisher, & S. C. Hayes (Eds.), *Cognitive behavior therapy: Applying empirically supported techniques in your practice* (pp. 229–237). Hoboken, NJ: Wiley.

Linehan, M. M., Schmidt, H., Dimeff, L. A., Craft, J. C., Kanter, J., & Comtois, K. A. (1999). Dialectical behavior therapy for clients with borderline personality disorder and drug-dependence. *American Journal on Addictions, 8*, 279–292.

Lynch, T. R. (in press). *Radically open dialectical behavior therapy: Treating disorders of overcontrol.* New York: Guilford Press.

Lynch, T. R., & Bronner, L. L. (2006). Mindfulness and dialectical behavior therapy: application with depressed older adults with personality disorders. In R. A. Baer (Ed.), *Mindfulness-based treatment approaches: A clinician's guide to evidence base and applications.* Burlington, MA: Elsevier.

Lynch, T. R., Chapman, A. L., Rosenthal, M. Z., Kuo, J. R., & Linehan, M. M. (2006). Mechanisms of change in dialectical behavior therapy: Theoretical and empirical observations. *Journal of Clinical Psychology, 62*, 459–480.

Lynch, T. R., & Cheavens, J. S. (2008). Dialectical behavior therapy for co-morbid personality disorders. *Journal of Clinical Psychology, 64*, 1–14.

Lynch, T. R., Cheavens, J. S., Cukrowicz, K. C., Thorp, S., Bronner, L., & Beyer, J. (2007). Treatment of older adults with co-morbid personality disorder and depression: A dialectical behavior therapy approach. *International Journal of Geriatric Psychiatry, 22*, 131–143.

Lynch, T. R., Gray, K. L. H., Hempel, R. J., Titley, M., Chen, E. Y., & O'Mahen, H. A. (2013). Radically open-dialectical behavior therapy for adult anorexia nervosa: Feasibility and outcomes from an inclient program. *BMC Psychiatry, 13*, 293

Lynch, T. R., Hempel, R. J., & Dunkley, C. (in press). Remembering our tribal nature: Radically open-dialectical behavior therapy for disorders of overcontrol. *American Journal of Psychotherapy.*

Lynch, T. R., Morse, J. Q., Mendelson, T., & Robins, C. J. (2003). Dialectical behavior therapy for depressed older adults: A randomized pilot study. *American Journal of Geriatric Psychiatry, 11*, 33–45.

Lynch, T. R., Robins, C., Morse, J. Q., & Krause, E. D. (2001). A mediational model relating affect intensity, emotion inhibition, and psychological distress. *Behavior Therapy, 32*, 519–536.

Lynch, T. R., Trost, W. T., Salsman, N., & Linehan, M. M. (2007). Dialectical behavior therapy for borderline personality disorder. *Annual Review of Clinical Psychology, 3*, 181–205.

Meeus, W., Van de Schoot, R., Klimstra, T., & Branje, S. (2011). Personality types in adolescence: Change and stability and links with adjustment and relationships: A five-wave longitudinal study. *Developmental Psychology, 47*(4), 1181–1195

Mennin, D. S., Holaway, R., Fresco, D. M., Moore, M. T., & Heimberg, R. G. (2007). Delineating components of emotion and its dysregulation in anxiety and mood psychopathology. *Behavior Therapy, 38*, 284–302.

Miller, A. L., Rathus, J. H., & Linehan, M. M. (2007). *Dialectical behavior therapy with suicidal adolescents.* New York: Guilford Press

Moffitt, T. E., Arseneault, L., Belsky, D., Dickson, N., Hancox, R. J., Harrington, H., et al. (2011). A gradient of childhood self-control predicts health, wealth, and public safety. *PNAS Proceedings of the National Academy of Sciences of the United States of America, 108*(7), 2693–2698.

Newton, T. L., & Contrada, R. J. (1994). Alexithymia and repression: Contrasting emotion-focused coping styles. *Psychosomatic Medicine, 56*(5), 457–462.

Philippot, P., Schaefer, A., & Herbette, G. (2003). Consequences of specific processing of emotional information: Impact of general versus specific autobiographical memory priming on emotion elicitation. *Emotion, 3*, 270–283.

Riso, L. P., Blandino, J. A., Penna, S., Dacey, S., Grant, M. M., Du Toit, P. L., et al. (2003). Cognitive aspects of chronic depression. *Journal of Abnormal Psychology, 112*(1), 72–80.

Rosenthal, M. Z., Gratz, K. L., Kosson, D. S., Cheavens, J. S., Lejuez, C. W., & Lynch, T. R. (2008). Borderline personality disorder and emotional responding: A review of the research literature. *Clinical Psychology Review, 28*, 75–91.

Sanislow, C. A., Grilo, C. M., & McGlashan, T. H. (2000). Factor analysis of the DSM-III-R borderline personality disorder criteria in psychiatric inclients [Research Support, U.S. Gov't, P.H.S.]. *American Journal of Psychiatry, 157*(10), 1629–1633.

Segal, Z. V., Williams, J. M. G., & Teasdale, J. D. (2002). *Mindfulness-based cognitive therapy for depression*. New York: Guilford Press.

Skodol, A. E., Gunderson, J. G., Pfohl, B., Widiger, T. A., Livesley, W. J., & Siever, L. J. (2002). The borderline diagnosis I: Psychopathology, comorbidity, and personaltiy structure. *Biological Psychiatry, 51*(12), 936–950.

Skodol, A. E., Siever, L. J., Livesley, W. J., Gunderson, J. G., Pfohl, B., & Widiger, T. A. (2002). The borderline diagnosis II: Biology, genetics, and clinical course. *Biological Psychiatry, 51*(12), 951–963.

Toussulis, Y. (2010). *Sufism and the way of blame: Hidden sources of a sacred psychology*. Wheaton, IL: Quest Books.

Turner, R. M. (2000). Naturalistic evaluation of dialectical behavior therapy-oriented treatment for borderline personality disorder. *Cognitive and Behavioral Practice, 7*, 413–419.

Verheul, R., van den Bosch, L. M. C., Koeter, M. W. J., de Ridder, M. A., Stijnen, T., & van den Brink, W. (2003). Dialectical behaviour therapy for women with borderline personality disorder: 12-month, randomised clinical trial in the Netherlands. *British Journal of Psychiatry, 182*, 135–140.

Zucker, N. L., Losh, M., Bulik, C. M., LaBar, K. S., Piven, J., & Pelphrey, K. A. (2007). Anorexia nervosa and autism spectrum disorders: Guided investigation of social cognitive endophenotypes. *Psychological Bulletin, 133*(6), 976–1006.

CHAPTER 19

Mindfulness-Based Cognitive Therapy for Chronic Depression

Julie Anne Irving, Norman A. S. Farb, and Zindel V. Segal

Background and Development

Mindfulness-based cognitive therapy (MBCT) was developed against a backdrop of growing awareness of the challenges inherent in effectively treating depressive illness. Research has revealed major depressive disorder (MDD) as one of the most common, costly, and chronic current epidemiological concerns. Prevalence rates for MDD range from 3 to 13% worldwide (Gelenberg, 2010; Richards, 2011), with lifetime risk estimated at 17–19% in the United States (Kessler et al., 1994). Depressive illness represents one of the most costly medical conditions worldwide and is predicted by the World Health Organization to become the second most common cause of medical disability by 2020. Despite the establishment of efficacious treatments for the disorder, such as antidepressant medication and cognitive-behavioral therapies, MDD is thought to be rising in prevalence (Richards, 2011). Moreover, the chronic nature of depressive illness is a major contributing factor to the challenge of tackling this daunting public health concern. Numerous studies have demonstrated the risk of relapse that increases with each subsequent episode of depression. Individuals who have recovered from a major depressive episode are 50–60% more likely to have a second episode. For those with a history of two or more episodes, relapse rates become as high as 70–80% (Judd, 1997; Solomon et al., 2000).

Medication and psychotherapy are currently considered to be the most effective first-line treatments for the acute phase of depressive illness, with recovery rates hovering at approximately 46% for both (Casacalenda, Perry, & Looper, 2002). Until recently, however, maintenance pharmacotherapy was the most widely supported and implemented approach to prophylaxis (Kupfer et al., 1992). The continuation of antidepressant medication in the periods following recovery, at times indefinitely, has been widely adopted as a best practice to circumvent future episodes. Cognitive therapy (CT) has also been shown to effect long-lasting protective benefits posttreatment (Fava, Rafanelli, Grandi, Canestrari, & Morphy, 1998; Paykel et al., 1999). This early evidence base for CT hinted that a maintenance version of CT could potentially offer an alternative to the standard practice of maintenance pharmacotherapy. Rather than modifying existing CT formats, Segal, Williams, and Teasdale (2012) sought to expand upon existing CT techniques, keeping in mind the growing literature on how cognitive vulnerabilities influence depressive relapse (Kendler, Thornton, & Gardner, 2000; Post, 1992; Post & Weiss, 1998).

Risk for Depressive Relapse and Recurrence: Reactivity Matters

It has been well established that numerous, interacting determinants of susceptibility and onset of MDD include genetic, socioeconomic, physiological, and psychological factors. While studies examining heritability suggest that MDD has a strong genetic component, the preponderance of risk arises from environmental factors, which account for 60–70% of variance within families (Sullivan, Neale, & Kendler, 2000). Interestingly, while such environmental stressors hold strong predictive value for initial episodes, dysphoric moods and dysfunctional thinking styles incur greater influence with recurrent episodes. Teasdale's (1988) differential activation hypothesis (DAH) maintains that the repeated association of dysphoric moods and cognitive reactivity/negative thinking common to depressive episodes contributes to an increased likelihood of triggering dysfunctional thinking in the face of negative affective states during times of wellness. This dysfunctional thinking has been shown to perpetuate dysphoric moods, thereby creating a vicious cycle wherein relatively minor environmental triggers provoke relapse. The recurrence of negativistic thinking patterns, activated by mild to moderate emotional challenges, can serve to drive depressive episodes and sensitize individuals to future relapse.

Cognitive reactivity to emotional challenge has been operationalized and demonstrated to hold significant predictive value for individuals with a history of depressive illness in several studies. In 2006, Segal and colleagues measured formerly depressed individuals' engagement in negative automatic thinking with the Dysfunctional Attitude Scale (DAS; Weissman, 1979) pre- and postexposure to a sad mood paradigm. They found that individuals with the greatest magnitude of mood-induced reactivity were those most apt to relapse, and in the shortest amount of time. In a neuroimaging (functional magnetic resonance imaging [fMRI]) study published in 2011, Farb, Anderson, Bloch, and Segal provided an elaborated picture of cognitive reactivity. Individuals recruited from a clinical trial comparing MBCT to maintenance antidepressant medication (Segal et al., 2010) were exposed to sad and neutral film clips during fMRI scanning to provide a neural picture of reactivity. Following exposure to the mood challenge, increased activity was observed in the medial prefrontal cortex (mPFC), which is associated with self-evaluative and task-oriented processing. This increase was coupled with decreased activity in the visual cortex, suggesting that a tradeoff was occurring between sensory information and elaborative processing.

Moreover, those individuals with the greatest discrepancies between prefrontal and visual reactivity were most likely to relapse during an 18-month follow-up period. The authors concluded that there may be a prophylactic role of attending to sensory information in individuals when encountering negative emotion, which appears to become hijacked by ruminative cognitive reactivity in those individuals most at risk for relapse.

Taken together, these findings suggest differentiated mechanisms of relapse from the factors that contribute to initial onset and perpetuation of depression during the acute phase, and support the process of recurrence posited by Teasdale's (1988) DAH. From a neural standpoint, rather than the amygdala hyperactivity and prefrontal hypoactivity that are observed during the acute phase of depressive illness, prefrontal hyperactivity appears to play a role in risk for relapse during periods of relative wellness (Farb, Segal, & Anderson, 2011). These findings imply that the effectiveness of interventions designed to prevent relapse would be enhanced by a somewhat differentiated approach to those found in standard CT interventions targeting depression. First, interventions aimed at reducing relapse risk should attenuate the provocation of negativistic cognitive reactivity by dysphoric mood states. This may be accomplished through (1) increased awareness of negative thinking in the face of emotional challenge and (2) development of psychological skills to enable a "stepping back" from ruminative thought streams. To practice such skills, individuals would be encouraged to face, and at times, actively explore experiences of negative mood. In this sense, individuals with a history of prior depression may benefit from opportunities to normalize and maintain attention to somatosensory information and patterns of thought activated by states of mild sadness, thereby preventing escalation into spreading activations of elaborative and self-referential rumination. In the section to follow, we discuss how MBCT can provide a scaffold for the development of such skills by combining elements of cognitive-behavioral therapy with mindfulness meditation.

Building on Traditional Models of CT

The capacity for CT to reduce rates of relapse for future depressive episodes has been well established. At the time that MBCT was under development by Segal and colleagues (2012), it was understood that one of the mechanisms through which CT achieved these effects was "decentering." Ingram and Hollon (1986) proposed that CT achieves prophylactic effects by enhancing an individual's ability to take a distanced, disidentified perspective from depressive thoughts, that is, the understanding that thoughts are not facts. This view was an important feature in Beck, Rush, Shaw, and Emery's (1979) cognitive model, which proposed that depressive vulnerability would be reduced by modifying underlying dysfunctional attitudes and core beliefs. While the concept of "decentering" was acknowledged in this original model, it was viewed as a means to end, toward the eventual goal of cognitive restructuring. An alternative view is that the act of decentering itself can help a person mitigate negativistic thoughts by viewing them as passing events in the broader landscape of the mind, as opposed to absolute truths about the self or reflections of reality.

Building upon the cognitive vulnerability model, and the potential for "decentering" to offer a protective mechanism, Segal and colleagues (2012) sought to develop a treatment that would focus on awareness of the types of negative thoughts triggered by dysphoric mood, and provide a means through which to develop a new relationship to those thoughts. This second emphasis on developing a different attitude to thoughts raised the possibility of considering interventions outside of CT, and Kabat-Zinn's (1990) mindfulness-based stress reduction (MBSR) program proved to be a valuable source. The program, originally conceived as a means to help individuals with chronic pain and illness, promoted a decentered relationship with thoughts, feelings, and body sensations through the practice of mindfulness meditation. Building upon this model, Segal and colleagues proposed the development of an integrated program, MBCT, that would combine CT with mindfulness meditation.

Review of Empirical Support for MBCT in Preventing Depressive Relapse

Early Trials

Results from two early randomized controlled trials established an initial evidence base for MBCT as an effective prophylactic treatment for depressive relapse (Ma & Teasdale, 2004; Teasdale, Segal, Williams, Ridgeway, Soulsby, & Lau, 2000). Teasdale and colleagues (2000) conducted an initial multicenter trial and a single-site replication was conducted by Ma and Teasdale in 2004. In both studies, remitted individuals who had experienced at least two previous episodes of depression were randomized to either MBCT or treatment as usual (TAU) conditions. In the TAU condition, participants were instructed to seek support from a primary care physician or other sources as they would normally if they experienced difficulties during the course of the study. Severity of depressive symptoms and relapse were determined with the Structured Clinical Interview for DSM-IV (SCID; Spitzer, Williams, Gibbon, & First, 1992) administered at bimonthly intervals over the course of the treatment and at a 15-month follow-up point. Individuals were then grouped according to the number of previous episodes of depression they had experienced (two vs. three or more). Results from the initial trial revealed a differentiated pattern of relapse between the two groups; for those individuals with only two previous episodes of depression, relapse rates at 15 months were similar across treatment conditions. However, in the sample of individuals who had experienced three or more episodes (representing 77% of the sample) a statistically significant effect was observed between MBCT and TAU conditions for those individual who had completed at least four treatment sessions. Relapse occurred in 66% of individuals in the TAU condition and in only 37% of those in the MBCT condition. Moreover, this difference remained significant when analyses were replicated with an intent-to-treat (ITT) sample, wherein relapse in the MBCT condition occurred in 40% of cases. Notably, individuals in the MBCT group used less medication than those enrolled in the TAU condition. These findings were replicated by Ma and Teasdale in 2004. In their sample of patients with three or more episodes of depression (73% of the sample), based on ITT analyses, relapse rates for the MBCT condition were approximately half (36%) of those in the TAU condition (78%). Interestingly, the finding that MBCT did not hold a prophylactic benefit for those with only two previous episodes of depression was reproduced as well.

Recent Trials and Comparison to Antidepressant Medication

In 2010, Segal and colleagues conducted a randomized trial comparing MBCT to maintenance antidepressant medication (M-ADM) and a placebo medication condition. Patients in this sample had been previously treated with 8 months of algorithm-informed antidepressant medication. Out of 165 candidates, 84 achieved remission and were assigned to one of the three study conditions. Individuals in this study were determined to have achieved "stable" (49%) versus "unstable" (51%) remission states during the acute phase of treatment for depression (those who had experienced "symptom flurries": occasional, transient symptom elevations on the Hamilton Rating Scale for Depression; Hamilton, 1960). Interestingly, ITT analyses revealed comparable rates of relapse across treatment conditions for unstable remitters (28% for MBCT and 27% for M-ADM) versus 71% relapse rates for unstable remitters enrolled in the placebo condition. For stable remitters, relapse rates were not different across treatments. As such, it was concluded that the provision of a long-term active treatment provided a significant prophylaxis to individuals with a history of unstable remission. Moreover, MBCT demonstrated protective benefits similar to those of maintenance pharmacotherapy.

Several independent controlled trials have determined the efficacy of MBCT in preventing relapse in formerly depressed individuals when compared to usual care. Outcomes such as lowered rates of relapse (in the range of 50%), longer periods of wellness between episodes of depression, reduced residual depressive symptoms in the short- and long-term, and improvements in health-related measures of well-being and experiences of momentary positive affect (measured through experience sampling self-reports during the 6 days before and after the intervention) have been observed in MBCT treatment groups (Bondolfi et al., 2010; Geschwind, Peeters, Drukker, van Os, & Wichers, 2011; Godfrin & van Heeringen, 2010; Kuyken et al., 2008, 2010).

Mechanisms of Change in MBCT

The assertion, made earlier, that MBCT enhances an individual's capacity to adopt a decentered position from negative thinking patterns associated with depressive relapse has been supported both in controlled trials that have included measures of change processes, and in several rigorous qualitative studies. One means through which decentering has been operationalized is through self-report assessment, such as the Measure of Awareness and Coping in Autobiographical Memory (MACAM; Moore, Hayhurst, & Teasdale, 1996). This measure taps the ability to see negative thoughts and feelings as passing mental events rather than as an aspect of self when faced with depression-related cues for autobiographical memory. Treatment with MBCT has been associated with increased metacognitive awareness (using the MACAM) in the face of negative cognitions and affective experiences (Teasdale et al., 2002). Recent investigations (e.g., Bieling et al., 2012) have further demonstrated that MBCT may be unique in its ability to engender increases in the ability to monitor thoughts immediately following treatment, and at 6-month follow-up, when compared with M-ADM. Furthermore, preliminary support for the specific importance of the mindfulness component of MBCT has been offered through two rigorous qualitative studies. Mason and Hargreaves (2001) interviewed seven participants from the first multicenter trial (Teasdale et al., 2000). In this cohort, the development of mindfulness skills was identified as one of MBCT's key elements that contributed to reduced relapse risk. Allen, Bromley, Kuyken, and Sonnenberg (2009) interviewed patients who had been enrolled in MBCT in the clinical trial of Kuyken and colleagues (2008). Themes derived from systematic analyses included heightened ability to be aware of body sensations and cognitive markers of low mood. Moreover, these participants identified being able to "objectify depression," seeing thoughts as thoughts, and depression as "not me." Collectively, several studies employing different research methods have contributed results that support the development of metacognitive awareness and a decentered perspective as key mechanisms of change that result from participation in MBCT (Kuyken et al., 2010).

MBCT Key Principles

The MBCT program is a hybrid of major elements of Kabat-Zinn's (1990) MBSR and aspects of CT designed to target relapse prevention for depression. Mindfulness practices comprise a significant component of the MBCT curriculum and include formal meditation exercises such as the body scan, sitting and walking meditations, and mindful movement in the form of gentle yoga and stretching. The generalization of mindfulness skills to aspects of everyday life is supported through informal practices such as mindful eating, noticing body sensations, affect, and thoughts during pleasant and unpleasant experiences, as well as taking a mindful approach to aspects of one's daily routine typically completed on "automatic pilot." The CT components of the program include psychoeducation surrounding depressive symptoms, as well as instruction regarding the cognitive model, including automatic thoughts, and how thoughts are impacted by situations and moods. Participants are also encouraged to identify activities generating a sense of pleasure or mastery in which to engage during times of low mood. They are also asked to identify key people whom they can enlist for support as part of their individualized relapse prevention plans. A novel aspect of MBCT is the addition of the "3-minute breathing space," a brief centering meditation exercise designed for use during times of emotional challenges or stress. The group-based inquiry process found in MBCT combines elements of Socratic questioning and the dialoging used in MBSR to explore thoughts, emotions, and body awareness that arise during meditation practice. The inquiry serves to facilitate meta-awareness of patterns and reactions to what is discovered during mindfulness practices. Additionally, the inquiry provides opportunities to reflect on how this awareness may have applications for staying well, particularly in the face of early warning signs of depressive relapse. Throughout the inquiry process, instructors are expected to model acceptance, compassion, openness, and kindness to whatever content arises. Taken together, skills drawn from MBSR and CT are aimed at promoting an accepting and compassionate attitude toward the negative thinking patterns that can contribute to depressive relapse. In what follows, we provide an outline of how these intentions are actualized over the course of the 8-week program.

Approaching Present Moment Experience with Acceptance

The first four sessions of the program provide a framework for patients to learn to approach present-moment experiences in a nonjudgmental way. This goal is accomplished tacitly through the formal meditation practices, which promote learning to focus (and refocus as needed) attentional resources to anchors such as the breath and bodily sensations. This process facilitates the ability to observe the structure of one's internal experience as it arises in a given moment, with the intention not to judge the content, knowing that the judgment of emotionally reactive component one's experience can be more detrimental that the raw experience itself. Experiences are parsed into body sensation, affective content, and thoughts that may arise in any given moment. The skills to deconstruct experience in this way are then specifically applied to depression, using exercises from CT that underscore how reactions to given situations can be colored by thought and interpretation. Thus, the understanding is cultivated that thoughts are not facts is cultivated, and that thoughts, feelings, and body sensations are often transient and dynamic aspects of experience.

Expanding Awareness of Depression-Related Experience

In the fourth session, psychoeducation specific to depressive illness is formally introduced. In addition to information surrounding the nature of commonly discussed depressive symptoms (neurovegetative and mood), the types of negative thinking associated with depression are also explored. Thus, individuals are encouraged to build on their ability to detect the early warning signs of relapse and to identify their unique "relapse signatures."

Promoting Flexible and Deliberate Responses at Times of Risk for Relapse

The latter four sessions of the program emphasize the development of a thoughtful and flexible response style for dealing with the signs and symptoms of relapse. The concept of acceptance, which was previously implicit to the meditation practices and embodied by instructors, is formally introduced. Acceptance is identified as an entry point from which informed decisions can be made for dealing with difficulties. Specific instructions for dealing with difficulties are introduced in the 3-minute breathing space, and embedded in sitting meditation practices. The theme "thoughts are not facts" is the focus in the sixth session, which employs a CT exercise to illustrate how readily mood can impact thoughts. Participants are encouraged to explore how, during times of low mood especially, thoughts may not coincide with reality. The practice of "taking a step back" from thoughts is promoted. In the seventh session, relapse prevention strategies drawn from CT are discussed. The groundwork is laid for an individualized relapse prevention plan for each participant that includes involving family members in an early warning system, keeping a list of highly effective pleasure and mastery activities, and noting habitual automatic thoughts and cognitive themes that have preceded relapse in the past.

Differences and Similarities among MBCT, MBSR, and CT

As illustrated earlier, MBCT is truly a hybrid of MBSR and standard CT for depression. However, an amalgam of the two approaches necessitates several subtle but important differences from the original interventions. MBCT and MBSR share many similar structural elements in terms of length and flow (moving seamlessly between experiential practices and didactics), as well as strong similarities with regard to the intensive home mindfulness practices that are assigned each week. However, MBSR was designed and originally implemented with heterogeneous groups of individuals facing a wide range of medical illnesses and day-to-day stressors. MBCT, with its specialized population of formerly depressed individuals, carries an explicit psychoeducational focus on depressive illness and relapse prevention.

Accordingly, MBCT draws heavily on traditional CT approaches to treating depression, including the identification of triggers, early warning signs, and the development of an individualized action plan. Psychoeducation relative to the role of automatic thoughts in perpetuating negative moods, as well as monitoring of pleasant and unpleasant events, and becoming aware of pleasure and mastery on a day-to-day basis, are also derived from CT. Nonetheless, MBCT diverges from CT in several ways. First, MBCT emphasizes an acceptance-based approach in contrast to CT's change-based orientation. For example, when working with negative automatic thoughts such as "I am a failure," the two interventions differ considerably. In a traditional CT approach, the goal might be to challenge thoughts, restructuring beliefs so as to move toward a more balanced or functional view of the self. In MBCT, individuals are encouraged to notice thoughts and to accept them as passing mental events. Thoughts, then, are less likely to be viewed as absolute truths and consequently are less likely to drive distressing emotions or automatic behaviors such as avoidance. As such, in MBCT, one's relationship to thoughts is a point of intervention rather than the particular thought itself (see also Szabo, Long, Villatte, & Hayes, Chapter 8, this volume). Additionally, in CT, individuals are often encouraged to expose themselves to challenging situations so as to practice their developing skills. In MBCT, skills are practiced naturalistically, with content that arises during meditation practices, and during the mundane, pleasant, or challenging events and experiences of a given week as they normally unfold. Finally, instructors of MBCT are expected to have a well-established mindfulness meditation practice of their own because personal experience is thought to provide a rich and meaningful source of experience on which to draw during the group inquiry process.

MBCT Preparation: Laying the Groundwork for an MBCT Course

Determining Eligibility for MBCT

Despite the current application of MBCT to novel populations (see "Extended Applications of MBCT" below), it is important to keep in mind that the program was designed specifically for individuals in remission from depression. As such, eligibility for participation in MBCT is determined in a presession clinical interview, bearing a number of considerations in mind. First, current depression status must be determined with a diagnostic interview such as the Structured Clinical Interview for Diagnosis for DSM-IV (SCID-IV), supplemented with symptom severity measures (Beck Depression Inventory–II [BDI-II]; Hamilton Rating Scale for Depression [HRSD]). Second, the commitment required when taking part in the program is described and the participants' ability to engage and persist in all aspects of the course over 8 weeks is assessed. Finally, clinical factors that would preclude taking part in the program at the present time are taken into consideration; individuals are not accepted into the program if they are actively suicidal and do not have outside support, or if they are currently abusing substances or experiencing intrusive symptoms of posttraumatic stress. Furthermore, although MBCT was designed to help remitted depressed persons stay well, this population remains at high risk for relapse. As such, MBCT instructors are encouraged to monitor participants' progress over the 8 weeks through verbal reports, or weekly tracking with formal measures of depressive symptoms such as the BDI-II. A comprehensive assessment at the end of the program (e.g., HRSD, SCID-IV) is also recommended. Should a significant return of symptoms occur during the course, a thorough assessment may also be appropriate and consideration given to whether mindfulness practice adaptations may be necessary (e.g., assigning less home practice or shortening the length of practices) or the participant should be referred to another type of intervention.

Prerequisite Training Required of MBCT Instructors

The combined emphasis upon mindfulness meditation and CT of the MBCT program carries with it a unique constellation of training requirements for instructors. Segal, Williams, and Teasdale (2012) have outlined the following basic requirements: (1) accreditation in counseling, psychotherapy, or as a mental health professional; (2) formal training in cognitive-behavioral therapy; (3) experience facilitating group psychotherapy or psychoeducational interventions; (4) training in MBCT through completion of a weeklong intensive teacher development workshop; and (5) critically, an established and ongoing meditation practice. One reason for this commitment to a steady practice rests in the dialectic tension between "doing" and "being" modes inherent in MBCT instruction. Crane, Kuyken, Hastings, Rothwell, and Williams (2010) have proposed detailed guidelines for teacher training, with an in-depth rationale for instructors' personal practice. The authors describe the *doing mode* as one of goal-oriented pushing for change in the way things are and the way the mind may wish them to be. The *being mode* is related to the capacity to accept and remain in the present moment with an attitude of nonstriving and "nondoing." They note that while this being mode is taught explicitly through the in-session and home practice experiential exercises, a second means of imparting an attitude of compassion and acceptance is via modeling. In MBCT, key elements of the program, such as self-compassion, are not explicitly taught but rather are tacitly embodied by instructors. If instructors are easily pulled into doing mode—for example, by abruptly shifting to the next set of exercises, rushing to "fix" a group member's problem, or demonstrating a lack of self-compassion during the inquiry—invaluable opportunities for transmitting core teaching points are lost. CT therapists may also struggle to step out of the directive, didactic, and change-oriented mode to which they are accustomed in standard CT treatments for depression. Cultivating a regular mindfulness practice carries the benefit of becoming more aware of and attuned to one's own "automatic pilot" mode as a therapist, which can be invaluable when teaching this novel intervention that often requires stepping out of the familiar ways of intervening associated with other types of clinical work.

Extended Applications of MBCT

MBCT for People with Co-Occurring Disorders

Individuals experiencing depression often suffer from a host of other comorbid issues (Richards, 2011). MBCT was designed to treat remitted depressed patients, and as such, in the original studies, individuals with active substance abuse, psychotic disorders, eating disorders, obsessive–compulsive disorder (OCD), and borderline personality disorder (BPD) were excluded. The rationale behind such exclusion criteria was manifold. Individuals with acute depression often experience compromised attention and concentration that may pose significant challenges when engaging in an already challenging practice. For those with OCD, BPD, and active substance abuse, engagement in lengthy formal practices may be particularly difficult due to intrusive thoughts, impulses, and cravings (Hayes, Strosahl, & Wilson, 1999; Linehan, 1993). Moreover, other effective treatments such as CT for acute depression, acceptance and commitment therapy (ACT) for OCD, and dialectical behavior therapy (DBT) for BPD have been well established (Beck et al., 1979; Hayes et al., 1999; Linehan, 1993).

Nonetheless, a growing body of research has demonstrated that individuals with co-occuring issues such as anxiety and bipolarity may derive significant benefits from engagement in MBCT. A strong theoretical rationale has been made for the application of mindfulness skills in the treatment of anxiety disorders, in light of the future-oriented nature of worry (Roemer & Orsillo, 2002). Results from pilot studies have suggested the promise of MBCT for treating anxiety and mood symptoms in individuals suffering from social anxiety disorder and generalized anxiety (Evans et al., 2008; Piet, Hougaard, Hecksher, & Rosenberg, 2010). Preliminary findings from several small randomized controlled trials have demonstrated positive outcomes associated with participation in MBCT for individuals in the remitted phase of bipolar disorder, such as decreased symptoms of anxiety and depression (Weber et al., 2010; Williams et al., 2008).

Despite such promising findings, clinicians and expert meditation teachers recommend caution when treating individuals with a history of trauma with mindfulness-based interventions. Germer (2005b) has posited the importance of using careful clinical judgment in such cases to determine suitability, while other authors have indicated the importance of establishing preexisting "grounding skills" for those patients who may be at risk of experiencing intrusive thoughts or are particularly cognitively reactive (Crane & Williams, 2010; Dobkin, Irving, & Amar, 2012). Patients planning to engage in this type of intensive mindfulness training require the skills necessary to redirect their attention should it become drawn into destabilizing memories or overwhelming affective states prior to commencing the MBCT program.

Additional Clinical Applications

Given the efficacy MBCT has demonstrated for reducing and keeping depressive symptoms at bay, a common question surrounds the potential impact of the program for individuals with acute depression. Several open (Finucane & Mercer, 2006; Kenny & Williams, 2007) and controlled (Kingston, Dooley, Bates, Lawlor, & Malone, 2007; Williams et al., 2008) trials yielded promising results when MBCT was investigated with acutely depressed patient samples, including significant decreases in symptoms of depression and anxiety according to clinical interview and self-reports. Eisendrath, Chartier, and McLane (2011) have developed a modified version of MBCT targeting treatment-resistant depression (TRD). These authors have identified a theoretical rationale for adopting the approach with TRD given that cognitive reactivity is thought to play a significant role in driving and maintaining depressogenic states in this population. The approach is currently under evaluation in a randomized controlled trial, while small pilot studies have demonstrated promising results (Barnhofer et al., 2009; Eisendrath et al., 2008).

MBCT has also been evaluated for the treatment of recurrent suicidal ideation. In keeping with the DAH, cognitive vulnerability for suicidal relapse and recurrence may be addressed with a modified MBCT protocol. Although individuals susceptible to chronic suicidality have been shown to have high rates of attrition in MBCT, it has been posited that they may "have the most to gain" from this intervention, which holds the promise to engender decentering from distressing and potentially lethal intrusive suicidal ideation (Crane & Williams, 2010, p. 10). Pilot work (Crane & Williams, 2010; Lau, Segal, & Williams, 2004; Williams, Duggan, Crane, & Fennell, 2006) has supported the application of MBCT for the prevention of recurrent suicidal behavior, and a large-scale clinical trial is under way to examine outcomes of MBCT with this population.

Individuals with other types of intrusive or overwhelming ruminative processes, such as those implicated in dealing with a chronic and potentially life-threatening illness, or the recursive negative appraisals of body sensations that underscore hypochondriasis, may also be suitable candidates for MBCT. Foley, Baillie, Huxter, Price, and Sinclair (2010) have tailored MBCT to treat the depressive and anxious symptoms that commonly arise following the diagnosis of cancer. In a randomized trial of MBCT versus wait-list controls, significant improvements in self-reported depressive and anxious symptoms, distress, and quality of life were observed in the MBCT condition, with moderate to large effect sizes. McManus and colleagues (2012) investigated the impact of an adapted version of MBCT plus customary unrestricted treatment versus unrestricted treatment alone for individuals with hypochondriasis. MBCT participants reported significantly lower health anxiety at 1-year follow-up. Further analyses indicated that increases in mindfulness practice skills on the Five Factor Mindfulness Scale (Baer, Smith, Hopkins, Krietemeyer, & Toney, 2006) significantly mediated the difference observed in health anxiety.

Additionally, novel applications of MBCT have included the development of adapted programs targeting populations at both ends of the lifespan. Semple, Lee, Rosa, and Miller (2010) developed mindfulness-based cognitive therapy for children (MBCT-C), targeting children ages 9–13. The program aims to increase socioemotional resiliency in children at risk for stress and anxiety tied to academic difficulties; initial findings indicate that the program increased attention capacities and led to lower rates of behavior problems and anxiety symptoms (Semple et al., 2010). Smith, Graham, and Senthinathan (2007) reported evidence for the effectiveness of MBCT for older adults (age 65 and older) with a previous history of anxious and depressive symptoms.

Future Directions for Research

The efficacy of MBCT for the prevention of depressive relapse has been supported by evidence from several randomized controlled clinical trials and by meta-analyses (Hofmann, Sawyer, Witt, & Oh, 2010; Piet & Hougaard, 2011). In addition, the mechanisms through which changes occur have been explored in open and controlled trials, as well as in a small number of rigorous qualitative investigations that highlighted components that patients described as being integral to their own changes during and after participation in MBCT. Research to elucidate the underlying neural mechanisms of change is under way, building on the qualitative accounts and self-report measures aimed at operationalizing change processes in MBCT.

Despite these advances, several prominent questions regarding MBCT's efficacy remain. MBCT has demonstrated a very specific prophylactic efficacy for chronic depression—that is, three or more episodes rather than a first or second episode of depression (e.g., Ma & Teasdale, 2004). This finding suggests that relapse mechanisms may change following repeated episodes, making them particularly amenable to the contemplative practices found in MBCT. Furthermore, pilot studies indicate that patients with chronic depression or TRD may benefit from MBCT even during the acute phase of depressive episodes (Barnhofer et al., 2009; Eisendrath et al., 2008), challenging the notion that MBCT is only efficacious in the contexts of low dysphoric severity found during remission. Together, these findings support the hypothesis that MBCT effects may be founded on engaging with the familiar patterns of thought brought about by dysphoric affect, irrespective of the intensity of the dysphoria. This is to say that because a primary focus of MBCT rests on building awareness of maladaptive patterns of cognitive reactivity to emotional distress, participants are most likely to respond to this treatment when such patterns are familiar and repeatedly experienced. Such knowledge may give participants a "handle" on their patterns of reactivity on which to affix fledgling skills of nonjudgmental acceptance of experience. This presents one potential explanation for MBCT's differential efficacy that is perhaps worthy of exploration.

A second issue lies in the comparable outcomes associated with MBCT and M-ADM therapy. The similar efficacies between the two prophylactic techniques have been best supported in cases of fluctuating or unstable remission (Segal et al., 2010). Thus, for physicians attempting to discern the optimal course of treatment for a patient, stability of mood during remission should be a chief consideration. The persistence of elevated emotional reactivity to stress following seemingly successful pharmacotherapy may indicate a partial or incomplete treatment effect, driven perhaps by maladaptive patterns of cognitive reactivity that are independent of baseline neurochemical imbalance. In such cases, M-ADM may impose a masking or stifling of cognitive habits otherwise addressed through more "top-down" interventions such as MBCT or CBT. If such a hypothesis is correct, studies with longer follow-up periods should be able to document a divergence between M-ADM and MBCT because the unaddressed cognitive habits in M-ADM are strengthened while drug tolerance lowers medication effects in some patients. As mentioned earlier, Bieling and colleagues (2012) found significant increases in decentering that were unique to participants who had received MBCT relative to those receiving M-ADM or placebo. One method that could further elucidate changes in patterns of cognitive reactivity and capacity for decentering is an experience-sampling method (ESM), which might provide closer proximity to reactivity relative to naturalistic stressors in real time. This method has afforded important insights about day-to-day mind wandering as it relates to happiness more generally (Killingsworth & Gilbert, 2010), and how positive affective experiences and reward responsiveness may be facilitated in individuals vulnerable to depressive relapse in the period immediately following treatment with MBCT (Geschwind et al., 2011).

Another potential explanation for the equivalence in efficacy of MBCT and M-ADM is the likely possibility that there exist two (or more) subtypes of chronic depression driven by distinct causes that are addressed most efficaciously by one or the other of these two techniques. Neuroimaging research indicates that at least some chronically depressed patients differ from healthy controls in their ability to direct executive resources to down-regulate affective responses (Johnstone, van Reekum, Urry, Kalin, & Davidson, 2007), suggesting a need to limit maladaptive cognitive control efforts in favor of the cultivation of skills for distress tolerance and acceptance that are practiced through MBCT. Another subset of patients may experience intense upswings of emotion that overwhelm cognitive resources, and that are best benefited by directly impacting chemical transmission in the brain. This suggests the use of M-ADM, which could be more efficacious than simply learning to accept the extremes of emotion accompanying chemical imbalances associated with depressive illness. Of course, in most cases, there are aspects of both maladaptive regulatory efforts and related chemical imbalance, with individual differences in the pervasiveness of both. Learning to evaluate the systemic determinants of depressive affect may help clarify these distinctions on an individual level, leading to more customized allocation of patients to prophylactic interventions, thereby raising the success rates of both MBCT and M-ADM.

Another area of future research interest lies in examining potential changes in the brain's intrinsic connectivity networks commensurate with participation in an MBCT intervention. Predictions about such changes may be informed by recent literature examining the correlation between resting-state networks and dispositional measures of mindfulness and depressive symptomology. In particular, it would be important to identify whether MBCT enhances the attention-orienting aspects of the posterior default network (cf. Prakash, De Leon, Klatt, Malarkey, & Patterson, 2013), while reducing the strength of activation of the ventromedial PFC (Way, Creswell, Eisenberger, & Lieberman, 2010), and increasing connectivity between prefrontal and sensory cortices (Kilpatrick et al., 2011). In the short term, such research can help inform whether MBCT is effecting trait-like changes in information processing; in the long-term, such research may serve as the foundation for biomarkers of depression vulnerability and help to predict the most efficacious course of treatment. In essence, if MBCT and competing alternative therapies really do target distinct mechanisms of dysphoric illness, then the dysfunction of each of these mechanisms should possess a distinct neural signature. For example, if we can form reliable metrics of sensory–frontal connectivity that relate to depressive symptomology, this could be one indicator for embodied awareness training associated with MBCT. In cases where sensory connectivity to the frontal cortices is preserved, yet patients still display inflexible dysphoric self-schemas, CBT may be most appropriate. Finally, patients who demonstrate hyperactivity in limbic cortices but preserved sensory integration may be best served through M-ADM.

Conclusion

Initial support establishing MBCT as an effective treatment for the prevention of depressive relapse has been significantly bolstered in recent years, with effects demonstrated to be commensurate to those of the traditional first-line treatment for depressive relapse, namely, M-ADM (Kuyken et al., 2008; Segal et al., 2010). This finding suggests that MBCT represents a viable option for individuals who have difficulty tolerating M-ADM, such as women who are pregnant, or for those who have experienced tachyphylaxis. MBCT may also follow medication as a part of a sequential treatment approach to depression (Fava, Ruini, & Rafanelli, 2005). Examinations of several promising applications of MBCT are under way, including adapted protocols for clinical issues such as chronic refractory depression, recurrent suicidality, and comorbid anxiety disorders, as well as protocols tailored to child and elder populations. Future adaptations may also consider populations for whom accessibility issues are at play, calling for Web-based intervention formats that could make MBCT available to those in remote locations or for whom mobility is limited. Studies including long-term follow-up will likely be necessary to extend our understanding of the prophylactic effects of MBCT, incorporating a diversity of methods, such as experience sampling, in addition to reliance on self-report measures and clinical interviews. Collaboration with the fields of cognitive and affective neuroscience holds promise for uncovering neural markers of cognitive reactivity, and triangulating changes in self-reported symptom change and behavioral data with evidence of neuroplasticity following engagement in MBCT. Findings from such studies will further refine our understanding of whom MBCT may be best suited for and most effective.

ACKNOWLEDGMENTS

We would like to thank Ms. Safa Ali for her editorial assistance on this chapter and her ongoing commitment to the Mood Balance project at the Centre for Addiction and Mental Health. We would also like to acknowledge colleagues Adam K. Anderson, Lance Hawley, and Emily Blake for thoughtful comments that facilitated the writing of this chapter.

REFERENCES

Allen, M., Bromley, A., Kuyken, W., & Sonnenberg, S. J. (2009). Participants' experiences of mindfulness-based cognitive therapy: "It changed me in just about every way possible." *Behavioral and Cognitive Psychotherapy, 37*, 413–430.

Barnhofer, T., Crane, C., Hargus, E., Amarasinghe, M., Winder, R., & Williams, J. M. (2009). Mindfulness-based cognitive therapy as a treatment for chronic depression: A preliminary study. *Behaviour Research and Therapy, 47*(5), 366–373.

Baer, R., Smith, G., Hopkins, J., Krietemeyer, J., & Toney, L. (2006) Using self-report assessment methods to exploring facets of mindfulness. *Assessment, 13*(1), 27–45.

Beck, A. T., Rush, A. J., Shaw, B. F., & Emery, G. (1979). *Cognitive therapy of depression.* New York: Guilford Press.

Bieling, P. J., Hawley, L. L., Bloch, R. T., Corcoran, K. M., Levitan, R. D., Young, L. T., et al. (2012). Treatment-specific changes in decentering following mindfulness-based cognitive therapy versus antidepressant medication or placebo for prevention of depressive relapse. *Journal of Consulting and Clinical Psychology, 80*(3), 365–372.

Bondolfi, G., Jermann, F., Van der Linden, M., Gex-Fabry, M., Bizzini, L., Rouget, B. W., et al. (2010). Depression relapse prophylaxis with mindfulness-based cognitive therapy: Replication and extension in the Swiss health care system. *Journal of Affective Disorders, 122*, 224–231.

Casacalenda, N., Perry, J. C., & Looper, K. (2002). Remission in major depressive disorder: A comparison of pharmacotherapy, psychotherapy, and control conditions. *American Journal of Psychiatry, 159*(8), 1354–1360.

Crane, R. S., Kuyken, W., Hastings, R. P., Rothwell, N., & Williams, G. (2010). Training teachers to deliver mindfulness-based interventions: Learning from the UK experience. *Mindfulness, 1*, 74–86.

Crane, C., & Williams, J. M. G. (2010). Factors associated with attrition from mindfulness based cognitive therapy for suicidal depression. *Mindfulness, 1*, 10–20.

Dobkin, P. L., Irving, J. A., & Amar, S. (2012). For whom may participation in a mindfulness-based stress reduction program be contraindicated? *Mindfulness, 3*(1), 44–50.

Eisendrath, S., Chartier, M., & McLane, M. (2011). Adapting mindfulness-based cognitive therapy for treatment-resistant depression. *Cognitive and Behavioural Practice, 18,* 362–370.

Eisendrath, S. J., Delucchi, K., Bitner, R., Fenimore, P., Smit, M., & McLane, M. (2008). Mindfulness-based cognitive therapy for treatment-resistant depression: A pilot study. *Psychotherapy and Psychosomatics, 77*(5), 319–320.

Evans, S., Ferrando, S., Findler, M., Stowell, C., Smart, C., & Haglin, D. (2008). Mindfulness-based cognitive therapy for anxiety. *Journal of Anxiety Disorders, 22,* 716–721.

Farb, N. A. S., Anderson, A. K., Bloch, R. T., & Segal, Z. V. (2011). Mood-linked responses in medical prefrontal cortex predict relapse in patients with recurrent unipolar depression. *Biological Psychiatry, 70*(4), 366–372.

Farb, N. A. S., Segal, Z. V., & Anderson, A. K. (2011). Towards a neuroimaging biomarker of depression vulnerability. *Translational Neuroscience, 2*(4), 281–292.

Fava, G. A., Rafanelli, C., Grandi, S., Canestrari, R., & Morphy, M. A. (1998). Six-year outcome for cognitive behavioral treatment of residual symptoms in major depression. *American Journal of Psychiatry, 155*(10), 1443–1445.

Fava, G. A., Ruini, C., & Rafanelli, C. (2005). Sequential treatment of mood and anxiety disorders. *Journal of Clinical Psychiatry, 66*(11), 1392–1400.

Finucane, A., & Mercer, S. W. (2006). An exploratory mixed-methods study of the acceptability and effectiveness of mindfulness-based cognitive therapy for patients with active depression and anxiety in primary care. *BMC Psychiatry, 6*(14).

Foley, E., Baillie, A., Huxter, M., Price, M., & Sinclair, E. (2010). Mindfulness-based cognitive therapy for individuals whose lives have been affected by cancer: A randomized controlled trial. *Journal of Consulting and Clinical Psychology, 78*(1), 72–79.

Gelenberg, A. J. (2010). The prevalence and impact of depression. *Journal of Clinical Psychiatry, 71*(3)

Germer, C. K. (2005a). Mindfulness: What is it? What does it matter? In C. K. Germer, R. D. Siegel, & P. R. Fulton (Eds.), *Mindfulness and psychotherapy* (pp. 3–27). New York: Guilford Press.

Germer, C. K. (2005b). Teaching mindfulness in therapy. In C. K. Germer, R. D. Siegel, & P. R. Fulton (Eds.), *Mindfulness and psychotherapy* (pp. 113–129). New York: Guilford Press.

Geschwind, N., Peeters, F., Drukker, M., van Os, J., & Wichers, M. (2011). Mindfulness training increases momentary positive emotions and reward experience in adults vulnerable to depression: A randomized controlled trial. *Journal of Consulting and Clinical Psychology, 79*(5), 618–628.

Godfrin, K. A., & van Heeringen, C. (2010). The effects of mindfulness-based cognitive therapy on recurrence of depressive episodes, mental health and quality of life: A randomized controlled study. *Behaviour Research and Therapy, 48,* 738–746.

Hamilton, M. (1960). A rating scale for depression. *Journal of Neurology, Neurosurgery and Psychiatry, 23,* 56–62.

Hayes, S. C., Strosahl, K. D., & Wilson, K. G. (1999). *Acceptance and commitment therapy: An experiential approach to behavior change.* New York: Guilford Press.

Hofmann, S. G., Sawyer, A. T., Witt, A. A., & Oh, D. (2010) The effect of mindfulness-based therapy on anxiety and depression: A meta-analytic review. *Journal of Consulting and Clinical Psychology, 78,* 169–183.

Ingram, R. E., & Hollon, S. D. (1986). Cognitive therapy of depression from an information processing perspective. In R. E. Ingram (Ed.), *Information processing approaches to clinical psychology* (pp. 259–281). San Diego, CA: Academic Press.

Johnstone, T., van Reekum, C. M., Urry, H. L., Kalin, N. H., & Davidson, R. J. (2007). Failure to regulate: Counterproductive recruitment of top-down prefrontal-subcortical circuitry in major depression. *Journal of Neuroscience, 27*(33), 8877–8884.

Judd, L. J. (1997). The clinical course of unipolar major depressive disorders. *Archives of General Psychiatry, 54*, 989–991.

Kabat-Zinn, J. (1990). *Full catastrophe living: Using the wisdom of your mind to face stress, pain and illness.* New York: Dell.

Kendler, K. S., Thornton, L. M., & Gardner, C. O. (2000). Stressful life events and previous episodes in the etiology of major depression in women: An evaluation of the "kindling" hypothesis. *American Journal of Psychiatry, 157*(8), 1243–1251.

Kenny, M. A., & Williams, J. M. G. (2007). Treatment-resistant depressed patients show a good response to mindfulness-based cognitive therapy. *Behaviour Research and Therapy, 45*(3), 617–625.

Kessler, R. C., McGonagle, K. A., Zhao, S., Nelson, C. B., Hughes, M., Eshlerman, S., et al. (1994). Lifetime and twelve-month prevalence of DSM-III-R psychiatric disorders in the United States: Results from the National Comorbidity Study. *Archives of General Psychiatry, 51*, 8–19.

Killingsworth, M. A., & Gilbert, D. T. (2010). A wandering mind is an unhappy mind. *Science, 330*, 932.

Kilpatrick, L. A., Suyenobu, B. Y., Smith, S. R., Bueller, J. A., Goodman, T., Creswell, J. D., et al. (2011). Impact of mindfulness-based stress reduction training on intrinsic brain connectivity. *NeuroImage, 56*(1), 290–298.

Kingston, T., Dooley, B., Bates, A., Lawlor, E., & Malone, K. (2007). Mindfulness-based cognitive therapy for residual depressive symptoms. *Psychology and Psychotherapy: Theory, Research and Practice, 80*(2), 193–203.

Kupfer, D. J., Frank, E., Perel, J. M., Cornes, C., Mallinger, A. G., Thase, M. E., et al. (1992). Five-year outcomes for maintenance therapies in recurrent depression. *Archives of General Psychiatry, 49*, 769–773.

Kuyken, W., Byford, S., Taylor, R. S., Watkins, E., Holden, E., White, K., et al. (2008). Mindfulness-based cognitive therapy to prevent relapse in recurrent depression. *Journal of Consulting and Clinical Psychology, 76*(6), 966–978.

Kuyken, W., Watkins, E., Holden, E., White, K., Taylor, R. S., Byford, S., et al. (2010). How does mindfulness-based cognitive therapy work? *Behaviour Research and Therapy, 48*, 1105–1112.

Lau, M. A., Segal, Z. V., & Williams, J. M. G. (2004). Teasdale's differential activation hypothesis: Implications for mechanisms of depressive relapse and suicidal behaviour. *Behaviour Research and Therapy, 42*, 1001–1017.

Linehan, M. M. (1993). *Cognitive-behavioral treatment of borderline personality disorder.* New York: Guilford Press.

Ma, S. H., & Teasdale, J. D. (2004). Mindfulness-based cognitive therapy for depression: Replication and exploration of differential relapse prevention effects. *Journal of Consulting and Clinical Psychology, 72*, 31–40.

Mason, O., & Hargreaves, I. (2001). A qualitative study of mindfulness-based cognitive therapy for depression. *British Journal of Medical Psychology, 74*, 197–212.

McManus, F., Surawy, C., Muse, K., Vazquez-Montes, M., & Williams, J. M. G. (2012). A randomized clinical trial of mindfulness-based cognitive therapy versus unrestricted services for health anxiety (hypochondriasis). *Journal of Consulting and Clinical Psychology, 80*(5), 817–828.

Moore, R. G., Hayhurst, H., & Teasdale, J. D. (1996). *Measure of awareness and coping in autobiographical memory: Instructions for administering and coding.* Unpublished manuscript, Department of Psychiatry, University of Cambridge, Cambridge, UK.

Paykel, E. S., Scott, J., Teasdale, J. D., Johnson, A. L., Garland, A., Moore, R., et al. (1999). Prevention of relapse in residual depression by cognitive therapy: A controlled trial. *Archives of General Psychiatry, 56*(9), 829–835.

Piet, J., & Hougaard, E. (2011). The effect of mindfulness-based cognitive therapy for prevention of relapse in recurrent major depressive disorder: A systematic review and meta-analysis. *Clinical Psychology Reviews, 31*(6), 1032–1040.

Piet, J., Hougaard, E., Hecksher, M. S., & Rosenberg, N. K. (2010). A randomized pilot study of mindfulness-based cognitive therapy and group cognitive-behavioral therapy for young adults with social phobia. *Scandinavian Journal of Psychology, 51*(5), 403–410.

Post, R. M. (1992). Transduction of psychosocial stress into the neurobiology of recurrent affective disorder. *American Journal of Psychiatry, 149,* 999–1010.

Post, R. M., & Weiss, S. R. B. (1998). Sensitization and kindling phenomena in mood, anxiety, and obsessive–compulsive disorders: The role of serotonergic mechanisms in illness progression. *Biological Psychiatry, 44,* 193–206.

Prakash, R. S., De Leon, A. A., Klatt, M., Malarkey, W., & Patterson, B. (2013). Mindfulness disposition and default-mode network connectivity in older adults. *Social Cognitive and Affective Neuroscience, 8*(1), 112–117.

Richards, D. (2011). Prevalence and clinical course of depression: A review. *Clinical Psychology Review, 31*(7), 1117–1125.

Roemer, L., & Orsillo, S. M. (2002). Expanding our conceptualization of and treatment for generalized anxiety disorder: Integrating mindfulness/acceptance-based approaches with existing cognitive-behavioral models. *Clinical Psychology: Science and Practice, 9,* 54–68.

Semple, R. J., Lee, J., Rosa, D., & Miller, L. F. (2010). A randomized trial of mindfulness-based cognitive therapy for children: Promoting mindful attention to enhance social-emotional resilience in children. *Journal of Child and Family Studies, 19,* 218–229.

Segal, Z. V., Bierling, P., Young, T., MacQueen, G., Cooke, R., Martin, L., et al. (2010). Antidepressant monotherapy versus sequential pharmacotherapy and mindfulness-based cognitive therapy, or placebo, for relapse prophylaxis in recurrent depression. *Archives of General Psychiatry, 67*(12), 1256–1264.

Segal, Z. V., Kennedy, S., Gemar, M., Hood, K., Pederson, R., & Buis, T. (2006). Cognitve reactivity to sad mood provocation and the prediction of depressive relapse. *Archives of General Psychiatry, 63,* 749–755.

Segal, Z. V., Williams, J. M. G., & Teasdale, J. D. (2012). *Mindfulness-based cognitive therapy for depression: A new approach for preventing relapse* (2nd ed.). New York: Guilford Press.

Solomon, D. A., Keller, M. B., Leon, A. C., Mueller, T. I., Lavori, P. W., Shea, M. T., et al. (2000). Multiple recurrences of major depressive disorder. *American Journal of Psychiatry, 157,* 229–233.

Smith, A., Graham, L., & Senthinathan, S. (2007). Mindfulness based cognitive therapy for recurring depression in older people: A qualitative study. *Aging and Mental Health, 11,* 346–357.

Spitzer, R. L., Williams, J. B. W., Gibbon, M., & First, M. B. (1992). The Structured Clinical Interview for DSM-III-R (SCID): I. History, rationale, and description. *Archives of General Psychiatry, 49,* 624–629.

Sullivan, P. F., Neale, M. C., & Kendler, K. S. (2000). Genetic epidemiology of major depression: Review and meta-analysis. *American Journal of Psychiatry, 157*(10), 1552–1562.

Teasdale, J. (1988). Cognitive vulnerability to persistent depression. *Cognition and Emotion, 2*, 247–274.

Teasdale, J. D., Moore, R. G., Hayhurst, H., Pope, M., Williams, S., & Segal, Z. V. (2002). Metacognitive awareness and prevention of relapse in depression: Empirical evidence. *Journal of Consulting and Clinical Psychology, 70*, 275–287.

Teasdale, J. D., Segal, Z. V., Williams, J. M. G., Ridgeway, V. A., Soulsby, J. M., & Lau, M. A. (2000). Prevention of relapse/recurrence in major depression by mindfulness-based cognitive therapy. *Journal of Consulting and Clinical Psychology, 68*, 615–623.

Way, B. M., Creswell, J. D., Eisenberger, N. I., & Lieberman, M. D. (2010). Dispositional mindfulness and depressive symptomatology: Correlations with limbic and self-referential neural activity during rest. *Emotion, 10*(1), 12–24.

Weber, B., Jermann, F., Gex-Fabry, M., Nallet, A., Bondolfi, G., & Aubry J. M. (2010). Mindfulness-based cognitive therapy for bipolar disorder: A feasibility trial. *European Psychiatry, 25*(6), 334–337.

Weissman, A. N. (1979). *Assessing depressogenic attitudes: A validation study.* Unpublished thesis, University of Pennsylvania.

Williams, J. M. G., Alatiq, Y., Crane, C., Barnhofer, T., Fennell, M. J. V., Duggan, D. S., et al. (2008). Mindfulness-based cognitive therapy (MBCT) in bipolar disorder: Preliminary evaluation of immediate effects on between-episode functioning. *Journal of Affective Disorders, 107*(1–3), 275–279.

Williams, J. M. G., Duggan, D. S., Crane, C., & Fennell, M. J. V. (2006). Mindfulness-based cognitive therapy for prevention of recurrence of suicidal behaviour. *Journal of Clinical Clinical Psychology, 62*, 201–210.

CHAPTER 20

Mindfulness in the Treatment of Anxiety

Sarah A. Hayes-Skelton and Lauren P. Wadsworth

Anxiety is a normal part of the human experience. We, as humans, experience adaptive anxiety when we are anticipating a job interview, meeting our partner's parents for the first time, or standing at the top of a tall building. However, for some, anxiety leads to significant interference in life and emotional distress, becoming what is considered to be an anxiety disorder. As a group, anxiety disorders are characterized by individuals' reactions to perceived threats in the environment; a narrowed, reactive, and judgmental view of these reactions; and in turn, a desire not to experience these reactions. This typically leads individuals to avoid situations, objects, people, and internal experiences that may trigger anxiety, thus constraining life and decreasing well-being (American Psychiatric Association, 2013). The specific types of stimuli that trigger the anxiety response depend partly on the type of anxiety a person experiences. For example, for panic disorder, the trigger may be a racing heart; for social anxiety disorder, it may be being called on in class; for claustrophobia, it may be a small elevator; or for obsessive–compulsive disorder (OCD), it may be a dirty bathroom. As a class, anxiety disorders are the most common mental health diagnoses (Kessler, Berglund, et al., 2005), with 28.8% of members of the population meeting criteria for an anxiety disorder in their lifetime (Kessler, Berglund, et al., 2005) and 18.1% meeting criteria in the 12 months prior to the survey (Kessler, Chiu, Demler, Merikangas, & Walters, 2005). Based on this survey, specific phobias had the highest lifetime prevalence (13.2%), followed by social anxiety disorder (12.6%), posttraumatic stress disorder (PTSD; 8.7%), generalized anxiety disorder (GAD; 8.3%), panic disorder (6.0%), and agoraphobia without panic (1.6%) (Kessler, Berglund, et al., 2005). Anxiety disorders have been associated with a chronic course, in that they do not typically remit without treatment (Hirschfeld, 1996), and people with anxiety disorders have higher rates of financial dependence and unemployment

(Leon, Portera, & Weissman, 1995), increased disability and lower quality of life (Alonso et al., 2004), and increased risk for suicide (Cougle, Keough, Riccardi, & Sachs-Ericsson, 2009).

According to an acceptance-based behavioral model of anxiety (Roemer & Orsillo, 2009), anxiety is characterized by a narrowed, reactive, and judgmental relationship with the internal anxiety responses, a rigid desire not to experience anxiety, and a restricted number of activities as a way to avoid anxiety. In this model, cultivating mindfulness that broadens and opens awareness to the full range of experiences with an attitude of compassion may reduce the problematic relationship with internal experiences that characterizes anxiety, thus reducing avoidance and anxiety. Therefore, it is perhaps no surprise that there has been a rise in interventions that incorporate mindfulness or mindfulness-based principles for anxious individuals. As described below, the amount of focus specifically on mindfulness and the types of mindfulness practices can vary widely across these interventions. While mindfulness by itself shows some promise in the treatment of anxiety, it is more typically incorporated alongside other behavior therapy elements into multicomponent treatment packages. Mindfulness practice may by itself decrease anxiety; however, increasing mindful awareness may also enhance the efficacy of other behavioral interventions, such as exposure exercises. Mindfulness-based treatments may also be helpful when the cognitive responses to a situation are not irrational or maladaptive, such as when one's social anxiety is related to acts of racism or other forms of marginalization, or when anxiety and worry about finances are warranted given someone's current financial situation.

In this chapter we briefly review Roemer and Orsillo's acceptance-based behavioral model of anxiety, which places a major emphasis on mindfulness, and shows how increasing mindful awareness may be an adaptive response to anxiety (see Figure 20.1). We then briefly review the current literature on mindfulness-based treatments for anxiety. In our final section we focus on emerging applications of mindfulness-based approaches, including ways that mindful awareness can be enhanced in both mindfulness-based and non-mindfulness-based interventions for anxiety.

An Acceptance-Based Model of Anxiety

According to an acceptance-based behavioral model of anxiety (Roemer, & Orsillo, 2014), anxiety is characterized by a fused, narrowed, reactive, and judgmental relationship with internal experiences (e.g., thoughts, feelings, images, urges), and simultaneously a strong desire to push away these anxious experiences, which only serves to increase the problematic relationship with them. As a result, it is only natural to then avoid future situations and limit experiences that increase anxiety. In other words, anxiety is maintained by (1) a problematic relationship with internal experiences; (2) experiential avoidance, or the internal strategies aimed at suppressing anxious thoughts, feelings, or sensations, decreasing their frequency or changing their form (Hayes, Strosahl, & Wilson, 2012); and (3) behavioral constriction and avoidance. While this model was originally developed specifically for GAD, it is broadly

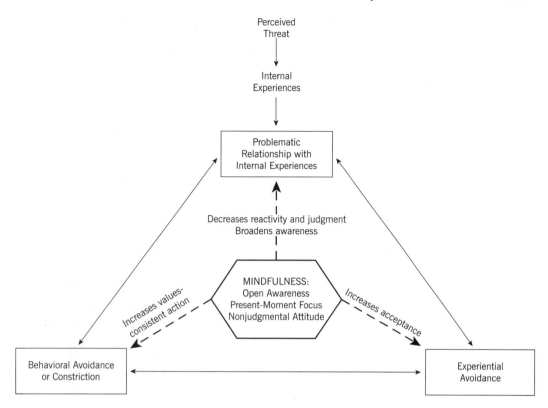

FIGURE 20.1. Impact of mindfulness on an acceptance-based behavioral model of anxiety. In this model, anxiety is maintained by a problematic relationship with internal experiences, by experiential avoidance, and by behavioral avoidance. Mindfulness is theorized to impact each stage of the anxiety maintenance model by providing increased acceptance, decreased reactivity, and broadened awareness, allowing the individual to engage in greater value-consistent action.

applicable to anxiety in general and is consistent with disorder-specific acceptance and mindfulness-based models of social anxiety disorder (Herbert & Cardaciotto, 2005), panic disorder (Levitt & Karekla, 2005), OCD (Twohig, 2009), and PTSD (Batten, Orsillo, & Walser, 2005).

Problematic Relationship with Internal Experiences

Because anxiety is an adaptive response to a potentially dangerous situation, when an individual enters or anticipates an anxiety-provoking situation, he or she experiences a cascade of thoughts and physical experiences adapted to assess danger. For example, the person may experience an increased heart rate, so that he or she is better able to flee the situation, and a narrowed attentional focus that aides in searching for threat. While these responses are often adaptive, or even necessary for survival, they can also be problematic, particularly when they are rigidly reacted to with judgment.

In other words, we become entangled (Germer, 2005), "hooked" (Chodron, 2007), or fused (Herzberg et al., 2012) with our experiences. Based on this model, it is not the thoughts, feelings, or sensations that are problematic, but rather the way people respond to them that exacerbates anxiety.

In support of this model's hypothesis that it is our reactions to experiences that are problematic rather than the experiences themselves, GAD is characterized as worry about worry (Wells, 1995), and panic disorder is characterized by the fear of panic rather than the panic itself (American Psychiatric Association, 2013). Research has shown that individuals with generalized anxiety are more reactive toward and judgmental of their emotions and negative thoughts than those without significant anxiety (e.g., Lee, Orsillo, Roemer, & Allen, 2010; Mennin, Heimberg, Turk, & Fresco, 2005; Wells & Carter, 1999). Similarly, changes in reactivity to emotions (measured as fear of emotions and anxiety sensitivity) predict anxiety and depression outcomes above and beyond changes in the frequency of negative emotions following treatment with the transdiagnostic Unified Protocol (Sauer-Zavala et al., 2012).

However, in addition to the reactivity and judgment of internal experiences that arise (e.g., thoughts, feelings, sensations, images, urges), anxiety also leads to a hypervigilance toward signs of threat or a narrowed focus on threat-relevant information. For example, one of the key criteria for PTSD is this hypervigilance to threat (American Psychiatric Association, 2013). Similarly, research indicates that self-focused attention characterizes social anxiety disorder (Bögels & Mansell, 2004). This self-focus is characterized by negative self-images that one believes to be accurate (Hofmann & Heinrichs, 2003). At the same time, the attentional resources are directed inward, so that positive cues from the environment are missed (Flory, Räikkönen, Matthews, & Owens, 2000). Together, these narrowed attentional processes maintain anxiety by continuing the focus on potential threat cues.

The final way in which anxiety is maintained by a problematic relationship with internal experiences occurs when the individual becomes fused or entangled with the internal representations of anxiety, so that the experiences are seen as constant signs of reality rather than passing events in the mind. This concept of fusion comes from relational frame theory (Hayes et al., 2012), which suggests that we, as humans, derive relationships among events, feelings, images, and experiences as we interact with others and the environment. The result is that our internal stimuli (thoughts, feelings, images, etc.) take on the function of the events to which they are linked. This tendency to mistake these transient experiences as permanent can lead to further reactivity toward internal experiences and can lead to avoidance of potentially anxiety-provoking situations (Blackledge, 2007).

Experiential Avoidance

When anxiety is experienced as all-encompassing and as a negative indication of self-worth, then it is only natural to want to avoid the internal experiences that have become signs of anxiety. This desire to push away, escape, or change distressing internal experiences has been termed *experiential avoidance* (Hayes et al., 2012) and is considered the opposite of acceptance or willingness. We know from the thought suppression literature (Purdon, 1999) that the more effort one makes to push away an internal experience, the stronger its return. For example, Roemer and Borkovec (1994) found that when individuals were asked to suppress specific thoughts, they subsequently reported increased anxiety in response to these thoughts. Similarly, Campbell-Sills, Barlow, Brown, and Hofmann (2006) found that participants who were instructed to suppress their emotions reported more negative affect following an emotion-provoking film, and an increase in heart rate during the film, than did individuals instructed to accept their emotions. Therefore, when individuals try to push away the internal experiences that fuel anxiety, they are often unable to do so, which only serves to increase the fusion and self-judgment about their inability to rid themselves of anxiety. This then increases the experiential avoidance further, perpetuating the cycle. Experiential avoidance has been associated with excessive worry and GAD diagnosis (Buhr & Dugas, 2012) and anxiety in general (Salters-Pedneault & Diller, 2013). Experiential avoidance has also differentiated individuals with social anxiety disorder from non-anxious controls (Kashdan et al., 2013).

Behavioral Avoidance or Constriction

When situations are perceived to lead to troubling internal experiences and subsequent experiential avoidance, then it is only natural that individuals avoid those situations. Individuals with anxiety often constrict their lives in an effort to avoid these experiences. For example, individuals with GAD are less likely than individuals without GAD to engage in behaviors that are important to them, which results in a diminished quality of life (Michelson, Lee, Orsillo, & Roemer, 2011). However, when one avoids a situation or experience, he or she misses opportunities for new learning, for finding evidence that the situation does not need to be feared (see Craske et al., 2008), which reinforces the avoidance and makes it more difficult to approach similar situations in the future. This avoidance of feared situations and triggers is a major part of the criteria for most anxiety disorders and is often a major contributor to the interference and distress of anxiety disorders.

Mindful Awareness as an Adaptive Response to Anxiety

If anxiety is characterized by this reactive, fused, judgmental, and narrowed relationship with internal experience that can then trigger experiential and behavioral avoidance, then the cultivation of a cognitive stance characterized by accepting, nonjudgmental, nonreactive, open awareness—in other words, cultivating mindfulness, or an "openhearted, moment-to-moment, nonjudgmental awareness" (Kabat-Zinn, 2005, p. 24)—should decrease this anxiety response. Three components of mindfulness training (open awareness, present-moment focus, and a nonjudgmental/compassionate attitude) together should reduce the reactive, fused, and judgmental reaction to internal experiences, thus decreasing experiential and behavioral avoidance.

The *open awareness* characteristic of mindfulness training should expand and broaden awareness to counter the narrowed, threat-focused attention. Rather than scanning the self and the environment for signs of threat, bringing mindful awareness to bear involves broadening awareness to take in the full context, including neutral and positive cues. This should provide a more balanced view of the situation at hand as opposed to the narrowed, threat-focused perspective. This increased awareness provides the opportunity for individuals to make choices about how they want to respond (Teasdale et al., 2000). In other words, it is theorized that the open awareness of mindfulness helps to increase awareness regarding the reasons to take or avoid action, making individuals more conscious of times they want to override the urge to avoid or to take an action. Similarly, the *present-moment focus* counters the rumination and anticipatory anxiety that characterizes anxiety disorders. For example, the focus on what is happening in the moment provides an alternative for the anxious focus on the future. Finally, the *nonjudgmental/compassionate focus* provides a strong alternative to the negative biases that are characteristic of anxiety. For example, the practice of experiencing thoughts as just thoughts (instead of "good" or "bad" thoughts) may help an individual to recognize the biases in his or her view of internal and external events. Mindfulness may also provide distance, or *decentering*, from our internal experiences in a nonjudgmental manner. Internal experiences can be entangled or fused with anxious experiences, so that the anxious experiences seem to be constant and defining features of oneself. Mindfulness can help the individual step back, decenter, and see the transience of these internal experiences in a nonjudgmental way rather than as indicators of a permanent, unchanging truth. In this way, mindfulness-based therapies can help teach participants that thoughts are not facts (Baer, 2003; Segal, Williams, & Teasdale, 2002). Viewing these thoughts, feelings, and sensations as transient mental events may help to reduce reactivity toward them, thus decreasing experiential avoidance, followed by a decrease in anxiety. Similarly, learning to respond to internal experiences and the self more generally with compassion can help to promote acceptance of these internal experiences, which may serve to reduce the experiential avoidance characteristic of anxiety.

Supporting this model, research has highlighted that lower levels of mindfulness are associated with GAD and worry (Roemer et al.,, 2009), social anxiety symptoms, fear of negative evaluation (Burton, Schmertz, Price, Masuda, & Anderson, 2013; Hayes-Skelton & Graham, 2012), and anxiety and distress more generally (Brown & Ryan, 2003; Desrosiers, Vine, Klemanski, & Nolen-Hoeksema, 2013). Several recent studies provide preliminary evidence that decentering (Hayes-Skelton & Graham, 2012), cognitive appraisal of the probability and cost of the social outcome (Schmertz, Masuda, & Anderson, 2012), and affective reactivity (Ostafin, Brooks, & Laitem, in press) at least partially account for the relationship between mindfulness and anxiety. However, much more research is needed to understand better the mechanisms through which mindfulness is associated with lowered anxiety.

Mindfulness-Based Interventions for Anxiety Disorders

A number of mindfulness-based treatment approaches have been developed. While not originally designed for anxiety, mindfulness-based cognitive therapy (MBCT; Segal et al., 2002) and mindfulness-based stress reduction (MBSR; Kabat-Zinn, 1982) have been applied to social anxiety disorder (Goldin, Ramel, & Gross, 2009; Koszycki, Benger, Shlik, & Bradwejn, 2007), GAD (Craigie, Rees, & March, 2008;

Evans et al., 2008), panic disorder (Kim et al., 2010), and mixed anxiety samples (Kim et al., 2009; Yook et al., 2008). MBSR is a group-based psychoeducational program that focuses on in-session and between-session mindfulness exercises. MBCT, which was derived from MBSR, also includes exercises specifically aimed at increasing awareness of and disengaging from negative cognitive processes.

Similarly, acceptance approaches such as acceptance and commitment therapy (ACT; Hayes, Strosahl, et al., 2012) and dialectical behavior therapy (DBT; Linehan, 1993) incorporate mindfulness-based principles. For example, ACT uses mindfulness and acceptance principles to enhance behavioral and experiential psychotherapy techniques, encouraging individuals to approach (rather than avoid) their anxious thoughts with a nonjudgmental and nonreactive stance. ACT has been applied to social anxiety disorder (e.g., Dalrymple & Herbert, 2007; Ossman, Wilson, Storassli, & McNeill, 2006), OCD (e.g., Twohig et al., 2010), and mixed anxiety samples (e.g., Arch et al., 2012). While DBT has not been applied specifically for anxiety disorders, in a trial of DBT for recurrently suicidal women with borderline personality disorder, 39% of clients with secondary anxiety diagnoses had symptoms remit by the end of treatment (Harned et al., 2008).

In addition to the previously mentioned treatment approaches that were designed more broadly and then applied to anxiety disorders, there have been a few mindfulness-based treatment approaches designed specifically for anxiety disorders, such as acceptance-based behavioral therapy (ABBT; Roemer & Orsillo, 2014) developed for GAD, and mindfulness and acceptance-based group therapy for social anxiety disorder (MAGT; Kocovski, Fleming, & Rector, 2009). These treatments specifically incorporate mindfulness practices with additional behavioral interventions for anxiety disorders, such as a focus on decreasing experiential and behavioral avoidance. These treatments also focus on using mindfulness- and acceptance-based strategies to help clients engage in previously avoided valued actions.

Efficacy of Mindfulness-Based Interventions

A growing body of research has supported mindfulness-based interventions for anxiety disorders. In a meta-analysis focusing on MBCT and MBSR, there was a large effect size (Hedges's $g = 0.97$) for change in anxiety symptoms across treatments targeting GAD, GAD and panic, and social anxiety disorder (Hofmann, Sawyer, Witt, & Oh, 2010). To broaden the previous meta-analyses of mindfulness- and acceptance-based interventions to include more anxiety disorders, Vøllestad, Nielsen, and Nielsen (2012) conducted a meta-analysis that included studies of MBCT, MBSR, ACT, ABBT, and MAGT for anxiety disorders. Of the 19 studies included, the majority (14) were based on MBCT/MBSR, with two on ACT, two on ABBT, and one on MAGT. Most of the studies (7) focused on social anxiety disorder, with four focused on GAD, one on panic disorder, four on mixed anxiety disorders, and three on mixed anxiety and depression. Overall, there were large pre- to posttreatment effect sizes for anxiety outcomes (Hedges's $g = 1.08$). In that review, there was some evidence that treatments with specific psychotherapeutic content had stronger effects than those that were more purely focused on mindfulness training; however, this should be interpreted cautiously given the small number of studies included.

Overall, evidence indicates that these mindfulness-based interventions increase trait mindfulness (Carmody & Baer, 2008; Keng, Smoski, & Robins, 2011; Nyklíček & Kuijpers, 2008). While these studies indicate that mindfulness changes over treatment, more research is needed to determine whether it is in fact the change in mindfulness that leads to the changes in symptoms. Because these treatments have multiple components, dismantling studies are needed to determine the relative contribution of different components in changing mindfulness.

The Practice of Mindfulness in Anxiety Interventions

Within the Eastern spiritual and religious traditions, mindfulness has been taught in myriad ways. Similarly, within mindfulness-based treatments, mindfulness skills have been incorporated in several ways that vary in the structure, form, and intensity of practice, while sharing the goal of raising present-focused, nonjudgmental awareness. For example, MBSR involves a series of guided meditation practices completed in group sessions; then participants are requested to practice the meditative exercises for approximately 45 minutes a day between sessions (Kabat-Zinn, 1990). In contrast, DBT focuses on practicing mindfulness skills in the context of daily life through teaching components of mindfulness in combination with other behavioral skills rather than through formal meditation practice (Linehan, 1993). Treatment approaches such as ABBT fall somewhere in the middle. In ABBT, there is a more flexible application of both formal meditation in and out of session and an application of mindfulness skills throughout daily life in combination with behavioral principles (Roemer & Orsillo, 2009).

These practices differ in their structure and form. Throughout these therapies, mindfulness practices are taught as formal meditation practices, informal practices, or both. Here, *formal mindfulness practice* refers to a discrete, time-delineated practice of sitting meditation, mindful yoga, body scans, or formal walking meditations (Kabat-Zinn, 1990). However, because of the episodic nature of anxiety, a mindfulness-based treatment for anxiety also needs to have a way to teach an application-based mindfulness skill that can be practiced in the moment because it is not always possible to engage in a formal practice in the midst of an anxiety-provoking situation. Therefore, these treatments often also focus on *informal mindfulness practice*, or the experience of intentionally drawing mindful attention to whatever activities are taking place in the moment, with the intent of helping individuals move toward being able to apply mindfulness skills in difficult situations during daily life (Kabat-Zinn, 1990). These informal practices can take many forms, such as washing the dishes, eating, folding laundry, or having a difficult conversation with a loved one, and can be planned and scheduled into one's daily life. They can serve as a bridge between engaging in the formal meditation practices and the application of mindfulness skills to spontaneous situations (Roemer & Orsillo, 2009). Combined, these practices may have the effect of generally increasing the natural, or spontaneous, state of mindful awareness, which may generally decrease stress and anxiety.

Additionally, several practices focus specifically on applying mindfulness in the midst of anxiety-provoking or otherwise distressing situations. These *applied mindfulness practices* are intended to be used in the moment to bring mindful awareness to the current situation. For example, the 3-minute breathing space (Segal et al., 2002) is a brief exercise designed to help an individual become aware of all that is occurring in the present, to center attention on the breath, and to expand attention back out to the world as a whole. This exercise can be applied in the midst of an anxiety-inducing situation to encourage an expanded, nonjudgmental awareness of all of the internal and external stimuli that may be contributing to anxiety. Learning to bring this kind of mindful awareness to distressing situations may help the individual understand the natural urge to avoid and may help him or her recognize why he or she may want to move forward with an action even in the face of anxiety. Behavioral engagement is a cornerstone of many approaches to reducing the interference and distress associated with anxiety.

The majority of the mindfulness-based interventions for anxiety incorporate additional techniques and practices along with the mindfulness practices. As mentioned in the meta-analysis of mindfulness-based treatments for anxiety (Vøllestad et al., 2012), there is some evidence that approaches including additional content along with mindfulness may be more effective than treatments using only mindfulness. In addition to the effects of mindfulness alone, mindful awareness and skills may also help clients engage in other aspects of therapy. For example, in ABBT (Roemer & Orsillo, 2009) and MAGT (Fleming & Kocovski, 2013), there is an explicit focus on using mindfulness to help a client build awareness of then engage in actions and activities that are meaningful to him or her. This focus on taking values-consistent action (see Wilson & Murrell, 2004, for a discussion of valued action in therapy) is the primary focus of the second half of these treatments. Based on these treatment models, it is the mindful awareness that promotes clarity about what these activities should be, then promotes a tool (e.g., 3-minute breathing space) to enhance nonjudgmental awareness to make these behavioral actions possible when the anxiety arises.

Empirical Support for Mindfulness Practice

There is much written about the amount and role of mindfulness practice; however, we are far from reaching a consensus on the relationship between mindfulness practice and outcome. For example, a meta-analysis of MBSR and MBCT (Vettese, Toneatto, Stea, Nguyen, & Wang, 2009) found that less than one-fourth of the reviewed studies reported on the relationship between practice and outcome. Of the 24 studies that analyzed the association between practice and outcome, approximately one-half (13) reported a significant association between practice and outcome, while the remaining 11 studies did not find this association. These mixed findings may have to do with the ways that mindfulness practice and mindfulness skills were measured and assessed or with (lack of) variability in the amount or quality of practice. For example, Morgan, Graham, Hayes-Skelton, Orsillo, and Roemer (in press) found that for clients with GAD receiving ABBT, the amount of informal mindfulness practice was related to longer-term improvements in GAD severity, worry, and quality of life; however, formal mindfulness practice was not related to outcome. This finding of the importance of informal practice is encouraging for clinical practice because informal mindfulness practices may be more culturally congruent for some clients (see Sobczak & West, 2013). Additionally, most of the previous studies on mindfulness practice have examined the frequency and duration of practice and not the *quality* of practice. More recently, del Re, Flückiger, Goldberg, and Hoyt (2013) developed a measure of mindfulness practice quality and found that practice quality was related to more favorable outcome. However, this self-report measure relies on participants' ability to assess the quality of their mindfulness practice accurately. More work is needed to figure out how best to assess mindfulness practice to determine what kind, how much, and what quality of practice is needed for most effective outcomes.

Increasing Mindful Awareness through Non-Mindfulness-Based Therapies

While the preceding studies highlight how mindfulness-based therapies that incorporate formal and informal mindfulness practice help to reduce the suffering and symptoms of anxiety, other intervention strategies may also foster increased mindful awareness as a mechanism to decreased anxiety. Paying attention to the ways that these interventions already foster mindful awareness and intentionally increasing the mindful components inherent in these interventions may help further to promote efficacy. For example, does the efficacy of applied relaxation improve if mindful awareness is fostered in the relaxation practice? Do exposure exercises become more effective when mindfulness exercises are used to enhance awareness? Similarly, do cognitive restructuring exercises inherently enhance mindful awareness? If so, would there be benefit to increasing mindfulness intentionally during these practices? Rather than treating these as separate approaches to treating anxiety, it is possible that they may be combined either formally by adding mindfulness practices to these therapies or by drawing further attention to the practices in these therapies that already enhance mindful awareness. These questions have not been adequately studied; therefore, the following comments should be read as hypotheses to be tested further.

Mindfulness and Applied Relaxation

Applied relaxation (AR) involves relaxation training, increased awareness of early signs of anxiety, and applying relaxation at the first sign of anxiety (Bernstein, Borkovec, & Hazlett-Stevens, 2000). AR is considered an empirically-supported treatment for GAD (Chambless & Ollendick, 2001), although it has also been used to treat panic disorder (Öst, 1987) and specific phobia (Öst, Johansson, & Jerremalm, 1982). As described in Hayes-Skelton, Roemer, Orsillo, and Borkovec (2013), there is considerable overlap between AR and mindfulness-based therapies. For example, the self-monitoring involved in noticing early signs of anxiety likely increases awareness similarly to mindfulness exercises because self-monitoring requires an individual to develop a more objective and curious approach to his or her experience. Simply paying attention to anxiety cues and writing them down and/or reporting on them naturally shifts the pattern of experiential avoidance characteristic of anxiety toward one of curiosity and approach. Additionally, these self-monitoring activities create an opportunity for a more objective experience toward thoughts. Saying thoughts out loud or writing them down often reduces the reactivity associated with thoughts. Similarly, the relaxation techniques at the center of AR are functionally similar to mindfulness (Borkovec & Sharpless, 2004) in that they cultivate a present-moment awareness as participants are encouraged to focus their attention on sensations in the body. Within the relaxation exercises, using language that specifically encourages curiosity, decentering, and compassion may further enhance the mindful awareness that may naturally accompany these exercises. While the role of mindfulness in relaxation-based treatments has not been empirically examined, a case series focused on clients receiving AR for GAD demonstrated ways that relaxation treatment may enhance mindfulness (Hayes-Skelton, Usmani, Lee, Roemer, & Orsillo, 2012).

Mindfulness and Exposure-Based Therapies

Exposure-based procedures have been a hallmark of anxiety treatments (Barlow, 2002). These exposure-based procedures involve the individual repeatedly confronting a feared stimulus while resisting avoidance tendencies (Craske, 1999). Theories of exposure procedures highlight the importance of staying engaged with the feared stimulus either to incorporate disconfirming evidence into the fear network (Foa, Huppert, & Cahill, 2006) or to promote inhibitory learning and increase fear tolerance (Craske et al., 2008). Whether the mechanism of exposure is through the incorporation of disconfirming evidence or through increasing fear tolerance, mindfulness may be particularly beneficial in promoting this new learning (Treanor, 2011).

There are several ways that bringing mindful awareness to an exposure exercise may enhance extinction learning and fear tolerance. For example, mindfulness may foster a greater engagement with the feared stimulus and an increased willingness to experience the anxiety (Hayes, Wilson, Gifford, Follette, & Strosahl, 1996), thus increasing tolerance of the anxious response, which all should lead to less avoidance in the future. Similarly, the broadened awareness that comes from mindful attention may also help one to take in the full complement of current experiences, which may increase the likelihood of noticing the disconfirming evidence that may facilitate extinction learning. As Treanor (2011) describes, extinction learning should be more effective when multiple anxious stimuli are present during the exposure, in that the discrepancy between what is predicted and what occurs should increase with more of the feared stimuli present. Therefore, the broadened awareness that mindfulness practice provides may help the individual to be aware of these multiple conditioned stimuli in context. This increased mindful awareness may come from intentional, formal mindfulness exercises practiced prior to the exposure or from informal or applied practices in the midst of the exposure. However, even in the absence of this potential increased awareness, the enhanced attentional capacities seen in mindfulness practice may be beneficial to extinction learning (Treanor, 2011). Indeed, mindfulness meditation has been shown to improve sustained attention and the processing of distracter stimuli without losing focus (Lutz et al., 2009).

While mindfulness may enhance learning during exposures, mindfulness itself may be a form of exposure, in that it encourages contact with avoided stimuli (Baer, 2003). For example, one hypothesis behind GAD is that worry serves an avoidant function by serving as a distraction from more emotional topics (Borkovec & Roemer, 1995). Therefore, the act of drawing mindful awareness to present experience may in fact expose the individual to the underlying emotional stimuli. In this way, mindfulness practice in and of itself may be an exposure exercise.

Mindfulness and Cognitive Therapy

There is much debate about whether the most effective treatments for anxiety should focus on changing the *content* of thoughts versus changing the person's *relationship* with his or her thoughts (e.g., Hayes, 2008; Hofmann & Asmundson, 2008; Longmore & Worrell, 2007). However, it is possible that the two approaches may be more similar than distinct (e.g., Arch & Craske, 2008; Heimberg & Ritter, 2008; Orsillo, Roemer, Lerner, & Tull, 2004). For example, intentionally enhancing mindful awareness around the cognitive restructuring procedures that are the focus of traditional cognitive therapy may improve the depth of restructuring. Mindfulness may increase awareness of the automatic thoughts and distressing internal experiences that are driving anxiety and may increase one's ability to evaluate the thoughts through cognitive restructuring and also foster compassion and nonreactivity toward these thoughts. This may lead to the beliefs being held more loosely, which may provide more space and decentering, so that the content of the thoughts may change. In fact, some have cited the same mechanisms, such as decentering, as underlying both change-based (e.g., Beck, Rush, Shaw, & Emery, 1979; Heimberg & Ritter, 2008) and relationship-based approaches (e.g., Bishop et al., 2004), and others have referred to decentering as a common key change process (Mennin, Ellard, Fresco, & Gross, 2013).

Taken together, there is ample evidence that mindful awareness, with its non-reactive, nonjudgmental stance, is helpful for anxiety. However, more research is needed to understand further the ways that formal, informal, and applied mindfulness practices may be incorporated along with existing treatments to further improve outcomes.

Mindfulness and Anxiety in Stigmatized Populations

To date, most clinical research on anxiety has focused on intrapersonal and interpersonal issues. Yet there is growing evidence that societal experiences, such as discrimination, can increase anxiety. Prevalence and/or persistence rates of anxiety disorders are higher in marginalized populations, such as people of minority sexual orientations (Cochran, 2001), minority gender identities (Budge, Adelson, & Howard, 2013), and minority races and ethnicities (Breslau, Kendler, Su, Gaxiola-Aguilar, & Kessler,

2005). Specifically, recent research has found links between experiences of racial discrimination and GAD in African Americans (Soto, Dawson-Andoh, & Belue, 2011), and relations between perceived racism and worry in a black sample (Rucker, West, & Roemer, 2009). Research on lesbians and on gay men has found a relationship between experiences of discrimination and social anxiety (Burns, Kamen, Lehman, & Beach, 2012; Feinstein, Goldfried, & Davila, 2012). While our societal context means that, unfortunately, individuals from marginalized groups will continue to face these experiences, developing ways to separate from and cope with the pain of marginalization may be important in reducing subsequent anxiety.

Mindfulness may be useful as a coping skill to buffer the effects of stigmatization on anxiety (Fuchs, Lee, Roemer, & Orsillo, 2013; Graham, West, & Roemer, 2013). Mindful awareness could be useful in helping the individual acknowledge that the marginalization is a systemic problem and not rooted within him- or herself. In support of this, Graham and colleagues (2013) found that trait mindfulness moderated the relationship between frequency of recent racist experiences and anxious arousal. Specifically, metaphors, often used in mindfulness approaches, may be helpful in discussing psychological difficulties that are rejected in certain populations/cultures. The emphasis on understanding a client's context contributes to the cultural competence of mindfulness approaches (Fuchs et al., 2013). However, there may be culture-specific difficulties in using mindfulness strategies with marginalized groups that should be explored and considered in future research and clinical work. Sobczak and West (2013) discuss challenges of instruction on mindfulness practices with individuals from nondominant groups, including encouraging acceptance in the face of adversity, acceptability of mindfulness itself, and differences in perspective between the therapist/instructor and client. They recommend that therapists consider power differentials both within the therapeutic relationship and in metaphors used in mindfulness exercises. Furthermore, mindfulness strategies that include a welcoming of, or curiosity about, distressing thoughts may be difficult for someone who is experiencing heightened contextual distress, such as racism or homophobia. Validating the difficulty of a client's experiences is crucial in building a relationship wherein the painful process of engaging with difficult emotions can safely take place.

Conclusions

Mindful awareness appears to be an important process in reduction of symptoms and increased coping with anxiety. The nonjudgmental, nonreactive awareness that can be cultivated through mindfulness practice helps one not only to step back from internal experiences but also to broaden awareness to a full range of experiences rather than focusing narrowly on threat-relevant cues. Similarly, this nonreactivity decreases experiential avoidance, making it less likely for the cycle of anxiety to continue. As a result, mindful awareness makes it more likely that effective actions are taken. Additionally, mindfulness may also enhance the individual's awareness of avoidance behaviors and provide an avenue for recognizing when to move forward with a behavioral action, even when it may lead to anxiety. Mindful awareness can be cultivated in mindfulness-based interventions through the use of formal, informal, and applied practices, both as a stand-alone treatment and, more commonly, incorporated with other behavioral strategies in the treatment of anxiety disorders. Paying attention to ways that existing interventions can foster mindfulness may improve the efficacy of these treatments. However, research is needed that explicitly examines the role of mindfulness alone and in combination with other approaches. Focusing on the principles supporting mindfulness and looking for ways to incorporate these principles more broadly within treatments and across contexts is likely to continue to enhance the effectiveness of current treatments for anxiety.

REFERENCES

Alonso, J., Angermeyer, M. C., Bernert, S., Bruffaerts, R., Brugha, T. S., Bryson, H., et al. (2004). Disability and quality of life impact of mental disorders in Europe: Results from the European Study of the Epidemiology of Mental Disorders (ESEMeD) project. *Acta Psychiatrica Scandinavica 109*, 38–46.

American Psychiatric Association. (2013). *Diagnostic and statistical manual of mental disorders* (5th ed.). Arlington, VA: Author.

Arch, J. J., & Craske, M. G. (2008). Acceptance and commitment therapy and cognitive behavioral therapy for anxiety disorders: Different treatments, similar mechanisms. *Clinical Psychology: Science and Practice, 15*, 263–279.

Arch, J. J., Eifert, G. H., Davies, C., Vilardaga, J. C. P., Rose, R. D., & Craske, M. G. (2012). Randomized clinical trial of cognitive behavioral therapy (CBT) versus acceptance and commitment therapy (ACT) for mixed anxiety disorders. *Journal of Consulting and Clinical Psychology, 80*, 750–765.

Baer, R. A. (2003). Mindfulness training as a clinical intervention: A conceptual and empirical review. *Clinical Psychology: Science and Practice, 10*, 125–143.

Barlow, D. H. (2002). *Anxiety and its disorders: The nature and treatment of anxiety and panic* (2nd ed.). New York: Guilford Press.

Batten, S. V., Orsillo, S. M., & Walser, R. D. (2005). Acceptance and mindfulness-based approaches to the treatment of posttraumatic stress disorder. In S. M. Orsillo & L. Roemer (Eds.), *Acceptance and mindfulness-based approaches to anxiety* (pp. 241–269). New York: Springer.

Beck, A. T., Rush, A. J., Shaw, B. F., & Emery, G. (1979). *Cognitive therapy of depression*. New York: Guilford Press.

Bernstein, D. A., Borkovec, T. D., & Hazlett-Stevens, H. (2000). *New directions in progressive relaxation training: A guidebook for helping professionals*. Westport, CT: Praeger.

Bishop, S. R., Lau, M., Shapiro, S., Carlson, L., Anderson, N. D., Carmody, J., et al. (2004). Mindfulness: A proposed operational definition. *Clinical Psychology: Science and Practice, 11*, 230–241.

Blackledge, J. T. (2007). Disputing verbal processes: Cognitive diffusion in acceptance and commitment therapy and other mindfulness-based psychotherapies. *Psychological Record, 57*, 555–576.

Bögels, S. M., & Mansell, W. (2004). Attention processes in the maintenance and treatment of social phobia: Hypervigilance, avoidance and self-focused attention. *Clinical Psychology Review, 24*, 827–856.

Borkovec, T. D., & Roemer, L. (1995). Perceived functions of worry among generalized anxiety disorder subjects: Distraction from more emotionally distressing topics? *Journal of Behavior Therapy and Experimental Psychiatry, 26*, 25–30.

Borkovec, T. D., & Sharpless, B. (2004). Generalized anxiety disorder: Bringing cognitive-behavioral therapy into the valued present. In S. C. Hayes, V. M. Follette, & M. Linehan (Eds.), *Mindfulness and acceptance: Expanding the cognitive-behavioral tradition* (pp. 209–242). New York: Guilford Press.

Breslau, J., Kendler, K. S., Su, M., Gaxiola-Aguilar, S., & Kessler, R. C. (2005). Lifetime risk and persistence of psychiatric disorders across ethnic groups in the United States. *Psychological Medicine: A Journal of Research in Psychiatry and the Allied Sciences, 35*, 317–327.

Brown, K. W., & Ryan, R. M. (2003). The benefits of being present: Mindfulness and its role in psychological well-being. *Journal of Personality and Social Psychology, 84*, 822–848.

Budge, S. L., Adelson, J. L., & Howard, K. S. (2013). Anxiety and depression in transgender individuals: The roles of transition status, loss, social support, and coping. *Journal of Consulting and Clinical Psychology, 81*, 545–557.

Buhr, K., & Dugas, M. J. (2012). Fear of emotions, experiential avoidance, and intolerance of uncertainty in worry and generalized anxiety disorder. *International Journal of Cognitive Therapy, 5*, 1–17.

Burns, M. N., Kamen, C., Lehman, K. A., & Beach, S. R. H. (2012). Minority stress and attributions for discriminatory events predict social anxiety in gay men. *Cognitive Therapy and Research, 36*, 25–35.

Burton, M., Schmertz, S. K., Price, M., Masuda, A., & Anderson, P. L. (2013). The relation between mindfulness and fear of negative evaluation over the course of cognitive behavioral therapy for social phobia. *Journal of Clinical Psychology, 69*, 222–228.

Campbell-Sills, L., Barlow, D. H., Brown, T. A., & Hofmann, S. G. (2006). Effects of suppression and acceptance on emotional responses of individuals with anxiety and mood disorders. *Behaviour Research and Therapy, 44*, 1251–1263.

Carmody, J., & Baer, R. A. (2008). Relationships between mindfulness practice and levels of mindfulness, medical and psychological symptoms and well-being in a mindfulness-based stress reduction program. *Journal of Behavioral Medicine, 31*, 23–33.

Chambless, D. L., & Ollendick, T. H. (2001). Empirically supported psychological interventions: Controversies and evidence. *Annual Review of Psychology, 52*, 685–716.

Chodron, P. (2007). *Practicing peace in times of war*. Boston: Shambhala.

Cochran, S. D. (2001). Emerging issues in research on lesbians' and gay men's mental health: Does sexual orientation really matter? *American Psychologist, 56*, 929–947.

Cougle, J. R., Keough, M. E., Riccardi, C. J., & Sachs-Ericsson, N. (2009). Anxiety disorders and suicidality in the National Comorbidity Survey–Replication. *Journal of Psychiatric Research, 43*, 825–829.

Craigie, M. G., Rees, C. S., & Marsh, A. (2008). Mindfulness-based cognitive therapy for generalized anxiety disorder: A preliminary evaluation. *Behavioral and Cognitive Psychotherapy, 36*, 553–568.

Craske, M. G. (1999). *Anxiety disorders: Psychological approaches to theory and treatment*. New York: Basic Books.

Craske, M. G., Kircanski, K., Zelikowsky, M., Mystkowski, J., Chowdhury, N., & Baker, A. (2008). Optimizing inhibitory learning during exposure therapy. *Behaviour Research and Therapy, 46*, 5–27.

Dalrymple, K. L., & Herbert, J. D. (2007). Acceptance and commitment therapy for generalized social anxiety disorder: A pilot study. *Behavior Modification, 31*, 543–568.

del Re, A. C., Flückiger, C., Goldberg, S. B., & Hoyt, W. T. (2013). Monitoring mindfulness practice quality: An important consideration in mindfulness practice. *Psychotherapy Research, 23,* 54–66.

Desrosiers, A., Vine, V., Klemanski, D. H., & Nolen-Hoeksema, S. (2013). Mindfulness and emotion regulation in depression and anxiety: common and distinct mechanisms of action. *Depression and Anxiety, 30,* 654–661.

Evans, S., Ferrando, S., Findler, M., Stowell, C., Smart, C., & Haglin, D. (2008). Mindfulness-based cognitive therapy for generalized anxiety disorder. *Journal of Anxiety Disorders, 22,* 716–721.

Feinstein, B. A., Goldfried, M. R., & Davila, J. (2012). The relationship between experiences of discrimination and mental health among lesbians and gay men: An examination of internalized homonegativity and rejection sensitivity as potential mechanisms. *Journal of Consulting and Clinical Psychology, 80*(5), 917–927.

Fleming, J. E., & Kocovski, N. L. (2013). *The mindfulness and acceptance workbook for social anxiety and shyness.* Oakland, CA: New Harbinger.

Flory, J. D., Räikkönen, K., Matthews, K. A., & Owens, J. F. (2000). Self-focused attention and mood during everyday social interactions. *Personality and Social Psychology Bulletin, 26,* 875–883.

Foa, E. B., Huppert, J. D., & Cahill, S. P. (2006). Emotional processing theory: An update. In B. O. Rothbaum (Ed.), *Pathological anxiety: Emotional processing in etiology and treatment* (pp. 3–24). New York: Guildford Press.

Fuchs, C., Lee, J. K., Roemer, L., & Orsillo, S. M. (2013). Using mindfulness- and acceptance-based treatments with clients from nondominant cultural and/or marginalized backgrounds: Clinical considerations, meta-analysis findings, and introduction to the special series—clinical considerations in using acceptance- and mindfulness-based treatments with diverse populations. *Cognitive and Behavioral Practice, 20,* 1–12.

Germer, C. K. (2005). Anxiety disorders: Befriending fear. In C. K. Germer, R. D. Siegel, & P. R. Fulton (Eds.), *Mindfulness and psychotherapy* (pp. 152–172). New York: Guilford Press.

Goldin, P. R., Ramel, W., & Gross, J. J. (2009). Mindfulness meditation training and self-referential processing in social anxiety disorders: Behavioral and neural effects. *Journal of Cognitive Psychotherapy, 23,* 242–257.

Graham, J. R., West, L. M., & Roemer, L. (2013). The experience of racism and anxiety symptoms in an African-American sample: Moderating effects of trait mindfulness. *Mindfulness, 4,* 332–341.

Harned, M. S., Chapman, A. L., Dexter-Mazza, E. T., Murray, A., Comtois, K. A., & Linehan, M. M. (2008). Treating co-occurring Axis I disorders in chronically suicidal women with borderline personality disorder: A 2-year randomized trial of dialectical behavior therapy versus community treatment by experts. *Journal of Consulting and Clinical Psychology, 76,* 1068–1075.

Hayes, S. C. (2008). Climbing our hills: A beginning conversation on the comparison of acceptance and commitment therapy and traditional cognitive behavioral therapy. *Clinical Psychology: Science and Practice, 15,* 286–295.

Hayes, S. C., Strosahl, K. D., & Wilson, K. G. (2012). *Acceptance and commitment therapy: The process and practice of mindful change* (2nd ed.). New York: Guilford Press.

Hayes, S. C., Wilson, K. G., Gifford, E. V., Follette, V. M., & Strosahl, K. (1996). Experiential avoidance and behavioral disorders: A functional dimensional approach to diagnosis and treatment. *Journal of Consulting and Clinical Psychology, 64,* 1152–1168.

Hayes-Skelton, S., & Graham, J. (2012). Decentering as a common link among mindfulness, cognitive reappraisal, and social anxiety. *Behavioural and Cognitive Psychotherapy, 1,* 1–12.

Hayes-Skelton, S. A., Roemer, L., Orsillo, S. M., & Borkovec, T. D. (2013). A contemporary view of applied relaxation for generalized anxiety disorder. *Cognitive Behaviour Therapy, 42,* 292–302.

Hayes-Skelton, S. A., Usmani, A., Lee, J., Roemer, L., & Orsillo, S. M. (2012). A fresh look at potential mechanisms of change in applied relaxation: A case series. *Cognitive and Behavioral Practice, 19,* 451–462.

Heimberg, R. G., & Ritter, M. R. (2008). Cognitive behavioral therapy and acceptance and commitment therapy for the anxiety disorders: Two approaches with much to offer. *Clinical Psychology: Science and Practice, 15,* 296–298.

Herbert, J. D., & Cardaciotto, L. (2005). An acceptance and mindfulness-based perspective on social anxiety disorder. In S. M. Orsillo & L. Roemer (Eds.), *Acceptance and mindfulness-based approaches to anxiety* (pp. 189–212). New York: Springer.

Herzberg, K. N., Sheppard, S. C., Forsyth, J. P., Credé, M., Earleywine, M., & Eifert, G. H. (2012). The Believability of Anxious Feelings and Thoughts Questionnaire (BAFT): A psychometric evaluation of cognitive fusion in a nonclinical and highly anxious community sample. *Psychological Assessment, 24,* 877–891.

Hirschfeld, R. M. A. (1996). Panic disorder: Diagnosis, epidemiology, and clinical course. *Journal of Clinical Psychiatry, 57,* 3–8.

Hofmann, S. G., & Asmundson, G. J. (2008). Acceptance and mindfulness-based therapy: New wave or old hat? *Clinical Psychology Review, 28,* 1–16.

Hofmann, S. G., & Heinrichs, M. (2003). Differential effect of mirror manipulation on self-perception in social phobia subtypes. *Cognitive Therapy and Research, 27,* 131–142.

Hofmann, S. G., Sawyer, A. T., Witt, A. A., & Oh, D. (2010). The effect of mindfulness-based therapy on anxiety and depression: A meta-analytic review. *Journal of Consulting and Clinical Psychology, 78,* 169–183.

Kabat-Zinn, J. (1982). An outpatient program in behavioral medicine for chronic pain patients based on the practice of mindfulness meditation: Theoretical considerations and preliminary results. *General Hospital Psychiatry, 4,* 33–47.

Kabat-Zinn, J. (1990). *Full catastrophe living: Using the wisdom of your body and mind to face stress, pain, and illness.* New York: Delta.

Kabat-Zinn, J. (2005). *Coming to our senses: Healing ourselves and the world through mindfulness.* New York: Hyperion.

Kashdan, T. B., Farmer, A. S., Adams, L. M., Ferssizidis, P., McKnight, P. E., & Nezlek, J. B. (2013). Distinguishing healthy adults from people with social anxiety disorder: Evidence for the value of experiential avoidance and positive emotions in everyday social interactions. *Journal of Abnormal Psychology, 122,* 645–655.

Keng, S.-L., Smoski, M. J., & Robins, C. J. (2011). Effects of mindfulness on psychological health: A review of empirical studies. *Clinical Psychology Review, 31,* 1041–1056.

Kessler, R. C., Berglund, P., Demler, O., Jin, R., Merikangas, K. R., & Walters, E. E. (2005). Lifetime prevalence and age-of-onset distributions of DSM-IV disorders in the National Comorbidity Survey Replication: Erratum. *Archives of General Psychiatry, 62,* 593–602.

Kessler, R. C., Chiu, W. T., Demler, O., Merikangas, K. R., & Walters, E. E. (2005). Prevalence, severity, and comorbidity of 12-month DSM–IV disorders in the National Comorbidity Survey Replication. *Archives of General Psychiatry, 62,* 617–627.

Kim, Y. W., Lee, S., Choi, T. K., Young, S. Y., Kim, B., Kim, C. M., et al. (2009). Effectiveness of mindfulness-based cognitive therapy as an adjunct to pharamacotherapy in patients with panic disorder or generalized anxiety disorder. *Depression and Anxiety*, 26, 601–606.

Kim, Y. W., Lee, S., Kim, Y. W., Choi, T. K., Yook, K., Suh, S. Y., et al. (2010). Effectiveness of a mindfulness-based cognitive therapy program as an adjunct to pharamacotherapy in patients with panic disorder. *Journal of Anxiety Disorders*, 24, 590–595.

Kocovski, N. L., Fleming, J. E., & Rector, N. A. (2009). Mindfulness and acceptance-based group therapy for social anxiety disorder: An open trial. *Cognitive Behavioral Practice*, 16, 276–289.

Koszycki, D., Benger, M., Shlik, J., & Bradwejn, J. (2007). Randomized trial of a meditation-based stress reduction program and cognitive behavior therapy in generalized social anxiety disorder. *Behaviour Research and Therapy*, 45, 2518–2526.

Lee, J. K., Orsillo, S. M., Roemer, L., & Allen, L. B. (2010). Distress and avoidance in generalized anxiety disorder: Exploring the relationships with intolerance of uncertainty and worry. *Cognitive Behaviour Therapy*, 39, 126–136.

Leon, A. C., Portera, L., & Weissman, M. M. (1995). The social cost of anxiety disorders. *British Journal of Psychiatry*, 166, 19–22.

Levitt, J. T., & Karekla, M. (2005). Integrating acceptance and mindfulness with cognitive behavioral treatment for panic disorder. In S. M. Orsillo & L. Roemer (Eds.), *Acceptance and mindfulness-based approaches to anxiety* (pp. 165–188). New York: Springer.

Linehan, M. M. (1993). *Cognitive-behavioral treatment of borderline personality disorder.* New York: Guilford Press.

Longmore, R. J., & Worrell, M. (2007). Do we need to challenge thoughts in cognitive behavior therapy? *Clinical Psychology Review*, 27, 173–187.

Lutz, A., Slagter, H. A., Rawlings, N. B., Francis, A. D., Greischar, L. L., & Davidson, R. J. (2009). Mental training enhances attentional stability: Neural and behavioral evidence. *Journal of Neuroscience*, 29, 13418–13427.

Mennin, D. S., Ellard, K. K., Fresco, D. M., & Gross, J. J. (2013). United we stand: Emphasizing commonalities across cognitive-behavioral therapies. *Behavior Therapy*, 44, 234–248.

Mennin, D. S., Heimberg, R. G., Turk, C. L., & Fresco, D. M. (2005). Preliminary evidence for an emotion dysregulation model of generalized anxiety disorder. *Behaviour Research and Therapy*, 43, 1281–1310.

Michelson, S. E., Lee, J. K., Orsillo, S. M., & Roemer, L. (2011). The role of values-consistent behavior in generalized anxiety disorder. *Depression and Anxiety*, 28, 358–366.

Morgan, L., Graham, J., Hayes-Skelton, S. A., Orsillo, S. M., & Roemer, L. (in press). Relationships between amount and type of post-treatment mindfulness practice and follow-up outcome in an ABBT for GAD. *Journal of Contextual Behavioral Science*.

Nyklíček, I., & Kuijpers, K. F. (2008). Effects of mindfulness-based stress reduction intervention on psychological well-being and quality of life: Is increased mindfulness indeed the mechanism? *Annals of Behavioral Medicine*, 35, 331–340.

Orsillo, S. M., Roemer, L., Lerner, J., & Tull, M. T. (2004). Acceptance, mindfulness, and cognitive-behavioral therapy: Comparisons, contrasts, and application to anxiety. In S. C. Hayes, V. M. Follette, & M. M. Linehan (Eds.), *Mindfulness and acceptance: Expanding the cognitive-behavioral tradition* (pp. 66–95). New York: Guilford Press.

Ossman, W. A., Wilson, K. G., Storaasli, R. D., & McNeill, J. W. (2006). A preliminary investigation of the use of acceptance and commitment therapy in group treatment for social phobia. *International Journal of Psychology and Psychological Therapy*, 6, 397–416.

Öst, L. G. (1987). Applied relaxation: Description of a coping technique and review of controlled studies. *Behaviour Research and Therapy, 25,* 397–409.

Öst, L. G., Johansson, J., & Jerremalm, A. (1982). Individual response patterns and the effects of different behavioral methods in the treatment of claustrophobia. *Behaviour Research and Therapy, 20,* 445–460.

Ostafin, B. D., Brooks, J. J., & Laitem, M. (in press). Affective reactivity mediates an inverse relation between mindfulness and anxiety. *Mindfulness.*

Purdon, C. (1999). Thought suppression and psychopathology. *Behaviour Research and Therapy, 37,* 1029–1054.

Roemer, L., & Borkovec, T. D. (1994). Effects of suppressing thoughts about emotional material. *Journal of Abnormal Psychology, 103,* 467–474.

Roemer, L., Lee, J. K., Salters-Pedneault, K., Erisman, S. M., Orsillo, S. M., & Mennin, D. S. (2009). Mindfulness and emotion regulation difficulties in generalized anxiety disorder: Preliminary evidence for independent and overlapping contributions. *Behavior Therapy, 40,* 142–154.

Roemer, L., & Orsillo, S. M. (2009). *Mindfulness- and acceptance-based behavioral therapies in practice.* New York: Guilford Press.

Roemer, L., & Orsillo, S. M. (2014). An acceptance-based behaviorial therapy for generalized anxiety disorder. In D. H. Barlow (Ed.), *Clinical handbook of psychological disorders* (5th ed., pp. 206–236). New York: Guilford Press.

Rucker, L. S., West, L. M., & Roemer, L. (2010). Relationships among perceived racial stress, intolerance of uncertainty, and worry in a black sample. *Behavior Therapy, 41,* 245–253.

Salters-Pedneault, K., & Diller, J. W. (2013). A preliminary study of anxiety, negative affect, experiential avoidance, and delaying of aversive events. *Behaviour Change, 30,* 241–248.

Sauer-Zavala, S., Boswell, J. F., Gallagher, M. W., Bentley, K. H., Ametaj, A., & Barlow, D. H. (2012). The role of negative affectivity and negative reactivity to emotions in predicting outcomes in the unified protocol for the transdiagnostic treatment of emotional disorders. *Behaviour Research and Therapy, 50,* 551–557.

Schmertz, S. K., Masuda, A., & Anderson, P. L. (2012). Cognitive processes mediate the relation between mindfulness and social anxiety within a clinical sample. *Journal of Clinical Psychology, 68,* 362–371.

Segal, Z. V., Williams, J. M. G., & Teasdale, J. D. (2002). *Mindfulness-based cognitive therapy for depression: A new approach to preventing relapse.* New York: Guilford Press.

Sobczak, L. R., & West, L. M. (2013). Clinical considerations in using mindfulness- and acceptance-based approaches with diverse populations: Addressing challenges in service delivery in diverse community settings. *Cognitive Behavioral Practice, 20,* 13–22.

Soto, J., Dawson-Andoh, N., & Belue, R. (2011). The relationship between perceived discrimination and generalized anxiety disorder among African American, Afro-Caribbeans, and non-Hispanic whites. *Journal of Anxiety Disorders, 25,* 258–265.

Teasdale, J. D., Segal, Z. V., Williams, J. M. G., Ridgeway, V. A., Soulsby, J. M., & Lau, M. A. (2000). Prevention of relapse/recurrence in major depression by mindfulness-based cognitive therapy. *Journal of Consulting and Clinical Psychology, 68,* 615–623.

Treanor, M. (2011). The potential impact of mindfulness on exposure and extinction learning in anxiety disorders. *Clinical Psychology Review, 31,* 617–625.

Twohig, M. P. (2009). The application of acceptance and commitment therapy to obsessive compulsive disorder. *Cognitive Behavioral Practice, 16,* 18–28.

Twohig, M. P., Hayes, S. C., Plumb, J. C., Pruitt, L. D., Collins, A. B., Hazlett-Stevens, H., et al. (2010). A randomized clinical trial of acceptance and commitment therapy versus progressive relaxation training for obsessive–compulsive disorder. *Journal of Consulting and Clinical Psychology, 78*(5), 705–716.

Vettese, L. C., Toneatto, T., Stea, J. N., Nguyen, L., & Wang, J. J. (2009). Do mindfulness meditation participants do their homework? And does it make a difference?: Review of the empirical evidence. *Journal of Cognitive Psychotherapy: An International Quarterly, 23*, 198–225.

Vøllestad, J., Nielsen, M. B., & Nielsen, G. H. (2012). Mindfulness- and acceptance-based interventions for anxiety disorders: A systematic review and meta-analysis. *British Journal of Clinical Psychology, 51*, 239–260.

Wells, A. (1995). Meta-cognition and worry: A cognitive model of generalized anxiety disorder. *Behavioural and Cognitive Psychotherapy, 23*, 301–320.

Wells, A., & Carter, K. (1999). Preliminary tests of a cognitive model of generalized anxiety disorder. *Behaviour Research and Therapy, 37*, 585–594.

Wilson, K. G., & Murrell, A. R. (2004). Values work in acceptance and commitment therapy: Setting a course for behavioral treatment. In S. C. Hayes, V. M. Follette, & M. M. Linehan (Eds.), *Mindfulness and acceptance: Expanding the cognitive-behavioral tradition* (pp. 120–151). New York: Guilford Press.

Yook, K., Lee, S.-H., Ryu, M., Kim, K.-H., Choi, T. K., Suh, S. Y., et al. (2008). Usefulness of mindfulness-based cognitive therapy for treating insomnia in patients with anxiety disorders: A pilot study. *Journal of Nervous and Mental Disease, 196*, 501–503.

CHAPTER 21

A Mindfulness-Based Approach to Addiction

Sarah Bowen, Cassandra Vieten, Katie Witkiewitz,
and Haley Carroll

Addictive behaviors have tremendous individual and societal costs, and present a notoriously difficult and ongoing battle for millions of individuals worldwide. While therapies for addictive behaviors such as substance abuse, problem gambling, and binge eating have certainly made strides over recent decades, treatment effectiveness still lags behind that of interventions for other medical and psychological disorders. Some of this may be due to the complex etiology and processes underlying addiction, which we are only beginning to uncover.

Despite recent advances in both medical and behavioral understandings and treatment approaches to addictive disorders, treatment remains primarily symptom-focused, lacking a more comprehensive understanding of the basic human tendencies that drive these patterns. Buddhist and mindfulness-based views of addiction may illuminate some of the underlying mechanisms that perpetuate these often devastating cycles of behavior. In this chapter we discuss the varied definitions of and perspectives on addiction, with a deeper exploration of the theory underlying mindfulness-based addictions treatment. We then highlight recent randomized trials of this treatment approach before addressing future directions for this emerging field of study.

What Is Addiction?

Addiction has been defined in numerous ways and from varied perspectives over past centuries (Alexander & Schweighofer, 1988; Davies, 1998; Reinarman, 2005). The root Latin word *addico* appears first to have come into usage in ancient Rome, and means to "sentence" or assign as an indentured servant or slave to another. In the late 19th century, addiction came to be defined as a habitual or compulsive devotion to an object or activity (*Webster's Ninth New Collegiate Dictionary*, 1988). In the late 20th century, there was a movement to define addiction narrowly as physiological dependence on a chemical substance, necessitating increasing amounts of the substance to achieve the same effects (tolerance), and distress or discomfort when the substance is discontinued (withdrawal) (Akers, 1991).

Today, DSM-5 (American Psychiatric Association, 2013) defines addiction to drugs or alcohol as substance use disorders (SUDs). Diagnosis is made on a continuum from mild to severe depending on the number of symptoms endorsed from an 11-item list: (1) using greater amounts of a substance for a longer period of time than intended; (2) wanting to cut down or discontinue use but being unable to do so; (3) spending excessive amounts of time getting, using, or recovering from use of the substance; (4) the presence of cravings and urges to use the substance; (5) not managing work, home or school responsibilities due to substance use; (6) continuing to use despite it causing problems in relationships; (7) giving up important activities due to substance use; (8) using substances repeatedly even when doing so puts one in danger; (9) continued use despite physical or psychological problems caused or made worse by the substance; (10) development of tolerance; (11) withdrawal. Endorsing two to three symptoms indicates a mild SUD, four to five indicate a moderate SUD, and six or more symptoms indicate a severe SUD.

DSM-5 identifies SUDs in 10 categories of substances (e.g., alcohol use disorder, stimulant use disorders), though recent critiques challenge the notion that the addictiveness lies within use of a specific substance, and instead frame these as varying manifestations of an underlying addictive syndrome (Shaffer et al., 2004). However, others are promoting a return to the definition of *addiction* as "the loss of control over the intense urges to take the drug even at the expense of adverse consequences" (O'Brien, Volkow, & Li, 2006). There appears to be a movement once again toward defining addiction in terms of behaviors (Holden, 2001). Currently, gambling is the only recognized behavioral addiction in DSM-5, and "Internet gaming disorder" is listed as requiring further research before being included as a formal disorder.

While the definition is continually evolving, the enduring behavioral elements across perspectives seem to include (1) consuming substances or engaging in behaviors at a level or in a manner that causes harm to oneself and potentially to others, (2) significant interference with daily functioning, and (3) repeated unsuccessful attempts to refrain from engagement in the behavior. Although "addiction" is not currently a technical diagnosis, for purposes of our discussion, *addiction* refers to the broader class of addictive behaviors, including but not limited to substance abuse or dependence. We focus in this chapter primarily on SUDs but acknowledge the relevance of other addictive behaviors with common underlying processes.

Etiology of Addiction

Ideas about the causes of addiction are as varied as attempts to define it. Historically, addiction was viewed as arising from moral shortcomings or a weakness in character

(Hart, 1998). The concept of an "addictive personality" was popular for a period of time (Nelson, 1983), but evidence failed to support this idea (Berglund et al., 2011). With the rise of behaviorism (Skinner, 1953), addiction came to be seen as a result of learned associations, wherein a substance exerts control over behavior, often beginning with casual use in which the drug has a modest influence on behavior, then moving to the extreme (i.e., addiction) in which drug use dominates the individual's behavior (Bozarth, 1990). Addictive behaviors are positively reinforced by pleasant effects of a substance, or negatively reinforced by the alleviation of distress or pain. As addiction progresses, this negative reinforcement often becomes more prominent as the distress of withdrawal symptoms is alleviated through use of the substance, until substance use crowds out other self-care behaviors and becomes difficult to extinguish.

As neuropsychological and biopsychological sciences have garnered empirical support and gained popularity as leading explanations for behavioral disorders, addiction is often framed primarily as a brain disorder (or "disease") resulting from a combination of genetic and environmental factors (Nestler, 2001). Based on data from twin and family studies, genetic factors appear to constitute about 50% of the risk for substance dependence (Crabbe, 2002). As a brain disorder, addiction can be viewed as "hijacking" the brain's dopamine reward system, involving the dysregulation of multiple neurotransmitters and corresponding hedonic dysregulation that leads to a strong subjective craving for increasing amounts of the substance to attempt to reestablish homeostasis (Hyman, 2007; Koob, 2011; Nestler, 2001; Wise, 1996).

Although addictive behaviors have strong brain correlates, there are limits to a solely biological explanation. Despite millions of dollars spent on development of pharmacological treatments, the few drugs that target addiction are minimally effective at best, often have significant side effects, or may be addictive themselves (Kranzler, 2006; Soyka & Rosner, 2010). Despite a significant body of research, no single identified genetic allele explains more than approximately 10% of the variance in addiction (other than a protective allele responsible for a flushing response to alcohol that is prevalent in individuals of Asian descent). Likewise, several psychologically oriented treatments that have shown promise for addictive disorders are also only partially effective (Group, 1997), and mechanisms of action in these treatments remain unclear.

Addiction comprises a complex set of behaviors, with multiple etiologies, diverse manifestations, and varying neurobiological explanations (Pihl, 2009). Although psychological, behaviorist, genetic and neurobiological, and even moral perspectives have each contributed to our understanding, a biopsychosocial approach may best explain the complex mechanisms underlying addition (Baker, Stockwell, Barnes, & Holroyd, 2011), offering an umbrella theory (Donovan & Marlatt, 2005; Griffiths, 2005; Moos, 2003) under which biological, psychological, and social factors are all players in the etiology, maintenance, and successful treatment of addiction. A mindfulness-based approach may offer a unique perspective on understanding and treating addictive disorders: one that targets these psychological, neurobiological, and social elements of addiction, goes beyond a symptom focus to address root causes, and is compatible with many other leading psychological and biological treatment approaches.

A Mindfulness Perspective on Addictive Behaviors

Mindfulness, often defined in the psychological literature as moment-to-moment, non-judgmental awareness of one's experience as it unfolds (Kabat-Zinn, 2005), has become increasingly prominent in Western medicine and psychology. Mindfulness has its roots in a number of the world's contemplative traditions, most notably Buddhism. Although mindfulness practices are typically secularized for use in clinical populations, and therefore extracted from these cultural roots, the underlying philosophy remains particularly relevant, providing an innovative and potentially enriched perspective on the conceptualization and treatment of SUDs and other addictive behaviors.

Mindfulness practices were originally part of a recommended method for observing the "Four Noble Truths," or fundamental realities about human life that are said to have been discovered by the historical Buddha through disciplined self-inquiry. These can be summarized briefly as follows: (1) Suffering is a fundamental part of life; (2) suffering is caused by *aversion* or resistance to unpleasant experiences, and *attachment* to, or craving for, pleasurable ones; (3) cessation of suffering is possible; and (4) there is a path toward cessation of suffering not based on chasing pleasant or avoiding unpleasant experiences. Instead, this path involves eight recommendations for living that include cultivation of wisdom, ethics, and mental training, including training in mindfulness (Rahula, 1974). It can be argued that the experiential core of addictive behaviors is the suffering that arises from craving of, or attachment to, pleasurable experiences, and the aversion to, and desire to escape from, distressing ones (Marlatt, 2002).

A fast-growing body of research supports the effectiveness of mindfulness-based interventions for addictive behaviors (see Zgierska et al., 2009, for review), as well as a number of chronic conditions that co-occur with and give rise to addictive behaviors, including pain, stress, depression, and anxiety (see Fjorback, Arendt, Ørnbøl, Fink, & Walach, 2011, for review). Evidence suggests that these approaches are useful for treating fundamental aspects of addiction, such as craving and emotion regulation (Carmody, Vieten, & Astin, 2007; Davis, Fleming, Bonus, & Baker, 2007; Hayes, Wilson, et al., 2004; Witkiewitz, Bowen, & Donovan, 2011; Witkiewitz, Bowen, Douglas, & Hsu, 2013), increasing protective factors such as awareness and acceptance, and decreasing risk factors such as avoidance and expectations, directly targeting the problematic and often deeply engrained cognitive and behavioral patterns of addiction. There are several aspects of mindfulness-based approaches that may be particularly important for working with addictive behaviors.

Awareness

A mindfulness-based perspective on addictive behaviors first recognizes the key role of *awareness* in the recovery process. Recovery from addictive behaviors begins with a fundamental first step of recognizing that one's patterns of substance use behaviors have become problematic. *Denial*, or refusing to acknowledge the existence or severity of substance abuse and its consequences, is a well-recognized hallmark of addiction. Those with addictive disorders often go to great lengths to hide the addiction and resulting consequences, both from themselves and from loved ones and colleagues.

Thus, capacities fostered through mindfulness practice, such as paying attention to experience, seeing things as they are, and engaging in honest examination of inner experiences, are essential. In fact, *vipassanā*, the traditional practice from which many of the mindfulness-based practices in contemporary psychology are drawn, is often translated as "seeing clearly" (Hart, 1987). Enlightenment or liberation (a goal of Buddhist practice) is often described as simply "being awake." "Waking up," however, may require significant commitment and diligent practice.

One aspect of mindfulness-based interventions for addictive behaviors that differentiates them from other interventions is the strong emphasis placed on direct, repeated, practical training in metacognitive awareness of cognitive processes that often lead to relapse. Lack of awareness or metacognitive capacity to recognize high-risk situations, to notice when one's inner resources are becoming depleted, and to see the mistruths one might tell oneself (e.g., "It's OK, I can have just one drink") are common patterns seen in addiction and relapse. Clinicians working with addiction have inevitably heard clients describe their relapse process with astonishment or confusion, saying, "I don't know what happened. I went to the bar for one drink and before I knew it, I was being arrested again."

Increasing awareness, particularly metacognitive awareness, is an important element in preventing relapse. The ability to identify cues in the environment, to monitor risky situations, and to engage in cognitive and behavioral course corrections requires that a client first become aware of the cognitions that can often facilitate drug-seeking and drug-taking behaviors. In other words, clients need to be trained to be aware of a tendency to go on "automatic pilot" in the presence of cues that have previously been paired with addictive behaviors. Simply becoming aware, and seeing things more clearly, is a crucial initial step for those struggling with addictive behaviors.

Mindfulness practice may also foster an uncoupling, or *defusion*, from identifying too closely with thoughts, feelings, and sensations. For example, in addition to experiencing sensations of craving (which are often experienced as urgent), individuals in mindfulness-based addictions treatment develop greater *awareness* of the sensations of craving, and even the response (e.g., frustration or fear) to these sensations, creating a metacognitive distancing from the experience. The more they are able to locate themselves in the awareness of the experience, as opposed to the experience itself, the more they are able to make more skillful choices about how to respond that align with their values and goals, as opposed to falling into an "automatic" conditioned response. Mindfulness practice may therefore extinguish conditioned behavior through bringing the nature and experience of conditioning itself into conscious awareness.

Acceptance-Based Coping

A second common precipitant of relapse is *negative affect* (Marlatt & Gordon, 1985; Sinha, 2007)—specifically, an inability to tolerate and regulate behavior in response to cognitive, affective, or somatic distress (Brady & Sonne, 1999; Breslin, Zack, & McMain, 2002; Brown, 1993). This distress intolerance is often combined in early abstinence with hedonic dysregulation that can heighten the acuity of distress and simultaneously prevent the rewarding qualities of healthier activities, such as taking a walk or talking to a friend. Whether the result of a major disruptive event, such as the loss of a loved one, or a relatively small event, such as a critical comment from a boss, distress that is experienced as intolerable is often followed by an immediate search for a way to alleviate or escape it. Experiential avoidance, avoidant coping, and attempts at suppression are particularly predominant in those with addictive behaviors (Hayes, Wilson, Gifford, Follette, & Strosahl, 1996). In fact, addiction might be understood as an incorrect understanding of the addictive behavior as a refuge from, or avoidance of, suffering (Marlatt, 2002) that paradoxically causes greater suffering.

Individuals struggling with addictive behaviors are often told by well-meaning loved ones and treatment professionals to "work harder," to engage willpower to suppress cravings, and to reframe negative thought patterns. While potentially effective in the short term, attempts to control or suppress negative affect or craving may in the longer term keep clients embattled with their internal experience, reinforcing the notion that such mental–emotional–bodily states are intolerable and must be changed rather than simply treated as part of ordinary human existence. Some evidence suggests that the unwillingness to remain in contact with negatively evaluated events, or what has been termed *experiential avoidance* (Hayes et al., 1996), and chronic attempts to alter the form of these events or the contexts in which they arise, may be a stronger predictor of psychological distress and psychopathology than the actual content of such aversive internal events (Kashdan, Barrios, Forsyth, & Steger, 2006; Keogh, Bond, Hanmer, & Tilston, 2005).

A growing body of experimental evidence suggests that acceptance-based strategies for coping with aversive experience may be more effective than strategies that emphasize change and control. Laboratory studies, for example, have demonstrated that subjects instructed in approach-based coping, which emphasizes acceptance of uncontrollable events or symptoms in response to an anxiogenic stimulus (i.e., inhaled carbon dioxide), compared to those instructed to control such experiences through the use of standard cognitive-behavioral techniques, reported less fear, appeared less behaviorally avoidant, and reported fewer catastrophic thoughts during the noxious experience (Eifert & Heffner, 2003). Studies also suggest that the use of acceptance as opposed to control- or change-based strategies is frequently more effective in helping subjects cope with laboratory-induced pain (e.g., a cold pressor test; Feldner et al., 2006; Keogh et al., 2005) and chronic pain (McCracken, Vowles, & Eccleston, 2004). In relation to addiction, evidence suggests that attempts to suppress unwanted thoughts (vs. the frequency with which these thoughts occur) is significantly related to substance use following a period of abstinence, and that mindfulness meditation lessens the suppression attempts (Bowen, Witkiewitz, Dillworth, & Marlatt, 2007).

Central to a mindfulness perspective is the shift from attempting to change the *content* of one's experience to changing one's *relationship to* that content. This often begins with practicing the simple observation of the sensations of breathing, followed by expanding awareness to observation of body sensations, emotions, and thoughts, and eventually examining the nature of the mind itself. During mindfulness practice, clients are instructed to notice when they are evaluating, criticizing, or lost in thought altogether. They practice acceptance of whatever arises in the field of consciousness, attending to the relationship to what arises rather than its meaning or content.

Exposure

A primarily behavioral mechanism underlying mindfulness-based treatments across all maladies and populations may be an "exposure with response prevention" process, similar to that used to treat obsessive-compulsive and other disorders (Foa & Kozak, 1996). Mindfulness practitioners learn to encounter the flow of experiences repeatedly, often including unpleasant or "triggering" stimuli, without engaging in change-based coping responses or avoidant behaviors. The aversive stimuli in addictions are often internal experiences (e.g., negative affect, craving) rather than the external triggers common in phobias (e.g., spiders). Instructions in mindfulness-based approaches are to notice the arising of these aversive experiences, observe the tendency either to cling to pleasant sensations or resist or escape distressing ones, and to delay reactive responses.

A client recovering from addiction might also be instructed to pay attention to evaluation of the experience, or of self, as "good" or "bad." When one notices appraisal or evaluation, or clinging and resistance, the instruction is to simply be aware of this and return to a neutral focus of breath or body sensations. Usually done in a quiet sitting posture, the practice prevents immediate behavioral reactions and encourages the meditator to "sit with" and observe with curiosity whatever arises. The intention is to help clients gradually enlarge the internal "container" for distressing experiences, allowing them to arise and pass rather than fixate on them or engage in unhealthy behaviors in an attempt to make them change or stop. Through this process, clients gradually increase their tolerance of distressing experience, developing a sense of self-efficacy in relation to these challenges, and beginning to retrain conditioned responses.

A further intention of mindfulness practice is to illuminate, through observation, the temporary nature of all experiences. For individuals struggling with addiction, this can be practiced through the practice of "urge surfing" (Marlatt & Gordon, 1985), or allowing a craving to arise, peak, and pass away while using the sensations of breathing to stay steady. By "riding" the wave of sensations, thoughts, or emotions rather than attempting to resist or avoid them, clients "meet" the experience and allow it to naturally pass without reacting. With repeated practice, they become increasingly confident in the ability to relate to discomfort with acceptance, trusting that it will pass, rather than engaging in avoidance-based coping.

Harm Reduction

While mindfulness training can be consistent with abstinence-based approaches, such as 12-step programs, a person with a mindfulness-based approach might view lapses and even full-blown relapses as he or she would any other experience—by meeting the situation as it is, without judgment or recrimination, inquiring with compassion and curiosity about how the situation came to be, observing the results of the behavior pattern, and returning to the practice of mindful awareness. This may help to avoid "abstinence violation effects" (Marlatt & Gordon, 1985), when thoughts such as "I already blew it" or feelings of shame and defeat follow an initial lapse in abstinence, increasing the probability of continued substance use and full-blown relapse. The vast majority of those with addictive behaviors require repeated attempts at reduction or abstinence, even when they receive formal treatment. This compassionate and realistic view of addiction, far from being passive or permissive, is a courageous approach that involves unyielding honesty with oneself and others, but without recrimination. The practice of mindfulness meditation, in which the practitioner becomes aware that the mind has wandered from the intended focus and gently returns it once again to present experience, lays the foundation for such an approach to lapses in abstinence.

Mindfulness-Based Treatments for Addictions

Incorporation of mindfulness into treatment of addictive behaviors, including substance use, binge eating, gambling, and sex and Internet addiction, has taken several forms. Perhaps the most widely known contemporary mindfulness-based treatment in Western psychology is mindfulness-based stress reduction (MBSR), an 8-week mindfulness-based intervention initially developed by Kabat-Zinn (1990) for the treatment of chronic pain. A handful of studies have modified MBSR to suit the clinical needs of a substance-abusing population (e.g., Britton et al., 2012; Davis et al., 2007).

Mindfulness-Based Relapse Prevention

Mindfulness-based relapse prevention (MBRP; Bowen et al., 2009; Bowen, Chawla, & Marlatt, 2010; Witkiewitz, Marlatt, & Walker, 2005), an 8-week program specifically designed for treatment of addictive behaviors, integrates practices from MBSR and mindfulness-based cognitive therapy (MBCT; Segal, Williams, & Teasdale, 2002) with Marlatt's cognitive-behavioral approach to relapse prevention (Marlatt & Gordon, 1985). MBRP incorporates formal (e.g., body scan) and informal (e.g., urge surfing) practices to cultivate mindful awareness, while also including cognitive-behavioral coping skills training. As demonstrated in an initial randomized feasibility trial (Bowen et al., 2009), individuals ($N = 168$) who received MBRP aftercare treatment for SUDs had significantly fewer days of substance use than individuals who received treatment as usual (TAU), until 4-month follow-up, at which point levels were no longer significantly different. Additionally, compared to TAU, the MBRP group showed significantly less craving and an increase in scores on acceptance, as measured by the Acceptance and Action Questionnaire (Hayes, Strosahl, et al., 2004) and on the Acting with Awareness component of the Five Facet Mindfulness Questionnaire (Baer, Fischer, & Huss, 2006).

A recent, larger trial examined the efficacy of MBRP in comparison to TAU and relapse prevention (RP) without mindfulness training (Bowen et al., 2014).

Participants (N = 286) were 71.5% male and represented diverse races and ethnicities. They were using a range of substances (49.1% alcohol, 14.7% cocaine, 13.7% heroin or other opiates, 11.9% stimulants, 9.5% marijuana, and 1.1% "other"). Participants were randomized to one of the three aftercare treatment conditions (MBRP, TAU, or RP) after completing an initial inpatient or intensive outpatient treatment program at a community treatment center. The TAU condition (n = 95) was the standard aftercare provided by the treatment center, which comprised primarily 12-step process-oriented psychoeducational groups (see Bowen et al., 2009, for more details). MBRP (n = 103) and RP (n = 88) were both manualized group treatment programs with similar format (led by two facilitators), length (2 hours per week for 8 weeks), and activities (both treatments included a variety of homework exercises). MBRP was the same intervention used in the feasibility trial noted earlier (Bowen et al., 2009). The RP program was based on the Daley and Marlatt (2006) RP manual, adapted to match the format of MBRP and to incorporate the RP content and activities that were part of the MBRP program (e.g., identifying substance use triggers, psychoeducation about the relapse process).

Preliminary results from the 12-month follow-up assessment suggest that both treatments have superior substance-related outcomes compared to TAU, and that MBRP may be more effective than both RP and TAU in delaying relapse to drinking. Specifically, individuals randomized to both RP and MBRP had fewer days of drug use than the TAU group across the entire study period when researchers controlled for treatment hours and baseline days of drug use. Across the 12-month follow-up, individuals in both MBRP and RP used drugs an average of 12 days (RP: M = 12.1; SD = 34.6; MBRP: M = 12.3; SD = 49.0) and drank an average of 9 days (RP: M = 9.9; SD = 22.2; MBRP: M = 8.8; SD = 24.7), compared to 21 days (SD = 54.3) of drug use and 17.5 drinking days (SD = 46.0) in TAU. Among those who were abstinent from drugs at the beginning of treatment (n = 209), only 21% of those assigned to MBRP reported any drug use across the 12-month follow-up, as compared to 30% in RP and 37% in TAU, although this difference did not reach statistical significance. Individuals in MBRP also reported fewer negative substance-related consequences at 12-month follow-up (M = 1.7, SD = 3.9) than those in RP (M = 2.1, SD = 4.5) or TAU (M = 3.2, SD = 5.2).

Survival analyses indicated that treatment had a significant effect on the probability of relapse to drug use and to drinking. Receiving either MBRP or RP significantly reduced the probability of any drug or drinking relapse in comparison to TAU. Over the 365 days following baseline, the mean survival rates for any drug/drinking lapses were 255 days for TAU, 273 days for RP, and 274 days for MBRP. To better understand for whom and how these treatments may be effective, future analyses will focus on factors that may predict who is better matched to which treatment, and both common and unique mechanisms of action in MBRP and standard RP.

Studies of modified or adapted versions of MBRP have found improvements in drinking behavior, mindfulness, craving, and depression (Zgierska et al., 2008), and decreased cigarette smoking when compared to standard best practices for smoking cessation (Brewer et al., 2011). Similarly, studies of treatments incorporating mindfulness-based practices for SUDs have found promising cognitive, physiological, and substance use outcomes (Garland, Boettiger, Gaylord, Chanon, & Howard, 2011; Garland, Gaylord, Boettiger, & Howard, 2010) and decreased negative affect, stress, emotional reactivity, and increased positive affect and mindfulness (Vieten, Astin, Buscemi, & Galloway, 2010).

In addition to treatment protocols that have formal and informal meditation practices as their foundation, other cognitive and behavioral treatment approaches integrate mindfulness practices and approaches as a component of a multifaceted treatment, such as acceptance and commitment therapy (ACT; Hayes, Strosahl, & Wilson, 1999) and dialectical behavior therapy (DBT; Linehan, 1993). These therapies, while not initially developed for treatment of substance use, have been adapted and applied in several trials for treatment of addictive behaviors, with preliminary evidence supporting efficacy (e.g., Gifford et al., 2004; Hayes, Wilson, et al., 2004; Linehan et al., 1999, 2002; Wilson, Hayes, & Byrd, 2000).

Alongside studies of mindfulness-based or mindfulness-informed treatments for substance abuse, mindfulness has shown promise for treatment of other addictive behaviors, such as gambling (de Lisle, Dowling, & Allen, 2011; Toneatto, Vettese, & Nguyen, 2007), and binge eating (Courbasson, Nishikawa, & Shapira, 2011; Kristeller & Wolever, 2011).

In summary, the growing field of mindfulness-based treatment for addictive behaviors shows promise as both a complementary and an alternative option for treatment of substance abuse and other addictive behaviors. As is typical of early-stage research, the current body of literature includes studies with methodological limitations, including limited sample sizes and a no standardized measurement of both therapist fidelity and outcomes measurement issues. Results, too, are mixed, with some studies showing shifts in purported change mechanisms but not in subsequent relapse rates. Others show short-term reductions in relapse but lack evidence for longer-term sustainability of treatment gains. These limitations notwithstanding, we see consistent evidence of posttreatment shifts in mechanisms associated with addictive behavior, such as craving (Bowen et al., 2009; Zgierska et al., 2008), emotional reactivity, (Vieten et al., 2010), and/or the target behaviors themselves. This calls for continued exploration of the integration of mindfulness and acceptance-based practices into the more traditional cognitive-behavioral interventions. Larger-scale randomized trials are clearly necessary at this stage to discern whether these effects are reliable across addiction populations and treatment settings (e.g., inpatient care, court-mandated programs, private treatment centers), and to test which treatment structures and protocols are most beneficial. Such trials would also allow a more nuanced look at potential moderating and mediating factors that might distinguish between two active treatment conditions, such as cognitive-behavioral therapy (CBT) and mindfulness-based treatment, identifying for whom which treatment may be better suited, and the unique and common mechanisms underlying effectiveness of the interventions.

Neurobiological and Physiological Correlates

As these studies grow in number, scientists are increasingly interested in understanding better the underlying mechanisms of change. As the study of mindfulness-based treatment for addictions is still in its early stages, so too are studies of the possible underlying neurological and physiological correlates of the changes seen following such interventions. Although there is a significant body of research detailing the neurological effects of addiction, and a burgeoning literature on neural correlates of mindfulness and training in it (e.g., Hölzel et al., 2011), to our knowledge there are no published studies investigating the neurological effects of mindfulness in individuals with addiction.

However, Brewer, Bowen, Smith, Marlatt, and Potenza (2010) outlined the theoretical application of mindfulness for dual diagnoses of depression and SUDs from a neuroscience perspective. Based on research detailing the neurobiological effects of mindfulness, they hypothesized that the attention and acceptance mechanisms of mindfulness training may benefit those with dual diagnoses of depression and substance use. Regarding attention networks, Brewer and colleagues presented evidence suggesting that activity in the "default network" of the brain (midline prefrontal cortical structures) decreases when attending to present-moment thoughts without elaboration (e.g., Farb et al., 2007). Based on these findings, Brewer and colleagues hypothesized that mindfulness training may help individuals identify ruminative thought cycles, perhaps even reducing the frequency and intensity of these maladaptive thought patterns. They therefore operationally define acceptance processes as nonelaborative and nonattached types of processing. Regarding acceptance processes, several studies show mindfulness training to be associated with a decoupling of the insula from the ventromedial prefrontal cortex (vmPFC), and increased coupling with the dorsolateral prefrontal cortex (dlPFC; e.g., Farb et al., 2007), as well as increased insular thickness (e.g., Hölzel et al., 2008). Because increased thickness in the insula has also been associated with activation in the midline of the PFC, such as the vmPFC relation to self-referential experiences, the decoupling of the insula from the vmPFC may represent a transition to more objective observation of subjective experience and behavior. Furthermore, activation in the dlPFC has been associated with better stress task performance in the laboratory; thus, the increased insular dlPFC coupling may represent greater task-oriented processing. Ultimately, Brewer and colleagues suggested that the increased coupling of the insula with the dlPFC, combined with decreased coupling with the vmPFC, may be evidence of a transition from self-referential observation to more objective and task-specific processing. They further hypothesized that these changes may be related to reduced stress and substance use severity.

Studies investigating effects of mindfulness on psychophysiology in individuals with substance use disorders are similarly scant. Given the importance of stress in relapse and addiction, understanding psychophysiological patterns of responding can be an important marker of recovery. Brewer and colleagues (2009) compared cardiac vagal control in 36 participants receiving treatment for alcohol or cocaine dependence randomized to either 12 weeks of CBT or 9 weeks of mindfulness training (MT) based on a modified version of MBRP. Within 2 weeks of treatment completion, participants were exposed to neutral and stress-inducing imagery scripts while physiological data were recorded. Electrocardiography (ECG) was used to record heart rate (HR), and cardiac vagal control was calculated with a ratio difference of sympathetic and vagal tone (S/V ratio). Galvanic skin response (GSR) was also recorded.

The results revealed no significant differences between CBT and MT in GSR or HR. However, the MT group showed a significant decrease in the S/V ratio (indicative of increased cardiac vagal control, considered to be a marker of self-regulation) compared to the CBT group, which showed a significant increase in S/V ratio. These results suggest that those who have undergone mindfulness training for smoking may engage the stressor without getting "wrapped up" in stress-related thinking. A related study (Garland et al., 2010) compared cardiac vagal control in 53 adult adults receiving treatment for alcohol dependence, randomly assigned to either mindfulness-oriented recovery enhancement (MORE) or an alcohol support group. Participants completed a laboratory paradigm measuring cardiac vagal control in response to alcohol cue-induced stress pre-, mid-, and post-treatment. ECG was used to calculate the vagal index of the root mean square of successive differences (RMSSD) of heart-beat (R-R) intervals. Results revealed that during the postcourse test, the MORE participants displayed higher, albeit not statistically significant, RMSSD during the stressor, which then decreased during recovery (again indicative of cardiac vagal tone), whereas the alcohol skills group showed lower RMSDD during the stressor, which then increased during the recovery. These results also suggest that MT may allow individuals to engage in a stressful task without becoming overly involved in the stressor.

In another study, Libby, Worhunsky, Pilver, and Brewer (2012) measured vagal control in a sample of 31 adult treatment-seeking smokers by recording high-frequency heart rate variability (HF-HRV) via pressure transducer, while participants were undergoing a functional magnetic resonance imaging (fMRI) scan during which they received meditation instructions. Results showed that 28% of participants who had increased cardiac vagal control maintained smoking abstinence at a 17-week follow-up as opposed to 12.5% of participants who experienced decreased cardiac vagal control during the task. These results support the literature suggesting that mindfulness meditation is associated with cardiac vagal control, and suggest that cardiac vagal control is related to favorable substance use outcomes.

Finally, Lustyk and colleagues (2012) compared cardiac vagal control following a cognitive laboratory stressor in a community-based treatment facility for adults in treatment for SUDs who had been randomized to MBRP, RP, or TAU in a community agency. Within 2 months of group completion, participants ($N = 34$) completed a laboratory appointment in which ECG was used to record HF-HRV in response to a cognitive challenge. Preliminary evidence suggests that the participants in the MBRP group show greater HF-HRV at baseline and increased HF-HRV during the stressor, which is indicative of cardiac vagal control. This study also demonstrates increased cardiac vagal control in the face of a stressor when individuals have received mindfulness training for the treatment of SUDs. Ultimately, these physiological findings are of particular significance in the context of the role of stress in relapse and recovery given that cardiac vagal control is considered a marker of self-regulation. These findings suggest that participants may be engaging in emotion regulation techniques in the presence of a stressor, such that they are accepting the stressful situation, allowing it to occur without resisting or becoming overly involved, and are therefore able to respond in a more appropriate and skillful manner. However, evidence is still preliminary and further investigation is warranted.

Conclusion

Addiction is costly and tremendously difficult to treat, and it impacts afflicted individuals, family and friends, and communities at large. The development of addiction is complex, with multiple etiologies and manifestations of symptoms, but a central factor in developing and maintaining addiction is behavioral choice in response to internal and external stimuli. All addictive drugs and behaviors have in common qualities of positive reinforcement (e.g., feelings of euphoria) and negative reinforcement (e.g., alleviation of distress). While genetic, environmental, and neurobiological factors play a significant role in determining who will become addicted and remain addicted, the ultimate outcome is one in which an individual trapped by his or her own mind and behavior.

Long-standing tradition and a growing body of evidence in many health domains point to the promise of mindfulness practices for treating addiction. Research assessing the paradigm-shifting potential of these practices for alleviation of the suffering caused by addiction is clearly under way. The basic science and clinical protocols integrating mindfulness training into a contemporary framework are still in early stages, however. While there is considerable and warranted excitement, we must exercise caution to not get ahead of the evidence. There remains at this point a paucity of well-designed trials; lasting behavior change remains elusive in many studies; and very little is known about the neurobiological, behavioral, or cognitive mechanisms of successful behavior changes following mindfulness-based treatments for addictions. However, as in other targets of mindfulness-based treatments, there appear to be consistent and robust improvements in emotion regulation, affect and mood, cognitive processes, and self-efficacy, as well as findings demonstrating similar increases in functioning and quality of life when symptoms are approached with acceptance, gentleness, and compassion rather than with attempts to control or eliminate them.

The current literature points toward several potentially fruitful research questions. Do the underlying premises and practices of mindfulness-based treatments for addictive behaviors suggest a transdiagnostic approach, targeting common underlying mechanism across, for example, binge eating, substance abuse, and gambling? Or do these treatments need to be tailored to specific disorders, and further, perhaps to different subtypes of substance abuse, such as methamphetamine versus alcohol addiction?

Also potentially exciting is the interdisciplinary nature of inquiry and study. Findings in basic science that illuminate neurobiological or physiological substrates of addiction and of effective interventions may help clinicians to understand better, and target with better precision, the processes necessary for change. For example, through better understanding of mechanisms underlying craving, we may be better able to structure specific practices within treatment to target this experience. Evidence on effects of duration or type of exposure to triggers on the craving response could have immediate applicability to clinical practices.

As a newcomer to the field of addiction treatment, the study of mindfulness-based interventions has some ground to cover to catch up with the volume and sophistication of research in other, longer-standing areas of addiction treatment, such as motivational interviewing or contingency management. Offering a unique and promising approach, however, the research is growing and will undoubtedly continue to improve in methodological rigor and scope of application, and therefore the ability to answer more sophisticated questions and ultimately decrease the suffering of those struggling with addictive behaviors.

When confronted with a problem, many of us are inclined to fix it, eradicate it, distract ourselves from it, or hide it from others. The approach of accepting a distressing feeling, allowing it to be as it is, quietly observing it, and not reactively "fixing" it is quite antithetical and uncomfortable to most contemporary Western adults. Yet wisdom dating back several thousand years and recent evidence both suggest that "fighting" and "fixing" may not be the way out of the cycle of addiction. Perhaps bringing an accepting, curious, and compassionate attitude to cravings and urges to engage in substance use behaviors, and learning to stay when we most want to run, is where freedom from addiction begins.

REFERENCES

Akers, R. L. (1991). Addiction: The troublesome concept. *Journal of Drug Issues, 21,* 777–793.

Alexander, B. K., & Schweighofer, R. F. (1988). Defining "addiction." *Canadian Psychology/Psychologie Canadienne, 29,* 151–162.

American Psychiatric Association. (2013). *Diagnostic and statistical manual of mental disorders* (5th ed.). Arlington, VA: Author.

Baer, R. A., Fischer, S., & Huss, D. B. (2006). Mindfulness and acceptance in the treatment of disordered eating. *Journal of Rational-Emotive and Cognitive-Behavior Therapy, 23,* 281–300.

Baker, T. E., Stockwell, T., Barnes, G., & Holroyd, C. B. (2011). Individual differences in substance dependence: At the intersection of brain, behaviour and cognition. *Addiction Biology, 16*(3), 458–466.

Berglund, K., Roman, E., Balldin, J., Berggren, U., Eriksson, M., Gustavsson, P., et al. (2011). Do med with excessive alcohol consumption and societal stability have an addictive personality? *Scandanavian Journal of Psychology, 52*(3), 257–260.

Bowen, S., Chawla, N., Collins, S. E., Witkiewitz, K., Hsu, S., Grow, J., et al. (2009). Mindfulness-based relapse prevention for substance use disorders: A pilot efficacy trial. *Substance Abuse: Official Publication of the Association for Medical Education and Research in Substance Abuse, 30,* 295–305.

Bowen, S., Chawla, N., & Marlatt, G. A. (2010). *Mindfulness-based relapse prevention for addictive behaviors: A clinician's guide.* New York: Guilford Press.

Bowen, S., & Vieten, C. (2012). A compassionate approach to the treatment of addictive behaviors: The contributions of Alan Marlatt to the field of mindfulness-based interventions. *Addiction Research and Theory, 20*(3), 243–249.

Bowen, S., Witkiewitz, K., Clifasefi, S. L., Grow, J., Chawla, N., Hsu, S. H., et al. (2014). Relative efficacy of mindfulness-based relapse prevention, standard relapse prevention, and treatment as usual for substance use disorders: A randomized clinical trial. *JAMA Psychiatry, 71*(5), 547–556.

Bowen, S., Witkiewitz, K., Dillworth, T. M., & Marlatt, G. A. (2007). The role of thought suppression in the relationship between mindfulness mediation and alcohol use. *Addictive Behaviors, 32*(10), 2324–2328.

Bozarth, M. A. (1990). Drug addiction as a psychobiological process. In D. M. Warburton (Ed.), *Addiction controversies* (pp. 112–134). Amsterdam: Harwood Academic

Brady, K. T., & Sonne, S. C. (1999). The role of stress in alcohol use, alcoholism treatment, and relapse. *Alcohol Research and Health, 23,* 263–271.

Breslin, F. C., Zack, M., & McMain, S. (2002). An information-processing analysis of mindfulness: Implications for relapse prevention in the treatment of substance abuse. *Clinical Psychology: Science and Practice, 9,* 275–298.

Brewer, D. D., Catalano, R. F., Haggerty, K., Gainey, R. R., & Fleming, C. B. (1998). A meta-analysis of predictors of continued drug use during and after treatment for opiate addiction. *Addiction, 93*(1), 73–92.

Brewer, J. A., Bowen, S., Smith, J. T., Marlatt, G. A., & Potenza, M. N. (2010). Mindfulness-based treatments for co-occurring depression and substance use disorders: What can we learn from the brain? *Addiction, 105*(10), 1698–1706.

Brewer, J. A., Mallik, S., Babuscio, T. A., Nich, C., Johnson, H. E., Deleone, C. M., et al. (2011). Mindfulness training for smoking cessation: Results from a randomized controlled trial. *Drug and Alcohol Dependence, 119*(1–2), 72–80.

Brewer, J. A., Sinha, S., Chen, J., Michaelsen, R. N., Babuscio, T. A., Nich, C., et al. (2009). Mindfulness training and stress reactivity in substance abuse: Results from a randomized, controlled stage I pilot trial. *Substance Abuse, 30,* 1–12.

Britton, W. B., Bootzin, R. R., Cousins, J. C., Hasler, B. P., Peck, T., & Shapiro, S. L. (2012). The contribution of mindfulness practice to a multicomponent behavioral sleep intervention following substance abuse treatment in adolescents: A treatment development study. *Substance Abuse, 31,* 86–97.

Brown, S. A. (1993). *Recovery patterns in adolescent substance abuse.* London: Sage.

Carmody, T. P., Vieten, C., & Astin, J. A. (2007). Negative affect, emotional acceptance, and smoking cessation. *Journal of Psychoactive Drugs, 39,* 499–508.

Courbasson, C. M., Nishikawa, Y., & Shapira, L. B. (2011). Mindfulness-action based cognitive behavioral therapy for concurrent binge eating disorder and substance use disorders [Clinical trial]. *Eating Disorders, 19*(1), 17–33.

Crabbe, J. C. (2002). Genetic contributions to addiction. *Annual Review of Psyhology, 53,* 435–462.

Daley, D. C., & Marlatt, G. A. (2006). *Overcoming your alcohol or drug problem: Effective recovery strategies: Therapist guide* (2nd ed.). New York: Oxford University Press.

Davies, J. B. (1998). Pharmacology versus social process: Competing or complementary views on the nature of addiction? *Pharmacology and Therapeutics, 80*(3), 265–275.

Davis, J. M., Fleming, M. F., Bonus, K. A., & Baker, T. B. (2007). A pilot study on mindfulness based stress reduction for smokers. *BMC Complementary and Alternative Medicine, 7,* 2.

de Lisle, S. M., Dowling, N. A., & Allen, J. S. (2011). Mindfulness and problem gambling: A review of the literature. *Journal of Gambling Studies, 10,* 210–228.

Donovan, D. M., & Marlatt, G. A. (2005). *Assessment of addictive behaviors* (2nd ed.). New York: Guilford Press.

Eifert, G. H., & Heffner, M. (2003). The effects of acceptance versus control contexts on avoidance of panic-related symptoms. *Journal of Behavior Therapy and Experimental Psychiatry, 34*(3–4), 293–312.

Farb, N. A., Segal, Z. V., Mayberg, H., Bean, J., McKeon, D., Fatima, Z., et al. (2007). Attending to the present: Mindfulness meditation reveals distinct neural modes of self-reference. *Social Cognitive and Affective Neuroscience, 2,* 313–322.

Feldner, M. T., Hekmat, H., Zvolensky, M. J., Vowles, K., E., Secrist, Z., & Leen-Feldner, E.

W. (2006). The role of experiential avoidance in acute pain tolerance: A laboratory test. *Journal of Behavior Therapy and Experimental Psychiatry, 37*, 146–158.

Fjorback, L. O., Arendt, M. M., Ørnbøl, E. E., Fink, P. P., & Walach, H. H. (2011). Mindfulness-based stress reduction and mindfulness-based cognitive therapy—A systematic review of randomized controlled trials. *Acta Psychiatrica Scandinavica, 124*(2), 102–119.

Foa, E. B., & Kozak, M. J. (1996). Psychological treatment for obsessive-compulsive disorder. In M. R. Mavissakalian & R. F. Prien (Eds.), *Long-term treatments of anxiety disorders* (pp. 285–309). Arlington, VA: American Psychiatric Association.

Freud, S. (1898). Sexuality in the aetiology of the neuroses. In J. Strachey (Ed. & Trans.), *The standard edition of the complete psychological works of Sigmund Freud* (Vol. III, 1893–1899). London: Hogarth.

Garland, E. L., Boettiger, C. A., Gaylord, S., Chanon, V. W., & Howard, M. O. (2011). Mindfulness is inversely associated with alcohol attentional bias among recovering alcohol-dependent adults. *Cognitive Therapy and Research, 36*, 441–450.

Garland, E. L., Gaylord, S. A., Boettiger, C. A., & Howard, M. O. (2010). Mindfulness training modifies cognitive, affective, and physiological mechanisms implicated in alcohol dependance: Results of a randomized controlled pilot trial. *Journal of Psychoactive Drugs, 42*, 177–192.

Gifford, E. V., Kohlenberg, B. S., Hayes, S. C., Antonuccio, D. O., Piasecki, M. M., Rasmussen-Hall, M. L., et al. (2004). Acceptance-based treatment for smoking cessation. *Behavior Therapy, 35*(4), 689–705.

Griffiths, M. (2005). The biopsychosocial approach to addiction. *Psyke and Logos, 26*(1), 9–26.

Group, P. M. R. (1997). Matching alcoholism treatments to client heterogeneity: Project MATCH post-treatment drinking outcomes. *Journal of Studies on Alcohol, 58*, 7–29.

Hart, P. D. (1998). The Road to Recovery: A landmark study on public perceptions of alcoholism and barriers to treatment. Carpinteria, CA: Rush Recovery Institute.

Hart, W. (1987). *The art of living: Vipassanā meditation.* New York: HarperOne.

Hayes, S. C., Strosahl, K. D., & Wilson, K. G. (1999). *Acceptance and commitment therapy: An experiential approach to behavior change.* New York: Guilford Press.

Hayes, S. C., Strosahl, K., Wilson, K. G., Bissett, R. T., Pistorello, J., Toarmino, D., et al. (2004). Measuring experiential avoidance: A preliminary test of a working model. *Psychological Record, 54*, 553–578.

Hayes, S. C., Wilson, K. G., Gifford, E. V., Bissey, R., Piasecki, M., Batten, S., et al. (2004). A preliminary trial of twelve-step facilitation and acceptance and commitment therapy with polysubstance-abusing methadone-maintained opiate addicts. *Behavior Therapy, 35*, 667–688.

Hayes, S. C., Wilson, K. G., Gifford, E. V., Follette, V. M., & Strosahl, K. D. (1996). Experiential avoidance and behavioral disorders: A functional dimensional approach to diagnosis and treatment. *Journal of Consulting and Clinical Psychology, 64*(6), 1152–1168.

Holden, C. (2001). "Behavioral" addictions: Do they exist? *Science, 294*, 980–982.

Hölzel, B. K., Lazar, S. W., Gard, T., Schuman-Olivier, Z., Vago, D. R., & Ott, U. (2011). How does mindfulness meditation work?: Proposing mechanisms of action from a conceptual and neural perspective. *Perspectives on Psychological Science, 6*(6), 537–559.

Hölzel, B. K., Ott, U., Gard, T., Hempel, H., Weygandt, M., Morgen, K., et al. (2008). Investigation of mindfulness meditation practitioners with voxel-based morphometry. *Social Cognitive and Affective Neuroscience, 3*(1), 55–61.

Hyman, S. E. (2007). The neurobiology of addiction: Implications for voluntary control of behavior. *American Journal of Bioethics, 7,* 8–11.

Kabat-Zinn, J. (1990). *Full catastrophe living.* New York: Bantam/Dell.

Kabat-Zinn, J. (2005). *Full catastrophe living: Using the wisdom of your body and mind to face stress, pain, and illness* (15th anniversary ed.). New York: Delta Trade Paperback/ Bantam/Dell.

Kashdan, T. B., Barrios, V., Forsyth, J. P., & Steger, M. F. (2006). Experiential avoidance as a generalized psychological vulnerability: Comparisons with coping and emotion regulation strategies. *Behaviour Research and Therapy, 9,* 1301–1320.

Keogh, E., Bond, F. W., Hanmer, R., & Tilston, J. (2005). Comparing acceptance and control-based coping instructions on the cold-pressor pain experiences of healthy men and women. *European Journal of Pain, 9,* 591–598.

Koob, G. F. (2011). Neurobiology of addiction. *Focus, 9,* 55–65.

Kranzler, H. (2006). Medications to treat heavy drinking: are we there yet? *Addiction, 101*(2), 153 –154.

Kristeller, J. L., & Wolever, R. Q. (2011). Mindfulness-based eating awareness training for treating binge eating disorder: The conceptual foundation. *Eating Disorders, 19*(1), 49–61.

Libby, D. J., Worhunsky, P. D., Pilver, C. E., & Brewer, J. A. (2012). Meditation-induced changes in high-frequency heart rate variability predict smoking outcomes. *Frontiers in Human Neuroscience, 6,* 54.

Linehan, M. M. (1993). *Skills training manual for treating borderline personality disorder.* New York: Guilford Press.

Linehan, M., Dimeff, L. A., Reynolds, S. K., Comtosis, K. C., Welch, S. S., Heagerty, P., et al. (2002). Dialectical behavior therapy versus comprehensive validation therapy plus 12-step for the treatment of opioid dependent women meeting criteria for borderline personality disorder. *Drug and Alcohol Dependence, 67,* 13–26.

Linehan, M., Schmidt, H., Dimeff, L. A., Craft, J. C., Kanter, J., & Comtosis, K. A. (1999). Dialectical behavior therapy for patients with borderline personality disorder and drug-dependence. *American Journal on Addictions, 8,* 279–292.

Lustyk, M. K. B., Douglas, H., Shilling, B., Witkiewitz, K., Chawla, N., & Bowen, S. (2012). *Cardiovascular responses to a laboratory stressor in substance abusers after treatment with mindfulness-based relapse prevention.* Unpublished manuscript.

Marlatt, G. A. (2002). Buddhist philosophy and the treatment of addictive behavior. *Cognitive and Behavioral Practice, 9,* 44–49.

Marlatt, G. A., & Gordon, J. R. (1985). *Relapse prevention: Maintenance strategies in the treatment of addictive behaviors.* New York: Guilford Press.

McCracken, L. M., Vowles, K. E., & Eccleston, C. (2004). Acceptance of chronic pain: Component analysis and a revised assessment method. *Pain, 107*(1–2), 159–166.

Moos, R. H. (2003). Addictive disorders in context: Principles and puzzles of effective treatment and recovery. *Psychology of Addictive Behaviors, 17*(1), 3–12.

Nelson, B. (1983, January 18). The addictive personality: Common traits are found. *New York Times,* p. C1.

Nestler, E. J. (2001). Molecular neurobiology of addiction. *American Journal on Addictions, 10,* 201–217.

O'Brien, C. P., Volkow, N., & Li, T.-K. (2006). What's in a word?: Addiction versus dependence in DSM-V. *American Journal of Psychiatry, 163*(5), 764–765.

Pihl, R. O. (2009). *Substance abuse: Etiological considerations.* Oxford, UK: Oxford University Press.

Rahula, W. (1974). *What the Buddha taught.* New York: Grove Press.

Reinarman, C. (2005). Addiction as accomplishment: The discursive construction of disease. *Addiction Research and Theory, 13,* 307–320.

Segal, Z. V., Williams, J. M. G., & Teasdale, J. D. (2002). *Mindfulness-based cognitive therapy for depression: A new approach to preventing relapse.* New York: Guilford Press.

Shaffer, H. J., LaPlante, D. A., LaBrie, R. A., Kidman, R. C., Donato, A. N., & Stanton, M. V. (2004). Toward a syndrome model of addiction: Multiple expressions, common etiology. *Harvard Review of Psychiatry, 12*(6), 367–374.

Sinha, R. (2007). The role of stress in addiction relapse. *Current Psychiatry Reports, 9,* 388–395.

Skinner, B. F. (1953). *Science and human behavior.* New York: Macmillan.

Soyka, M., & Rosner, S. (2010). Nalmefene for treatment of alcohol dependence. *Expert Opinion on Investigational Drugs, 19*(11), 1451–1459.

Toneatto, T., Vettese, L., & Nguyen, L. (2007). The role of mindfulness in the cognitive-behavioural treatment of problem gambling. *Journal of Gambling Issues, 19,* 91–100.

Vieten, C., Astin, J. A., Buscemi, R., & Galloway, G. P. (2010). Development of an acceptance-based coping intervention for alcohol dependence relapse prevention. *Substance Abuse, 31*(2), 108–116.

Webster's ninth new collegiate dictionary. (1988). Springfield, MA: Merriam-Webster.

Wilson, K. G., Hayes, S. C., & Byrd, M. (2000). Exploring compatibilities between acceptance and commitment therapy and 12-step treatment for substance abuse. *Journal of Rational-Emotive and Cognitive-Behavior Therapy, 18,* 209–234.

Wise, R. A. (1996). Neurobiology of addiction. *Current Opinion in Neurobiology, 6,* 243–251.

Witkiewitz, K., Bowen, S., & Donovan, D. M. (2011). Moderating effects of a craving intervention on the relation between negative mood and heavy drinking following treatment for alcohol dependence. *Journal of Consulting and Clinical Psychology, 79*(1), 54–63.

Witkiewitz, K., Bowen, S., Douglas, H., & Hsu, S. H. (2013). Mindfulness-based relapse prevention for substance craving. *Addictive Behaviors, 38*(2), 1563–1571.

Witkiewitz, K., Marlatt, G. A., & Walker, D. (2005). Mindfulness-based relapse prevention for alcohol and substance use disorders. *Journal of Cognitive Psychotherapy: An Interntational Quarterly, 19*(3), 211–228.

Zgierska, A., Rabago, D., Chawla, N., Kushner, K., Koehler, R., & Marlatt, A. (2009). Mindfulness meditation for substance use disorders: A systematic review. *Substance Abuse, 30,* 266–94.

Zgierska, A., Rabago, D., Zuelsdorff, M., Coe, C., Miller, M., & Fleming, M. (2008). Mindfulness meditation for alcohol relapse prevetion: A feasability pilot study. *Journal of Addictive Medicine, 2*(3), 165–173.

CHAPTER 22

Mindfulness-Based Interventions for Physical Conditions

A Selective Review

Linda E. Carlson

This chapter reviews and integrates the growing literature investigating the application of mindfulness-based interventions (MBIs) for people coping with a wide array of physical diseases and conditions. MBIs in this area include mindfulness-based stress reduction (MBSR), mindfulness-based cognitive therapy (MBCT), acceptance and commitment therapy (ACT), and other modifications or variations on these that incorporate mindfulness training and have been applied to physical health conditions. Although sometimes including mindfulness training, studies of yoga interventions alone were excluded, due primarily to the large volume of work in that area.

The aim of this chapter is not to provide a comprehensive summary of the voluminous research in this area (for this, see Carlson, 2012). Rather, the approach here addresses a series of key questions relevant to this area of inquiry: What might a wide variety of medical conditions have in common that makes them amenable to mindfulness training influences? Could there be underlying mechanisms by which the application of mindfulness training may be helpful across such a diverse array of problems? What does the research tell us about what works best for which symptoms and in which physical conditions? There may not be one unifying, underlying explanation for treatment effects, but several possibilities merit exploration. Hence, in the first part of this chapter I discuss common issues across many medical conditions that MBIs may address, followed by a summary of selected research in this broad area, and conclude with commentary and recommendations for further research.

Why Mindfulness Training?

The question arises as to why mindfulness training might impact a broad range of difficult psychosocial and physical issues in medical populations. Receiving a diagnosis of a serious and potentially life-threatening disease inevitably challenges one's view of oneself and the world in which one lives. Practically, disease treatment and management also poses many limitations, such as having to take time away from career and family for debilitating and often mutilating acute and ongoing treatments, and lifestyle changes that may have to be permanent. On an existential level, people are forced to confront their own mortality more directly than ever before. Whatever the diagnosis, the possibility of one's death becomes real and potentially imminent, and substantial and perhaps permanent changes in functional abilities may follow, as well as having to face ongoing symptoms including pain and fatigue. On a psychological level, diagnosis and treatment often produce a sense of unpredictability, loss of control, and feelings of anxiety and fear. Life plans and priorities may have to change in unwanted and unpredictable ways.

Training in mindfulness practices can help to address these issues in a number of ways. The core training in MBIs is the development of stable and kind mindful attention, through repetitive and consistent application of attention to facilitate awareness of present-moment experience, with a kind, curious, and nonjudgmental attitude. This typically begins with training in focused attention on the breath or bodily sensation through body scanning, sitting meditation, and mindful movement. Once stability of attention has been established through ongoing practice, a broadening of attention ("bare awareness" or "open monitoring") is applied, which allows people to directly experience the nature of mind for what it is: transient, impersonal (e.g., having a "mind of its own"), and constantly changing. Through observation, participants can also directly experience how grasping at certain outcomes or states of being causes suffering, and through that insight learn to let go of clinging and the personalization of experience.

A mindfulness approach is eminently adaptable to a wide array of illness circumstances. Simply absorbing the general understanding that the only certainty in life is change, and that sometimes the best thing to do to solve a problem is to accept it, can be extremely relieving and even liberating to people who are desperately and often frantically trying to fix things that are uncontrollable. Realizing that in fact they can slow down and see things as they are, without "cognitive blinders," and learn ways to hold the strong emotions and sensations that arise can be transformative. The further realization that although specific symptoms may be unpleasant, they are tolerable and are also constantly in flux, can provide further liberation from suffering. Stepping back and seeing the racing thoughts, worries, and self-blame as just thoughts, and not necessarily the truth, provide yet another degree of freedom. Hence, change occurs not only by training the mind through formal mindfulness practice but also via a shift in attitude and perspective that allows people to see their illness in a new light, without allowing distress to consume their thoughts and to drive their behavior.

We have formalized this process theoretically by suggesting several mechanisms of action of MBIs that may promote change, including exposure to difficult inner experience, acceptance of experience, practicing emotion regulation strategies, adoption of psychological (emotional, cognitive, and behavioral) flexibility in response to difficult experience, and clarifying one's values about what is important in life (Shapiro & Carlson, 2009). For example, in terms of emotion regulation, which has garnered an increasing amount of research attention, our recent work shows MBSR participants ruminate on the past and worry about the future less, and engage in less experiential avoidance of difficult feelings and situations (Labelle, 2012). Mediation analysis shows this is possible through the application of mindfulness skills, particularly present-moment, nonjudgmental awareness. The effects of these changes in the way that people engage with their inner experience are subsequent decreases in specific disease symptomatology, as well as improvements in a broad range of psychological outcomes (Labelle, 2012).

Despite some promising work, few other studies within this area examine how change happens over the course of mindfulness training because the focus to date primarily has been on quantifying the nature and extent of benefits. Some qualitative studies that shed additional light on processes of change in physical health populations are summarized later in this review.

Summary of the Literature

The strategy employed here in reviewing research on MBI effects of physical health outcomes is to add to other comprehensive reviews (Carlson, 2012; Shapiro & Carlson, 2009, Chapter 6) by highlighting more recent, well-designed studies that may deepen our understanding of efficacy and mechanisms of action. The literature is summarized by disease type rather than by outcomes, since a broad range of outcomes have been studied, many of which are specific to the populations of interest.

Clinical Populations

Cancer

Cancer is a leading cause of morbidity and mortality worldwide, with 13 million new cases and 7.6 million deaths recorded in 2008 alone (Boyle & Levin, 2008). In the United States, for example, about 1.67 million new cancer cases were diagnosed in 2014, and over 585,000 people died from cancer. However, due to improvements in treatments and increasing incidence rates, growing numbers of people are also living for longer periods after having been treated for cancer: An estimated 14.48 million Americans with a history of cancer were alive in 2014 (American Cancer Society, 2014). Yet cancer treatments and disease processes often leave survivors with symptoms and side effects such as lingering fatigue, sleep difficulties, pain, anxiety, depression, and worries about cancer recurrence (Carlson, Angen, et al., 2004). Hence, there is a significant need for psychosocial interventions to help people cope with the difficulties of cancer diagnosis and treatment.

As a response to this high level of need, there is now a large body of work investigating the efficacy of MBIs for patients with various types of cancer. This literature has been reviewed on several occasions since 2006 (Lamanque & Daneault, 2006; Ledesma & Kumano, 2009; Matchim & Armer, 2007; Matchim, Armer, & Stewart, 2011; Musial, Bussing, Heusser, Choi, & Ostermann, 2011; Shennan, Payne, & Fenlon, 2011). A meta-analysis of 10 MBI studies (Ledesma & Kumano, 2009) found a medium-sized effect on psychosocial outcome variables (d = 0.48) but only a small effect on the handful of physical biomarker variables measured up to that point (d = 0.18). In a more recent meta-analysis of 19 studies, Musial and colleagues (2011) reported similar effect sizes on mood (d = 0.42) and distress (d = 0.48) but did not report on biological outcomes.

The first MBI study in a cancer population was published in Canada by Speca, Carlson, Goodey, and Angen (2000): In a randomized controlled trial (RCT), 89 patients with a variety of cancer diagnoses were randomized to MBSR or a wait-list control condition. Patients in the MBSR program improved significantly more on mood states and symptoms of stress than did controls, with large improvements of approximately 65% on mood and 35% on stress symptoms; these changes were maintained at a 6-month follow-up point (Carlson, Ursuliak, Goodey, Angen, & Speca, 2001). The greatest treatment improvements were seen on anxiety, depression, and irritability, and more home practice was associated with greater decreases in overall mood disturbance. Since that time, many pre- and posttreatment observational studies without comparison groups and RCTs with usual care or wait-list control groups have been published, citing improvements in a range of outcomes including quality-of-life (QL) domains such as emotional, social, role, and physical functioning, and psychological improvements on measures including stress symptoms, anxiety, depression, fear, and avoidance (for reviews, see Ledesma & Kumano, 2009; Matchim et al., 2011; Musial et al., 2011; Shennan et al., 2011).

Although there is now a substantial number of RCTs that compare MBIs to wait-list or usual care controls, some with quite large sample sizes (Branstrom, Kvillemo, & Moskowitz, 2012; Foley, Baillie, Huxter, Price, & Sinclair, 2010; Hoffman et al., 2012; Lengacher et al., 2009), still very few studies have included randomization to active comparison groups. A notable exception is a three-arm trial in which Henderson and colleagues (2012) randomized 172 early-stage breast cancer patients to MBSR, into a nutrition education program matched on contact time, or into a usual care control condition, and included follow-up assessments postprogram (4 months) and 1 and 2 years later. The MBSR group improved more than the other two conditions on a wide range of measures at the 4-month postprogram assessment, including QL, active behavioral and cognitive coping, avoidance, and spirituality, as well as depression, hostility, anxiety, unhappiness, meaningfulness, and several measures of emotional control. These group differences eroded somewhat over time, however, as participants in the other two groups continued to improve more slowly, such that at 12 months, MBSR was only superior on measures of Spirituality, Behavioral Coping, and the sense of coherence subscale Comprehensibility (i.e., making sense of one's predicament). At 24 months, the only apparent group differences were on measures of anxiety, unhappiness, and emotional control, still favoring MBSR over usual care, but not the other active, nutrition education intervention. From this study, it appears that MBSR participation may not only help speed up the natural course of cancer recovery across many domains but also may add a shift in perspective and enhanced skills in emotion regulation that appear lasting.

Carlson and colleagues (2013) reported the largest trial to date, randomizing 272 distressed breast cancer survivors to either a variant of MBSR (called mindfulness-based cancer recovery; MBCR), supportive–expressive therapy (matched on contact time), and a minimal treatment control condition. Postprogram, MBSR produced greater improvements in mood, stress, and QL relative to the two comparison programs. These findings represent the most well-controlled test to date of an MBI in the cancer context and suggest benefits of a condition-tailored MBI over other active interventions immediately posttreatment; however, 6- and 12-month follow-up data have not yet been reported.

One other relatively recent trial focused specifically on sleep disorders. In a partially blinded RCT (patients did not know what the specific treatments were when they enrolled in the study), Garland, Carlson, Antle, Samuels, and Campbell (2011) specifically compared MBSR and cognitive-behavioral therapy (CBT) for the treatment of insomnia in cancer survivors. Immediately postintervention, insomnia outcomes favored CBT, but by 3 months postintervention, MBSR was not inferior to this "gold standard" treatment, and both groups showed clinically meaningful improvements in insomnia severity (Garland, Carlson, Antle, Samuels, & Campbell, 2014).

Another area of focus in cancer populations has been assessment of the impact of MBIs on biomarkers such as salivary cortisol and measures of immune functioning relevant to stress and cancer progression. For example, Carlson and colleagues (Carlson, Speca, Patel, & Faris, 2007; Carlson, Speca, Patel, & Goodey, 2003, 2004) measured immune and endocrine function pre- and post-MBSR treatment in 59 breast and prostate cancer survivors. T cell production of interleukin 4 (IL-4; an anti-inflammatory cytokine) increased when stimulated, while interferon gamma (IFN-gamma) and natural killer (NK) cell production of IL-10 decreased. Carlson and colleagues (2007) found that patterns of change in cytokines over 1 year of follow-up also supported a continued reduction in proinflammatory cytokine production.

Lengacher and colleagues (2013) additionally reported increased response of T cells to antigen stimulation and an improved ratio of T cell (Th1/Th2) cytokines in early stage breast cancer patients after a 6-week MBSR program. They also found decreases in both cortisol and IL-6 pre- to postsession, and decreases in baseline levels across sessions in patients with advanced cancer and their caregivers (Lengacher et al., 2012). The interpretation of these results is complex, but, in general, an anti-inflammatory environment is thought to be more favorable to cancer outcomes than one with elevated Th2 (proinflammatory) cytokines (Armaiz-Pena, Lutgendorf, Cole, & Sood, 2009).

Salivary cortisol profiles also shifted pre- to postintervention, with fewer evening cortisol elevations post-MBSR, and some normalization of abnormal diurnal salivary cortisol profiles (Carlson, Speca, et al., 2004). Over a year of follow-up, continuing decreases in overall diurnal cortisol levels were seen, mostly due to further decreases in evening cortisol (Carlson et al., 2007). This shift in cortisol slopes was replicated in a recent RCT comparing MBSR to a control condition (Carlson et al., 2013) in which steeper slopes and lower evening cortisol levels were reported post-MBSR compared to controls. This is significant because higher cortisol levels, particularly in the evening, are considered a potential marker of dysregulated cortisol secretion patterns and poorer clinical outcomes, such as shorter survival times in metastatic breast cancer patients (Sephton, Sapolsky, Kraemer, & Spiegel, 2000).

Measures of autonomic system function have also been of interest, since cancer survivors are at high risk for cardiovascular disease due to the toxicity of their cancer treatments. In a group of 72 women with various forms of cancer, weekly home blood pressure (BP) monitoring showed significant decreases in systolic blood pressure over the course of a MBSR program for women with higher premorbid BP, compared to those in a comparable naturalistic wait-list group (Campbell, Labelle, Bacon, Faris, & Carlson, 2012).

In summary, the literature on cancer and MBIs is substantial and continues to grow, with improving quality of research design through the application of active control groups, larger samples, more diverse patient groups, longer follow-up periods, and a wide range of outcomes. Outcomes consistently favor MBSR over usual care and other active interventions immediately postprogram across a range of psychological and QL outcomes. Its superiority over other active interventions over a longer period of time has yet to be demonstrated definitively, though some specificity of effect is emerging. Associations between home practice of mindfulness and outcomes have not been adequately investigated. The value of MBIs in improving cancer-related biomarkers also requires further investigation.

Chronic Pain and Low Back Pain

Chronic pain affects approximately 13% of the population and is defined as an unpleasant sensory and emotional experience associated with actual or potential tissue damage that persists beyond the expected time frame for healing, or that occurs in disease processes in which healing may never occur (Ospina & Harstall, 2002). The earliest reported application of MBSR was for patients with chronic pain (Kabat-Zinn, 1982), and work has continued to grow in this area. Specific pain conditions have also been studied, including low back pain, fibromyalgia, rheumatoid arthritis, and migraine. This literature has been reviewed in depth on several occasions (Chiesa & Serretti, 2011; Elabd, 2011; McCracken & Thompson, 2011; Patil, 2009; Veehof, Oskam, Schreurs, & Bohlmeijer, 2011). Chiesa and Serretti (2011) systematically reviewed all controlled studies (*n* = 10) and concluded that MBIs could have nonspecific effects on mood, coping, and pain symptoms in chronic pain patients, but that studies often suffered from small sample sizes, lack of randomization, and the use of nonspecific control groups. Veehof and colleagues (2011) conducted a meta-analysis of both controlled and uncontrolled studies (*n* = 22) and found small effect sizes of 0.37 for pain improvements and 0.32 for depressive symptomatology reductions. Veehof and colleagues suggested that while MBSR and ACT interventions for chronic pain may be viable alternatives to standard CBT for pain, they have not been shown to be superior to it.

While many early studies of MBIs and chronic pain utilized pre- to posttreatment designs and showed improvements across a wide range of outcomes, including ratings of pain, psychiatric symptoms, depression, pain-related anxiety, disability, medical visits, work status, and acceptance of physical performance limits (see Veehof et al., 2011, for a review), only two studies employed randomized comparison groups. In one, Plews-Ogan, Owens, Goodman, Wolfe, & Schorling(2005) evaluated MBSR for the management of chronic musculoskeletal pain in 30 pain patients randomly assigned to MBSR, massage, or a no-intervention control condition. Immediately postintervention, the massage group had more pain reduction and improved mental health status compared to the usual care group, whereas the MBSR group showed greater 1-month postintervention improvements in mental health outcomes than did the usual care and the massage conditions. Thus, MBSR was more effective for enhancing mood in the long term, but massage provided more immediate pain relief.

In the second study, completed in Hong Kong, Wong and colleagues (2011) conducted the largest trial to date in chronic pain, comparing two active interventions—MBSR versus a multidisciplinary pain intervention that comprised primarily psychoeducation with sessions on physiotherapy for pain and nutrition—for 99 patients with chronic pain. In both groups, patients who completed the interventions improved similarly on measures of pain intensity and pain-related distress over time. However, without usual care or no-treatment control groups, it is difficult to conclude whether these improvements are due to the interventions themselves or simply fluctuations in symptomatology due to natural healing over time, historical trends, regression toward average pain and distress, or expectancy effects.

For low back pain, Carson and colleagues (2005) applied a variant of MBSR with an extended focus on loving-kindness practice (cultivating feelings of kindness and friendliness toward the self and others) with 43 patients randomly assigned to the loving kindness-integrated program or treatment as usual (TAU). Whereas MBI participants showed improvements in pain perception and psychological distress, the control group demonstrated no improvements. Morone, Greco, and Weiner (2008) randomized 37 pain-affected older adult participants (average age 75 years) to MBSR or a wait-list control condition. Compared to the wait-list, MBSR participants showed significantly greater improvements on measures of chronic pain acceptance, engagement in activities, and overall physical functioning.

Although sample sizes in the RCTs in this area remain small, the support for MBSR as a helpful intervention to improve coping with pain symptoms and overall adjustment in patients with chronic low back pain continues to mount, but superiority to comparison programs (e.g., standard CBT) for pain has not been established.

Fibromyalgia

In fibromyalgia (FM), a pain-related condition associated with overall bodily stiffness, soreness, pain trigger points throughout the body, fatigue, and sleep disturbance, symptoms seem to be exacerbated by stress (Grossman, Tiefenthaler-Gilmer, Raysz, & Kesper, 2007). Earlier pre- to posttreatment studies and some wait-list or usual care MBI RCTs (Goldenberg et al., 1994; Grossman et al., 2007; Weissbecker et al., 2002) have shown improved pain, sleep, FM impact, severity of psychological symptoms, coping, QL, anxiety, depression, somatic complaints, and sense of coherence.

In the most rigorous study to date (Schmidt et al., 2011), 177 female patients were randomized to MBSR, to an active control condition, or to a wait-list condition. The active control was matched to MBSR on format, instructors, contact time, and homework, with the focus on progressive muscle relaxation and stretching rather than mindfulness practices per se. There were no significant differences between groups on the primary outcome of health-related QL (HRQL) 2 months posttreatment; patients improved in all three conditions over time. Yet post hoc analyses of within-group changes showed that only MBSR resulted in a significant pre- to postintervention improvement in HRQL (with an effect size of 0.39) and on six of eight secondary outcome variables (e.g., depressive symptoms, anxiety and sleep problems) compared to improvements on three measures for the active control group, and two in the wait-list condition.

Hence, MBSR seems to be an effective intervention for alleviating symptoms common in FM such as pain, depression, and a range of psychological outcomes, although, as with chronic pain, it has not proven superior to other active comparison programs. MBIs have also not yet been compared to proven efficacious treatments such as CBT, which would provide a more rigorous test of overall efficacy.

Rheumatoid Arthritis

There are two RCTs investigating the effect of MBSR on *rheumatoid arthritis* (RA), a painful autoimmune condition caused by swelling of the joints. In the first (Pradhan et al., 2007), 63 participants were randomized to MBSR or to a wait-list control condition. After 2 months, there were no differences between the groups on measures of depressive symptoms, psychological distress, well-being, mindfulness, and RA disease activity, as evaluated by a physician masked to treatment status. However, at a 6-month follow-up point, there were significant improvements across these self-reported outcomes in the MBSR group.

The second study in this area employed multimodal outcome measures and compared 144 participants randomly assigned to one of three conditions: CBT for pain; mindfulness meditation and emotion regulation therapy; or education only, which served as an attention placebo control (Zautra et al., 2008). This is one of the first published studies to compare an MBI directly with a proven efficacious CBT intervention, so it has the potential to inform conclusions about specificity of treatment effects and mechanisms. The greatest improvements in pain control and reductions in inflammatory cytokines were observed in participants in the CBT pain group, whereas both the CBT and mindfulness groups improved more in coping efficacy compared to the education control group. Patients with a positive history of depression benefited more from mindfulness training on both negative and positive affect, and physicians' ratings of joint tenderness, suggesting that MBSR might be preferable to CBT for treating individuals with RA who also struggle with depression; however, overall, the mindfulness–emotion regulation treatment did not prove to be a superior intervention.

In summary, in controlled trials with active comparison groups, only with secondary analyses did RA-relevant outcomes emerge that consistently favored MBSR. For RA pain control itself, it may be that standard CBT remains the most effective treatment, whereas MBIs emphasizing acceptance may be more effective to increase the ability to tolerate ongoing pain, and for people who struggle with depression in addition to pain. The qualitative work reviewed later sheds further light on this question.

Cardiovascular Diseases

Cardiovascular disorders are the most prevalent diseases in North America and include a range of conditions such as hypertension (high blood pressure), coronary artery disease, heart failure, and angina. The effect of MBIs on cardiovascular disease outcomes and clinical markers has been reviewed elsewhere (Ospina et al., 2007), so here the focus is on recent applications of MBIs in participants diagnosed with either hypertension or heart disease.

In addition to recent pre- to posttreatment studies indicating improvements on a range of psychological outcomes in people with heart disease (Chang, Casey, Dusek, & Benson, 2010; Delaney, Barrere, & Helming, 2011; Olivo, Dodson-Lavelle, Wren, Fang, & Oz, 2009), two very small RCTs comparing MBSR to waitlist control groups reported benefits in anxiety, emotion regulation, and reduced use of reactive coping styles in MBSR participants (Robert McComb, Tacón, Randolph, & Caldera, 2004; Tacón, McComb, Caldera, & Randolph, 2003).

Sullivan and colleagues (2009) conducted a novel prospective cohort study in which they geographically assigned 208 patients with chronic heart failure to an MBI that comprised mindfulness meditation practice, coping skills and group discussion for those who lived close enough to attend, or a usual care control condition for those living further away from the medical center. Patients in the MBI had greater decreases in anxiety, depression, and cardiac symptoms postintervention and at 3 and 6 months. However, after 1 year of follow-up, group differences were no longer apparent, as all participants showed increased symptoms. This pattern is similar to that seen in studies of other conditions, where MBSR provides an initial benefit that erodes somewhat over time. Again, home practice over the follow-up period was not reported, but one speculation is that continued practice may be important to maintain psychological and physical benefits.

Diabetes

Diabetes impacts about 7% of the North American population and is due to the body's inability to produce and/or use insulin sufficiently. It is characterized by symptoms of fatigue, lack of energy, frequent infections, easy bruising, tingling and pain in extremities, and weight changes (Public Health Agency of Canada, 2012). A number of MBI studies have been reported in this area recently, many of which have monitored biomarkers, as well as psychological functioning. Several studies have compared MBIs to control conditions in RCTs. One such small RCT compared MBSR to nutrition education control in 20 patients (Teixeira, 2010) and reported greater improvements on QL related to pain and symptoms in the MBSR group.

In the largest study to date (Hartmann et al., 2012) 110 patients with type 2 diabetes were assigned to either MBSR or a TAU control, and followed for 5 years on both psychological and biological outcome markers. At the first year of follow-up, MBSR participants improved more on overall health status, depression, and stress symptoms relative to controls. Thus, there is initial evidence that MBIs can improve psychological functioning and possibly gylcemic control associated with type 2 diabetes. However, MBIs have been compared only to usual care or education at this point, and studies are still few in number.

HIV/AIDS

In 2010, 34 million people worldwide (3 million in North America) were reported to be living with HIV, which typically causes flu-like symptoms and puts a person at risk for opportunistic infections (World Health Organization, 2012). Untreated, HIV progresses to full-blown AIDS, characterized by symptoms such as fatigue, shortness of breath, fever, chronic cough, weight loss, and eventual death (World Health Organization, 2012). MBSR research in this area has increased substantially in the last 4 years. For example, a recent RCT sought to assess the potential for MBSR to help patients cope with common side effects of antiretroviral medication, including gastrointestinal problems such as diarrhea, nausea, and vomiting, neuropathic pain, and dermatological problems including rashes (Duncan et al., 2012). Seventy-six people living with HIV were assigned to MBSR or wait-list control and assessed postprogram and over a 6-month follow-up period. The MBSR group had fewer symptoms related to antiretroviral therapies at both postprogram and follow-up, as well as less symptom-related distress.

Some studies have also investigated the impact of MBSR on immune measures in HIV-positive (HIV+) participants. Creswell, Myers, Cole, and Irwin (2009) assigned 48 HIV-infected adults to either an 8-week MBSR class or a 1-day stress reduction education seminar control condition. Peripheral counts of CD4+ T lymphocytes decreased substantially in the control group but remained stable in the MBSR group. Class attendance mediated the effects of MBSR on buffering CD4+ T lymphocyte decreases over time, such that participants who attended more classes showed more stability in their counts, accounting for up to two-thirds of the effect on T cell counts. In the largest study to date, 173 Iranian HIV+ patients not yet receiving antiretroviral therapy were randomized to either MBSR or a brief 2-hour education support group (SeyedAlinaghi et al., 2012). In the MBSR condition, the mean CD4+ lymphocyte count increased up to 9 months posttreatment, then returned to baseline levels at 12 months. Control group counts remained relatively stable over the full year. Physical and psychiatric symptomatology also remained stable for control patients, but for MBSR participants, improvements were seen postprogram across all domains. However, only physical symptoms (e.g., pain, fatigue) and HIV-related items such infections remained lower than those of controls over follow-up.

In summary, MBSR in HIV-infected men may help to improve psychological well-being and symptom control, as well as measures of immune system functioning that are important predictors of disease progression, but research has not used evidence-based active control groups matched on intervention duration, which might potentially have the same benefits.

Irritable Bowel Syndrome

Irritable bowel syndrome (IBS), a functional disorder of the lower gastrointestinal (GI) tract, is defined by the presence of chronic or recurring symptoms that include abdominal pain, flatulence, bloating, and altered bowel habits (Drossman, 1994). Prior to 2010, there were no reports in the literature on the application of MBIs for treating symptoms and improving the well-being of people with IBS, but since that time, several research groups have reported large, well-designed RCTs. The first treatment results were published by Ljottson, Andersson, and colleagues (2011) in Sweden. The intervention they evaluated was a 10-session group focusing on three themes: cognitive awareness and education around stress and coping; mindfulness training; and exposure to noxious IBS symptoms. They conducted an RCT of an online adapted version of their acceptance- and mindfulness-based intervention with 61 patients, comparing it to wait-list controls. The intervention was conducted online largely by patients on their own at home, following a structured program of education and practice, with weekly Internet contact with therapists via e-mail. There was also a closed discussion forum for patients to share questions or progress with one another (Ljotsson, Andersson, et al., 2011). Compared to those on the wait list, participants improved more over time on self-reported IBS symptom severity, QL, and IBS-related fear and avoidance behaviors, which were maintained over 12 months.

This research group has also investigated the impact of the online MBI against an active control group, randomly assigning 86 patients to either the online acceptance and mindfulness intervention or an online discussion forum wait list (Ljotsson et al., 2010). In this case, participants in the treatment condition reported a 42% decrease (compared to a 12% increase in the control group) in self-reported primary IBS symptoms, and they improved on GI-specific anxiety, depression, and general functioning, with large effect sizes. These participants were followed up 16 months later after they had all completed the intervention (Ljotsson, Hedman, Lindfors, et al., 2011). Treatment gains were maintained on all outcome measures, including IBS symptoms, QL, and anxiety related to GI symptoms, again with large effect sizes (most $d > 1.0$).

Finally, in a very well-designed RCT, this group investigated their online mindfulness intervention compared to online stress management matched in time and format with 195 patients, and also measured credibility of the treatments, expectancy for improvement, and therapeutic alliance (Ljotsson, Hedman, Andersson, et al., 2011). At posttreatment and at 6-month follow-up, the MBI group improved more than stress management controls on IBS symptom severity, IBS QL, visceral sensitivity, and the Cognitive Scale for Functional Bowel Disorders. Both groups improved similarly on the Perceived Stress Scale and Hospital Anxiety and Depression Scale subscales. There were also no group differences on the Treatment Credibility Scale or the Working Alliance Inventory. This impressive series of studies provides strong support for the efficacy of the online MBI for improving both physical symptoms and

QL in IBS patients but showed that other active interventions can also successfully treat stress, anxiety, and depression.

Two North American groups have also evaluated in-person traditional MBSR for IBS. In an RCT of MBSR compared to a wait list for 90 patients with IBS, Zernicke, Campbell, Speca, and colleagues (2013) found that whereas both groups exhibited a decrease in IBS symptom severity scores over time, the improvement in the MBSR group was greater than that in the controls and was clinically meaningful, with symptom severity decreasing from constantly to occasionally present, which was maintained in the MBSR group 6 months later. In an active comparison trial, 75 women were randomized to MBSR or to a support group matched for time and other nonspecific factors (Gaylord et al., 2011). Women in MBSR, compared to the support group, showed greater reductions in IBS symptom severity posttraining (26.4 vs. 6.2% reduction) and at 3-month follow-up (38.2 vs. 11.8%). Changes in QL, psychological distress, and visceral anxiety favoring MBSR emerged only at the 3-month follow-up. Path analysis suggested that MBSR worked by promoting nonreactivity to gut-focused anxiety and less catastrophic appraisals of the significance of abdominal sensations, as well as refocusing attention onto interoceptive data without the high levels of emotional reactivity often characteristic of the disorder (Garland, Gaylord, et al., 2011).

Considered together, this body of well-designed and executed studies provides consistent evidence for the efficacy of both in-person and online versions of MBIs for IBS sufferers, showing greater improvements specifically in IBS symptoms over other credible treatments, including stress management and social support.

Organ Transplant

A series of well-designed studies was conducted by Gross and colleagues (2010; Kreitzer, Gross, Ye, Russas, & Treesak, 2005) for organ transplant recipients, who often cope with a host of medical symptoms, side effects of antirejection drugs, and symptoms associated with recovery from complicated surgeries (Gross et al., 2010; Kreitzer, Gross, Ye, Russas, & Treesak, 2005). In a large RCT, 138 recipients of kidney, kidney–pancreas, liver, heart, or lung transplants were randomized to either MBSR or a health education control group (Gross et al., 2010). MBSR participants had greater reductions in anxiety and sleep symptoms compared to the controls, with medium-sized effects up to 1-year follow-up. Within the MBSR group, self-reported anxiety, depression, and sleep symptoms decreased and QL improved by 8 weeks; these benefits were maintained at 1 year. Hence, this initial evidence suggests that MBSR may be an effective treatment for psychological symptoms in organ transplant recipients.

Qualitative Studies

Qualitative research is valuable in that it helps to better understand the lived experience of MBI participants and has the potential to help explain salutary effects in a descriptive way. Through interviews and focus groups, participants can describe deeply and in rich language the process of engagement and how they perceive beneficial change from learning mindfulness practices.

Several early qualitative studies set the groundwork for this line of inquiry. In the first study with cancer patients, Mackenzie, Carlson, Munoz, and Speca (2007) interviewed nine cancer patients who had participated in the 8-week MBSR program, and who continued to attend weekly drop-in MBSR sessions for 1 to 6 years. With individual semistructured interviews and a focus group, five major themes were identified: (1) opening to change; (2) self-regulation; (3) shared experience; (4) personal growth; and (5) spirituality. The interviews were used to develop specific theory concerning mechanisms whereby MBSR effects change for cancer patients. In this theory, initial participation in the 8-week program was seen as only the beginning of an ongoing process of self-discovery. The MBSR program taught concrete tools for self-regulation, and introduced to participants ways to perceive themselves and their lives that they previously may not have considered. Underlying this process was a theme of personal transformation and, specifically, of feeling part of a larger whole. With this came the development of positive qualities of personal growth and positive health orientations, often beyond the symptom reduction documented over the course of the initial 8-week program. A growing spirituality based on finding meaning and purpose in one's life and feeling increasingly interconnected with others was part of this personal transformation. The participants also described the development of gratitude, compassion, and equanimity.

Similarly, Dobkin (2008) interviewed 13 women who had completed breast cancer treatment The women reported taking better care of themselves and viewing life as more meaningful and manageable. Themes identified in focus groups included (1) acceptance; (2) regaining and maintaining mindful control; (3) taking responsibility for what could change; and (4) cultivating a spirit of openness and connectedness. These map well onto the themes of opening to change, connecting with others, and self-control identified by Mackenzie and colleagues (2007).

More recent international qualitative work also highlighted similar themes in 28 Japanese participants after just two mindfulness meditation sessions (Ando, Morita, Akechi, & Ifuku, 2011). However, they highlighted that the concepts around spirituality and self-control were not as predominant in their Japanese group compared to previous Western samples. The focus was on adaptive coping, personal growth, and finding positive meaning in their cancer experience.

Kvillemo and Branstrom (2010) reported on 18 Swedish cancer patients who participated in an 8-week MBSR program; interestingly, interviewees expressed not only positive outcomes, but several also struggled with particular practices, and some expressed that they received little benefit. This may be interpreted as suggesting that the program may not be for everyone, although it may also suggest the importance of adapting to meet individual needs. Nonetheless, to date, it is rare to find "negative" results discussed in most research reports.

In a qualitative study, Hsu, Bluespruce, Sherman, and Cherkin (2010) interviewed 18 chronic low back pain patients participating in MBSR and identified themes specific to chronic pain: changes in ways of thinking about pain (as impermanent and changing rather than permanent and constant) that helped to increase feelings of hope. Similarly, in FM sufferers, a changing relationship to pain was described, in that it no longer dominated their life, overwhelmed them, or restricted their activities as before (Hawtin & Sullivan, 2011). Instead, more responsive approaches to pain were described, including engaging with, approaching, and exploring pain rather than trying to resist or deny its existence.

Similarities across these studies and across medical conditions are apparent, including the importance of sharing deep experiences with people suffering from similar medical conditions and knowing that one is not alone in one's suffering. Also, a shift in perspective, better emotional control, openness to experience, and acceptance of circumstances as they are emerge are important factors for participants. It also highlights that this approach may not be for everyone, and raises further questions about who is best suited for MBIs.

One drawback of the qualitative work is that non-MBSR participants with similar medical conditions were not interviewed. This raises the possibility that many of the changes described could be part of the natural process of "working through" or coming to terms with having to live with a chronic medical condition. Indeed, the phenomenon of "posttraumatic growth" has been identified as often occurring without intervention in people facing life-threatening circumstances (Calhoun & Tedeschi, 1999), including chronic medical conditions and aggressive medical treatments. So while participants did credit the mindfulness training in their improvements, it is also possible that people may use other means to achieve personal growth. Future qualitative studies would benefit from comparing participants' lived experiences in MBIs with those of other active group treatment programs to understand unique qualitative mechanisms of change.

Summary and Mechanisms

This chapter began with a brief description of how MBIs might help people with a broad range of physical conditions. This was followed by a short review of the specific conditions with the most empirical evidence to support their efficacy. Generally, MBIs seem effective for short-term relief of symptoms across conditions, but the longer-term effects are not yet well studied, and there are suggestions that benefits erode over time without ongoing practice. However, some studies also indicated that benefits took time to accrue, not demonstrating the full value for symptom reduction until several months postprogram. This issue has scarcely been investigated. Comparisons with active interventions, particular CBT-based modalities, suggest they may be comparable in some ways for outcomes such as pain control or insomnia treatment.

As evidence mounts supporting the efficacy of MBIs across a range of conditions, process questions around what happens to facilitate improvement are increasingly being addressed. Proposed mechanisms, such as the development of mindfulness, exposure, acceptance, emotion regulation, psychological (emotional, cognitive and behavioral) flexibility, and values clarification, have been identified as important (Shapiro & Carlson, 2009). Other factors highlighted in the qualitative work include the importance of the group format for feeling a sense of universality in the illness experience, support for change and a shift in one's worldview. Researchers and theorists have termed this shift in worldview *decentering, reperceiving,* and *cognitive defusion* (Shapiro & Carlson, 2009). The application of mindfulness skills and practice through an MBI program is thought to support this shift, but studies have not looked into how or when this may happen.

Considering the illness experience itself, it is possible that developing and applying mindful attention and the subsequent exposure to arising thoughts and feelings are important mechanisms of change. Learning to identify the stress response and associated symptoms, and to respond mindfully rather than react with aversion, can result in acceptance and relaxation, which may then result in symptom attenuation. For diagnoses that are the cause of considerable worry, anxiety, and life threat, processes such as acceptance and emotion regulation that result in reduction in worry and rumination are likely important. Indeed, many studies have now measured improvements in mindfulness skills and have found that these can mediate changes in some psychological and physical symptomatology outcomes (for reviews, see Labelle, 2012; Labelle, Campbell, & Carlson, 2010).

Future Research Directions

Comparisons to "gold standard" active interventions constitute rigorous tests of the specificity of MBIs, and more of these are needed. As seen in some pain studies in particular, and for treating insomnia in cancer, MBIs may not prove superior to other cognitive-behavioral approaches. Nonspecific factors, such as group support, the therapeutic alliance, expectancy for improvement, psychoeducation, self-monitoring, and self-empowerment, are likely also important drivers of change, as may be the specific targets of CBT: altering dysfunctional thoughts and behaviors directly relating to the presenting problem.

In terms of understanding processes of change, we know that enhancing emotion regulation strategies that help to decrease worry and rumination, and the development of certain facets of mindfulness, including nonjudging and present-moment awareness, are important to improve symptomatology in medical patients. Further dismantling research evaluating other postulated mechanisms of change, timing of changes as interventions progress, and mediating factors would help to improve our understanding of active ingredients within the typically multidimensional MBIs.

As suggested by some qualitative studies in this review, not everyone benefits from mindfulness-based approaches. Indeed, some studies suggest that other behavioral treatments (e.g., CBT) may produce better outcomes than MBIs (e.g., Zautra et al., 2008). Moreover, it is possible that some patients may benefit from CBT training first, followed by a mindfulness approach for maintenance of effects, or the timing of treatment effects may be different across treatment modalities. This latter possibility is hinted at in our study wherein CBT had a more rapid effect than MBSR for treating insomnia, but the MBSR group "caught up" 3 months after program completion (Garland et al., 2014). Perhaps a combined approach would be the "best of both worlds" with an early response and maintenance of benefit.

A focus on tailoring interventions to individuals would also be helpful for potentially improving program retention and maximizing outcomes. Given that there is always attrition in MBIs, better understanding of the motivations for taking programs, reasons for dropping out, and barriers to developing and maintaining home practice would be helpful. The identified barriers could potentially be addressed either programmatically or on a case-by-case basis. Further adapting MBIs to single-person interventions, home study programs, Internet-based programs, and shorter programs would also be beneficial in reaching a larger number of underserved patients in rural and remote locations (see, e.g., Zernicke, Campbell, Blustein, et al., 2013). These alternative formats and lengths have scarcely been investigated, but they hold great potential.

Additionally, investigating the impact of patient preferences and treatment credibility on outcomes in RCTs would approximate more real-world scenarios wherein patients choose interventions of their liking that they think will work. For example, in a subanalysis of RCT data, patients who were assigned to their preferred treatment (MBSR or support group) improved more on social support regardless of which treatment they received (Carlson et al., 2013). This suggests that bolstering the credibility of treatments may be important to harness expectancy effects. Utilizing pragmatic or preference-based trial designs in which patients with a preference are assigned to their preferred intervention, while those with no preference are randomized to one of two treatments, is an interesting way to investigate these influences.

Finally, the principles of training facilitators who themselves are grounded in mindfulness practice and receive adequate training and supervision are widely considered to be essential, but little research has been conducted in this area. Studies should empirically investigate the role of facilitator experience on treatment outcome, adherence, compliance, and related issues. If, as most MBI leaders believe, training and personal practice is essential to successfully facilitate MBIs, this element is likely to be of increased importance as various MBI adaptations in form and delivery continue to appear.

ACKNOWLEDGMENTS

Linda E. Carlson holds the Enbridge Research Chair in Psychosocial Oncology, cofunded by the Alberta Cancer Foundation and the Canadian Cancer Society Alberta/NWT Division. She is also an Alberta Innovates–Health Solutions Health Scholar. Many thanks to Dale Dirkse for help with literature searches and referencing.

REFERENCES

American Cancer Society. (2014). *Cancer facts and figures, 2014.* Atlanta: Author.

Ando, M., Morita, T., Akechi, T., & Ifuku, Y. (2011). A qualitative study of mindfulness-based meditation therapy in Japanese cancer patients. *Support Care Cancer, 19*(7), 929–933.

Armaiz-Pena, G. N., Lutgendorf, S. K., Cole, S. W., & Sood, A. K. (2009). Neuroendocrine modulation of cancer progression. *Brain, Behavior, and Immunity, 23*(1), 10–15.

Boyle, P., & Levin, B. (2008). *World cancer report 2008*. Geneva: WHO Press.

Branstrom, R., Kvillemo, P., & Moskowitz, J. T. (2012). A randomized study of the effects of mindfulness training on psychological well-being and symptoms of stress in patients treated for cancer at 6-month follow-up. *International Journal of Behavioral Medicine, 19*(4), 535–542.

Calhoun, L. G., & Tedeschi, R. G. (1999). *Facilitating post-traumatic growth: A clinician's guide*. Mahwah, NJ: Erlbaum.

Campbell, T. S., Labelle, L. E., Bacon, S. L., Faris, P., & Carlson, L. E. (2012). Impact of mindfulness-based stress reduction (MBSR) on attention, rumination and resting blood pressure in women with cancer: A waitlist-controlled study. *Journal of Behavioral Medicine, 35*(3), 262–271.

Carlson, L. E. (2012). Mindfulness-based interventions for physical conditions: A narrative review evaluating levels of evidence. *ISRN Psychiatry, 2012*, Article No. 651583.

Carlson, L. E., Angen, M., Cullum, J., Goodey, E., Koopmans, J., Lamont, L., et al. (2004). High levels of untreated distress and fatigue in cancer patients. *British Journal of Cancer, 90*(12), 2297–2304.

Carlson, L. E., Doll, R., Stephen, J., Faris, P., Tamagawa, R., & Speca, M. (2013). Randomized-controlled multi-site trial of mindfulness-based cancer recovery (MBCR) versus supportive expressive group therapy (SET) for distressed breast cancer survivors (MINDSET): Effects on mood, stress symptoms, quality of life and diurnal salivary cortisol. *Journal of Clinical Oncology, 31*(25), 33119–3126.

Carlson, L. E., Speca, M., Patel, K. D., & Faris, P. (2007). One year pre-post intervention follow-up of psychological, immune, endocrine and blood pressure outcomes of mindfulness-based stress reduction (MBSR) in breast and prostate cancer outpatients. *Brain, Behavior, and Immunity, 21*(8), 1038–1049

Carlson, L. E., Speca, M., Patel, K. D., & Goodey, E. (2003). Mindfulness-based stress reduction in relation to quality of life, mood, symptoms of stress, and immune parameters in breast and prostate cancer outpatients. *Psychosomatic Medicine, 65*(4), 571–581.

Carlson, L. E., Speca, M., Patel, K. D., & Goodey, E. (2004). Mindfulness-based stress reduction in relation to quality of life, mood, symptoms of stress and levels of cortisol, dehydroepiandrosterone sulfate (DHEAS) and melatonin in breast and prostate cancer outpatients. *Psychoneuroendocrinology, 29*(4), 448–474.

Carlson, L. E., Ursuliak, Z., Goodey, E., Angen, M., & Speca, M. (2001). The effects of a mindfulness meditation based stress reduction program on mood and symptoms of stress in cancer outpatients: Six month follow-up. *Supportive Care in Cancer, 9*, 112–123.

Carson, J. W., Keefe, F. J., Lynch, T. R., Carson, K. M., Goli, V., Fras, A. M., et al. (2005). Loving-kindness meditation for chronic low back pain: Results from a pilot trial. *Journal of Holistic Nursing, 23*(3), 287–304.

Chang, B. H., Casey, A., Dusek, J. A., & Benson, H. (2010). Relaxation response and spirituality: Pathways to improve psychological outcomes in cardiac rehabilitation. *Journal of Psychosomatic Research, 69*(2), 93–100.

Chiesa, A., & Serretti, A. (2011). Mindfulness-based interventions for chronic pain: A systematic review of the evidence. *Journal of Alternative and Complementary Medicine, 17*(1), 83–93.

Creswell, J. D., Myers, H. F., Cole, S. W., & Irwin, M. R. (2009). Mindfulness meditation training effects on CD4+ T lymphocytes in HIV-1 infected adults: A small randomized controlled trial. *Brain, Behavior, and Immunity, 23*(2), 184–188.

Delaney, C., Barrere, C., & Helming, M. (2011). The influence of a spirituality-based intervention on quality of life, depression, and anxiety in community-dwelling adults with cardiovascular disease: A pilot study. *Journal of Holistic Nursing, 29*(1), 21–32.

Dobkin, P. L. (2008). Mindfulness-based stress reduction: What processes are at work? *Complementary Therapies in Clinical Practice, 14*(1), 8–16.

Drossman, D. A. (1994). Irritable bowel syndrome. *Gastroenterologist, 2*(4), 315–326.

Duncan, L. G., Moskowitz, J. T., Neilands, T. B., Dilworth, S. E., Hecht, F. M., & Johnson, M. O. (2012). Mindfulness-based stress reduction for HIV treatment side effects: A randomized, wait-list controlled trial. *Journal of Pain and Symptom Management, 43*(2), 161–171.

Elabd, S. (2011). Mindful meditation for chronic pain sufferers may have positive effect. *Topics in Pain Management, 27*(4), 9.

Foley, E., Baillie, A., Huxter, M., Price, M., & Sinclair, E. (2010). Mindfulness-based cognitive therapy for individuals whose lives have been affected by cancer: A randomized controlled trial. *Journal of Consulting and Clinical Psychology, 78*(1), 72–79.

Garland, E. L., Gaylord, S. A., Palsson, O., Faurot, K., Douglas Mann, J., & Whitehead, W. E. (2011). Therapeutic mechanisms of a mindfulness-based treatment for IBS: Effects on visceral sensitivity, catastrophizing, and affective processing of pain sensations. *Journal of Behavioral Medicine, 35*(6), 591–602.

Garland, S. N., Carlson, L. E., Antle, M. C., Samuels, C., & Campbell, T. (2011). I-CAN SLEEP: Rationale and design of a non-inferiority RCT of mindfulness-based stress reduction and cognitive behavioral therapy for the treatment of insomnia in CANcer survivors. *Contemporary Clinical Trials, 32*(5), 747–754.

Garland, S. N., Carlson, L. E., Antle, M. C., Samuels, C., & Campbell, T. S. (2014). Mindfulness-based stress reduction compared to cognitive-behavioral therapy for the treatment of insomnia comorbid with cancer: A randomized, partially blinded, non-inferiority trial. *Journal of Clinical Oncology, 32*(5), 449–457.

Gaylord, S. A., Palsson, O. S., Garland, E. L., Faurot, K. R., Coble, R. S., Mann, J. D., et al. (2011). Mindfulness training reduces the severity of irritable bowel syndrome in women: Results of a randomized controlled trial. *American Journal of Gastroenterology, 106*(9), 1678–1688.

Goldenberg, D. L., Kaplin, K. H., Nadeau, M. G., Brodeur, C., Smith, S., & Schmid, C. H. (1994). A controlled study of a stress-reduction, cognitive-behavioral treatment program in fibromyalgia. *Journal of Musculoskeletal Pain, 2*(2), 53–66.

Gross, C. R., Kreitzer, M. J., Thomas, W., Reilly-Spong, M., Cramer-Bornemann, M., Nyman, J. A., et al. (2010). Mindfulness-based stress reduction for solid organ transplant recipients: A randomized controlled trial. *Alternative Therapies in Health and Medicine, 16*(5), 30–38.

Grossman, P., Tiefenthaler-Gilmer, U., Raysz, A., & Kesper, U. (2007). Mindfulness training as an intervention for fibromyalgia: Evidence of postintervention and 3-year follow-up benefits in well-being. *Psychotherapy and Psychosomatics, 76*(4), 226–233.

Hartmann, M., Kopf, S., Kircher, C., Faude-Lang, V., Djuric, Z., Augstein, F., et al. (2012). Sustained effects of a mindfulness-based stress-reduction intervention in type 2 diabetic patients: Design and first results of a randomized controlled trial (the heidelberger diabetes and stress-study). *Diabetes Care, 35*(5), 945–947.

Hawtin, H., & Sullivan, C. (2011). Experiences of mindfulness training in living with rheumatic disease: An interpretative phenomenological analysis. *British Journal of Occupational Therapy, 74*(3), 137–142.

Henderson, V. P., Clemow, L., Massion, A. O., Hurley, T. G., Druker, S., & Hebert, J. R. (2012). The effects of mindfulness-based stress reduction on psychosocial outcomes and quality of life in early-stage breast cancer patients: A randomized trial. *Breast Cancer Research and Treatment, 131*(1), 99–109.

Hoffman, C. J., Ersser, S. J., Hopkinson, J. B., Nicholls, P. G., Harrington, J. E., & Thomas, P. W. (2012). Effectiveness of mindfulness-based stress reduction in mood, breast- and endocrine-related quality of life, and well-being in stage 0 to III breast cancer: A randomized, controlled trial. *Journal of Clinical Oncology, 30*(12), 1335–1342.

Hsu, C., Bluespruce, J., Sherman, K., & Cherkin, D. (2010). Unanticipated benefits of CAM therapies for back pain: An exploration of patient experiences. *Journal of Alternative and Complementary Medicine, 16*(2), 157–163.

Kabat-Zinn, J. (1982). An outpatient program in behavioral medicine for chronic pain patients based on the practice of mindfulness meditation: Theoretical considerations and preliminary results. *General Hospital Psychiatry, 4*, 33–47.

Kreitzer, M. J., Gross, C. R., Ye, X., Russas, V., & Treesak, C. (2005). Longitudinal impact of mindfulness meditation on illness burden in solid-organ transplant recipients. *Progress in Transplantation, 15*(2), 166–172.

Kvillemo, P., & Branstrom, R. (2011). Experiences of a mindfulness-based stress-reduction intervention among patients with cancer. *Cancer Nursing, 34*(1), 24–31.

Labelle, L. E. (2012). *How does mindfulness-based stress reduction (MBSR) improve psychological functioning in cancer patients?* Unpublished doctoral dissertation, University of Calgary, Calgary, Alberta, Canada.

Labelle, L. E., Campbell, T. S., & Carlson, L. E. (2010). Mindfulness-based stress reduction in oncology: Evaluating mindfulness and rumination as mediators of change in depressive symptoms. *Mindfulness, 1*(1), 28–40.

Lamanque, P., & Daneault, S. (2006). Does meditation improve the quality of life for patients living with cancer? *Canadian Family Physician Medecin De Famille Canadien, 52*, 474–475.

Ledesma, D., & Kumano, H. (2009). Mindfulness-based stress reduction and cancer: A meta-analysis. *Psycho-Oncology, 18*(6), 571–579.

Lengacher, C. A., Johnson-Mallard, V., Post-White, J., Moscoso, M. S., Jacobsen, P. B., Klein, T. W., et al. (2009). Randomized controlled trial of mindfulness-based stress reduction (MBSR) for survivors of breast cancer. *Psycho-Oncology, 18*(12), 1261–1272.

Lengacher, C. A., Kip, K. E., Barta, M. K., Post-White, J., Jacobsen, P., Groer, M., et al. (2012). A pilot study evaluating the effect of mindfulness-based stress reduction on psychological status, physical status, salivary cortisol, and interleukin-6 among advanced-stage cancer patients and their caregivers. *Journal of Holistic Nursing, 30*(3), 170–185.

Lengacher, C. A., Kip, K. E., Post-White, J., Fitzgerald, S., Newton, C., Barta, M., et al. (2013). Lymphocyte recovery after breast cancer treatment and mindfulness-based stress reduction (MBSR) therapy. *Biological Research for Nursing, 15*(1), 37–47.

Ljotsson, B., Andersson, G., Andersson, E., Hedman, E., Lindfors, P., Andreewitch, S., et al. (2011). Acceptability, effectiveness, and cost-effectiveness of internet-based exposure treatment for irritable bowel syndrome in a clinical sample: A randomized controlled trial. *BMC Gastroenterology, 11*, 110.

Ljotsson, B., Falk, L., Vesterlund, A. W., Hedman, E., Lindfors, P., Ruck, C., et al. (2010). Internet-delivered exposure and mindfulness based therapy for irritable bowel syndrome—a randomized controlled trial. *Behaviour Research and Therapy, 48*(6), 531–539.

Ljotsson, B., Hedman, E., Andersson, E., Hesser, H., Lindfors, P., Hursti, T., et al. (2011). Internet-delivered exposure-based treatment vs. stress management for irritable bowel syndrome: A randomized trial. *American Journal of Gastroenterology, 106*(8), 1481–1491.

Ljotsson, B., Hedman, E., Lindfors, P., Hursti, T., Lindefors, N., Andersson, G., et al. (2011). Long-term follow-up of internet-delivered exposure and mindfulness based treatment for irritable bowel syndrome. *Behaviour Research and Therapy, 49*(1), 58–61.

Mackenzie, M. J., Carlson, L. E., Munoz, M., & Speca, M. (2007). A qualitative study of self-perceived effects of mindfulness-based stress reduction (MBSR) in a psychosocial oncology setting. *Stress and Health, 23*(1), 59–69.

Matchim, Y., & Armer, J. M. (2007). Measuring the psychological impact of mindfulness meditation on health among patients with cancer: A literature review. *Oncology Nursing Forum, 34*(5), 1059–1066.

Matchim, Y., Armer, J. M., & Stewart, B. R. (2011). Mindfulness-based stress reduction among breast cancer survivors: A literature review and discussion. *Oncology Nursing Forum, 38*(2), E61–E71.

McCracken, L. M., & Thompson, M. (2011). Psychological advances in chronic pain: A concise selective review of research from 2010. *Current Opinion in Supportive and Palliative Care, 5*(2), 122–126.

Morone, N. E., Greco, C. M., & Weiner, D. K. (2008). Mindfulness meditation for the treatment of chronic low back pain in older adults: A randomized controlled pilot study. *Pain, 134*(3), 310–319.

Musial, F., Bussing, A., Heusser, P., Choi, K. E., & Ostermann, T. (2011). Mindfulness-based stress reduction for integrative cancer care: A summary of evidence. *Forschende Komplementärmedizin, 18*(4), 192–202.

Olivo, E. L., Dodson-Lavelle, B., Wren, A., Fang, Y., & Oz, M. C. (2009). Feasibility and effectiveness of a brief meditation-based stress management intervention for patients diagnosed with or at risk for coronary heart disease: A pilot study. *Psychology, Health and Medicine, 14*(5), 513–523.

Ospina, M., & Harstall, C. (2002). *Prevalence of chronic pain: An overview* (Health Technology Assessment No. 29). Edmonton, Alberta, Canada: Alberta Heritage Foundation for Medical Research.

Ospina, M. B., Bond, T. K., Karkhaneh, M., Tjosvold, L., Vandermeer, B., Liang, Y., et al. (2007). *Meditation practices for health: State of the research* (Evidence Report/Technology Assessment No. 155). Rockville, MD: Agency for Healthcare Research and Quality.

Patil, S. G. (2009). Effectiveness of mindfulness meditation (vipassanā) in the management of chronic low back pain. *Indian Journal of Anaesthesia, 53*(2), 158–163.

Plews-Ogan, M., Owens, J. E., Goodman, M., Wolfe, P., & Schorling, J. (2005). A pilot study evaluating mindfulness-based stress reduction and massage for the management of chronic pain. *Journal of General Internal Medicine, 20*(12), 1136–1138.

Pradhan, E. K., Baumgarten, M., Langenberg, P., Handwerger, B., Gilpin, A. K., Magyari, T., et al. (2007). Effect of mindfulness-based stress reduction in rheumatoid arthritis patients. *Arthritis and Rheumatism, 57*(7), 1134–1142.

Public Health Agency of Canada. (2012). Diabetes. Retrieved from *www.phac-aspc.gc.ca/cd-mc/diabetes-diabete/index-eng.php.*

Robert McComb, J. J., Tacón, A., Randolph, P., & Caldera, Y. (2004). A pilot study to examine the effects of a mindfulness-based stress-reduction and relaxation program on levels of stress hormones, physical functioning, and submaximal exercise responses. *Journal of Alternative and Complementary Medicine, 10*(5), 819–827.

Schmidt, S., Grossman, P., Schwarzer, B., Jena, S., Naumann, J., & Walach, H. (2011). Treating fibromyalgia with mindfulness-based stress reduction: Results from a 3-armed randomized controlled trial. *Pain, 152*(2), 361–369.

Sephton, S. E., Sapolsky, R. M., Kraemer, H. C., & Spiegel, D. (2000). Diurnal cortisol rhythm as a predictor of breast cancer survival. *Journal of the National Cancer Institute, 92*(12), 994–1000.

SeyedAlinaghi, S., Jam, S., Foroughi, M., Imani, A., Mohraz, M., Djavid, G. E., et al. (2012). Randomized controlled trial of mindfulness-based stress reduction delivered to human immunodeficiency virus-positive patients in iran: Effects on CD4(+) T lymphocyte count and medical and psychological symptoms. *Psychosomatic Medicine, 74*(6), 620–627.

Shapiro, S. L., & Carlson, L. E. (2009). *The art and science of mindfulness: Integrating mindfulness into psychology and the helping professions.* Washington, DC: American Psychological Association.

Shennan, C., Payne, S., & Fenlon, D. (2011). What is the evidence for the use of mindfulness-based interventions in cancer care?: A review. *Psycho-Oncology, 20*(7), 681–697.

Speca, M., Carlson, L. E., Goodey, E., & Angen, M. (2000). A randomized, wait-list controlled clinical trial: The effect of a mindfulness meditation-based stress reduction program on mood and symptoms of stress in cancer outpatients. *Psychosomatic Medicine, 62*(5), 613–622.

Sullivan, M. J., Wood, L., Terry, J., Brantley, J., Charles, A., McGee, V., et al. (2009). The support, education, and research in chronic heart failure study (SEARCH): A mindfulness-based psychoeducational intervention improves depression and clinical symptoms in patients with chronic heart failure. *American Heart Journal, 157*(1), 84–90.

Tacón, A. M., McComb, J., Caldera, Y., & Randolph, P. (2003). Mindfulness meditation, anxiety reduction, and heart disease: A pilot study. *Family and Community Health, 26*, 25–33.

Teixeira, E. (2010). The effect of mindfulness meditation on painful diabetic peripheral neuropathy in adults older than 50 years. *Holistic Nursing Practice, 24*(5), 277–283.

Veehof, M. M., Oskam, M. J., Schreurs, K. M., & Bohlmeijer, E. T. (2011). Acceptance-based interventions for the treatment of chronic pain: A systematic review and meta-analysis. *Pain, 152*(3), 533–542.

Weissbecker, I., Salmon, P., Studts, J. L., Floyd, A. R., Dedert, E. A., & Sephton, S. E. (2002). Mindfulness-based stress reduction and sense of coherence among women with fibromyalgia. *Journal of Clinical Psychology in Medical Settings, 9*, 297–307.

Wong, S. Y., Chan, F. W., Wong, R. L., Chu, M. C., Kitty Lam, Y. Y., Mercer, S. W., et al. (2011). Comparing the effectiveness of mindfulness-based stress reduction and multidisciplinary intervention programs for chronic pain: A randomized comparative trial. *Clinical Journal of Pain, 27*(8), 724–734.

World Health Organization. (2012). Global health observatory data repository. Retrieved from *http://apps.who.int/ghodata*.

Zautra, A. J., Davis, M. C., Reich, J. W., Nicassario, P., Tennen, H., Finan, P., et al. (2008). Comparison of cognitive behavioral and mindfulness meditation interventions on adaptation to rheumatoid arthritis for patients with and without history of recurrent depression. *Journal of Consulting and Clinical Psychology, 76*(3), 408–421.

Zernicke, K. A., Campbell, T. S., Blustein, P. K., Fung, T. S., Johnson, J. A., Bacon, S. L., et al. (2013). Mindfulness-based stress reduction for the treatment of irritable bowel syndrome symptoms: A randomized wait-list controlled trial. *International Journal of Behavioral Medicine, 20*(3), 385–396.

Zernicke, K. A., Campbell, T. S., Speca, M., McCabe-Ruff, K., Flowers, S., Dirkse, D. A., et al. (2013). The eCALM trial-eTherapy for cancer appLying mindfulness: Online mindfulness-based cancer recovery program for underserved individuals living with cancer in Alberta: Protocol development for a randomized wait-list controlled clinical trial. *BMC Complementary and Alternative Medicine, 13*, 34.

CHAPTER 23

Biological Pathways Linking Mindfulness with Health

J. David Creswell

This handbook is testament to the impressive growth in research and scholarship in mindfulness science. Over the past decade, there has been a proliferation of methods developed for measuring and inducing mindfulness, and mindfulness training has been linked with a broad range of outcomes in healthy and patient populations. Some of the most well-publicized findings in this emerging literature have focused on how mindfulness interventions improve mental and physical health outcomes (for reviews, see Brown, Ryan, & Creswell, 2007; Ludwig & Kabat-Zinn, 2008). For example, randomized controlled trials (RCTs) indicate that mindfulness interventions reduce risk for major depression relapse in at-risk participants (Ma & Teasdale, 2004; Teasdale et al., 2000), improve immune system function (Barrett et al., 2012; Davidson et al., 2003; Rosenkranz et al., 2013), reduce pain (Zeidan et al., 2011), improve skin-clearing rates in psoriasis (Kabat-Zinn et al., 1998), and delay clinical markers of disease pathogenesis in HIV infection (Creswell, Myers, Cole, & Irwin, 2009; SeyedAlinaghi et al., 2012), to name just a few examples. There has been a lot of recent theorizing about the psychological mechanisms of mindfulness training (e.g., emotion regulation, acceptance, decentering, self-awareness), predominantly for explaining improvements in clinical symptoms, such as psychological distress (e.g., Baer, 2003; Brown et al., 2007; E. N. Carlson, 2013; Hölzel et al., 2011). In this chapter I consider a complementary question: What are the biological pathways linking mindfulness with these health outcomes?

In order to consider how this capacity of the mind ("mindfulness") impacts our biology, I have divided this chapter into three parts. First, I formalize an account for how mindfulness might affect health, the *mindfulness stress-buffering hypothesis*, then consider the available evidence for this account. Second, I ground this stress-buffering account in an evidence-based biological model (Miller, Chen, & Cole,

2009) depicting how mindfulness influences stress-related neural and peripheral biological pathways, which in turn might explain a broad range of stress-related mental and physical health outcomes. I conclude with thoughts about how this account stimulates new questions that might be fruitfully explored in subsequent research.

How Does Mindfulness Affect Health?: The Mindfulness Stress-Buffering Hypothesis

The stress-buffering hypothesis was first described formally in the social support literature as a potential explanation for how social support improves health outcomes (Cohen & Wills, 1985; Dean & Lin, 1977). In an influential review, Cohen and Wills (1985) argued that the effects of social support on health may be explained by two possible pathways—either social support has direct effects on the physiological processes that cause disease (a direct effect model), or social support protects individuals from the adverse effects of stressful events, which in turn impact health (a stress-buffering model). Consistent with the stress-buffering model, Cohen and Wills described how the perceived availability of interpersonal resources (i.e., the perception of social support) can act as a stress buffer by muting stress appraisals and reducing stress reactivity responses.

In parallel fashion, *the mindfulness stress-buffering hypothesis posits that mindfulness mitigates stress appraisals and reduces stress reactivity responses, and that these stress reduction effects partly or completely explain how mindfulness affects mental and physical health outcomes.* At first blush, it may not seem all that novel to suggest stress-buffering pathways for mindfulness–health effects. After all, Jon Kabat-Zinn (1990) described his well-known mindfulness training program as mindfulness-based *stress reduction* (MBSR), and many people report using meditation practices to foster relaxation and stress reduction (cf. Barnes, Bloom, & Nahin, 2008). Thus, I do not present this basic mindfulness stress-buffering hypothesis as new here, but I believe a deeper look at this hypothesis hints at some more provocative predictions and implications. First, the stress-buffering account suggests that the most pronounced effects of mindfulness on health are observed in contexts in which participants carry high-stress burdens (e.g., unemployed adults, participants high in psychological distress) and, by contrast, that mindfulness training interventions are unlikely to have much impact on health outcomes in low-stress participants. Second, the stress-buffering hypothesis suggests that mindfulness effects on health are present in populations in which stress is known to trigger the onset or exacerbation of disease pathogenic processes, or to alter health behaviors (e.g., smoking) that in turn impact disease. Again, by contrast, mindfulness interventions are unlikely to affect disease pathogenic processes that are less affected by stress. Notably, some health conditions and diseases have been shown to be quite sensitive to stress. For example, stress is thought to be an important trigger for the onset of posttraumatic stress disorder (PTSD) and major depression, and stress is known to exacerbate disease pathogenic processes in HIV infection, inflammatory and cardiovascular diseases, diabetes, obesity, and cancer tumor growth and metastasis. For a recent review of the human literature linking stress to disease, see Cohen, Janicki-Deverts, and Miller (2007). As I discuss below, these stress-sensitive health conditions and diseases are the same types of health outcomes that have been shown to be altered by mindfulness interventions (Brown et al., 2007; Ludwig & Kabat-Zinn, 2008).

Does the current research base support the mindfulness stress-buffering hypothesis? Two lines of evidence offer preliminary support. First, initial studies indicate that mindfulness reduces psychological and biological stress reactivity to stressor exposures. For example, studies indicate that participants higher in basic forms of dispositional mindfulness have reduced self-reported psychological stress reactivity to laboratory stressors (Arch & Craske, 2010; Weinstein, Brown, & Ryan, 2009), and lower daily life stress perceptions (e.g., Brown & Ryan, 2003; Ciesla, Reilly, Dickson, Emanuel, & Updegraff, 2012; Tamagawa et al., 2013). Mindfulness training studies indicate similar stress reduction benefits (cf. Baer, 2003; Speca, Carlson, Goodey, & Angen, 2000). Notably, several initial mindfulness training studies suggest that the training reduces biological stress reactivity, particularly with use of a standardized social stress laboratory paradigm (called the Trier Social Stress Test; TSST) in which participants complete a 5-minute speech, then perform 5 minutes of difficult mental arithmetic calculations in front of evaluative panelists (Kirschbaum, Pirke, & Hellhammer, 1993). Specifically, these studies show that 8-week MBSR training reduces blood pressure reactivity to the TSST in high-stress community adults (Nyklíček, Van Beugen, & Van Boxtel, 2013) and MBSR reduces anxiety and distress responses to the TSST in a sample of patients with generalized anxiety disorder (Hoge et al., 2013). Moreover, as the stress-buffering hypothesis might predict, these studies are consistent with the notion that mindfulness stress-buffering effects are present or most pronounced in high-stress populations (e.g., Arch & Craske, 2010).

In the most direct test of the mindfulness stress-buffering hypothesis to date, Brown, Weinstein, and Creswell (2012) measured undergraduate participants' basic dispositional mindfulness (using the Mindful Attention Awareness Scale; MAAS), then manipulated whether participants completed a high- or low-stress challenge task. Specifically, participants were asked to perform the standard TSST speech and math performance tasks in front of evaluators (high-stress condition) or the same tasks alone into an audiorecorder (low-stress condition). Consistent with the stress-buffering hypothesis, we found that higher levels of dispositional mindfulness were associated with lower stressor-evoked cortisol reactivity in the high-stress condition, whereas there was no association between mindfulness and cortisol reactivity in the low-stress condition (Brown et al., 2012).

Although studies provide initial support for the first part of the stress-buffering hypothesis (i.e., mindfulness buffers stress reactivity), no studies have yet tested the more provocative stress–health predictions suggested by this hypothesis, namely, that stress-buffering effects partially or completely account for mindfulness effects on improving clinically relevant biological markers of mental and physical health. But the current mindfulness training literature suggests that this hypothesis might be worth pursuing for three reasons. First, an initial study indicates that mindful individuals have reduced stress appraisals and better coping under stress, which in turn mediates improvements in self-reported well-being at follow-up (Weinstein et al., 2009). Second, the most provocative demonstrations of mindfulness interventions on health outcomes have been observed almost exclusively in stress-sensitive mental and physical health outcomes, such as in HIV infection, depression, and inflammation (Creswell et al., 2009; Ma & Teasdale, 2004; Malarkey, Jarjoura, & Klatt, 2013; Rosenkranz et al., 2013; Teasdale et al., 2000). A detailed review of the elegant stress–health physiology literature is beyond the scope of this chapter, but this basic stress literature suggests that these mindfulness health effects may be explained by stress (buffering) pathways. For example, stress has been shown to accelerate HIV viral replication (Cole, Kemeny, Fahey, Zack, & Naliboff, 2003; Cole, Korin, Fahey, & Zack, 1998) and HIV-related mortality (Capitanio, Mendoza, Lerche, & Mason, 1998), and to increase the likelihood major depressive episodes (Gold, Goodwin, & Chrousos, 1988) and inflammation (Steptoe, Hamer, & Chida, 2007).

Finally, some mindfulness training researchers appear implicitly to assume that a stress-buffering pathway drives mindfulness effects on biology and health, as mindfulness studies commonly recruit high-stress populations (e.g., Creswell et al., 2009; Malarkey et al., 2013) or measure mindfulness training effects on biological markers of health after acute stress exposures (e.g., Nyklíček et al., 2013; Rosenkranz et al., 2013). Although these initial studies are consistent with a stress-buffering account, future mindfulness training studies might more specifically measure stress reduction pathways and test whether they might account for mindfulness training effects on these stress-related mental and physical health outcomes using established methods for testing intervening or mediating variable effects (for methodological reviews, see Baron & Kenny, 1986; Jo, 2008; Lockhart, MacKinnon, & Ohlrich, 2011).

Using the Mindfulness Stress-Buffering Hypothesis to Build a Biological Model of Mindfulness and Health

If mindfulness buffers stress, and this stress buffering helps explain how mindfulness gets under the skin to influence mental and physical health, what are the underlying biological stress reduction pathways? Here I draw from recent findings in my laboratory, and those of others, to sketch a testable biological account for mindfulness, stress buffering, and health. Specifically, this account offers some initial evidence on how mindfulness affects stress processing in the brain, which in turn is likely to change peripheral stress responses in the body and subsequent risk for stress-related disorders and disease outcomes over time. Figure 23.1 depicts a model of these brain, peripheral physiology, and stress-related disease outcomes, which I describe below.

The biology of mindfulness and stress buffering begins with the assumption that mindfulness will alter stress processing in the brain (for reviews of the neurobiology of stress, see Arnsten, 2009; Ulrich-Lai & Herman, 2009). It is important to note that emerging studies suggest that mindfulness can significantly change multiple brain networks (see Zeidan, Chapter 10, this volume), but here I focus on mindfulness and plausible alterations in neural stress processing. There is evidence for two promising neural stress-buffering pathways in recent mindfulness studies: Mindfulness may increase the recruitment of top-down regulatory regions of prefrontal cortex, which

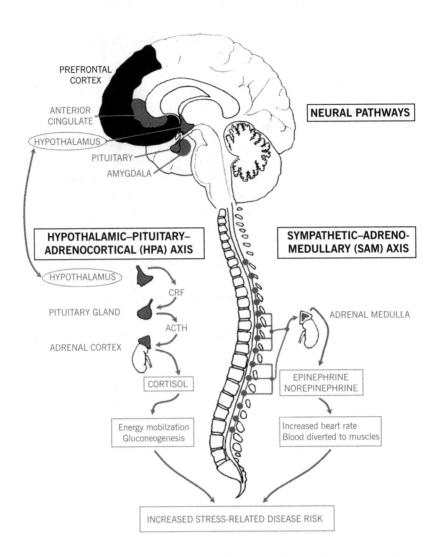

FIGURE 23.1. A conceptual model of the biological pathways linking mindfulness, stress-buffering, and stress-related disease outcomes. Black shaded regions depict regulatory pathways that are activated in mindful individuals or after mindfulness training, whereas grey shaded regions depict stress reactivity pathways that are reduced in mindful individuals or after mindfulness training interventions. The brain regions depicted in the neural pathways highlight how mindfulness increases the regulatory activity of areas in prefrontal cortex (in black), while turning down reactivity in areas such as the perigenual and subgenual anterior cingulate cortex, the amygdala, and corresponding brain regions implicated in HPA (hypothalamus, pituitary gland) and SAM (sympathetic nerve fibers in the brainstem and spinal cord) axis responses (in grey). Note that this diagram does not include parasympathetic nervous system projections or interactions, which may play an important regulatory role for SAM axis responding. Mindfulness is posited to decrease stress-related HPA axis activation, which results in cortisol production and release from the adrenal cortex. Mindfulness may also decrease activation of the SAM axis, reducing the release of norepinephrine from sympathetic nerve endings and epinephrine release from the adrenal medulla. Cortisol and epinephrine–norepinephrine are important chemical messengers for mobilizing energy and engaging bodily organ systems for fight-or-flight, but when these biological stress responses become recurrent, excessive, or dysregulated, they can increase stress-related disease risk.

may inhibit the reactivity of stress-processing regions (a top-down regulation pathway); studies also suggest that mindfulness may have direct effects on modulating the reactivity of stress-processing regions (a "bottom-up" reduced reactivity pathway). (My colleagues and I have recently written about top-down vs. bottom-up accounts in a related article on mindfulness and craving; see Westbrook et al., 2013.)

Neural Stress Reduction Pathways

Top-Down Regulation by the Prefrontal Cortex

In support of the top-down regulatory pathway, both basic dispositional mindfulness and mindfulness training interventions have been shown to increase the recruitment of regulatory regions of the prefrontal cortex (e.g., ventral and dorsal regions of lateral prefrontal cortex), particularly in contexts in which participants are asked to engage in active emotion regulatory tasks (e.g., affect labeling, reappraisal; Creswell, Way, Eisenberger, & Lieberman, 2007; Farb et al., 2007; Hölzel et al., 2013; Modinos, Ormel, & Aleman, 2010). Moreover, we have recently found that mindfulness meditation training (relative to a structurally matched relaxation training intervention) increases the coupling of individuals' resting state default mode network with regulatory regions of the prefrontal cortex (e.g., bilateral dorsolateral prefrontal cortex), and we find that this increased coupling statistically explains how mindfulness meditation training reduces inflammation at follow-up in a sample of stressed, unemployed community adults (Creswell, Pacilio, Lindsay, & Brown, 2014). It is important to note that little research has evaluated whether activation (or increased connectivity) in these regions of prefrontal cortex describe actual stress regulation pathways per se, but some work suggests that activation of these top-down regulatory pathways fosters the reduction of both pain and distress (e.g., Eisenberger, Lieberman, & Williams, 2003; Lieberman et al., 2004; Riva, Lauro, DeWall, & Bushman, 2012; Wager, Davidson, Hughes, Lindquist, & Ochsner, 2008).

Reduced Central Reactivity (of the Amygdala)

Regardless of whether top-down regulation pathways are recruited, mindfulness stress-buffering effects would be expected to occur if there is reduced reactivity in central stress-processing brain regions responsible for signaling peripheral stress response cascades (e.g., amygdala, anterior cingulate cortex, ventromedial prefrontal cortex, hypothalamus, parabrachial pons; for a review, see Ulrich-Lai & Herman, 2009). There is initial evidence that mindfulness might directly affect neural stress-processing dynamics. For example, research suggests that mindfulness alters amygdala function and structure, a region that is important for gating fight-or-flight stress responses (Arnsten, 2009; Gianaros et al., 2008; Hölzel et al., 2010). We have found that more mindful individuals have reduced resting-state amygdala activity (Way, Creswell, Eisenberger, & Lieberman, 2010) and smaller right amygdala volumes (Taren, Creswell, & Gianaros, 2013). These mindfulness-related alterations in amygdala function and structure may be accompanied by changes in the resting state functional connectivity of the amygdala with other stress processing regions. We have recently found that both basic dispositional mindfulness and mindfulness training reduce stress-related right amygdala resting-state functional connectivity with the subgenual anterior cingulate cortex, suggesting that mindfulness may reduce the strength of connectivity of brain networks driving stress reactivity (Taren et al., 2013).

Peripheral Stress Pathways: The Sympathetic–Adrenomedullary and Hypothalamic–Pituitary–Adrenocortical Stress Response Systems

So far I have described several of our own and others' initial neuroimaging studies that suggest mindfulness may increase stress regulatory signals from the prefrontal cortex, and also reduce activity and functional connectivity in stress-processing regions (e.g., amygdala) responsible for gating fight-or-flight stress response cascades (Arnsten, 2009). How might these changes in central stress processing change peripheral (bodily) stress responses? There are two well-characterized peripheral biological stress response systems: the sympathetic–adrenomedullary (SAM) and hypothalamic–pituitary–adrenocortical (HPA) stress response axes. It is possible that mindfulness might alter SAM axis activation (1) by reducing sympathetic nervous system activation and its principal stress effectors (secretion of the catecholamines—norepinephrine and epinephrine) or (2) by counterregulatory systems known to alter SAM axis activation, for example, by increasing activity in the parasympathetic nervous system, which can brake sympathetic nervous system fight-or-flight stress responses via the vagus nerve (Thayer & Lane, 2000). No studies to my knowledge have evaluated whether mindfulness alters the secretion of epinephrine and norepinephrine in stressed populations (an interesting direction for future research), although there is some research suggesting that mindfulness meditation may increase parasympathetic nervous system activation (Ditto, Eclache, & Goldman, 2006), which in turn might foster greater SAM axis stress regulation over time (Thayer & Lane, 2000).

There is evidence that mindfulness may alter stress-related HPA axis activation, which results in the release of glucocorticoids, most notably the stress hormone cortisol (Matousek, Dobkin, & Pruessner, 2010). Several studies suggest that mindfulness may reduce (or potentially normalize) diurnal cortisol secretion (Brand, Holsboer-Trachsler, Naranjo, & Schmidt, 2012; Carlson et al., 2013; Carlson, Speca, Faris, & Patel, 2007; Carlson, Speca, Patel, & Goodey, 2003; Jacobs et al., 2013; Matousek et al., 2010). Although these studies provide an initial indication of an effect of mindfulness on changes in diurnal HPA axis alterations, it is important to note that several published and unpublished reports do not support a mindfulness–diurnal cortisol link (e.g., Gex-Fabry et al., 2012), and it is unclear whether mindfulness would be expected to alter morning or evening cortisol secretion (or both) from this body of research. As mentioned earlier, my colleagues and I have published some initial research indicating that more mindful individuals show reduced cortisol reactivity to a high stress challenge task (Brown et al., 2012), lending support to the idea that mindfulness can buffer stress-related cortisol secretion. In summary, this brief review of the studies examining mindfulness and changes in SAM and HPA axis activation provides some initial support for peripheral stress-buffering effects, and more work is needed to evaluate these stress signaling pathways and their role in stress-related mental and physical health outcomes.

Stress Buffering and Disease Outcomes

If mindfulness buffers central (e.g., amygdala) and peripheral (SAM and HPA axis) stress response cascades, then how might these stress-buffering effects impact disease pathogenic processes? Here, a biological model of mindfulness and health diverges into specific biological disease-specific pathways for both mental (e.g., depression, generalized anxiety) and physical (e.g., HIV pathogenesis, inflammatory disease risk) outcomes. Critically, the assessment of stress–disease pathways depend on identifying the proximal biological processes driving disease pathogenesis, then evaluating how biological stress mediators (e.g., epinephrine, cortisol) interact with these specific disease pathogenic processes (e.g., Miller et al., 2009). In many diseases, the stress–disease links are increasingly well characterized— which permits the building of biological disease-specific models for mindfulness, stress buffering, and health. As just one example of this approach, one of our previous studies (Creswell et al., 2009) focused on recruiting a moderate to high stress HIV-positive sample and testing how mindfulness meditation training (using 8-week MBSR) might delay disease pathogenic processes in a small RCT. This work was guided by a biologically informed model. We first identified the proximal biological processes driving disease pathogenesis: HIV viral particles replicate and attack specific compartments of the immune system, reducing CD4+ T lymphocyte counts and increasing risk for opportunistic infections and death (Sloan, Collado-Hidalgo, & Cole, 2007). We then considered the role of stress in accelerating HIV replication and CD4+ T lymphocyte declines, noting an established literature showing that stress mediators (e.g., norepinephrine, cortisol, and perceived stress) can accelerate HIV replication and CD4+ T lymphocyte declines (Capitanio et al., 1998; Cole et al., 1998, 2003; Ironson et al., 2005). Our mindfulness training results were consistent with a stress-buffering account, in that the 8-week MBSR program reduced stress and buffered CD4+ T lymphocyte declines in our sample of high-stress HIV-positive (HIV+) community adults, providing one of the first controlled demonstrations that mindfulness training can directly impact a biological (and clinically relevant) disease process (Creswell et al., 2009).

The stress-buffering account and a consideration of the underlying biological stress-buffering pathways can inform future research aimed at evaluating whether mindfulness affects biological health and disease outcomes. What stress-related disease outcomes might one test in mindfulness intervention studies? Recent studies indicate that dysregulated glucocorticoid signaling increases inflammatory disease risk (Barnes & Adcock, 2009; Cohen et al., 2012) and risk for depression relapse (Zobel et al., 2001), and catecholamines have been implicated in fostering tumor growth and metastasis in ovarian carcinoma (Thaker et al., 2006). To the degree that the stress-buffering model is accurate, it suggests that mindfulness would alter neural stress processing dynamics in high-stress volunteers, reduce SAM or HPA axis reactivity (or normalize dysregulated stress signaling in these systems), and subsequently impact stress-related disease-specific biological processes (e.g., reduce tumor growth and metastasis in some cancers).

Open Questions and Future Research Directions

This chapter is designed to shed new light on the question of how the capacity to pay attention to one's experience moment-by-moment (mindfulness) affects underlying biological systems that drive mental and physical health outcomes. The emerging research described here suggests initial progress in addressing this big question, but many open questions remain. One central question is whether the stress-buffering account best captures how mindfulness affects most health outcomes. I believe the extant evidence strongly supports the idea that mindfulness may serve as a protective factor against the catabolic effects stress can have on disease pathogenic processes (the stress-buffering account). It is also possible that mindfulness may have direct effects on disease processes independent of stress reduction pathways (a direct effects account). As just one example of a direct effects pathway, mindfulness may have salutary effects, like those observed in the aerobic exercise literature, which suggest that aerobic exercise interventions directly increase central and peripheral growth factors (e.g., brain-derived neurotrophic factor [BDNF]) known to foster neuroplasticity and positive health in older adults (Cotman & Berchtold, 2002; Cotman, Berchtold, & Christie, 2007).

There are also open questions about the psychological processes that might foster mindfulness stress-buffering effects. It is reasonable to step back and ask why this attentional capacity would buffer stress responses in the first place. If mindfulness is about fostering greater attention toward one's present-moment experience, one may argue that mindfulness might *increase* stress appraisals and reactivity under stress. I suspect that mindfulness is not simply about enhanced attention but about fostering a capacity to observe stressors receptively as they arise with equanimity (cf. Anālayo, 2003), which in turn would alter initial stress appraisals. Consistent with this idea, Brown, Goodman, and Inzlicht (2013) found that more dispositionally mindful individuals show neural (electroencephalographic) patterns consistent with reduced threat appraisals to threatening and other emotionally evocative images, an effect that was observed within the first second of viewing the threatening images. Not only is it important to consider the psychological processes linking mindfulness with initial stress appraisals but also downstream effects on how mindfulness alters stress responses and coping efforts under stress. There are many anecdotal reports of how mindfulness training alters psychological and behavioral coping responses; for example, participants' reported changes in their response to stressors after 8 weeks of MBSR training, "I began living my life more consciously, for example, in regard to how I coped with stress. I started to ask myself: how do I want to deal with this? How am I reacting to my environment? In stressful situations I could sometimes take a step back and pause before I responded" (in Majumdar, Grossman, Dietz-Waschkowski, Kersig, & Walach, 2002). Although more research is needed to clarify how mindfulness affects one's response to stress, participant experiences highlight how mindfulness fosters greater awareness into how one is reacting to stress (e.g., perhaps via meta-awareness or decentering), which may in turn reduce rumination (Ciesla et al., 2012; Jain et al., 2007) and buffer working memory declines (Jha, Stanley, Kiyonaga, Wong, & Gelfand, 2010), and enable more effective approach-oriented coping (Weinstein et al., 2009).

In framing of the mindfulness and the stress-buffering hypothesis, mindfulness has at times been depicted as a static trait via measures of dispositional mindfulness or via consideration of extensive mindfulness training intervention effects (e.g., 8-week MBSR). But mindfulness is a capacity that can vary by situations and be developed over time with appropriate training—hence, mindfulness is probably best described as a dynamic process. This consideration of the dynamic nature of mindfulness also has implications for the mindfulness stress-buffering hypothesis. For example, there are open questions about whether mindfulness training might initially make individuals more sensitive to stress exposures. For example, in contrast to stress-buffering effects observed in 8-week mindfulness training studies or in dispositionally mindful individuals (e.g., Brown et al., 2012; Nyklíček et al., 2013), my colleagues and I found that a relatively brief, three-session mindfulness training intervention not only buffered psychological stress perceptions but also *increased* cortisol reactivity to the TSST (Creswell et al., 2014). One potential implication of these findings is that mindfulness training in the early stages of skills development may be more effortful to sustain, leading to greater biological stress reactivity. With greater amounts of practice, the capacity to be mindful under stress may become more automatic, reducing stress reactivity. We do not have good models of mindfulness training effects over time but, clearly, these models (and future studies in this area) would be helpful for understanding how the stress-buffering effects of mindfulness might change over time.

Conclusions

The mindfulness stress-buffering account provides an initial theoretical and biologically based approach for relating mindfulness to mental and physical health. I believe it has the potential to clarify *when* and *how* mindfulness affects not only psychological adjustment but also health and disease outcomes. Specifically, the *when* refers to high-stress populations with health conditions that are known to be triggered or exacerbated by stress (e.g., people who report recent significant life stressors or high levels of perceived stress). The *how* refers to the underlying biological stress pathways by which mindfulness gets under the skin to influence health. Herein I have offered some initial ideas on some promising central (brain) and peripheral (HPA and SAM axes) stress-buffering pathways in mindfulness studies. Finally, I conclude with the hope that formally describing the mindfulness stress-buffering hypothesis is generative. Future studies can be developed to test the psychological and biological pathways and mechanisms underlying mindfulness stress-buffering effects, helping to explain how the capacity to be mindful produces such a broad range of beneficial effects for health and well-being.

ACKNOWLEDGMENT

I thank Emily Lindsay for creating Figure 23.1.

REFERENCES

Anālayo. (2003). *Satipaṭṭhāna: The direct path to realization.* Cambridge, UK: Windhorse.

Arch, J. J., & Craske, M. G. (2010). Laboratory stressors in clinically anxious and non-anxious individuals: The moderating role of mindfulness. *Behaviour Research and Therapy, 48*(6), 495–505.

Arnsten, A. F. T. (2009). Stress signalling pathways that impair prefrontal cortex structure and function. *Nature Reviews Neuroscience, 10*(6), 410–422.

Baer, R. A. (2003). Mindfulness training as a clinical intervention: A conceptual and empirical review. *Clinical Psychology: Science and Practice, 10*(2), 125–143.

Barnes, P. J., & Adcock, I. M. (2009). Glucocorticoid resistance in inflammatory diseases. *Lancet, 373,* 1905–1917.

Barnes, P. M., Bloom, B., & Nahin, R. L. (2008). *Complementary and alternative medicine use among adults and children: United States, 2007.* Washington, DC: U.S. Department of Health and Human Services, Centers for Disease Control and Prevention, National Center for Health Statistics.

Baron, R. M., & Kenny, D. A. (1986). The moderator–mediator variable distinction in social psychological research: Conceptual, strategic, and statistical considerations. *Journal of Personality and Social Psychology, 51*(6), 1173–1182.

Barrett, B., Hayney, M. S., Muller, D., Rakel, D., Ward, A., Obasi, C. N., et al. (2012). Meditation or exercise for preventing acute respiratory infection: A randomized controlled trial. *Annals of Family Medicine, 10*(4), 337–346.

Brand, S., Holsboer-Trachsler, E., Naranjo, J. R., & Schmidt, S. (2012). Influence of mindfulness practice on cortisol and sleep in long-term and short-term meditators. *Neuropsychobiology, 65*(3), 109–118.

Brown, K. W., Goodman, R. J., & Inzlicht, M. (2013). Dispositional mindfulness and the attenuation of neural responses to emotional stimuli. *Social, Cognitive, and Affective Neuroscience, 8*(1), 93–99.

Brown, K. W., & Ryan, R. M. (2003). The benefits of being present: Mindfulness and its role in psychological well-being. *Journal of Personality and Social Psychology, 84*(4), 822–848.

Brown, K. W., Ryan, R. M., & Creswell, J. D. (2007). Mindfulness: Theoretical foundations and evidence for its salutary effects. *Psychological Inquiry, 18*(4), 211–237.

Brown, K. W., Weinstein, N., & Creswell, J. D. (2012). Trait mindfulness modulates neuroendocrine and affective responses to social evaluative threat. *Psychoneuroendocrinology, 37*(12), 2037–2041.

Capitanio, J. P., Mendoza, S. P., Lerche, N. W., & Mason, W. A. (1998). Social stress results in altered glucocorticoid regulation and shorter survival in simian acquired immune deficiency syndrome. *Proceedings of the National Academy of Sciences, 95*(8), 4714–4719.

Carlson, E. N. (2013). Overcoming the barriers to self-knowledge mindfulness as a path to seeing yourself as you really are. *Perspectives on Psychological Science, 8*(2), 173–186.

Carlson, L. E., Doll, R., Stephen, J., Faris, P., Tamagawa, R., Drysdale, E., et al. (2013). Randomized controlled trial of mindfulness-based cancer recovery versus supportive expressive group therapy for distressed survivors of breast cancer. *Journal of Clinical Oncology, 31*(25), 3119–3126.

Carlson, L. E., Speca, M., Faris, P., & Patel, K. D. (2007). One year pre–post intervention follow-up of psychological, immune, endocrine and blood pressure outcomes of mindfulness-based stress reduction (MBSR) in breast and prostate cancer outpatients. *Brain Behavior and Immunity, 21*(8), 1038–1049.

Carlson, L. E., Speca, M., Patel, K. D., & Goodey, E. (2003). Mindfulness-based stress reduction in relation to quality of life, mood, symptoms of stress, and immune parameters in breast and prostate cancer outpatients. *Psychosomatic Medicine, 65*(4), 571–581.

Ciesla, J. A., Reilly, L. C., Dickson, K. S., Emanuel, A. S., & Updegraff, J. A. (2012). Dispositional mindfulness moderates the effects of stress among adolescents: rumination as a mediator. *Journal of Clinical Child and Adolescent Psychology, 41*(6), 760–770.

Cohen, S. E., Janicki-Deverts, D., Doyle, W. J., Miller, G. E., Frank, E., Rabin, B. S., et al. (2012). Chronic stress, glucocorticoid receptor resistance, inflammation, and disease risk. *Proceedings of the National Academy of Sciences, 109*(16), 5995–5999.

Cohen, S. E., Janicki-Deverts, D., & Miller, G. E. (2007). Psychological stress and disease. *Journal of the American Medical Association, 298*(14), 1685–1687.

Cohen, S. E., & Wills, T. A. (1985). Stress, social support, and the buffering hypothesis. *Psychological Bulletin, 98*(2), 310–357.

Cole, S. W., Kemeny, M. E., Fahey, J. L., Zack, J. A., & Naliboff, B. D. (2003). Psychological risk factors for HIV pathogenesis: Mediation by the autonomic nervous system. *Biological Psychiatry, 54*(12), 1444–1456.

Cole, S. W., Korin, Y. D., Fahey, J. L., & Zack, J. A. (1998). Norepinephrine accelerates HIV replication via protein kinase A-dependent effects on cytokine production. *Journal of Immunology, 161*(2), 610–616.

Cotman, C. W., & Berchtold, N. C. (2002). Exercise: A behavioral intervention to enhance brain health and plasticity. *Trends in Neurosciences, 25*(6), 295–301.

Cotman, C. W., Berchtold, N. C., & Christie, L.-A. (2007). Exercise builds brain health: Key roles of growth factor cascades and inflammation. *Trends in Neurosciences, 30*(9), 464–472.

Creswell, J. D., Myers, H. F., Cole, S. W., & Irwin, M. R. (2009). Mindfulness meditation training effects on CD4+ T lymphocytes in HIV-1 infected adults: A small randomized controlled trial. *Brain Behavior and Immunity, 23*(2), 184–188.

Creswell, J. D., Pacilio, L. E., Lindsay, E. K., & Brown, K. W. (2014). Brief mindfulness meditation training alters psychological and neuroendocrine responses to social evaluative stress. *Psychoneuroendocrinology, 44*, 1–12.

Creswell, J. D., Way, B. M., Eisenberger, N. I., & Lieberman, M. D. (2007). Neural correlates of dispositional mindfulness during affect labeling. *Psychosomatic Medicine, 69*(6), 560–565.

Davidson, R. J., Kabat-Zinn, J., Schumacher, J., Rosenkranz, M., Muller, D., Santorelli, S. F., et al. (2003). Alterations in brain and immune function produced by mindfulness meditation. *Psychosomatic Medicine, 65*(4), 564–570.

Dean, A., & Lin, N. (1977). The stress-buffering role of social support: Problems and prospects for systematic investigation. *Journal of Nervous and Mental Disease, 165*(6), 403–417.

Ditto, B., Eclache, M., & Goldman, N. (2006). Short-term autonomic and cardiovascular effects of mindfulness body scan meditation. *Annals of Behavioral Medicine, 32*(3), 227–234.

Eisenberger, N. I., Lieberman, M. D., & Williams, K. D. (2003). Does rejection hurt?: An fMRI study of social exclusion. *Science, 302,* 290–292.

Farb, N. A. S., Segal, Z. V., Mayberg, H., Bean, J., McKeon, D., Fatima, Z., et al. (2007). Attending to the present: Mindfulness meditation reveals distinct neural modes of self-reference. *Social Cognitive and Affective Neuroscience, 2*(4), 313–322.

Gex-Fabry, M., Jermann, F., Kosel, M., Rossier, M. F., Van der Linden, M., Bertschy, G., et al. (2012). Salivary cortisol profiles in patients remitted from recurrent depression: One-year follow-up of a mindfulness-based cognitive therapy trial. *Journal of Psychiatric Research, 46*(1), 80–86.

Gianaros, P. J., Sheu, L. K., Matthews, K. A., Jennings, J. R., Manuck, S. B., & Hariri, A. R. (2008). Individual differences in stressor-evoked blood pressure reactivity vary with activation, volume, and functional connectivity of the amygdala. *Journal of Neuroscience, 28*(4), 990–999.

Gold, P. W., Goodwin, F. K., & Chrousos, G. P. (1988). Clinical and biochemical manifestations of depression: Relations to the neurobiology of stress. *New England Journal of Medicine, 319,* 348–353.

Hoge, E. A., Bui, E., Marques, L., Metcalf, C. A., Morris, L. K., Robinaugh, D. J., et al. (2013). Randomized controlled trial of mindfulness meditation for generalized anxiety disorder: Effects on anxiety and stress reactivity. *Journal of Clinical Psychiatry, 74*(8), 786–792.

Hölzel, B. K., Carmody, J., Evans, K. C., Hoge, E. A., Dusek, J. A., Morgan, L., et al. (2010). Stress reduction correlates with structural changes in the amygdala. *Social Cognitive and Affective Neuroscience, 5*(1), 11–17.

Hölzel, B. K., Hoge, E. A., Greve, D. N., Gard, T., Creswell, J. D., Brown, K. W., et al. (2013). Neural mechanisms of symptom improvements in generalized anxiety disorder following mindfulness training. *NeuroImage: Clinical, 2,* 448–458.

Hölzel, B. K., Lazar, S. W., Gard, T., Schuman-Olivier, Z., Vago, D. R., & Ott, U. (2011). How does mindfulness meditation work?: Proposing mechanisms of action from a conceptual and neural perspective. *Perspectives on Psychological Science, 6*(6), 537–559.

Ironson, G., O'Cleirigh, C., Fletcher, M. A., Laurenceau, J. P., Balbin, E., Klimas, N., et al. (2005). Psychosocial factors predict CD4 and viral load change in men and women with human immunodeficiency virus in the era of highly active antiretroviral treatment. *Psychosomatic Medicine, 67*(6), 1013–1021.

Jacobs, T. L., Shaver, P. R., Epel, E. S., Zanesco, A. P., Aichele, S. R., Bridwell, D. A., et al. (2013). Self-reported mindfulness and cortisol during a Shamatha meditation retreat. *Health Psychology, 32*(10), 1104–1109.

Jain, S., Shapiro, S. L., Swanick, S., Roesch, S. C., Mills, P. J., & Schwartz, G. E. (2007). A randomized controlled trial of mindfulness meditation versus relaxation training: Effects on distress, positive states of mind, rumination, and distraction. *Annals of Behavioral Medicine, 33*(1), 11–21.

Jha, A. P., Stanley, E. A., Kiyonaga, A., Wong, L., & Gelfand, L. (2010). Examining the protective effects of mindfulness training on working memory capacity and affective experience. *Emotion, 10*(1), 54–64.

Jo, B. (2008). Causal inference in randomized experiments with mediational processes. *Psychological Methods, 13*(4), 314–336.

Kabat-Zinn, J. (1990). *Full catastrophe living: Using the wisdom of your body and mind to face stress, pain, and illness.* New York: Delta.

Kabat-Zinn, J., Wheeler, E., Light, T., Skillings, A., Scharf, M. J., Cropley, T. G., et al. (1998). Influence of a mindfulness meditation-based stress reduction intervention on rates of skin clearing in patients with moderate to severe psoriasis undergoing phototherapy (UVB) and photochemotherapy (PUVA). *Psychosomatic Medicine, 60*(5), 625–632.

Kirschbaum, C., Pirke, K. M., & Hellhammer, D. H. (1993). The "Trier Social Stress Test"—a tool for investigating psychobiological stress responses in a laboratory setting. *Neuropsychobiology, 28,* 76–81.

Lieberman, M. D., Jarcho, J. M., Berman, S., Naliboff, B. D., Suyenobu, B. Y., Mandelkern, M., et al. (2004). The neural correlates of placebo effects: A disruption account. *NeuroImage, 22*(1), 447–455.

Lockhart, G., MacKinnon, D. P., & Ohlrich, V. (2011). Mediation analysis in psychosomatic medicine research. *Psychosomatic Medicine, 73*(1), 29–43.

Ludwig, D. S., & Kabat-Zinn, J. (2008). Mindfulness in medicine. *Journal of the American Medical Association, 300*(11), 1350–1352.

Ma, S. H., & Teasdale, J. D. (2004). Mindfulness-based cognitive therapy for depression: replication and exploration of differential relapse prevention effects. *Journal of Consulting and Clinical Psychology, 72*(1), 31–40.

Majumdar, M., Grossman, P., Dietz-Waschkowski, B., Kersig, S., & Walach, H. (2002). Does mindfulness meditation contribute to health?: Outcome evaluation of a German sample. *Journal of Alternative and Complementary Medicine, 8*(6), 719–730.

Malarkey, W. B., Jarjoura, D., & Klatt, M. (2013). Workplace based mindfulness practice and inflammation: A randomized trial. *Brain, Behavior, and Immunity, 27,* 145–154.

Matousek, R. H., Dobkin, P. L., & Pruessner, J. (2010). Cortisol as a marker for improvement in mindfulness-based stress reduction. *Complementary Therapies in Clinical Practice, 16*(1), 13–19.

Miller, G., Chen, E., & Cole, S. W. (2009). Health psychology: Developing biologically plausible models linking the social world and physical health. *Annual Review of Psychology, 60,* 501–524.

Modinos, G., Ormel, J., & Aleman, A. (2010). Individual differences in dispositional mindfulness and brain activity involved in reappraisal of emotion. *Social Cognitive and Affective Neuroscience, 5*(4), 369–377.

Nyklíček, I., Van Beugen, S., & Van Boxtel, G. J. (2013). Mindfulness-based stress reduction and physiological activity during acute stress: A randomized controlled trial. *Health Psychology, 32,* 1110–1113.

Riva, P., Lauro, L. J. R., DeWall, C. N., & Bushman, B. J. (2012). Buffer the pain away stimulating the right ventrolateral prefrontal cortex reduces pain following social exclusion. *Psychological Science, 23*(12), 1473–1475.

Rosenkranz, M. A., Davidson, R. J., MacCoon, D. G., Sheridan, J. F., Kalin, N. H., & Lutz, A. (2013). A comparison of mindfulness-based stress reduction and an active control in modulation of neurogenic inflammation. *Brain, Behavior, and Immunity, 27,* 174–184.

SeyedAlinaghi, S., Jam, S., Foroughi, M., Imani, A., Mohraz, M., Djavid, G. E., et al. (2012). Randomized controlled trial of mindfulness-based stress reduction delivered to human immunodeficiency virus–positive patients in Iran: Effects on CD4+ T lymphocyte count and medical and psychological symptoms. *Psychosomatic Medicine, 74*(6), 620–627.

Sloan, E., Collado-Hidalgo, A., & Cole, S. (2007). Psychobiology of HIV infection. In R. Ader, D. L. Felten, & N. Cohen (Eds.), *Psychoneuroimmunology* (pp. 1053–1076). San Diego, CA: Academic Press.

Speca, M., Carlson, L. E., Goodey, E., & Angen, M. (2000). A randomized, wait-list controlled clinical trial: The effect of a mindfulness meditation-based stress reduction program on mood and symptoms of stress in cancer outpatients. *Psychosomatic Medicine, 62*(5), 613–622.

Steptoe, A., Hamer, M., & Chida, Y. (2007). The effects of acute psychological stress on circulating inflammatory factors in humans: A review and meta-analysis. *Brain, Behavior, and Immunity, 21*(7), 901–912.

Tamagawa, R., Giese-Davis, J., Speca, M., Doll, R., Stephen, J., & Carlson, L. E. (2013). Trait mindfulness, repression, suppression, and self-reported mood and stress symptoms among women with breast cancer. *Journal of Clinical Psychology, 69*(3), 264–277.

Taren, A. A., Creswell, J. D., & Gianaros, P. J. (2013). Dispositional mindfulness co-varies with smaller amygdala and caudate volumes in community adults. *PLoS ONE, 8*(5), e64574.

Teasdale, J. D., Segal, Z. V., Mark, J., Ridgeway, V. A., Soulsby, J. M., & Lau, M. A. (2000). Prevention of relapse/recurrence in major depression by mindfulness-based cognitive therapy. *Journal of Consulting and Clinical Psychology, 68*(4), 615–623.

Thaker, P. H., Han, L. Y., Kamat, A. A., Arevalo, J. M., Takahashi, R., Lu, C., et al. (2006). Chronic stress promotes tumor growth and angiogenesis in a mouse model of ovarian carcinoma. *Nature Medicine, 12*(8), 939–944.

Thayer, J. F., & Lane, R. D. (2000). A model of neurovisceral integration in emotion regulation and dysregulation. *Journal of Affective Disorders, 61*(3), 201–216.

Ulrich-Lai, Y. M., & Herman, J. P. (2009). Neural regulation of endocrine and autonomic stress responses. *Nature Reviews Neuroscience, 10*(6), 397–409.

Wager, T. D., Davidson, M. L., Hughes, B. L., Lindquist, M. A., & Ochsner, K. N. (2008). Prefrontal–subcortical pathways mediating successful emotion regulation. *Neuron, 59*(6), 1037–1050.

Way, B. M., Creswell, J. D., Eisenberger, N. I., & Lieberman, M. D. (2010). Dispositional mindfulness and depressive symptomatology: Correlations with limbic and self-referential neural activity during rest. *Emotion, 10*(1), 12–24.

Weinstein, N., Brown, K. W., & Ryan, R. M. (2009). A multi-method examination of the effects of mindfulness on stress attribution, coping, and emotional well-being. *Journal of Research in Personality, 43*(3), 374–385.

Westbrook, C., Creswell, J. D., Tabibnia, G., Julson, E., Kober, H., & Tindle, H. A. (2013). Mindful attention reduces neural and self-reported cue-induced craving in smokers. *Social, Cognitive, and Affective Neuroscience, 8*, 73–84.

Zeidan, F., Martucci, K. T., Kraft, R. A., Gordon, N. S., McHaffie, J. G., & Coghill, R. C. (2011). Brain mechanisms supporting the modulation of pain by mindfulness meditation. *Journal of Neuroscience, 31*(14), 5540–5548.

Zobel, A. W., Nickel, T., Sonntag, A., Uhr, M., Holsboer, F., & Ising, M. (2001). Cortisol response in the combined dexamethasone/CRH test as predictor of relapse in patients with remitted depression: A prospective study. *Journal of Psychiatric Research, 35*(2), 83–94.

Author Index

Subject Index

455

Cognitive-behavioral therapy (CBT) *(cont.)*
    mindfulness research from the perspective of, 138,
        139–140
    mindfulness training and its benefits, 69
    overview, 131–132, 143
    physical conditions and, 409, 410, 412–413,
        418–419, 419
Comorbidity/co-occurring disorders, 357–358
Compassion
    addiction and, 393–394
    anxiety and, 372
    applied relaxation for anxiety and, 377
    effects of mindfulness training on, 316
Competence, 115
Computational modeling, 198, 201
Concentration, 12, 23–24, 32
Conceptual–evaluative processing mode, 97–98
Conceptualization of mindfulness, 151–155, 153*t*, 166.
        See also Science-based conceptualization
Concrete processing
    mindfulness training and, 105
    processing mode theory and, 100–102
    theoretical and empirical advances in the
        mindfulness science field, 3
Conflict monitoring
    attention and, 193
    cognitive system and, 191*f*
    effects of mindfulness training on, 313–314
    mindfulness-based stress reduction (MBSR) and, 273
    overview, 204
    See also Executive functioning
Consciousness
    attention and, 50–53
    cognitive awareness and, 46–50
    overview, 57
    study of, 42–43
Constriction, 369*f*, 371. *See also* Avoidance
Constructivist tendencies, 33
Contextual cognitive-behavioral therapy
    behavioral implications of mindfulness, 140–142
    overview, 131–132, 142–143
    See also Cognitive-behavioral therapy (CBT);
        Contextual perspectives
Contextual perspectives
    acceptance and commitment therapy (ACT) and,
        134–136
    behavioral implications of mindfulness, 140–142
    dialectical behavior therapy (DBT), 136
    metacognitive therapy (MCT) and, 133–134
    mindfulness research from, 137–140
    mindfulness-based cognitive therapy (MBCT) and,
        132–133
    overview, 130–131, 142–143
Control theory framework, 90–91, 98–102
Coping behaviors
    addiction and, 393
    metacognitive therapy (MCT) and, 133–134
    mindfulness and anxiety and, 379
Cortex, 234–235
Cortisol system
    biological model of mindfulness and health and,
        430*f*
    research regarding mindfulness-based interventions
        for physical conditions and, 409–410
Creativity
    free-association and, 228
    mind wandering and, 229–230
Cross-cultural cognitive science of mindfulness, 44–46,
    46

Curiosity
    addiction and, 393–394
    applied relaxation for anxiety and, 377
    presence and, 233–234
Darwinian evolutionary theory, 208
Deautomatization, 319
Decentered perspective, 71–72, 71*f*
Decentering
    anxiety and, 372
    applied relaxation for anxiety and, 377
    mindfulness-based cognitive therapy (MBCT) and,
        132–133
    overview, 319
    physical conditions and, 419
Decision making
    children and adolescents and, 285
    emotion contexts and, 208
    working memory and, 198
Default mode network, 180
Default networks, 397
Defusion, 135
Delusion, 34
Depression
    children and adolescents and, 301
    cognitive therapy (CT) and, 350–351
    MBCT and preventing depressive relapse, 351–353
    mindfulness-based cognitive therapy (MBCT) and,
        353–355, 357–361
    overview, 348–349
    physical conditions and, 412
    processing mode theory and, 94–96, 95*f*, 100–103
    risk for relapse and recurrence, 349–350
    See also Major depressive disorder (MDD)
Depressive relapse, 91
Description, 337
Detached mindfulness (DM), 134
Developmental processes, 83, 236–237
Dharma, 12, 32
Diabetes
    mindfulness stress-buffering hypothesis and,
        427–428
    research regarding mindfulness-based interventions
        for, 413–414
Diagnosis, 388
Dialectical behavior therapy (DBT)
    addiction and, 396
    anxiety and, 373–374, 374
    assumptions, 342–343
    borderline personality disorder (BPD) and, 357
    contextual CBT effects and, 139–140
    emotion dysregulation and, 331
    emotion regulation and, 330
    "how" skills in, 337–339
    mindfulness approaches in, 333–334
    overview, 132, 136, 142–143, 343–344
    research regarding, 339–341
    self-control to self-regulation and, 341–342
    states of mind, 334–336
    "what" skills in, 336–337
Differential activation hypothesis (DAH), 349–350
Discrimination, 378–379
Disease. *See* Health conditions; Physical conditions
Disidentification, 318–319
Dispositional mindfulness
    benefits of mindfulness for negative emotions and,
        210–211
    neurobiology of mindfulness meditation and,
        174–175